Health Care Ethics *in Canada*

Second Edition

Edited by

Françoise Baylis
Professor
Dalhousie University

Jocelyn Downie
Associate Professor
Dalhousie University

Barry Hoffmaster
Professor
University of Western Ontario

Susan Sherwin
University Research Professor
Dalhousie University

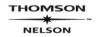

THOMSON

NELSON

Australia   Canada   Mexico   Singapore   Spain   United Kingdom   United States

THOMSON

NELSON

Health Care Ethics in Canada
Second Edition

Edited by Françoise Baylis, Jocelyn Downie,
Barry Hoffmaster, and Susan Sherwin

Editorial Director and Publisher:
Evelyn Veitch

Executive Editor:
Chris Carson

Marketing Manager:
Lenore Taylor

Developmental Editor:
Alwynn Pinard

Permissions Coordinator:
Nicola Winstanley

Production Editor:
Wendy Yano

Copy Editor:
Lisa Berland

Proofreader:
Carol J. Anderson

Production Coordinator:
Helen Locsin

Creative Director:
Angela Cluer

Interior Design:
Peter Papayanakis

Cover Design:
Katherine Strain

Cover Image:
Ryan McVay/PhotoDisc Red/
Gettty Images

Compositor:
Rachel Sloat

Printer:
Transcontinental

National Library of Canada Cataloguing in Publication Data

Health care ethics in Canada/ Françoise Baylis ... [et al.]. —2nd ed.

Includes bibliographical references.
ISBN 0-17-641553-X

1. Medical ethics—Canada. I. Baylis, Françoise, 1961–

R724.H38 2004   174'.2'0971
C2003-906961-3

Professor Benjamin Freedman was an editor of and contributor to the first edition of *Health Care Ethics in Canada*. In 1997, two years after the text was published, Benjamin Freedman died in only his forty-sixth year. Benjy's passing always will be felt most intensely and most irreparably by his family. They know better than anyone what he gave and what more he could have given as a husband, a father, and a man of consummate integrity who melded unshakable faith with calm reason and a passion for justice. His friends, his colleagues, and his students, among whom we are fortunate to count ourselves, know what he gave and what more he could have given to our profession. Benjy was an architect of health care ethics in Canada, but the impact of his writing was international. His distinguished corpus includes important contributions on informed consent, competence, and research ethics, work that is included and discussed in the second edition. In homage to Benjy's life and legacy, and in fidelity with his vision of and devotion to health care ethics, we dedicate the second edition to him.

Contents

Introduction

Much has changed since the first edition of *Health Care Ethics in Canada* appeared in 1995. Over the ensuing eight years health care ethics in Canada has flourished. Participation in the field, which has always been richly diverse and strongly committed, continues to grow, and both the quantity and quality of Canadian scholarship have become impressive. Consequently, the orientation of the second edition is decidedly and distinctively more Canadian. Whereas only 20 percent of the authors in the first edition were Canadian, over 50 percent of the authors in the second edition are Canadian. As a result, a number of the chapters are exclusively Canadian (Chapters 3 and 9), while others are predominantly Canadian (Chapters 4 and 10), and all but the first and last chapters contain seminal or important Canadian work. For the editors this is a welcome change.

As health care ethics has been maturing, its content and methodologies have continued to evolve. The core issues of health care ethics still exist, of course, but they regularly take new forms and acquire new meanings. For instance, questions of pluralism and multiculturalism now involve new conceptions of the meaning of culture when they are raised with respect to cochlear implants for deaf persons. Understanding the relationship between a health care professional and a patient is no longer just a matter of ascertaining who should decide what. The relationship must be conceived in a way that fosters genuine trust and communication — communication that is more than just a professional dispensing intelligible information and a patient accurately recalling that information. Determining competence no longer can be reduced to assessing a person's intellectual capacities; it must also recognize the cognitive dimensions of emotions. An ethical assessment of research involving humans is no longer limited to protecting participants, but must also consider the just distribution of the benefits, not merely the burdens, of research. In addition, given the development of governmental and university partnerships with private companies, the manifold ways in which economic incentives can create conflicts of interest and corrupt research now require careful scrutiny. As well, health care ethics is intimately implicated in the formation of public policy, which always is in flux. Matters related to the just allocation of health care resources, for example, now must be examined in the context of the Romanow report and judicial decisions about the responsibilities of provincial governments to fund particular health care services. Furthermore, scientific progress continually poses new challenges for health care ethics and policy. What is the proper response to stem cell research? What about the prospect of human cloning? The readings in the second edition raise the enduring issues of health care ethics, but they also recognize the new directions and new guises these issues have assumed.

Students coming to ethics want to know what they will be studying, so they naturally seek a definition of "ethics." Despite the concerted efforts of philosophers, however, a comprehensive, rigorous, and plausible definition remains elusive. Yet the desire to know what ethics is cannot be evaded – particularly in a robustly practical area such as health care ethics, where "doing ethics" can have momentous impacts on people's lives and deaths. Instead of searching for a definition, another way to try to understand ethics in general, and health care ethics in particular, is by examining its methodology. Contemporary health care ethics began in a familiar, seemingly uncontroversial manner. It was taken to be an instance of "applied" ethics: the application of general moral theories and their associated rules or principles to the facts of particular cases to yield decisions about what ought to be done. A version of this "top-down" approach continues to dominate the practice and the pedagogy of health care ethics. In fact, a canonical set of principles for health care ethics has emerged: principles directed at preventing harm (non-maleficence), promoting good (beneficence), protecting freedom (respect for autonomy), and ensuring fairness (justice). These principles are routinely applied to problems that arise for patients and health care professionals, the kinds of problems that themselves are widely regarded as constitutive of health care ethics because they implicate these principles.

As appealing as this methodological approach might be, it encounters serious difficulties. For a number of reasons, principles alone cannot always determine appropriate actions or justify decisions about how to resolve particular moral quandaries. Judgments have to be made about many crucial matters, including what features of a situation are morally salient; which principles are relevant to a situation; whether the specific features of a situation can be classified under the general terms of a principle; and which principle takes precedence when there is a conflict. Applying principles is by no means easy or straightforward, and the process requires resources beyond the principles themselves. That recognition has instigated considerable methodological development in health care ethics.

The first reaction to the difficulties inherent in a "top-down" approach to applied ethics was to shift from principles to particulars: to develop a "bottom-up" approach to health care ethics. Rather than beginning with principles and attempting to derive decisions from them, a "bottom-up" approach begins with cases and extrapolates decisions for new cases from decisions in previous cases. Its models are the operation of the doctrine of precedent in Anglo-American case law and the once influential tradition of moral casuistry. With this approach a case with a clear resolution is identified, and then a decision for a related case is reached via an argument by analogy. Proponents of a "bottom-up" approach have more confidence in our ability to decide what is right and wrong for concrete, specific cases than our ability to justify decisions in terms of general principles. Nevertheless, it is hard to jettison principles from a "bottom-up" approach. Constructing a strong argument by analogy requires that relevant similarities and dissimilarities between cases be identified, and that the comparative significance of those similarities and dissimilarities be evaluated. Unguided by theoretical commitments of the sort embodied in principles, decisions about those matters can appear capricious.

The goal of "top-down" and "bottom-up" methodologies is to provide moral guidance and justification for moral decisions. In a "top-down" approach the justification is a deductive argument; in a "bottom-up" approach the justification is an argument by analogy. The refractory problems with both approaches have prompted a more radical methodological move: the introduction of narrative ethics, which pursues the goal of understanding rather than justification. Narratives or stories connect events not in terms of temporal sequence, causation, or logical relationships, but in terms of meaning. Stories enable us to understand why a person or character perceived a matter in a certain way, felt and deliberated in a certain manner, and made a certain choice. They broaden our understanding of how other people live and what possibilities are open to us. It even has been proposed that we should regard our own lives as narratives and make decisions so as to create unified, coherent stories for ourselves. Narratives can convey the complexity, the quirkiness, and the messiness of life, can engage our emotions, and can reveal new sources of meaning. But how does the understanding they yield help us make moral decisions? How do we determine whether a story is true or whether one story is better than another? How does a story help us make a particular choice or adopt a way of life? Can concerns about justification simply be ignored?

The quest for understanding also has induced efforts to put moral issues in context. Principles are stated in spare and abstract terms, but the meanings those principles acquire and the moral problems on which they are brought to bear are dense and complicated. Those meanings are functions of the cultural, social, and historical backgrounds; the political, economic, and legal settings; the institutional and organizational structures; and the congeries of beliefs and values in which they are implicated. Real moral problems are complex, multi-layered, and ill-defined. Addressing them requires a perceptiveness that is informed by a variety of perspectives and that appreciates the realities that shape and constrain those problems. Feminist theories, for example, emphasize how the oppression of women (and other social groups) is located in and sustained by overlapping theoretical and practical contexts. The deeply contextual nature of moral problems makes moral progress a matter of social criticism and action, not just intellectual inquiry. But, again, concerns about justification are hard to ignore. What makes social criticism legitimate and telling? What vindicates movements for social reform? And what, ultimately, is the basis for determining that social change represents moral progress?

The methodological ferment in health care ethics is unlikely to abate. Providing accounts of what ethics is, and how ethics is done, remains a daunting theoretical and practical challenge. It is impossible to capture this challenge in a few readings, and Chapter 1 does not make that attempt. Rather, Chapter 1 offers a general orientation to ethics and health care ethics and presents conceptual terminology and tools that are helpful. It contains a range of methodological perspectives illustrating the diverse approaches that are taken to specific topics in the readings that follow.

Chapter 2 begins a move from theory to practice by locating central issues of health care ethics — making decisions about life support, telling the truth to patients, donating organs for transplantation, and understanding the relationship between patients and physicians — and various methodological approaches to these issues in an array of cultural contexts. Appreciating how these issues have developed and been addressed by people in Italy, by aboriginal people in Canada, and by people who are deaf, raises challenging questions about how the notion of culture should be understood and how it should influence moral decision making.

Still attending to context, Chapters 3 and 4 examine the Canadian health care system. Chapter 3 focuses on the overall design and structure of the system with respect to matters of justice, and Chapter 4 then raises concerns about justice for more specific problems of resource allocation. Beyond this, many of the classic problems of health care ethics concern decisions at the bedside. Chapter 5 situates that decision making within the roles, responsibilities, and relationships of the parties involved: patients, their families, and health care professionals.

The remaining chapters take up specific matters. Chapters 6 and 7 consider the two key components of decision making in health care: consent and competence. Chapter 8 examines research involving human subjects, the issue that inaugurated the contemporary field of health care ethics. Chapter 9 is devoted to topics in reproduction and Chapter 10 to topics in genetics. Chapter 11 considers challenges surrounding the end of life.

Since the publication of the first edition, there have been numerous judicial decisions in Canada related to health care ethics. Summaries of pertinent decisions appear at the end of most chapters. In addition, since the first edition, many resources in health care ethics have become available on the Internet. Brief descriptions of and directions to those resources, along with other helpful resources, are given at the end of the volume.

With its expanded Canadian content, its new organization, and its new resources, the second edition provides a comprehensive yet current introduction to health care ethics in Canada. We hope that this revised text will help health care ethics in Canada continue to grow and to flourish.

ACKNOWLEDGMENTS

Sincere thanks are owed to Carla Farmer, Thane Plantikow, and Natalie Ram for invaluable research assistance in the preparation of this book.

PART 1

The Nature and Context of Health Care Ethics in Canada

Chapter 1 THEORY AND METHOD

Practical Ethics

Peter Singer

… What is it to make a moral judgment, or to argue about an ethical issue, or to live according to ethical standards? How do moral judgments differ from other practical judgments? Why do we regard a woman's decision to have an abortion as raising an ethical issue, but not her decision to change her job? What is the difference between a person who lives by ethical standards and one who doesn't?

All these questions are related, so we only need to consider one of them; but to do this we need to say something about the nature of ethics. Suppose that we have studied the lives of a number of different people, and we know a lot about what they do, what they believe, and so on. Can we then decide which of them are living by ethical standards and which are not?

We might think that the way to proceed here is to find out who believes it wrong to lie, cheat, steal and so on, and does not do any of these things, and who has no such beliefs, and show no such restraints in their actions. Then those in the first group would be living according to ethical standards and those in the second group would not be. But this procedure mistakenly assimilates two distinctions: the first is the distinction between living according to (what we judge to be) the right ethical standards and living according to (what we judge to be) mistaken ethical standards; the second is the distinction between living according to some ethical standards, and living according to no ethical standards at all. Those who lie and cheat, but do not believe what they are doing to be wrong, may be

living according to ethical standards. They may believe, for any of a number of possible reasons, that it is right to lie, cheat, steal and so on. They are not living according to conventional ethical standards, but they may be living according to some other ethical standards.

This first attempt to distinguish the ethical from the non-ethical was mistaken, but we can learn from our mistakes. We found that we must concede that those who hold unconventional ethical beliefs are still living according to ethical standards, *if they believe, for any reason, that it is right to do as they are doing.* The italicized condition gives us a clue to the answer we are seeking. The notion of living according to ethical standards is tied up with the notion of defending the way one is living, of giving a reason for it, of justifying it. Thus people may do all kinds of things we regard as wrong, yet still be living according to ethical standards, if they are prepared to defend and justify what they do. We may find the justification inadequate, and may hold that the actions are wrong, but the attempt at justification, whether successful or not, is sufficient to bring the person's conduct within the domain of the ethical as opposed to the non-ethical. When, on the other hand, people cannot put forward any justification for what they do, we may reject their claim to be living according to ethical standards, even if what they do is in accordance with conventional moral principles.

We can go further. If we are to accept that a person is living according to ethical standards, the justification must be of a certain kind. For instance, a justification in terms of self-interest alone will not do. When Macbeth, contemplating the murder of Duncan, admits that only "vaulting ambition" drives him to do it, he is admitting that the act cannot be justified ethically. "So that I can be king in his place" is not a weak attempt at an ethical justification for assassination; it is not the sort of reason that counts as an ethical justification at all. Self-interested acts must be shown to be compatible with more broadly based ethical principles if they are to be ethically defensible, for the notion of ethics carries with it the idea of something bigger than the individual. If I am to defend my conduct on ethical grounds, I cannot point only to the benefits it brings me. I must address myself to a larger audience.

From ancient times, philosophers and moralists have expressed the idea that ethical conduct is acceptable from a point of view that is somehow *universal*. The "Golden Rule" attributed to Moses tells us to go beyond our own personal interests and "do unto others as we would have them do unto us." The same idea of putting oneself in the position of another is involved in the Christian commandment that we love our neighbour as ourself. The Stoics held that ethics derives from a universal natural law. Kant developed this idea into his famous formula: "Act only on that maxim through which you can at the same time will that it should become a universal law." Kant's theory has itself been modified and developed by R. M. Hare, who sees "universalizability" as a logical feature of moral judgments. The eighteenth-century British philosophers Hutcheson, Hume and Adam Smith appealed to an imaginary "impartial spectator" as the test of a moral judgment, and this theory has its modern version in the Ideal Observer Theory. Utilitarians, from Jeremy Bentham to J. J. C. Smart, take it as axiomatic that in deciding moral issues "each counts for one and none for more than one"; while John Rawls, a leading contemporary critic of utilitarianism, incorporates essentially the same axiom into his own theory by deriving basic ethical principles from an imaginary choice in which those choosing do not know whether they will be the ones who gain or lose by the principles they

select. Even Continental philosophers like the existentialist Jean-Paul Sartre and the Marxist Jürgen Habermas, who differ in many ways from their English-speaking colleagues—and from each other—agree that ethics is in some sense universal.

One could argue endlessly about the merits of each of these characterizations of the ethical; but what they have in common is more important than their differences. They agree that the justification of an ethical principle cannot be in terms of any partial or sectional group. Ethics takes a universal point of view. This does not mean that a particular ethical judgment must be universally applicable. Circumstances alter causes, as we have seen. What it does mean is that in making ethical judgments we go beyond our own likes and dislikes. From an ethical point of view the fact that it is I who benefit from, say, a more equal distribution of income and you, say, who lose by it, is irrelevant. Ethics requires us to go beyond "I" and "you" to the universal law, the universalizable judgment, the standpoint of the impartial spectator or ideal observer, or whatever we choose to call it.

Can we use this universal aspect of ethics to derive an ethical theory which will give us guidance about right and wrong? Philosophers from the Stoics to Hare and Rawls have attempted this. No attempt has met with general acceptance. The problem is that if we describe the universal aspect of ethics in bare, formal terms, a wide range of ethical theories, including quite irreconcilable ones, are compatible with this notion of universality; if, on the other hand, we build up our description of the universal aspect of ethics so that it leads us ineluctably to one particular ethical theory, we shall be accused of smuggling our own ethical beliefs into our definition of the ethical—and this definition was supposed to be broad enough, and neutral enough, to encompass all serious candidates for the status of "ethical theory." Since so many others have failed to overcome this obstacle to deducing an ethical theory from the universal aspect of ethics, it would be foolhardy to attempt to do so in a brief introduction to a work with a quite different aim. Nevertheless I shall propose something only a little less ambitious. The universal aspect of ethics, I suggest, does provide a persuasive, although not conclusive, reason for taking a broadly utilitarian position.

My reason for suggesting this is as follows. In accepting that ethical judgments must be made from a universal point of view, I am accepting that my own interests cannot, simply because they are *my* interests, count more than the interests of anyone else. Thus my very natural concern that my own interests be looked after must, when I think ethically, be extended to the interests of others. Now, imagine that I am trying to decide between two possible courses of action—any example would do. Imagine, too, that I am deciding in a complete ethical vacuum, that I know nothing of any ethical considerations. I am, we might say, in a pre-ethical stage of thinking. How would I make up my mind? One thing that would be still relevant would be how the possible courses of action will affect my interests. Indeed, if we define "interests" broadly enough, so that we count anything people desire as in their interests (unless it is incompatible with another desire or desires) then it would seem that at this pre-ethical stage, *only* one's own interests can be relevant to the decision.

Suppose I then begin to think ethically, to the extent of recognizing that my own interests cannot count for more, simply because they are my own, than the interests of others. In place of my own interests, I now have to take account of the interests of all those affected by my decision. This requires me to weigh up all these interests and adopt the course of action most likely to maximize the interests of those affected. Thus I must choose the course of action which has the best consequences, on balance, for all affected. This is a form of utilitarianism. It differs from classical utilitarianism in that "best consequences" is understood as meaning what, on balance, furthers the interests of those affected, rather than merely what increases pleasure and reduces pain. (It has, however, been suggested that classical uitilitarians like Bentham and John Stuart Mill used "pleasure" and "pain" in a broad sense which allowed them to include achieving what one desired as a "pleasure" and the reverse as a "pain." If this interpretation is correct, the difference between classical utilitarianism and utilitarianism based on interests disappears.)

What does this show? It does not show that utilitarianism can be deduced from the universal aspect of ethics. There are other ethical ideals—like individual rights, the sanctity of life, justice, purity and so on—which are universal in the required sense, and are, at least in some versions, incompatible with utilitarianism. It does show that we very swiftly arrive at an *initially* utilitarian position once we apply the universal aspect of ethics to simple, pre-ethical decision making. This, I believe, places the onus of proof on those who seek to go beyond utilitarianism. The utilitarian position is a minimal one, a first base which we reach by universalizing self-interested decision making. We cannot, if we are to think ethically, refuse to take this step. If we are to be persuaded that we should go beyond utilitarianism and accept non-utilitarian moral rules or ideals, we need to be provided with good reasons for taking this further step. Until such reasons are produced, we have some grounds for remaining utilitarians….

Foundations in Moral Theory

Ruth R. Faden, Tom L. Beauchamp, and Nancy M.P. King

PRINCIPLES, RULES, AND RIGHTS

Moral deliberation and justification rest on principles, rules, and rights, understood as abstract action-guides. These general guides and their relationships will be the focus of our attention in this section. However, before we turn directly to them, some background assumptions regarding the words "ethics," "morality," and "moral philosophy" deserve mention.

The Concept of Morality

The word "morality" has meanings that extend beyond philosophical contexts and professional codes of conduct. Morality is concerned with practices defining right and wrong that are usually transmitted within a culture or institution from generation to generation, together with other kinds of customs and rules. Morality denotes a social institution, composed of a set of standards pervasively acknowledged by the members of the culture. In this respect, it has an objective, ongoing status as a body of action guides. Like political constitutions and natural languages, morality exists prior to the acceptance (or rejection) of its rules and regulations by particular individuals. Its standards are usually abstract, uncodified, and applicable to behavior in many diverse circumstances.

The terms "ethical theory and "moral philosophy," by contrast, suggest *reflection* on the institution of morality. These terms refer to attempts to introduce clarity, substance, and precision of argument into the domain of morality. Moral philosophers seek to put moral beliefs and social practices of morality into a more unified and defensible package of action-guides by challenging presuppositions, assessing moral arguments, and suggesting modifications in existing beliefs. Their task often centers on "justifica-tion": Philosophers seek to justify a system of standards or some moral point of view on the basis of carefully analyzed and defended theories and principles, such as respect for autonomy, distributive justice, equal treatment, human rights, beneficence, nonmaleficence, and utility—some of the principles commonly employed in contemporary moral philosophy.

Despite these rough distinctions, we shall use the terms "moral" and "ethical" as synonymous, and "moral philosophy" and "ethical theory" will also be used interchangeably. "Morality," however, will be confined to social practice.

Reasoning by Principles

Philosophers try to exhibit how to avoid confusing a merely personal attitude or religious dogma with a reasoned and justified moral position. Accordingly, moral philosophy offers principles for the development and evaluation of moral arguments. Rights, duties, obligations, and the like derive from these principles. ("Values" is a still more general term, and one we shall rarely employ.) Such principles—the choice and analysis of which are controversial—constitute the heart of modern ethical theory.... Most of these principles are already embedded in public morality and policies, but only in a vague and imprecise form. The job of ethical theory is to lend precision without oversimplification. It should always be remembered that moral debate about a particular course of action or controversy is often rooted not only in disagreement about the proper interpretation of applicable moral principles, but also in the interpretation of factual information and in divergent assessments of the proper scientific, metaphysical, or religious description of a situation.

Although it is neither possible nor necessary to outline a full ethical theory in this volume, three moral principles relevant to our subject matter need to be addressed and briefly analyzed: respect for autonomy, beneficence, and justice. These broad principles provide the basis for the more specific rules and requirements found in professional codes of medical and research ethics…. We shall not here debate whether these three principles jointly form a *complete* moral system nor whether other moral principles are distinct or derivative from these three principles….

Rights as Correlative to Duties

Only recently has Western society emphasized the importance of human rights, and only recently have rights come to play an important role in public policy discussions…. Rights are powerful assertions of claims that demand respect and status, and they occupy a prominent place in moral theory and political documents. If someone appeals to rights, a response is demanded. We must accept the person's claim as valid, discredit it by countervailing considerations, or acknowledge the right but show how it can be overridden by competing moral claims.

Legal rights are widely acknowledged and codified, but the status of moral rights is more puzzling. Some thinkers are skeptical of their validity; others find absurd the profusion of rights and the conflicts resulting from their various claims. Absurd or otherwise, rights language has been extended to many controversial arenas—rights to privacy, rights to health care, rights of children, rights of animals, rights of the elderly, rights to confidential information, rights to shelter, and so on. How, then, are we to understand the language and basis of rights in moral discourse, and what is the relationship between one person's rights and another's duties?

A plausible claim is that a right always entails the imposition of a duty on others either not to interfere or to provide something, both the duty and the right being justified by the same overarching principle. Thus, if as a matter of justice a state promises or otherwise incurs a duty to provide such goods as influenza shots or other medical care to needy citizens, then citizens can claim an entitlement or right to that care if they meet the relevant criteria. The right to die, the right to privacy, the right to be free to make a decision, and all other so-called negative rights, which are often grounded in respect for autonomy, may be treated as entailing someone else's duty to abstain from interference with one's intended course in life.

If our treatment of the "correlativity thesis" is correct, little is distinctive about rights as a moral category. As with duties, the moral basis for their assertion simply rests in moral principles. Although it remains controversial in contemporary ethical theory whether rights are based on duties, duties based on rights, or neither based on the other, we have tried to circumvent this controversy by holding that the principles in a moral system both impose duties and confer rights….

THREE PRINCIPLES

Respect for Autonomy

Respect for autonomy is … conceived as a principle rooted in the liberal Western tradition of the importance of individual freedom and choice, both for political life and for personal development. "Autonomy" and "respect for autonomy" are terms loosely associated with several ideas, such as privacy, voluntariness, self-mastery, choosing freely, the freedom to choose, choosing one's own moral position, and accepting responsibility for one's choices….

Historically, the word "autonomy" is a legacy from ancient Greece, where *autos* (self) and *nomos* (rule or law) were joined to refer to political self-governance in the city-state. In moral philosophy, personal autonomy has come to refer to personal self-governance: personal rule of the self by adequate understanding while remaining free from controlling interferences by others and from personal limitations that prevent choice. "Autonomy," so understood, has been loosely analyzed in terms of external nonconstraint and the presence of critical internal capacities integral to self-governance.[1] But, again, major confusion can emerge over the precise analysis of autonomy if we move beyond the core idea that the autonomous person is not bound by controlling constraints and is in control of personal affairs.

Almost all existing analyses of autonomy focus on the autonomous *person*. Our central interest, however, is in autonomous *choice*—or, more generally, autonomous *action*. This distinction is between (1) persons who have the capacity to be independent and in control, and (2) the actions that reflect the exercise of those capacities. This distinction may be thought trivial because it might seem by definition that only autonomous persons act autonomously. However … the criteria of autonomous choices are not identical with the criteria of autonomous persons. Autonomous persons can and do make non-autonomous choices owing to temporary constraints such as ignorance or coercion….

It is one thing to be autonomous, and another to be *respected* as autonomous…. To respect an autonomous agent is to recognize with due appreciation that person's capacities and perspective, including his or her right to hold certain views, to make certain choices, and to take certain actions based on personal values and beliefs. Such respect has historically been connected to the idea that persons possess an intrinsic value independent of special circumstances that confer value. As expressed in Kantian philosophy, autonomous persons are ends in themselves, determining their own destiny, and are not to be treated merely as means to the ends of others.[2] Thus, the burden of moral justification rests on those who would restrict or prevent a person's exercise of autonomy.

The moral demand that we respect the autonomy of persons can be formulated as a *principle of respect for autonomy*: Persons should be free to choose and act without controlling constraints imposed by others. The principle provides the justificatory basis for the right to make autonomous decisions, which in turn takes the form of specific autonomy-related rights. For example, in the debate over whether autonomous, informed patients have the right to refuse self-regarding, life-sustaining medical interventions,[3] the principle of respect for autonomy suggests a morally appropriate response….

Beneficence

The welfare of the patient is the goal of health care and also of what is often called "therapeutic research." This welfare objective is medicine's context and justification: Clinical therapies are aimed at the promotion of health by cure or prevention of disease. This value of benefiting the person has long been treated as a foundational value—and sometimes as *the* foundational value—in medical ethics. For example, a celebrated principle in the history of medical codes of ethics is the maxim *primum non nocere*—"above all, do no harm"—commonly viewed as the fundamental maxim of the Hippocratic tradition in medicine. Recent scholarship has shown that in the Hippocratic writings the more precise formulation of the primary moral injunctions is "help, or at least do no harm,"[4] thus demanding the provision of benefit beyond mere avoidance of harm.

The principle of beneficence includes the following four elements, all linked through the common theme of promoting the welfare of others:[5] (1) one ought not to inflict evil or harm; (2) one ought to prevent evil or harm; (3) one ought to remove evil or harm; (4) one ought to do or promote good. Many philosophers have held that the fourth element may not, strictly speaking, be a duty; and some have claimed that these elements should be hierarchically arranged so that the first takes precedence over the second, the second over the third, and the third over the fourth.

There is a definite appeal to this hierarchical ordering internal to the principle of beneficence. In particular, good philosophical reasons exist for separating passive nonmaleficence (a so-called negative duty to avoid doing harm, as expressed in 1) and active beneficence (a so-called positive duty to afford assistance, as expressed in 2–4). Ordinary moral discourse and many philosophical systems suggest that negative duties not to injure others are more compelling than positive duties to benefit others.[6] For example, we do not consider it justifiable to kill a dying patient in order to use the patient's organs to save two others. Similarly, the duty not to injure a patient by abandonment seems to many stronger than the duty to prevent injury to a patient who has been abandoned by another (under the assumption that both are moral duties).

Despite the attractiveness of this hierarchical ordering rule, it is not firmly sanctioned by either morality or ethical theory. The duty expressed in (1) may not *always* outweigh those expressed in (2–4). For example, the harm inflicted in (1) may be negligible or trivial, while the harm to be prevented in (2) may be substantial. For instance, saving a person's life by a blood transfusion justifies the inflicted harms of venipuncture on the blood donor. One of the motivations for separating nonmaleficence from beneficence is that they themselves conflict when one must *either* avoid harm *or* bring aid. In such cases, one needs a decision rule to prefer one alternative to another. But if the weights of the two principles can vary, as they can, there can be no mechanical decision rule asserting that one principle must always outweigh the other.

In concrete cases, the conceptual distinctions between 1–4 begin to break down, at least in application. For example, if a physician prescribes morphine for a patient in extreme pain, is she providing a benefit (4) or removing a harm (3) or both? Similarly, when the state provides certain needed medical treatments to citizens, it can be argued that the state is not only providing a benefit (4), but also preventing and removing the harms of illness and death (2 and 3). To avoid running down a child playing in the street—that is, to refrain from doing harm (1)—requires positive steps of breaking, turning, warning, and the like.[7]

Such problems lead us to unify the moral demands that we should benefit and not injure others under a single principle of beneficence, taking care to distinguish, as necessary, between strong and weak requirements of this principle. The strength of these requirements corresponds only in some cases to the ordering of 1–4. In its general form, then, the principle of beneficence requires us to abstain from intentionally injuring others, and to further the important and legitimate interests of others, largely by preventing or removing possible harms.

There are several problems with the principle, so understood. For example, to what extent does the principle require the benefactor to assume personal risk or to suffer harm? Although it is widely agreed that we are obligated to act beneficently only if we can do so with minimal personal risk or inconvenience,[8] are there no conditions—special circumstances or role relationships—in which we are obligated to act beneficently even in the face of significant personal risk? Are not parents morally bound to sacrifice time and financial resources for their children? But would a stranger to the child be so bound?

A related problem is determining in any given instance to whom duties of beneficence are owed. Whose interests count, and whose count the most? The principle of beneficence should not, as a *principle*, be restricted to single parties even in special contests such as the patient-physician or subject-researcher relationship. Thus, the principle itself leaves open the question as to whom one's beneficence should be directed. For example, in the soliciting of consent to therapeutic research, there may be duties of beneficence to numerous third parties (future patients, employers, the state, endangered parties, etc.), even if the patient-subject's interests are the primary reason for an action. But third parties may not always have interests that should count.

Another vexing problem in ethical theory concerns the extent to which the principle of beneficence generates moral *duties*. Any analysis of beneficence that includes element (4) potentially demands severe sacrifice and extreme generosity in the moral life—for example, giving a kidney for transplantation or donating bone marrow. As a result, some philosophers have argued that this form of beneficent action is virtuous and a moral *ideal*, but not a duty. From this perspective, the positive benefiting of others is based on personal ideals that are supererogatory rather than obligatory: We are not morally *required* to promote the good of persons, even if we are in a position to do so, and even if the action is morally *justified*. The underlying problem is that actions such as sacrificing bodily parts and loving one's enemies may be more costly to the agent than morality demands.

Several proposals have been offered in moral philosophy to resolve this problem by showing that beneficence *is* a principle of duty, but these theoretical ventures are extraneous to our concerns here.[9] The scope or range of acts required by the duty of beneficence is an undecided issue, and perhaps an undecidable one. Fortunately, our arguments do not depend on its resolution. That we are morally obligated on *some* occasions to assist others is hardly a matter of moral controversy. Beneficent acts are demanded by the roles involved in fiduciary relationships between health care professionals and patients, lawyers and clients, researchers and subjects (at least in therapeutic research), bankers and customers, and so on. For example, physicians on duty in an emergency room are obligated to attend to injured, delirious, uncooperative patients, sometimes at considerable risk both to themselves and to the patient.

We will treat the basic roles and concepts that give substance to the principle of beneficence in medicine as follows: The positive benefit the physician is obligated to seek is the alleviation of disease and injury, if there is a reasonable hope of cure. The harms to be prevented, removed, or minimized are the pain, suffering, and disability of injury and disease. In addition, the physician is of course enjoined from *doing* harm if interventions inflict unnecessary pain and suffering on patients. While these considerations are all included under beneficence, we view the idea of a lexical ordering of sub-principles as an expendable overgeneralization.

In therapeutic research, the benefits and harms presented to subjects parallel those in medicine—the cure, removal, or prevention of pain, suffering, disability, and disease. In non-therapeutic research, the subjects' interests are less at center stage, because the positive benefit sought by the scientist is new knowledge. Often (but not necessarily) this knowledge is desired because it is expected to contribute to the resolution of important medical or social problems. Therapeutic and nontherapeutic research thus differ in the kinds of benefits each hopes to achieve. Although in both there is an equally strong imperative to avoid harming the subject, therapeutic research may legitimately present increased potential for harms if they are balanced by a commensurate possibility of benefits to the subject.

Those engaged in both medical practice and research know that risks of harm presented by interventions must constantly be weighed against possible benefits for patients, subjects, or the public interest. The physician who professes to "do no harm" is not pledging never to cause harm but rather to strive to create a positive balance of goods over inflicted harms. This is recognized in the Nuremberg Code, which enjoins: "The degree of risk to be taken should never exceed that determined by the humanitarian importance of the problem to be solved by the experiment."[10] Such a balancing principle is essential to any sound moral system: Beneficence assumes an obligation to weigh and balance benefits against harms, benefits against alternative benefits, and harms against alternative harms.

Health care professionals and research investigators often disagree over how to balance the various factors, and there may be no objective evidence that dictates one course rather than another.[11] In clinical contexts, this balancing can also present situations in which health care professionals and patients differ in their assessments of the professional's obligations. In some cases, benefit to another is involved—as, for example, when a pregnant woman refuses a physician's recommendation of fetal surgery. In other cases the refusal may be exclusively self-regarding. Some health care professionals will accept a patient's refusal as valid, whereas others are inclined to ignore the fact that an informed consent to treatment has not been given, and so try to "benefit" the patient through a medical intervention.

This problem of whether to override the decisions of patients in order to benefit them or prevent harm to them is one dimension of the problem of medical paternalism, in which a parental-like decision by a professional overrides an autonomous decision of a patient....

In health care, professionals and patients alike see the authority for some decisions as properly the patient's and authority for other decisions as primarily the professional's. It is widely agreed, for example, that the choice of a birth control method is properly the patient's but that the decision to administer a sedative to a panicked patient in an emergency room is properly the physician's. However, many cases in medicine exhibit no clear consensus about legitimate decisionmaking authority—for instance, who should decide which aggressive therapy, if any, to administer to a cancer victim or whether to prolong the lives of severely handicapped newborns by medical interventions? Similar disputes appear in the research context—for example, as to whether the researcher has the authority to use persons without their knowledge as subjects in low-risk research.

Decisions regarding who ought to serve as the legitimate authority—patient, subject, or professional—can turn decisively on what will maximally promote the patient's or subject's welfare. Standing behind the position that authority should rest with the patients or subjects may be the goal of benefiting patients and subjects by enabling them to make the decision that best promotes their welfare. Promotion of the value of autonomous choice in medical decision-making by patients is often justified by arguments from beneficence to the effect that decisional autonomy by patients enables them to survive, heal, or otherwise improve their own health. These arguments range from the simple contention that making one's own decisions promote one's psychological well-being to the more controversial observation that patients generally know themselves well enough to be the best

judges, ultimately, of what is most beneficial for them. Similar arguments are also used in research contexts where it is maintained that requiring the informed consent of subjects will serve as a curb on research risks. Here autonomous choice is valued extrinsically for the sake of health or welfare rather than intrinsically for its own sake.

Justice

Every civilized society is a cooperative venture structured by moral, legal, and cultural principles that define the terms of social cooperation. Beneficence and respect for autonomy are principles in this fabric of social order, but *justice* has been perhaps the subject of more treatises on the terms of social cooperation than any other principle. A person has been treated in accordance with the principle of justice if treated according to what is fair, due, or owed. For example, if equal political rights are due all citizens, then justice is done when those rights are accorded. Any denial of a good, service, or piece of information to which a person has a right or entitlement based in justice is an injustice. It is also an injustice to place an undue burden on the exercise of a right—for example, to make a piece of information owed to a person unreasonably difficult to obtain.

Many appeals to "justice" present a confused picture because they are not appeals to a *distinctive principle* of justice that is independent of other principles such as beneficence or respect for autonomy. These appeals to "what is just" use the term "just" in a broad and nonspecific sense to refer to that which is generally *justified*, or in the circumstances morally *right*. Claims of justice tend to emerge in literature on informed consent when it is believed that someone's legal or moral rights have been violated, and sometimes these claims also confuse justice with justification. For example, articles on psychological research involving deception often denounce the research as *unjustly* denying subjects information to which they are entitled. Yet, as the argument develops, it often turns out that the controlling moral principle in such a judgment is less one of justice per se than respect for autonomy. (The argument could, of course, involve appeal to both principles.) Similarly, proponents of a physician's obligation to withhold potentially harmful information from patients for therapeutic reasons sometimes argue that it would be *unjust* for the physician to provide less than the best possible medical treatment. Here the moral concern is one of beneficence rather than justice. Many complaints of "injustice" in the informed consent literature can be linked in this way to alleged violations of the principle of respect for autonomy or of the principle of beneficence.

However, not all issues of justice in biomedical ethics can be entirely accounted for by appeal to other principles. How to allocate scarce medical resources and the validity of claims to possess a right to health care are staple examples of justice-based problems. Although more difficult to isolate, various problems that plague the literature on informed consent also seem justice-based. For example, much of the controversy surrounding the use of prisoners as subjects in research centers less on whether prisoners can give valid informed consent in the coercive environment of incarceration than on whether justice permits creation of a ready pool of human volunteers out of the class of those incarcerated by the state, especially when the same pool of persons might be repeatedly used. This question turns on the just distribution of the burden of the risks of research participation in society and thus is *centrally* a problem about justice rather than beneficence or respect for autonomy. The issue is whether this burden could be warranted even if the public welfare is enhanced by the practice (a consideration of beneficence in the form of public utility) and even if the prisoners are capable of giving, and *do* give, a voluntary informed consent (a consideration of autonomy). The point of many analyses of research involving frequently used and vulnerable subjects is whether autonomous consent is sufficient to *override reservations based on justice* about approaching such persons to be research subjects in the first place.

It has also been argued that rules of informed consent can be motivated less by a concern to promote autonomous choice than by a concern to promote justice. Charles Lidz and his associates maintain that some who have argued for rules governing informed consent in psychiatry, including rules promoting increased disclosure in such areas as consent to electroconvulsive treatment (ECT), have been motivated by a concern over the *fairness* of subjecting patients to a potentially harmful treatment because of administrative convenience. They note that the advocates of strict disclosure "sought to use informed consent as a technique to minimize the use of ECT by using premises of equity and justice." However, as so often occurs, the persons Lidz has in mind were probably motivated by a *mixture* of moral concerns of respect for autonomy, beneficence, *and* justice. Lidz and others describe their *own* concerns in studying multiple problems of informed consent as motivated by the question whether a "more equal and mutual participatory relationship" can be established between health professionals and patients. They too seem motivated by a mixture of considerations of respect for autonomy, justice, *and* beneficence.[12] ...

BALANCING MORAL PRINCIPLES AND RIGHTS

Controversial problems about abstract moral principles such as "respect for autonomy" and "beneficence" inevitably arise over how much these principles demand and over how to handle situations of conflict with other moral principles, such as justice. Whatever the prominence of these principles, we must acknowledge that if they conflict—as they do on occasion—a serious weighting or priority problem is created. Successful novels and dramas often depict these moral principles in their baldest forms of conflict: A person steals in order to preserve a life, lies in order to protect a sworn secret, or breaks a duty to keep confidentiality in order to protect a person endangered by its maintenance. Under such conditions it must be decided which (if either) moral consideration has priority—a problem known in ethical theory as how to "weigh and balance moral principles." ...

The philosopher W. D. Ross is celebrated for his attempt to handle this problem of conflict.[13] Ross provides a list of several valid moral principles, including principles similar to the three we have had under examination. According to him, we must find "the greatest duty" in any circumstance of conflict by finding "the greatest balance" of right over wrong in that particular context. This metaphor of weights moving up and down on a balance scale is vivid, but crude and potentially misleading. Ross sought to give as much precision as possible to his ideas through a fundamental distinction between *prima facie* duties and *actual* duties: "Prima facie duty" refers to a duty always to be acted upon unless it conflicts on a particular occasion with an equal or stronger duty. A prima facie duty is always right and binding, all other things being equal. Although a firm duty, it is nonetheless conditional on not being overridden or outweighed by competing moral demands. One's actual duty, then, is determined by the balance of the respective weights of the competing prima facie duties.

Consider the following example:[14] A seventy-three-year-old man was mortally ill in a hospital and required a mechanical respirator. Although he had been judged competent, his request to have the respirator disconnected was refused. He then disconnected it himself, only to have the hospital staff reconnect it. The matter wound up in court. The patient contended that the hospital and his physicians had an obligation to allow him to make his own choices, even though his choice entailed his death. His physicians and legal representatives of the state of Florida argued that they had a duty to preserve life and to prevent suicide. Here the duty to preserve life is in direct conflict with the duty to respect the autonomous decisions of another person. Both are prima facie duties. A Florida court then had to fix the *actual* duty of the hospital and physicians. In a complicated balancing of the conflicting obligations, the court concluded that the patient's choice should be overriding because considerations of autonomy were *here* (though not *everywhere*) weightier. The court reasoned that "the cost to the individual" of refusing to recognize his choice in a circumstance of terminal illness could not be overridden by the duty to preserve life.

Partially as a result of Ross's arguments, moral philosophers have generally come to regard both duties and rights not as absolute trumps but, rather, as strong prima facie moral demands that may be validly overridden in circumstances where stringent opposing demands are presented by a competing moral principle. To call lying prima facie wrong means that if an act involves lying it *is* wrong, *unless* some more weighty moral consideration prevails in the circumstances. Moral principles and statements of rights thus have far greater moral importance than mere rules of thumbs, which do not have the same force of standing obligations.

As Ross admits, neither he nor any moral philosopher has yet been able to present a system of rules free of conflicts and exceptions. He argues that the nature of the moral life simply makes an exception-free hierarchy of rules and principles impossible. Contemporary moral philosophy has proved incapable of providing a solution to this problem of weighing and balancing that improves on Ross's approach. The metaphor of "weight" has not proved amenable to precise analysis, and no one has claimed to be able to arrange all moral principles in a hierarchical order that avoids conflicts.

Ross's thesis also applies to circumstances in which a single principle directs us to two equally attractive alternatives, only one of which can be pursued. For example, the principle of beneficence, when applied to problems of disclosing information to patients, could require both disclosure *and* nondisclosure; both options could lead to equally *beneficial*, albeit *different*, outcomes. Whether the conflict is of this sort or between two different principles, there may not be a *single* right action in some circumstances, because two or more morally acceptable actions may be unavoidably in conflict and prove to be of equal weight in the circumstances.

We assume ... that respect for autonomy is but a prima facie principle, and that it therefore has the same *but only the same* prima facie claim to override as other valid moral principles of comparable significance, such as beneficence or justice. Neither respect for autonomy nor any moral principle has an absolute standing that allows it on every occasion to override conflicting moral claims. Our analysis presupposes, as an inherent feature of the moral life, a pluralism of moral principles equally weighted in abstraction from particular circumstances. (Ross does not entirely accept this thesis of "equal weight.") Therefore, we hold that the moral principles of beneficence and justice—as well as more particular role responsibilities such as providing the best professional care—can have sufficient weight under *some* conditions to override respect for autonomy.

The moral view underlying this claim is not meant to diminish the standing of autonomy. Autonomy gives us respect, moral entitlement, and protection against invasions by others. Few matters of morals could be more important. But we should step back and ask, as Daniel Callahan has put it, "what it would be like to live in a community for which autonomy was the central value ... [and] sole goal."[15] There is an historical and cultural oddity about giving a standing of overriding importance to the autonomous individual. Moral communities—indeed morality itself—was founded at least as much on the other principles we have mentioned, and usually in a context of strong commitment to the public welfare.

Callahan has argued that making autonomy *the* moral value rather than *a* moral value, weighting it to trump every other moral value, buys the luxury of autonomy at too high a price, and we would agree. However, we would be well advised not to depress the value of autonomy relative to the other principles in our framework. Autonomy is almost certainly the most important value "discovered" in medical and research

ethics in the last two decades.... The pertinent point is that autonomy not be either overvalued or undervalued....

This analysis of plural prima facie *duties* applies to *rights* as well. It has often been assumed, owing perhaps to political statements about fundamental human rights, that certain rights are absolute trumps. However, decisive counterexamples can be mounted against this thesis. For example, it is sometimes proclaimed that the right to life is absolute, irrespective of competing claims or social conditions. The dubious validity of this thesis is evidenced by common moral judgments about capital punishment, international agreements about killing in war, and beliefs about the justifiability of killing in self-defense. Most writers in ethics now agree that we have an *exercisable right* not to have our life taken only if there is not a *sufficient moral justification* to override the right. The right to life—like the right to make an autonomous decision, the right to give an informed consent, or a parent's right to decide for a child—is legitimately exercisable and creates actual duties on others if and only if the right has an overriding status in the situation. Rights such as a right to an informed consent, a right to die, and a right to lifesaving medical technology thus must compete with other rights in many situations, producing protracted controversy and a need to balance with great discretion the competing rights' claims.

Numerous authors in biomedical and research ethics believe that if a person is acting autonomously and is the bearer of an autonomy right, then his or her choices morally ought *never* to be overridden by considerations of beneficence or proper care. This is not our assumption. Although the burden of moral proof will generally be on those who seek to intervene in another's choice, as the need to protect persons from harm becomes more compelling, thereby increasing the "weight" of moral considerations of beneficence in the circumstances, it becomes more likely that these considerations will validly override demands to respect autonomy. Similarly, because some autonomy rights are less significant than others, the demands to protect those rights are less weighty in the face of conflicting demands....

CONCLUSION

... Philosophy can provide a reasoned and systematic approach to moral problems, but it does not supply mechanical solutions or definitive procedures for decisionmaking. Practical wisdom and sound judgment are its indispensible allies in applied contexts. However, this lack of finality is no reason for skepticism. Moral philosophy can still yield well-constructed arguments and criticisms that advance our understanding. Moral dilemmas require a balancing of competing claims in untidy circumstances, and moral philosophy can make a significant if not decisive contribution. In these respects philosophy is neither surpassed by nor superior to legal reasoning and legal solutions....

Notes

1. See Isaiah Berlin, *Four Essays on Liberty* (London: Oxford University Press, 1969), 130.
2. For some reflections on what Kant's views do and do not show, see Arthur Flemming, "Using a Man as a Means," *Ethics* 88 (1978): 283–98.
3. See, for example, President's Commission for the Study of Ethical Problems in Medicine and Biomedical and Behavioral Research, *Deciding to Forego Life-Sustaining Treatment* (Washington, D.C.: U.S. Government Printing Office, 1983), 244ff; and, for the theoretical grounding of this claim in autonomy, *Making Health Care Decisions* (Washington, D.C.: U.S. Government Printing Office, 1982), Vol. 1, 44ff, esp. 47.
4. See Ludwig Edelstein, "The Hippocratic Oath: Text, Translation, and Interpretation," *Supplements to the Bulletin of the History of Medicine* 30, Supplement 1 (Baltimore: The Johns Hopkins University Press, 1943); reprinted in Owsei Temkin and C. Lilian Temkin, eds., *Ancient Medicine: Selected Papers of Ludwig Edelstein* (Baltimore: The Johns Hopkins Press, 1967). The translation provided here of the benefit injunction is from *Epidemics*, 1:11, in W.H.S. Jones, trans., *Hippocrates*, 4 vols. (Cambridge, MA: Harvard University Press, 1923), 1: 165.
5. See William K. Frankena, *Ethics*, 2nd ed. (Englewood Cliffs, N.J.: Prentice-Hall, Inc., 1973), esp. 47.
6. Perhaps the most important philosophical statement of this position is found in W.D. Ross, *The Right and the Good* (Oxford: Clarendon Press, 1930), 21.
7. For a discussion of such problems, see Joel Feinberg, *Harm to Others: The Moral Limits of the Criminal Law* (New York: Oxford University Press, 1984), 136–41; Richard Trammell, "Saving Life and Taking Life," *Journal of Philosophy* 72 (1975): 131–37, and "Tooley's Moral Symmetry Principle," *Philosophy and Public Affairs* 5 (1976): 305ff.
8. A widely held view is that one has a duty of beneficence only if one can prevent harm to others at minimal risk to oneself and if one's action promises to be of substantial benefit to the other person. This analysis of beneficence can be more tightly formulated as follows: X has a *duty* of beneficence toward Y only if each of the following conditions is satisfied: (1) Y is at risk of significant loss or damage, (2) X's action is needed to prevent this loss or damage, (3) X's action would probably prevent this loss or damage, and (4) the benefit that Y will probably gain outweighs any harms that X is likely to suffer and does not present significant risk to X. This formulation is indebted to Eric D'Arcy, *Human Acts: An Essay in Their Moral Evaluation* (Oxford: Clarendon Press, 1963), 56–57. Provision of benefit beyond these conditions would be to act generously but beyond the call of duty. Our formulation is only one plausible construal of the general duty of beneficence, but we believe it suffices for our purposes in this volume. For contrasting views, see Earl Shelp, "To Benefit and Respect Persons: A Challenge for Beneficence in Health Care," Allen Buchanan, "Philosophical Foundations of Beneficence," and Natalie Abrams, "Scope of Beneficence in Health Care," all in Earl Shelp, ed., *Beneficence and Health Care* (Dordrecht, Holland: D. Reidel Publishing Co., 1982).
9. See, for example, Frankena, *Ethics*, 47; Peter Singer, "Famine, Affluence, and Morality," *Philosophy and Public Affairs* 1 (1972): 229–43, and *Practical Ethics* (Cambridge: Cambridge University Press, 1979), 168ff; Marcus G. Singer, *Generalization in Ethics* (New York: Alfred A. Knopf, Inc., 1961), 180–89; and Michael A. Slote, "The Morality of Wealth," in William Aiken and Hugh LaFollette, eds., *World Hunger and Moral Obligation* (Englewood Cliffs, N.J.: Prentice-Hall, Inc., 1977), 125–47.

10. Nuremberg Code, Principle 6, from *Trials of War Criminals Before the Nuremberg Military Tribunals Under Control Council Law No. 10* (Military Tribunal I, 1947; Washington, D.C.: U.S. Government Printing Office, 1948–49).

11. A comprehensive treatment of this problem in the context of research is found in Robert J. Levine, *Ethics and Regulation of Clinical Research* (Baltimore: Urban & Schwarzenberg, 1981), chapter 3.

12. Charles W. Lidz, et al., *Informed Consent: A Study of Decisionmaking in Psychiatry* (New York: The Guilford Press, 1984), 7–8.

13. Ross, The Right and the Good, 19–42.

14. *Satz v. Perlmutter*, 362 S.2d 160 (Florida District Court of Appeals, 1978).

15. Daniel Callahan, "Autonomy: A Moral Good, Not a Moral Obsession," *The Hastings Center Report* 14 (October 1984): 40–42.

Metaphor and Analogy in Bioethics

James F. Childress

Many of our practices and much of our discourse in health care hinge on metaphors and analogies, whose significance is sometimes overlooked because they are considered merely decorative or escape notice altogether. Despite their relative neglect, they significantly shape our interpretations of what is going on as well as what should go on. In recent years they have received increasing attention, particularly from critics of principles-oriented approaches to bioethics who stress the role of imagination, emotion, and the like in morality and ethical reflection. I will examine metaphors before considering analogies, particularly in analogical reasoning, noting their overlap where appropriate....

METAPHORS IN BIOETHICS

The nature and function of metaphors. Perhaps because medicine and health care involve fundamental matters of life and death for practically everyone, frequently in mysterious ways, they are often described in metaphors. For instance, physicians may be viewed as playing God, or acting as parents, and nurses may be seen as advocates for patients; medicine itself may be interpreted as warfare against disease. Metaphors involve imagining something as something else, for example, viewing human beings as wolves or life as a journey. "The essence of a metaphor," according to Lakoff and Johnson, "is understanding and experiencing one thing through another."[1] More precisely, metaphors are figurative expressions that interpret one thing in terms of something else.[2]

In the large recent philosophical literature on metaphor, critics have challenged some traditional conceptions, contending that metaphors are more than merely ornamental or affective ways to state what could be stated in a more literal or comparative way and they can be and often are cognitively significant.[3] According to the traditional substitution view, a metaphorical expression is merely a substitute for some equivalent literal expression. For example, the metaphorical expression "John is a fox" substitutes for the literal expression "John is sly and cunning." One common version of the substitution view, what Max Black calls a comparison view (elements of which can be found in Aristotle), construes metaphor as the presentation of an underlying analogy or similarity. Hence, metaphor is a "condensed or elliptical simile,"[4] or it is a "comparison statement with parts left out."[5] "John is a fox," for example, indicates that "John is like a fox in that he is sly and cunning." According to such views, metaphors are dispensable ways to express what could be expressed differently, but they often appeal to the emotions more effectively than their equivalent literal expressions or comparisons would do.

By contrast many recent theories of metaphor stress its cognitive significance. For instance, in an early and very influential essay, philosopher Max Black defended an interaction view of metaphor, in which two juxtaposed thoughts interact to produce new meanings through the metaphor's "system of associated commonplaces" or "associated implications."[6] The metaphor—for instance, "wolf" in "man is a wolf"—serves as a "filter" for a set of associated implications that are transferred from the secondary subject ("wolf") to the principal subject ("man") in the sentence. (In a full interaction or interanimation view of metaphor, the transfer of meaning occurs both ways, not merely from the secondary subject to the principal subject.)[7]

Metaphors highlight and hide features of the principal subject, such as the physician who is viewed as a parent or as a friend, by their systematically related implications.[8] When argument is conceived as warfare, for example, the metaphor highlights the conflict involved in argument while it hides the cooperation and collaboration, involving shared rules, that are also indispensable to argument. Our metaphors thus shape how we think, what we experience, and what we do by what they highlight and hide. They use us, just as we use them.

Metaphors are often associated with models. For instance, we have both metaphors and models of the doctor–patient relationship. The physician may be viewed through the metaphor of father and the patient through the metaphor of child, and their relationship may be interpreted through the model of paternalism. Models, for our purposes, state the network of associated commonplaces and implications in more systematic and comprehensive ways—according to Max Black, "every metaphor is the tip of a submerged model."[9]

Metaphors and models may be good or bad, living or dead. Both metaphors and models can be assessed by how well they illuminate what is going on and what should go on. We can distinguish descriptive and normative uses of metaphors and models without admitting a sharp separation between fact and value. For instance, the metaphor of physician as father (or parent), and the model of paternalism (or parentalism), may accurately describe some relationships in medicine, or they may suggest ideal relationships in the light of some important principles and values.

Medicine as war, business, etc. The metaphor of warfare illuminates much of our conception of what is, and should be, done in health care. Consider the way this metaphor emerges in the day-to-day language of medicine: The physician as the captain leads the battle against disease; orders a battery of tests; develops a plan of attack; calls on the armamentarium or arsenal of medicine; directs allied health personnel; treats aggressively; and expects compliance. Good patients are those who fight vigorously and refuse to give up. Victory is sought; defeat is feared. Sometimes there is even hope for a "magic bullet" or a "silver bullet." Only professionals who stand on the firing line or in the trenches can really appreciate the moral problems of medicine. And they frequently have "war stories" to relate. Medical organization, particularly in the hospital, resembles military hierarchy, and medical training, particularly with its long, sleepless shifts in residencies, approximates military training more than any other professional education in our society.[10]

As medicine wages war against germs that invade the body and threaten its defenses, so the society itself may also declare war on cancer, or on AIDS, under the leadership of its chief medical officer, who in the United States is the Surgeon General. Articles and books even herald the "Medical-Industrial Complex: Our National Defense." As Susan Sontag notes, "Where once it was the physician who waged bellum contra morbum, the war against disease, now it's the whole society."[11]

The military metaphor first became prominent in the 1880s when bacteria were identified as agents of disease that threaten the body and its defenses. It both illuminates and distorts health care. Its positive implications are widely recognized—for instance, in supporting a patient's courageous and hopeful struggle against disease and in galvanizing societal support to fight against disease. But the metaphor is also problematic. Susan Sontag, who was diagnosed with cancer in the late 1970s, reports that her suffering was intensified by the dominance of the metaphor of warfare against cancer. Cancer cells do not just multiply; they are "invasive." They "colonize." The body's "defenses" are rarely strong enough. But since the body is under attack ("invasion"), by "alien" invaders, counterattack is justified. Treatments are also often described in military language:

> Radiotherapy uses the metaphors of aerial warfare; patients are "bombarded" with toxic rays. And chemotherapy is chemical warfare, using poisons. Treatment aims to "kill" cancer cells (without, it is hoped, killing the patient). Unpleasant side effects of treatment are advertised, indeed overadvertised. ("The agony of chemotherapy" is a standard phrase.) It is impossible to avoid damaging or destroying healthy cells (indeed, some methods used to treat cancer can cause cancer), but it is thought that nearly any damage to the body is justified if it saves the patient's life. Often, of course, it doesn't work. (As in: "We had to destroy Ben Suc in order to save it.") There is everything but the body count.[12]

Such "military metaphors," Sontag suggests, "contribute to the stigmatizing of certain illnesses and, by extension, of those who are ill." Other ill individuals have found the military metaphor unsatisfactory for other reasons. For instance, as a teenager, Lawrence Pray originally tried to conquer his diabetes, but his struggles and battles were futile and even counterproductive. Then over time he came to view his diabetes not as an "enemy" to be "conquered" but as a "teacher." Only then did he find a personally satisfactory way of living.[13]

Still others with illness, by contrast, have found the military metaphor empowering and enabling. In her wide-ranging study of pathographies, that is, autobiographical descriptions of personal experiences of illness, treatment, and dying, Anne Hunsaker Hawkins identifies several "metaphorical paradigms" that offer themes of "an archetypal, mythic nature."[14] In addition to illness as a battle, she concentrates on illness as a game or sport (a subset of the military metaphor), illness as a journey into a distant country, illness as rebirth or regeneration, and, on a somewhat different level, healthy-mindedness as an alternative to contemporary medicine. While pathographies are individualized statements, they provide "an immensely rich reservoir of the metaphors and models that surround illness in contemporary culture." These various metaphorical paradigms structure individuals' interpretations of their experiences of illness. Patterns emerge in individuals' selection of metaphors. They vary in part according to the illness involved—for example, the military metaphor is more common in descriptions of experiences with cancer and AIDS, while the rebirth metaphor is more common in descriptions of a critical life-threatening event, such as a heart attack. Furthermore, the military metaphor is generally more prevalent than the journey metaphor because it better fits the experience of modern medicine—for instance, it is easier to construe a physician as a "general" in a war than as a "guide" on a journey. Nevertheless, these various metaphors are often mixed and complementary. And they can be evaluated, Hawkins suggests, according to their capacity to enable and empower ill persons, for instance, by restoring a sense of personal dignity and worth. While expressing larger sociocultural patterns, the individual's choice of a particular metaphor is a creative act of assigning meaning to his or her illness.

The metaphor of warfare has been further challenged in modern medicine because of its apparent support for overtreatment, particularly of terminally ill patients, where death is the ultimate enemy and trauma, disease, or illness the immediate enemy. Physicians and families under the spell of this metaphor frequently find it difficult to let patients die. "Heroic" actions, with the best available weapons, befit the military effort that must always be undertaken against the ultimate enemy. Death signals defeat and forgoing treatment signals surrender. Some clinicians even feel more comfortable withholding (i.e., not starting) a treatment for cancer, for instance, than they do withdrawing (i.e., stopping) the same treatment, in part because withdrawing treatment implies retreat....

According to its critics, our invocation of the military metaphor often fails to recognize moral constraints on waging war. "Modern medicine," William F. May writes, "has tended to interpret itself not only through the prism of war but through the medium of its modern practice, that is, unlimited, unconditional war," in contrast to the just-war tradition.[15] In the spirit of modern total war, "hospitals and the physician-fighter wage unconditional battle against death." One result is that many patients seek assisted suicide or active euthanasia in order to escape from this warfare's terrorist bombardment. Traditional moral limits in the conduct of war include the principle of discrimination, which authorizes direct attacks on combatants but not on noncombatants. In medical care, the opposing combatant is the disease or death, not the patient. However, the patient is regularly the battleground and sometimes even becomes the enemy. This transformation into the enemy may occur if the patient betrays the military effort by not fighting hard enough or even by surrendering before the war ends. Finally, in accord with the just-war tradition's requirement of reasonable prospect of success and proportionality, the treatment should offer the patient a reasonable chance of success, and his or her suffering and other burdens must be balanced against the probable benefits of prolongation of life.[16]

Other problematic or ambiguous implications of the military metaphor appear in the allocation of resources for and within health care. It is not surprising that the two major terms for allocation and distribution of health care under conditions of scarcity emerged from, or were decisively shaped by, military experiences. These are triage and rationing. As Richard Rettig and Kathleen Lohr note,

> Earlier, policymakers spoke of the general problem of allocating scarce medical resources, a formulation that implied hard but generally manageable choices of a largely pragmatic nature. Now the discussion increasingly is of rationing scarce medical resources, a harsher term that connotes emergency—even war-time—circumstances requiring some societal triage mechanism.[17]

... I will only sketch some of the implications of the military metaphor for allocation, particularly macroallocation.

First, under the military metaphor, society's health care budget tends to be converted into a defense budget to prepare for and conduct war against disease, trauma, and death. As a consequence, the society may put more resources into health care in relation to other goods than it could justify, especially under a different metaphor, such as nursing or business (see below). Indeed, the society may overutilize health care, especially because technological care may contribute less to the national defense of health itself, through the reduction of morbidity and premature mortality, than other factors, such as the reduction of poverty.

Second, within the health care budget, the military metaphor tends to assign priority to critical care over preventive and chronic care. It tends to concentrate on critical interventions to cure disease, perhaps in part because it tends to view health as the absence of disease rather than as a positive state. It tends to neglect care when cure is impossible.

A third point is closely connected: In setting priorities for research and treatment, the military metaphor tends to assign priority to killer diseases, such as cancer and AIDS, over chronic diseases. Franz Ingelfinger once suggested that if we concentrated our research and treatment more on disabling diseases, such as arthritis, than on killer diseases, then national health expenditures would reflect the same values that individuals affirm: "It is more important to live a certain way than to die a certain way."[18] Anne R. Sommers has suggested that stroke is "a metaphor for the most difficult problems and challenges of geriatric medicine."[19] Although strokes are not limited to the elderly, they are more common among the elderly. Each year in the United States there are between 500,000 and 600,000 victims of stroke, 80 to 90 percent of them surviving their initial catastrophe, often with paralysis and aphasia, which have a terrible impact on both victims of stroke and their families. Approximately 2.5 million victims of stroke are alive today, 90 percent of them with varying degrees of incapacity and misery. Even though it has been called the single most costly disease in the United States, stroke received in 1979 only $18 million in research expenditures, in contrast to cancer, which received $937 million, and heart disease, which received $340 million. A major reason for this pattern of allocation is that, after the first acute phase, the stroke victim does not fit into the prevalent model of medical care, which emphasizes the specialist, who uses various technological weapons to fight specific problems. Hence this pattern continues.

Fourth, medicine as war concentrates on technological interventions over against non-technological modes of care and, within technologies, it tends to concentrate on more dramatic technologies, such as intensive care units and organ transplants, rather than less dramatic technologies, such as prostheses.

In short, the military metaphor has some negative or ambiguous implications for a moral approach to health care decisions: It tends to assign priority to health care (especially medical care) over other goods and, within health care, to critical interventions over chronic care, killer over disabling diseases, technological interventions over caring, and heroic treatment of dying patients rather than allowing them to die in peace.[20]

Some of the negative or ambiguous implications of the war metaphor for health care can be avoided if, as noted earlier, the metaphor is interpreted in accord with the limits set by the just-war tradition. However, the war metaphor may require supplementation as well as limitation. It is not the only prominent metaphor for health care, and since the early 1980s its dominance has been threatened by the language of economics and business, as reflected in the language of a health care industry: Providers deliver care to consumers, seek or are forced to seek productivity in light of cost-effectiveness or cost-benefit analyses, and may be concerned with "resource management, managed care systems, and market strategies."[21]

The business metaphor also highlights and hides various features of contemporary health care. Many critics of this metaphor worry that the language of efficiency will replace the language of care and compassion for the sick and equity in distribution of health care. Nevertheless, this metaphor has become more and more pervasive and persuasive as the structure of medicine and health care has changed and concerns about costs have become more central in societal discussions. Patients now often fear undertreatment as hospitals and professionals seek to reduce costs, in contrast to their fears of overtreatment under the war metaphor.

Both military and economic metaphors illuminate contemporary health care, but they may not be adequate, even together, to guide and direct health care. Whether any particular metaphor is adequate or not will depend in part on the principles and values it highlights and hides. Others have proposed nursing, a subset of health care, as a supplementary metaphor for the whole of health care, because of its attention to caring more than curing and to hands-on rather than technological care. Even though this metaphor of nursing—in contemporary discourse it is often more than a synecdoche—is also inadequate by itself, it could direct the society to alternative priorities in the allocation of resources for and within health care, particularly for chronic care….

Relationships between health care professionals and recipients of care. Relationships between physicians and other health care professionals, on the one hand, and patients, on the other, have been described and directed by a wide variety of metaphors and models.[22] For example, May has identified images of the physician as fighter, technician, parent, covenanter, and teacher, and Robert M. Veatch has identified several major competing models of physician-patient relationships: engineering, priestly (which includes the paternalistic model), collegial, and contractual models.[23] Other metaphors such as friend and captain of the ship have also been used.[24]

Some critics contend that such models are "whimsical gestalts," that many other arbitrary models could be invented—for example, bus driver or back-seat driver—and that moral points can and should be made more directly.[25] Such criticisms overlook how metaphors and models function in the interpretation and evaluation of interactions between physicians and patients. They miss the role of imagination, which can be defined as "reasoning in metaphors."[26] For example, opponents of paternalistic medical relationships usually do not eschew all use of metaphor; instead they offer alternative metaphors, such as partnership or contracts. And these various metaphors may be more or less adequate to describe what occurs and to direct what should occur in health care.

Metaphors and models highlight and hide features of the roles of physicians and other health care professionals by their various associated implications. For example, viewing the physician as a parent, or specifically as a father, based on the nineteenth-century model of the family, highlights some features of medical relationships, such as care and control, while hiding others, such as the payment of fees. The use of such metaphors to describe, interpret, and explain relationships is subject to criticism if they distort more than they illuminate. And when they are offered to guide relationships and actions, they are subject to criticism if they highlight only one moral consideration, such as the physician's duty to benefit the patient or to respect patient autonomy, while hiding or obscuring other relevant moral considerations. It is also appropriate to consider the feasibility of various ideal relationships in light of significant personal, professional, and institutional constraints.

Several metaphors may be necessary to interpret health care as it is currently structured and to guide and direct actions, practices, and policies in health care. Some metaphors may fit some relationships better than others; for example, relations in clinical research, family practice, and surgery may be illuminated respectively by the metaphors of partner, teacher–student, and technician–consumer. Furthermore, not all of these metaphors conflict with each other; some may even be mutually supportive as well as compatible, for example, contractor and technician. However, conflicts can be expected if a physician interprets and directs relationships paternalistically, while his or her patient interprets and directs the interaction through metaphors of negotiation and accommodation....

Nursing as advocacy. Major changes in the conception of nursing correlate with alterations in its primary metaphors. Whether situated within the military effort against disease or viewed as physicians' handmaidens and servants, nurses have traditionally been expected to cultivate passive virtues, such as loyalty and obedience. Their moral responsibility was primarily directed toward physicians and institutions, such as hospitals, and only secondarily toward patients. This interpretation of responsibility was shaped in part by nursing's military origins in the nineteenth century as well as by societal conceptions of gender.[27] Then in the 1970s, nursing was reconceived through the metaphor of advocacy. Nurses became advocates for "clients" and "consumers" (the term "patient" was often rejected as too passive). This legal metaphor, drawn from the advocate as one who pleads another's cause, especially before a tribunal of justice, highlights active virtues, such as courage, persistence, perseverance, and courage, and views the nurse as primarily responsible to the patient or client. This metaphor is explicit or implicit in formal nursing codes, and it is also featured in a large number of nurses' stories of advocacy and conflict in health care.[28]

Critics, such as Ellen Bernal, note that the metaphor of advocacy reduces the range of services traditionally offered by nurses; it is thus insufficiently comprehensive. In addition to distorting the human experience of illness, it distorts nursing by focusing almost exclusively on patients' or clients' rights, construed mainly in terms of autonomy, and it neglects positive social relationships in health care.[29] It highlights conflict among health care professionals because it implies that some of them do not adequately protect the rights of patients. Thus, the metaphor frequently supports a call for increased nursing autonomy as a way to protect patient autonomy. Because of its adversarial nature, many question whether the metaphor of advocacy can adequately guide relationships among health care professionals in the long run, even if it is useful in the short run. The metaphor may also assume that the nurse's responsibility to the patient/client is always clear-cut and overriding, even though nurses may face serious conflicts of responsibility involving patients, other individuals, associates, and institutions.[30] At the very least, sympathetic commentators call for further clarification of the metaphor of advocacy, while critics seek alternative metaphors and models, such as covenant, partnership, teamwork, or collegiality, which appear to offer more inclusive, cooperative ideals.

Playing God and other metaphors of limits. "Playing God" has been a common metaphor for both describing and (re)directing the activities of scientists, physicians, and other health care professionals. They have been criticized for usurping God's power—for instance, the power over life and death—by letting patients die or by using new reproductive technologies,

There are theological warrants for playing God in the Jewish and Christian traditions, which affirm the creation of human beings in God's image and likeness. Philosopher David Heyd builds on this idea of the image of God: "If indeed the capacity to invest the world with value *is* God's image, it elevates human beings to a unique (godly) status, which is not shared by any other creature in the world. This is playing God in a creative, 'human-specific' way."[31] And

Paul Ramsey calls on those who allocate health care to play God in a fitting way: "Men should then 'play God' in the correct way: he makes his sun rise upon the good and the evil and sends rain upon the just and the unjust alike." We should emulate God's indiscriminate care by distributing scarce lifesaving medical technologies randomly or by a lottery rather than on the basis of judgments of social worth.[32] ...

Despite a few such positive uses of the metaphor of "playing God," the metaphor is generally used to identify two aspects of divine activity that should not be imitated by humans: God's unlimited power to decide and unlimited power to act. On the one hand, users of this metaphor demand scientific and medical accountability over against unilateral decision making, for example, regarding life and death. On the other hand, they call for respect for substantive limits, for example, not creating new forms of life in violation of divinely ordained natural limits.[33] Critics frequently focus on human arrogance and rebellion in daring to "play God." In a more typical statement (in contrast to his positive use of the metaphor cited earlier), Ramsey writes: "Men ought not to play God before they learn to be men, and after they have learned to be men they will not play God."[34] Thus, critics of "playing God" usually demand scientific and medical accountability along with respect for substantive limits, such as not creating new forms of life. Objectors to negative uses of the metaphor of "playing God" often challenge the rationale for holding that a particular course of action, such as human genetic engineering, is wrong.

Edmund L. Erde contends that statements such as "doctors should not play God" are so unclear that they cannot function as commands and do not articulate a principle; thus, they cannot be followed because agents do not know how to conform their actions to them. Nor do they explain why certain actions should not be undertaken. Such phrases are, Erde argues, "metaphoric in that they tuck powerful feelings and images into descriptive language that cannot be understood literally." Any activity, such as mercy killing, that is "labeled 'playing god' carries the implication that it is clearly wrong." These phrases are used for situations in which agents face choices but one option is considered immoral and is rejected as arrogantly and presumptuously playing God. The background of intelligibility of this metaphor, according to Erde, is found in the Western idea of the great chain of being, which identifies appropriate responsibilities at each level and opposes the usurpation of power and the failure to respect limits.[35]

Other important and widespread metaphors of limits include the thin edge of the wedge and the slippery slope, both of which warn against undertaking certain actions because other unacceptable actions will inevitably follow. Examples regularly appear in debates about euthanasia. Such arguments about limits may take at least two different forms: (1) conceptual, and (2) psychological–sociological. The first focuses on the logic of moral reasoning, the hammer back of the wedge, and the other on what the wedge is driven into. Or, to shift to the slippery slope metaphor, the slope may be slippery for two different reasons. According to the first reason, the slope is slippery because the concepts and distinctions are vague, inadequately drawn, or ultimately indefensible. This first version derives its power from the principle of universalizability (discussed below), which commits us to treating relevantly similar cases in a similar way. Because of this principle of universalizability, Paul Ramsey argues, ethical (and legal) mistakes tend to replicate themselves: "It is quite clear that at the point of medical, legal, and ethical intersections at the edges of life … the so-called wedge argument is an excellent one. This is true because legal principles and precedents are systematically designed to apply to other cases as well. This is the way the law 'works,' and … also the way moral reasoning works from case to similar case."[36]

By contrast, the second version, which is more plausible in arguments against the legalization of physician-assisted suicide and euthanasia, considers the personal, social, institutional, and cultural context in order to determine the pos-

sible impact of changing rules or making exceptions. Even if certain distinctions between various acts are, in principle, clear and defensible, agents may not be able over time to draw them and act on them because of various psychological, social, institutional, and cultural forces, such as racisms, sexism, or ageism.[37]

Even though such metaphors of limits are often misused, they are appropriate in some contexts. In each use of these metaphor of limits, important moral questions require attention—the evaluation of the first action and subsequent actions—and important conceptual and empirical questions must be addressed in order to determine whether the putatively bad consequences will inevitably follow what might be innocuous first steps. (Similar points hold for analogies invoking moral limits.) …

Metaphors for bioethics and bioethicists. The role and function of the bioethicist have often been construed in metaphorical terms. The common langage of "applied ethics" invokes the metaphor of engineering as an application of basic science that does not contribute to basic science. The expertise of applied ethicists resides in their ability to apply general theories and principles to specific arenas of human activity. The metaphor of application has been widely challenged on the grounds that it is too narrow and distorts much that is important in bioethics. The term "applied" suggests that ethicists are problem solvers rather than problem setters, that they solve puzzles rather than provide perspectives, that they answer rather than raise questions, and that they begin from theory rather than from lived experience. It implies a limited technical or mechanical model of ethics.

The term "applied" distorts the numerous theoretical controversies in bioethics and neglects the way bioethics may help to resolve or recast some theoretical controversies. At the very least, the metaphor of application needs to be supplemented by various other metaphors for the task of practical ethics and the role of the practical ethicist: "Theoretician, diagnostician, educator, coach, conceptual policeman, and skeptic are also supplemental or alternative roles to that of the technician."[38] Some other metaphors are drawn from ancient religious roles, such as prophet or scribe. Yet another metaphor is "conversation," which is prominent in approaches to bioethics that emphasize interpretation, hermeneutics, and narrative. And the "stranger" has been proposed as the best metaphor for the ethicist in professional education because his or her outside perspective can challenge ordinary assumptions.[39]

No doubt several such metaphors are needed to interpret and direct the activities of ethicists. Which ones appear to fit best will depend in part on our operative conception of ethics and, in particular, on its breadth and richness….

Generative metaphors. Suggestions emerge at various times to retire all metaphors, not merely some metaphors, in some realm of discourse—for instance, Susan Sontag proposes retiring all metaphors for illness.[40] However, it is not possible to strip our discourse in science, medicine, and health care, or in biomedical ethics, of all metaphors. Instead, we must use metaphors with care and carefully assess their adequacy in their descriptive and normative functions.

For each use of metaphor, we have to ask whether, through highlighting and hiding features of subjects, it generates insights about what is or about what ought to be. A simple example of what Donald Schoen calls a generative metaphor, that is, one that generates insights, occurred when researchers were trying to improve the performance of a new paintbrush made with synthetic bristles. The new brush applied the paint to the surface in a "gloppy way." Nothing the researchers tried made the artificial bristles work as well as natural bristles. Then one day someone observed, " You know, a paintbrush is a kind of pump!" That was a generative metaphor: Pressing a paintbrush against a surface forces paint through the spaces or "channels" between the bristles, and painters sometimes even vibrate brushes to increase the flow. Once the researchers began to view the paintbrush as a kind of pump, they were able to improve the brush with synthetic bristles.[41] That is the kind of insight, both descriptive and directive, that we seek. Rarely, however, will it be so dramatic. In most issues confronted in biomedical ethics, the tests of adequacy of particular metaphors will be more complex and subtle. At the very least, tests of metaphors that function normatively to guide being and doing need to incorporate general moral considerations.

ANALOGIES IN BIOETHICS

Analogies and analogical reasoning. Often metaphors and analogies are presented in ways that indicate their substantial overlap. Indeed, in the comparison view of metaphor, there is little difference between them, because metaphors are compressed analogies. Some recent theories of metaphor have stressed, by contrast, that metaphors create similarities rather than merely expressing previously established and recognized similarities or analogies. According to Max Black, comparison views of metaphor fail because they reduce the ground for shifts of meaning (from the secondary subject to the primary subject) to similarity or analogy.[42] Nevertheless, there is a strong consensus that metaphorical statements presuppose some resemblance, even when they also create resemblance.[43] Black himself later conceded that metaphors "mediate an analogy or structural correspondence." Metaphor is, roughly speaking, "an instrument for drawing implications grounded in perceived analogies of structure between two subjects belonging to different domains."[44] And yet metaphor does not merely compare two things that are similar, but rather enables us to see similarities in what would be regarded as dissimilar.

Metaphors and analogies are thus closely related, with metaphors both expressing and creating similarities. In general, good metaphors function cognitively to generate new meaning and insight by providing new perspectives, while good analogies extend our knowledge by moving from the familiar to the unfamiliar, the established to the novel. In stretching language, concepts, and so forth for new situations, analogy does not involve the imaginative strain often evident in the use of metaphors.[45] Nevertheless, the differences in function between metaphors and analogies should not be exaggerated.

The term analogy derives from the Greek *analogia*, which referred to mathematical proportion. "An analogy in its original root meaning," Dorothy Emmet observes, "is a proportion, and primarily a mathematical ratio, e.g., 2:4::4:X." In such a ratio, given knowledge of three terms, and the nature of the proportionate relation, the value of the fourth term can be determined. Thus analogy is the repetition of the same fundamental pattern in two different contexts.[46]

Analogical reasoning thus proceeds inductively, moving from the known to the unknown. It appears prominently in problem solving and thus is featured in research in cognitive science and artificial intelligence.[47] For instance, computer problem-solving programs must search for analogous problems that have been successfully solved to generate solutions to new problems whether in highly structured domains such as law or in less structured domains.

Analogical reasoning has an important place in moral discourse, not only because of its importance in problem solving, but also because of the widely recognized moral requirement to treat similar cases in a similar way. Often stated as a principle of universalizability or of formal justice or formal equality, and dating back at least to Aristotle, the requirement to treat similar cases in a similar way also appears on the common law's doctrine of precedent. The basic idea is that one does not make an acceptable moral or legal judgment—perhaps not even a moral or legal judgment at all—if one judges that X is wrong but that a similar X is right, without adducing any relevant moral or legal difference between them. In general, analogical reasoning illuminates features of morally or legally problematic cases by appealing to relevantly similar cases that reflect a moral or legal consensus (precedent). Of course, much of the moral (or legal) debate hinges on determining which similarities and differences are both relevant and significant....

Analogy and casuistry. Over the last decade or so analogical reasoning has received renewed attention from philosophers and theologians focusing on case-oriented or casuistical judgments in bioethics and elsewhere, particularly in the wake of perplexities often associated with new technologies that appear, at least at first glance, to create or occasion unprecedented problems. In *The Abuse of Casuistry*, Albert R. Jonsen and Stephen Toulmin identify "the first feature of the casuistic method" in its classical formulations as "the ordering of cases under a principle by paradigm and analogy."[48] For instance, the rule prohibiting killing is set out in "paradigm cases" that illustrate its most manifest breaches according to its most obvious meaning. Moving from simple and clear cases to complex and uncertain ones, casuists examine various alternative circumstances and motives to determine whether those other cases violate the rule against killing. They seek analogies that permit the comparison of "problematic new cases and circumstances with earlier exemplary ones," that is, the similar type cases that constitute presumptions.[49]

Despite the claims of some modern casuists, it is not clear that analogical reasoning distinguishes casuistical from principlist approaches. For instance, in analyzing the novel microallocation problems of modern medicine, Ramsey, a strongly rule-oriented ethicist, appealed to the analogous "lifeboat" cases—when some passengers have to be thrown overboard to prevent the lifeboat from sinking—as a way to interpret the requirements of the principle of equality of opportunity in distributing such scarce lifesaving medical technologies as kidney dialysis.[50] Because principles and rules are indeterminate and because they sometimes conflict, analogical reasoning can be expected in case judgments—mere application cannot be sufficient in ethical frameworks that appeal to principles and rules....

Analogies are often divided into two main types, analogies of attribution and analogies of proportion.[51] The analogy of attribution involves a comparison of two terms or analogates, both of which have a common property, the analogon, that appears primarily in one and secondarily in the other. As Thomas Aquinas noted, "healthy" is used primarily for a person in a state of health (a "healthy" person) and secondarily for those medicines and practices that help to maintain or restore health (e.g., a "healthy" diet) or specimens that provide evidence of the body's health (e.g., "healthy" blood). By contrast, in the analogy of proportion, the analogates lack a direct relationship, but each of them involves a relationship that can be compared to a relationship in the other.[52] This second type is most common in analogical reasoning in biomedical ethics, as is evident in debates about maternal–fetal relations and abortion, where analogies of attribution also appear, particularly with reference to the fetus.

Analogical reasoning in debates about maternal–fetal relations. Debates about maternal–fetal relations, including pregnant women's decisions to abort and to decline caesarean sections, illustrate the pervasiveness and importance of analogical reasoning. Traditionally, abortion has been construed as directly killing the fetus, an innocent human being, in violation of the duty of nonmaleficence. Hence, in traditional Roman Catholic moral theology, direct abortions are tantamount to homicide. Sometimes the analogy of the "unjust aggressor" appears in situations where the pregnancy threatens the pregnant woman's life or health, but it has not been accepted in official Catholic thought the same way the similar analogy of the "pursuer" has been accepted in some Jewish thought to justify abortions when the pregnant woman's life or health is threatened.

Some feminists and others have attempted to recast the debate about abortion to focus on the basis and extent of the pregnant woman's obligation to provide bodily life support to the fetus. Often accepting, at least for purposes of argument, the premise that the fetus is a human being from the moment of conception (or at some time during the pregnancy), they argue that this premise does not entail that the pregnant woman always had a duty to sustain the fetus's life, regardless of the circumstances of pregnancy, the risks and inconveniences to the pregnant woman, and so forth. Their arguments often proceed through analogies to other hypothetical or real practices or cases, on the assumption that a judgment about those practices or cases will entail a similar judgement about abortion.

The fantastic abortion analogies introduced by Judith Jarvis Thomson have been particularly influential and controversial.[53] In one of her artificial cases, an individual with a rare blood type is kidnapped by the Society of Music Lovers and attached to a famous violinist who needs to purify his system because of his renal failure. Part of the debate is whether relevant analogies can be found in such fantastic, artificial cases, in contrast to actual real cases. For example, over against Thomson, John Noonan opposes abortion in part by appeal to a U.S. tort law case, in which the court held liable the hosts who had invited a guest for dinner but then put him out of the house into the cold night even though he had become sick and fainted and requested permission to stay.[54]

Some feminists and others contend that other analogous real-life legal and moral cases support the pregnant woman's free decision to continue or to discontinue her pregnancy. For many the relevant analogous cases concern living organ and tissue donation. Such donations are conceived as voluntary, altruistic acts that should not be forced by others even to save the potential recipient's life. They are "gifts of life." Requiring a pregnant woman to continue the pregnancy until birth imposes on her a heavier burden than others are expected to bear in analogous circumstances, such as a parent who could save a child's life by donating a kidney. Thus, the provision of bodily life support, whether through donating an organ or allowing the fetus to use the uterus, has been conceived as a gift of life that should not be legally enforced.[55]

According to Lisa Sowle Cahill, much analogical reasoning about pregnancy overlooks what is unique about maternal–fetal relations and thus obscures the morally relevant features of pregnancy or makes some relevant features more significant than they are. Many analogies problematically narrow our moral perspective on abortion by portraying the inception of pregnancy as accidental and the fetus as strange, alien, and even hostile. Furthermore, they often rely on the connotative meanings of their terms, particularly as embedded in a story, such as Thomson's case of kidnapping the unconscious violinist. Examples also appear in the rhetoric of abortion opponents who, for instance, speak of the fetus as a "child" and thereby distort the unique dependence of the fetus on the pregnant woman. Finally, Cahill contends, justifications of abortion based on analogy often rest on liberal convictions that special responsibilities derive only from free choice.[56]

For all these reasons, Cahill holds that analogical reasoning needs supplementation through direct examination of the unique features of maternal–fetal relations, particularly total fetal dependence, and of the ways these unique features qualify maternal, professional, and societal obligations. She argues that, as a category or class of moral relations, pregnancy "is unique among human relations at least because in it one individual is totally and exclusively dependent on a particular other within a relation which represents in its physical and social aspects what is *prima facie* to be valued positively."[57] Hence, she argues, most analogies hide what is distinctive and unique about pregnancy, even though they identify some morally relevant features of maternal–fetal relations.

With the emergence of other maternal–fetal conflicts, particularly regarding caesarean sections to benefit the fetus, similar debates have emerged about the appropriateness of the analogy with living organ and tissue donation. For instance, in the case of *In re A.C.* (No. 87–609, District of Columbia Court of Appeals, April 26, 1990), the majority of the court held that just as courts do not compel people to "donate" organs or tissue to benefit others, so they should not compel caesarean sections against the will of pregnant women to benefit potentially viable fetuses. The dissenting opinion rejected the analogy with organ and tissue donation, insisting that the pregnant woman "has undertaken to bear another human being, and has carried an unborn child to viability," that the "unborn child's" dependence upon the mother is unique and singular, and that the "viable unborn child is literally captive within the mother's body."

Even though analogies with organ and tissue donation are now widely invoked to oppose state control of pregnant women's decisions regarding both abortion and caesarean sections, there are important differences between these two sorts of issues in maternal–fetal relations. In the abortion debate, pregnancy is viewed as the provision of bodily life support and is itself analogous to the donated organ. In the debate about caesarean sections, the surgical procedure is analogous to organ donation—the potentially viable fetus is removed for its own benefit rather than to benefit some other party as in organ or tissue donation. In the abortion debate, the pregnancy is viewed as invasive; in the debate about caesarean sections, the surgical procedure is invasive. However, the central issue is whether state coercion to benefit the fetus is morally and legally acceptable in these cases, and the debate hinges in part on the appropriateness of living organ and tissue donation as an analogy. Even the critics of the analogy engage in analogical reasoning, but they deny that the similarities are more morally or legally relevant and significant than the dissimilarities. Defenders of governmental coercion could also hold that the moral or legal precedent is mistaken and that organs and tissues should sometimes be conscripted or expropriated from living persons.

Similar disputes appear in other areas of contemporary bioethics, for instance, in debates about whether mandatory testing or screening for antibodies to the human immunodeficiency virus, which causes AIDS, can be justified by analogy to accepted practices of mandatory testing or screening (and what precedents it would create for additional testing and screening, for example, for various genetic conditions), and in debates about whether transplantation experiments using human fetal tissue, following deliberate abortions, are analogous to the complicitous use of materials or data from the morally heinous Nazi experiments. In these cases, as in many others, the debates focus to a great extent on the relevance and significance of the proposed analogies....

CONCLUSIONS

Debates in biomedical ethics are often debates about which metaphors and analogies illuminate more than they distort. Far from being merely decorative or affective, metaphors and analogies are central to both discourse and practice, for framing our problems as well as for shaping our responses to them. They cannot be evaluated in general but rather must be evaluated specifically according to how well they function to describe and/or direct actions, relationships, and the like. Even though in recent bioethics they have sometimes been offered as ways to circumvent or transcend principles and rules, particularly through attention to cases, narratives, and aesthetic dimensions of experience, they are not necessarily incompatible with principles and rules. For instance, analogical reasoning is important within frameworks of principles and rules, as well as in casuistry, and metaphors and models often succeed or fail depending on how well they express the full range of relevant moral considerations....

Notes

1. George Lakoff and Mark Johnson, *Metaphors We Live By* (Chicago: University of Chicago Press, 1980), p. 5.
2. Janet Martin Soskice, *Metaphor and Religious Language* (Oxford: Clarendon Press, 1985).
3. See, for instance, Max Black, "Metaphor," in *Models and Metaphors: Studies in Language and Philosophy* (Ithaca: Cornell University Press, 1962), pp. 25–47; Paul Ricoeur, *The Rule of Metaphor,* trans. Robert Czerny (Toronto: University of Toronto Press, 1977); and Soskice, *Metaphor and Religious Language.*
4. Black, "Metaphor."
5. George Miller, "Images and Models, Similes and Metaphors," in *Metaphor and Thought,* ed. Andrew Ortony (Cambridge: Cambridge University Press, 1979), pp. 202–50.
6. Black, "Metaphor," and Black, "More about Metaphor," in *Metaphor and Thought,* ed. Ortony, pp. 19–43.
7. Soskice, *Metaphor and Religious Language.*
8. Black, "Metaphor," and Lakoff and Johnson, *Metaphors We Live By.*
9. Black, "More about Metaphor," p. 31.
10. Childress, *Who Should Decide?* chap. 1. See also Childress, *War as Reality and War as Metaphor: Some Moral Reflections,* The Joseph A. Reich, Sr., Distinguished Lecture, November 18, 1992 (Colorado Springs: U.S. Air Force Academy, 1993). For other discussions of military metaphors in health care, in addition to the ones that appear in these notes, see Virginia Warren, "A Powerful Metaphor: Medicine as War" (unpublished paper), and Samuel Vaisrub, *Medicine's Metaphors: Messages and Menaces* (Oradell, NJ: Medical Economics Company, 1977).
11. Susan Sontag, *Illness as Metaphor* and *AIDS and Its Metaphors* (New York: Doubleday Anchor Books, 1990), p. 72. Her essay "Illness as Metaphor" was first published separately in the *New York Review of Books* in 1978 and later that year by Farrar, Straus and Giroux, which also published the essay *AIDS and Its Metaphors* separately in 1989 before the combined edition appeared.
12. Ibid., p. 68.
13. Lawrence Pray, *Journey of a Diabetic* (New York: Simon and Schuster, 1983), and "How Diabetes Became My Teacher," *Washington Post,* July 31, 1983.
14. Anne Hunsaker Hawkins, *Reconstructing Illness: Studies in Pathography* (West Lafayette: Purdue University Press, 1993).
15. William F. May, *The Physician's Covenant* (Philadelphia: Westminster Press, 1983), p. 66.
16. For an explication of the just-war tradition, see James F. Childress, *Moral Responsibility in Conflicts* (Baton Rouge: Louisiana State University Press, 1982), esp. chap. 3 on "Just-War Criteria."
17. Richard Rettig and Kathleen Rohr, "Ethical Dimensions of Allocating Scarce Resources in Medicine: A Cross-National Study of End-Stage Renal Disease," unpublished manuscript (1981).
18. Franz Ingelfinger, Editorial, *New England Journal of Medicine* 287 (December 7, 1982): 1198–99.
19. Anne R. Somers, "The 'Geriatric Imperative' and Growing Economic Constraints," *Journal of Medical Education* 55 (February 1980): 89–90, which is also the source of the figures in the remainder of this paragraph.

20. For these points, see James F. Childress, "Ensuring Care, Respect, and Fairness for the Elderly," *Hastings Center Report* 14 (October 1984): 27–31.

21. Howard F. Stein, *American Medicine as Culture* (Boulder: Westview Press, 1990).

22. James F. Childress and Mark Siegler, "Metaphors and Models of Doctor-Patient Relationships: Their Implications for Autonomy," *Theoretical Medicine* 5 (1984): 17–30, which is reprinted below as chapter 3. See also Mark Siegler, "The Physician-Patient Accommodation: A Central Event in Clinical Medicine," *Archives of Internal Medicine* 142 (1982): 1899–1902.

23. May, *Physician's Covenant,* and Robert V. Veatch, "Models for Ethics in Medicine in a Revolutionary Age," *Hastings Center Report* 2 (June 1972): 5–7. See also May, "Code, Covenant, Contract, or Philanthropy," *Hastings Center Report* 5 (December 1975): 29–38.

24. Nancy M. P. King, Larry R. Churchill, and Alan W. Cross, eds., *The Physician as Captain of the Ship* (Dordrecht: D. Reidel, 1988).

25. K. Danner Clouser, "Veatch, May, and Models: A Critical Review and a New View," in *The Critical Encounter,* ed. Earl E. Shelp (Dordrecht: D. Reidel, 1983), pp. 89–103.

26. David Eerdman, "Coleridge as Editorial Writer," in *Power and Consciousness*, ed. Conor Cruise O'Brien and William Dean Vanech (New York: New York University Press, 1969), p. 197.

27. Gerald Winslow, "From Loyalty to Advocacy: A New Metaphor for Nursing," *Hastings Center Report* 14 (June 1984): 32–40; Ellen W. Bernal, "The Nurse as Patient Advocate," *Hastings Center Report* 22 (July/August 1992): 18–23.

28. Winslow, "From Loyalty to Advocacy," and Bernal, "Nurse as Patient Advocate."

29. Bernal, "Nurse as Patient Advocate."

30. Winslow, "From Loyalty to Advocacy."

31. David Heyd, *Genethics: Moral Issues in the Creation of People* (Berkeley: University of California Press, 1992), p. 4 (emphasis in original).

32. Paul Ramsey, *The Patient as Person* (New Haven: Yale University Press, 1970), chap. 7, esp. pp. 256 and 259. Ramsey waffles, sometimes holding that human beings should not play God, at other times (as in this context) suggesting that there are proper ways to play (and not to play) God.

33. See the discussion in the President's Commission for the Study of Ethical Problems in Medicine and Biomedical and Behavioral Research, *Splicing Life* (Washington, D.C.: U.S. Government Printing Office, 1983).

34. Paul Ramsey, *Fabricated Man: The Ethics of Genetic Control* (New Haven: Yale University Press, 1970), p. 138.

35. Edmund L. Erde, "Studies in the Explanation of Issues in Biomedical Ethics: (II) On 'On Playing God', Etc., *Journal of Medicine and Philosophy* 14 (1989): 593–615.

36. Paul Ramsey, *Ethics at the Edges of Life* (New Haven: Yale University Press, 1978), pp. 306–307.

37. For fuller analyses and assessments of wedge and slippery slope arguments, from which some of these points have been drawn, see Tom L. Beauchamp and James F. Childress, *Principles of Biomedical Ethics,* 4th ed. (New York: Oxford University Press, 1994), pp. 228–31.

38. Arthur L. Caplan, "Ethical Engineers Need Not Apply: The State of Applied Ethics Today," *Science, Technology and Human Values* 6 (1980): 30.

39. Larry Churchill, "The Ethicist in Professional Education," *Hastings Center Report* 8 (December 1978): 13–15.

40. Sontag, *Illness as Metaphor* and *AIDS and Its Metaphors.*

41. Donald Schoen, "Generative Metaphor: A Perspective on Problem-Setting in Social Policy," in *Metaphor and Thought*, ed. Ortony.

42. Black, "Metaphor."

43. Ricoeur, *The Rule of Metaphor.*

44. Black, "More about Metaphor."

45. Soskice, *Metaphor and Religious Language.*

46. Dorothy Emmet, *The Nature of Metaphysical Thinking* (New York: St. Martin's Press, 1945), p. 6

47. See David H. Helman, ed., *Analogical Reasoning: Perspectives of Artificial Intelligence, Cognitive Science, and Philosophy* (Dordecht: Kluwer, 1988); and Mark T. Keane, *Analogical Problem Solving* (Chichester: Ellis Norwood, 1988).

48. Albert R. Jonsen and Stephen Toulmin, *The Abuse of Casuistry: A History of Moral Reasoning* (Berkeley: University of California Press, 1988), p. 252.

49. Ibid., p. 316.

50. Ramsey, *Patient as Person*, chap. 7.

51. Lisa Sowle Cahill, "Abortion and Argument by Analogy," *Horizons* 9 (1982): 271–87.

52. Ibid.

53. Judith Jarvis Thomson, "A Defense of Abortion," *Philosophy and Public Affairs* 1 (1972): 47–66.

54. John T. Noonan, "How to Argue about Abortion," (New York: The Ad Hoc Committee in Defense of Life, 1974).

55. See Susan Mattingly, "Viewing Abortion from the Perspective of Transplantation: The Ethics of the Gift of Life," *Soundings* 67 (1984): 399–410; and Patricia Beattie Jung, "Abortion and Organ Donation: Christian Reflections on Bodily Life Support," *Journal of Religious Ethics* 16 (1988): 273–305.

56. Cahill, "Abortion and Argument by Analogy."

57. Ibid., p. 283.

Why a Feminist Approach to Bioethics?

Margaret Olivia Little

Those who work in feminist bioethics are all too familiar with the question, "Why think that feminism offers a distinctive contribution to bioethics?" When asked respectfully, I take it to be a fair question. After all, even if we were to stipulate that the tenets of feminism are profound and wise, it would not guarantee that they offer substantial illumination in every subject matter. However, while it is a good question to ask, it also has a good answer. In this essay, I outline why it is, and how it is, that feminist insights provide such a valuable theoretical aid to the study of bioethics.

First, however, certain misunderstandings need to be addressed. Some individuals seem to understand feminist bioethics to be talk about women's issues in bioethics or, again, to be women talking about bioethics. But while the subject bears some relation to each, it is equivalent to neither. Feminist bioethics is the examination of all sorts of bioethical issues from the perspective of feminist *theory*. The question of feminism's contribution to bioethics can be understood, then, as a question about how and why bioethics might benefit from excursions into this sort of theory. And here the potential for dialogue is too often stunted by a tendency, on the part of those who pose the question, to measure feminism's contribution solely in terms of any distinctive policy recommendations its advocates might give to familiar bioethical controversies. This tendency is often joined by frustration among those who have encountered the diversity within feminist thought, as they wonder how feminism's contribution to specific bioethical topics can be assessed until feminists resolve which camp—liberal, cultural, or radical, say—is correct. But this policy-oriented view of feminism, and of what would count as a "distinctive contribution," sets the stage for far too flat a conception of how feminist theory can enrich bioethics.

At its most general, feminist theory can be thought of as an attempt to uncover the ways in which conceptions of gender distort people's view of the world and to articulate the ways in which these distortions, which are hurtful to all, are particularly constraining to women. These efforts involve *theory*—and not merely benign protestations of women's value or equality—because the assumptions at issue are often so subtle or so familiar as to be invisible, and, crucially, because the assumptions about gender have shaped not only the ways in which we think about men and women, but also the contours of certain fundamental concepts—from "motherhood" to "rationality"—that constitute the working tools of theoretical analyses. According to feminist theory, that is, distorted and harmful conceptions of gender have come to affect the very ways in which we frame our vision of the world, affecting what we notice, what we value, and how we conceptualize what does come to attention.

If these claims are correct, then feminist theory will be useful to disciplines whose subject-matter or methods are appreciably affected by such distortions—and it will be useful in ways that far outstrip the particular policy recommendations that feminists might give to some standard checklist of topics. For one thing, feminist reflection may change the checklist—altering what questions people think to ask, what topics they regard as important, what strikes them as a puzzle in need of resolution. Or again, such reflection may change the analyses underlying policy recommendations—altering which assumptions are given uncontested status, which moves feel persuasive, what elements stand in need of explanation, and how substantive concepts are understood and deployed. If such reflections sometimes yield policies similar to those offered by nonfeminists, the differences in approach can still matter, and matter greatly, by influencing what precedent one takes oneself to have set, what dangers one is alerted to watch for, what would later count as reason to abandon or re-think the policy. And if such reflections are sometimes followed by diverse policy recommendations, we should not be surprised, much less frustrated; for the diagnostic work that forms the core enterprise of feminist theory leads to policy recommendations only in combination with commitments on a variety of other fronts, from economic theory to the empirical facts of the case, about which feminists will understandably disagree.

This, however, is so far rather abstract. To give a more concrete sense of how feminist theory might contribute to bioethics, we need to dip into the theory itself. Accordingly, I want to outline two central themes common to virtually all feminist reflection and use them to illustrate two quite different ways in which attention to feminist insight offers illumination in health care ethics.

ANDROCENTRISM

One of the central themes of feminist theory is that human society, to put it broadly, tends to be androcentric, or male-centered. Under androcentrism, man is treated as the tacit standard for human: he is the measuring stick, the unstated point of reference, for what is paradigmatic of or normal for humans. To start with an obvious example, man is used as the supposedly generic representative of humanity. That is, when we

want to refer to humans independently of gender, it is man that is cast for the job: in language ("Man does not live by bread alone"), in examples (such as the classic illustration of syllogistic reasoning, "All men are mortal, Socrates is a man, therefore Socrates is mortal"); in pictorial representations (according to the familiar depiction of evolution—still used in current biology texts—the indeterminate primate, gradually rising to bipedalism, is inevitably revealed in the last frame to be a man).

This depiction of "human" arguably places man in an unfairly privileged position, since he is not only a constituent, but the representative, of all humanity. But much deeper problems than this are at issue, for these supposedly neutral uses of man are not actually neutral. They are *false generics*, as revealed in our tendency to drop the so-called gender-neutral "he" in favor of "she" when speaking of professions (such as nanny) that are held mostly by women, or again by our difficulty in imagining the logic professor saying, "All men are mortal, Sally is a man (woman?), therefore Sally is mortal."

The first problem resulting from this hidden bias is that androcentrism has a disturbing cumulative effect on our understanding of "human": over time, our substantive conception of what is normal for humans has come to be filled in by what is normal for men (excellent discussions of this general theme can be found in Bem 1993, especially Chapters 3 and 6; Minow 1990; and MacKinnon 1987, Part I). Certain features of men—their experiences, their bodies, their values—have subconsciously come to be regarded as constituting the human norm. His psychology, for instance, tends to define the human mind. In a famous study (Broverman et al. 1970), when psychologists were canvassed and asked to describe the "healthy" man, the "healthy" woman, and the "healthy" human, the list for men and humans turned out to be virtually identical, the list for women divergent. His body tends to define the human body. A clear, if depressing, example can be found in the Supreme Court decision in *General Electric Co. v. Gilbert* (429 U.S. 125, 1976). In a decision finally superseded legislatively by the Pregnancy Discrimination Act, the Court decided that businesses could permissibly exclude pregnancy disabilities from general insurance coverage. Their reasoning was that "pregnancy-related disabilities constitute an additional risk, unique to women, and the failure to compensate them for this risk does not destroy the presumed parity of the benefits that accrue to both men and women," even though (as the Court was aware) the list of traditionally protected benefits included all manner of medical procedures that were unique to men, such as prostate operations and circumcisions. As Sandra Bem (1993, p. 76) puts it:

> The Court is androcentrically defining the male body as the standard human body; hence it sees nothing unusual or inappropriate about giving that standard human body full insurance coverage for each and every condition that might befall it. Consistent with this androcentric perspective, the Court is also defining equal protection as the granting to women of every conceivable benefit that this standard human body might require—which, of course, does not include disability coverage for pregnancy.

In addition, man's biography tends to define norms of practice in the work place. We need go no further than the academic tenure system for an example. Presumably, the idea of evaluating faculty for tenure after their first seven years of employment is premised on the supposition that job performance during those seven years provides some rough indication of performance over the remainder of academic life. But, while this may be true for men, the same cannot be said for women. Factoring in the average time spent at graduate school, those seven years precisely correspond to likely childbearing years for women faculty—years most likely to involve pregnancy, birth, and breast-feeding, and hence most likely to involve severe sleep deprivation and time pressure. Of all the years of her academic career, these will be the ones *least* likely to represent her overall potential.

Second, treating man as the human norm affects, in subtle but deep ways, our concept of "woman." Males and females obviously differ from one another in various ways. "Different from" is a relation, of course, and a symmetrical one at that: if x is different from y, it is just as true that y is different from x. Under androcentrism, however, we tend to anchor man as the reference point and view woman's nature as a departure from his. A subtle but powerful message is communicated when we always anchor one side of what is logically a symmetrical relation as the fixed point of reference: the anchored point gains the status of the center; the other receives the status of the margin. Because man has been fixed as the reference point for so long, part of our very conception of woman has become the conception of "other"—she is, as Simone de Beauvoir (1952) put it, the *second* sex. Instead of thinking that men differ from women who differ from men, a subtle conceptual shift occurs, and we begin to think of women as simply "different"—as though "different" were an intrinsic property that adheres to them, instead of a relational property men also instantiate (see Minow 1990, pp. 53–56). In the end, it is a short step to regarding aspects of woman's distinct nature as vaguely *deviant*.

Further, woman becomes closely defined by the *content* of her departure from man. The fundamental ways in which women and men differ are, of course, in certain biological features. But when man's body is regarded as the neutral "human" body, woman's biological sex becomes highlighted in such a way that, in the end, awareness of woman very often is awareness of her sex. The phenomenon is akin to one that occurs with race. In white-dominated societies, being white gets anchored as the tacit reference point; over time, the fact that whites have a race tends to fade from consciousness, while people of color are seen as somehow more intrinsically raced (think of how many Americans use the phrase "ethnic restaurants" to refer to non-European cuisine, as though Europeans had no ethnicity, or of how Western history books use the phrase "Ethnic Hoards" to refer, say, to the

Mongolian invaders of Europe, but not, say, to the United States' invasion of Okinawa). In a similar way, woman's sex comes to be seen as more essential to her nature than man's sex is to his. We are more likely to see woman as ruled by the whims of her reproductive system than man is by his; more subtly, if no less dangerously, we are simply more likely to think of and be concerned with reproductive issues when thinking of women than of men.[1]

Finally, under androcentrism, woman is more easily viewed in instrumental terms—in terms, that is, of her relation to others and the functions she can serve them. We tend, for instance, to specify a woman's identity in relation to the identity of some man (think of how traditional titles of respect for women indicate her marital status while those for men do not). Or again, the norms of a good woman, unlike those of a good man, tend to value her function for others: an excellent man is one who is self-directive and creative; an excellent woman is one who is nurturing of others and beautiful for them to behold. More concretely, women's legal status often reflects an instrumentalist interpretation of her being. In certain countries, indeed, the interpretation is still as stark as it was in early English common law's doctrine of coverture, which declared, as the legalist William Blackstone ([1765–1769] 1979, Vol. 1, p. 430) wrote:

> By marriage, the husband and wife are one person in law: that is, the very being or legal existence of the woman is suspended during the marriage, or at least incorporated and consolidated into that of the husband; under whose wing, protection, and cover, she performs everything.

Awareness of these general androcentric themes will give new food for thought on any number of topics in bioethics. The medicalization of childbirth, for instance—too often packaged as a tiresome debate between those generically loyal to and those generically suspicious of technology—takes on more suggestive tones when we consider it in light of the historical tendency to regard women as "other" or

deviant and hence in need of control (see, e.g., Rothman 1982). Certain patterns of research on women and AIDS emerge with greater clarity when viewed against our proclivity to view women instrumentally: until very recently such research focused almost entirely on women as transmitters of the disease to their fetuses, rather than on how the disease manifests itself, and might be treated, in the women themselves (Faden, Kass, and McGraw, in press). Let me develop in slightly more detail, though, an example that brings to bear the full range of androcentric themes outlined above.

Many people were taken by surprise when a 1990 U.S. Government Accounting Office report (GAO 1990) indicated that women seemed to be underrepresented in clinical trials. To give a few now-famous examples, the Physicians Health Study, which concluded in 1988 that an aspirin a day may help decrease the risk of heart disease, studied 22,000 men and no women; the Baltimore Longitudinal Study, one of the largest projects ever to study the natural processes of aging, included no women at its inception in 1958 and still had no data on women by 1984, although women constitute 60 percent of the population over age 65 in the United States (see Laurence and Weinhouse 1994, p. 61). It is difficult to be precise about women's overall representation in medical research because information on participants' sex often is not gathered; but there does seem to be legitimate cause for concern. For one thing, U.S. Food and Drug Administration (FDA) guidelines from 1977 to 1993 barred all women of childbearing potential from early clinical trials, which seems to have discouraged their representation in later stages of drug research (Merton 1994). More broadly, a review of medical studies published in JAMA in 1990 and 1992 revealed that, in studies on non-gender-specific diseases, women were underrepresented in 2.7 times as many studies than were men (Bird 1994; see also Laurence and Weinhouse 1994, pp. 64–67).

The possibility of significant underrepresentation has raised concerns that women are being denied equal opportunity to participate in something they may regard as valuable and that women may face compromised safety or efficacy in the drugs and procedures they receive (for instance, the difference in the average weights of women and men raises questions about the effects on women of drugs that are highly dosage-sensitive). Now, determining what policy we should advocate with respect to women's inclusion in medical research is a complicated matter—if only because adding sex as a variable in research protocols can significantly increase the cost of research.[2] What is clear, though, is that awareness of various androcentric motifs can highlight important issues that might otherwise remain hidden or camouflaged. Without the perspective of feminist theory, that is, certain concerns are likely not even to make it to the table to be factored in when policy questions arise (for a related discussion, see DeBruin 1994). Let me give some examples.

One argument against the inclusion of women commonly offered by those running clinical trials is that women's hormones represent a "complication": the cyclicity of women's hormonal patterns introduces a variable that can make it harder to discern the effects of the drug or procedure being studied. Now this is an interesting argument, for acknowledging the causal power of women's hormonal cyclicity might also suggest the very reason that it might be important to include women in studies, namely, the possibility that the cyclicity affects the underlying action of the drug or procedure. Medicine has only begun to consider and study this possibility in earnest (see Cotton 1990; Hamilton and Parry 1983). Early results include preliminary evidence that surgical treatment for breast cancer is more effective if done in the second, rather than the first, half of a woman's menstrual cycle, and that the effectiveness of antidepressants varies across a woman's menstrual cycle, suggesting that women currently receive too much for one half of the month and too little for the other (see Laurence and Weinhouse 1994, p. 71). Trust in all-male studies seems to reflect a broad confidence in the neutrality of treating the male body as the human norm and a familiar tendency

to regard that which is distinct to woman as a distortion—in this case, by regarding women's hormonal pattern as merely distorting the evidence concerning the true effect of a drug or procedure, and hence as something that is best ignored, rather than regarding it as an important factor in its own right, one influencing the actual effect of the object studied.

Another reason often given for the underrepresentation of women by those running clinical trials is that women are harder to find and to keep in studies. There is an important element of truth here: questionnaires reveal that women report greater problems navigating the logistics of participating in drug trials—they find it more difficult, for instance, to arrange for transportation and child care (Cotton 1993; Laurence and Weinhouse 1994, pp. 70–71). But if it is currently harder for women to participate than for men, it is not because of some natural or neutral ordering of things; it is in large part because drug trials are currently organized to accommodate the logistical structure and hassles of men's lives. Organizers routinely locate trials where men are, such as the military, for instance, and to organize activities around work schedules in the public economy. Again, there is a tendency to anchor what is normal for "participants" to features that are more typical of men. If women's distinctive needs show up on the radar screen at all, they appear as needs that would require "special" accommodation—and hence accommodation one may decline to make—as though accommodations for men have not already been made.

A different concern lay behind the now-defunct FDA guidelines barring women of childbearing potential from early clinical trials. Here the explicit rationale was fetal protection: the drugs women would be exposed to might harm fetuses they knowingly or unknowingly carried. A closer look, however, once again reveals the subtle presence of androcentrism: granting society's interest in fetal health, protective measures are applied quite differently to men and women. The guidelines in essence barred all fertile women from early trials—including single women not planning to have intercourse, women using reliable birth control, and women whose partners had had vasectomies (Merton 1994). In contrast, when trials were conducted on drugs suspected of increasing birth defects by affecting men's sperm (a possibility often forgotten), fertile men were simply required to sign a form promising to wear condoms during the trial (Laurence and Weinhouse 1994, pp. 72–73). The regulation was able to think of men under guises separate from their reproductive capacities, but, as Vanessa Merton (1994, p. 66) says, it "envisions all women as constantly poised for reproductive activity." Further, and again granting that fetal protection is important, one might argue that respect for parental autonomy argues in favor of allowing the individual to decide whether participation is worth the risk. But when respect for parental autonomy conflicts with protection for fetuses or children, society is much more willing to intrude on the autonomy if it belongs to a woman than to a man. Courts, for instance, have forced women to undergo cesarean sections in attempts to gain slight increases in a fetus's chance for survival, while they routinely deny requests to force fathers to donate organs—or even blood—to save the life of their children (see Daniels 1993).

GENDERED CONCEPTS

A second core theme of feminist theory maintains that assumptions about gender have, in subtle but important ways, distorted some of the broad conceptual tools that philosophers use. Certain key philosophical concepts, such as reason and emotion or mind and body, seem in part to be *gendered* concepts—that is, concepts whose interpretations have been substantively shaped by their rich historical associations with certain narrow conceptions of male and female.

One such distortion stems from the fact that, historically, that which is tightly and consistently associated with woman tends to become devalued. Throughout history, woman has been regarded as a deficient human: as a group, at least, she does not measure up to the standard set by man. (Indeed, it would be surprising if there

were not some such evaluation lurking behind the scenes of androcentrism, for it would otherwise be puzzling why it is man who is ubiquitously cast as the human norm.) Aristotle *defined* woman as "a mutilated male," placing her just above slaves in the natural hierarchy (*Generation of Animals*, Books I and II; *Politics*, Book I). In post-Darwinian Victorian society, when a theory emerged according to which "lower forms" of human remained closer to embryonic type, a flurry of studies claimed to demonstrate the child-like aspects of woman's anatomy. She was, as one chapter heading called her, "Undeveloped Man"; in the words of James Allan, a famous and particularly succinct anthropologist, "Physically, mentally, and morally, woman is a kind of adult child … Man is the head of creation" (both cited in Russett 1989, pp. 74, 55). Against this background, those things associated with woman can gradually inherit a depreciated status. "Womanly" attributes, or aspects of the world regarded as somehow "feminine," become devalued (which, of course, only serves to reinforce the poor judgment of women, as they are now associated with things of little value). To give just one illustration, think of the associations we carry about voice types and authority. A resonant baritone carries a psychological authority missing in a high squeaky voice. This is often cited as a reason women have trouble being viewed as authority figures; but it is also worth asking why authority came to be associated with a baritone rather than a soprano in the first place. Clearly, the association both reflects a prior conception of man as naturally more authoritative and reinforces that commitment, as women's voices then stand in the way of their meeting the "neutral" standard of authority.

Another common distortion stems from the fact that pairs of concepts whose members are associated with man and woman, respectively, tend to become interpreted in particularly dualistic ways. For much of Western history, but especially since the Scientific Revolution, men and women have been understood as having different appropriate spheres of function (see, e.g., Gatens

1991, Pateman 1989, Bordo 1986, Lloyd 1983, Okin 1979).[3] Man's central role was in the public sphere—economics, politics, religion, culture; woman's central role was in the private sphere—the domestic realm of care taking for the most natural, embodied, and personal aspects of humans. This separation of spheres was understood to constitute a complementary system in which each contributed something of value that, when combined, made an ideal whole—the marriage unit. Of course, given the devaluation of that which is associated with woman, it is not surprising that woman's sphere was regarded as less intrinsically valuable: it is man, and what is accomplished in the public sphere, that represents the human ideal (a view reflected in history books, which are histories of wars and political upheavals, not of hearth and home). In any event, because the division was understood as grounded in the natures of man and woman, the separation was a rigid one; the idea that either side of the division could offer something useful to the other's realm would simply not emerge as a possibility. This dualistic picture of the nature and function of women and men, with its subtle devaluing of women, can bleed over to concepts that have been tightly associated with the sexes. When abstract concepts, such as, say, mind and body, come to be paired with the concepts of male and female consistently enough, their substantive interpretations often become tainted with the dualism that characterizes the understanding of those latter concepts. The nature of each comes to be understood largely in opposition to the other, and, while the pair is understood as forming a complementary whole, the functions of the components are regarded as rigidly separated, and the one that is regarded as "male"—here, mind—is held in higher philosophical esteem.

These themes are mirrored in the interpretation of certain central philosophical concepts. An important instance is the traditional conception of reason and emotion, which plays a large role in moral philosophy. For all the hotly disputed debates in the history of ideas, one theme that emerges with remarkable consistency is an association of women with emotion and men with reason (see Tuana 1992, Chapters 2–4; Lloyd 1984). According to Aristotle (*Politics*, 1260a15), women have rationality "but without authority"; Rousseau (1979, p. 386) gives Sophie a different education from Emile because "the search for abstract and speculative truths, principles and axioms in the sciences, for everything that tends to general ideas, is not within the competence of women"; and according to Kant (1960, p. 79), "women's philosophy is not to reason but to sense." Science has contributed its support—for example, tracing woman's supposedly greater proclivity towards volatile emotions to disorders of the womb (hence "uterus" as the root of "hysteria") and her restricted intellect to the "hormonal hurricanes" of her menstrual cycle (see Smith-Rosenberg 1972; Russett 1989, especially Chapter 4; and Fausto-Sterling 1992, Chapter 4). As James Allan wrote, "In intellectual labor, man has surpassed, does now, and always will surpass woman for the obvious reason that nature does not periodically interrupt his thought in application" (cited in Russett 1989, p. 30). (Apparently Allan suffered no concern that man's rather more constant hormonal activity might be rather more constantly interrupting his thought!)

The conception of reason and emotion found in much of traditional ethical theory bears the mark of these entrenched associations (see Jaggar 1989, Lloyd 1983). There is a tendency to regard reason and emotion as having completely separate functions and to regard emotion, at best, as irrelevant to the moral enterprise and, at worst, as something that infects, renders impure, and constantly threatens to disrupt moral efforts. Emotion is conceptualized as something more to do with the body we have as animals than the mind we have as humans; it is viewed as a faculty of blind urges, akin to pains and tickles, rather than as responses that reflect evaluations of the world, and that hence can be "tutored" or developed into mature stances.

Thus, most traditional moral epistemology stresses that the stance appropriate to moral wisdom is a dispassionate one. To make considered, sound moral judgments, we are told to abstract from our emotions, feelings, and sentiments. Emotions are not part of the equipment needed to discern moral answers; indeed, only trouble can come of their intrusion into deliberations about what to do, for they "cloud" our judgment and "bias" our reasoning. To be objective is to be detached; to be clear-sighted is to achieve distance; to be careful in deliberation is to be cool and calm. Further, the tradition tends to discount the idea that experiencing appropriate emotion is an integral part of being moral. Moral theory tends to focus exclusively on questions about what actions are obligated or prohibited, or perhaps on what intention or motive one should have in acting, not on what emotional stance a moral agent should be feeling. Indeed, much of traditional moral theory has a positive suspicion of emotion as a basis for moral action. Emotions such as love or indignation, as opposed to some cerebral "respect for duty," are deemed fickle and unreliable (metaphors, of course, for the female); they "incite" and "provoke" us, rather than moving us by way of their reasonability. Finally, traditional moral theory vastly underplays the importance of the "emotional work" of life—of nurturing children, offering sympathetic support to colleagues, or displaying felt concern for patients. To the extent that the value of such work is recognized at all— as, for example, in treatises on "mother love"— it is often accorded a lesser status, regarded as reflective of instinct rather than skill, and hence not qualifying as moral work at all, or as relevant only in limited spheres of life, such as nursing or parenting, that are accorded lower value than other more impersonal enterprises.

Feminists argue that these presuppositions may not survive their gendered origins. Possession of appropriate emotion, for instance, arguably forms an indispensable component of a wise person's epistemic repertoire (see Little 1995). While our passions and inclinations can mislead us and distort our perceptions, they can also guide them. To give just one example, if one is deprived of felt concern for a patient, it is unlikely that one will be attuned to the subtle and unique nuances of his situation. Instead of discerning the contours of his particular needs, one

is likely to see his case as an instance of one's current favorite generality. Distance, that is, does not always clarify. Sometimes truth is better revealed, the landscape most clearly seen, from a position that has been called "loving perception" or "sympathetic thinking" (Lugones 1987, Jaggar 1989, Walker 1992b). And again, emotion arguably forms an integral part of being moral. Simply to perform a required action—while certainly better than nothing—is often not enough. Being moral frequently involves feeling appropriate emotions, including anger, indignation, and especially caring. The friend who only ever helps one out of a sense of duty rather than a feeling of generous reciprocity is not in the end a good friend; the citizen who gives money to the poor, but is devoid of any empathy, is not as moral as the one whose help flows from felt concern. This is not to say that we owe personal love to all who walk the earth—proper caring comes in different forms for different relationships. Nor is proper caring to be conflated with self-abnegation. Suspicions about the moral imperative to care often tacitly rely on self-sacrificial models of care, in which the boundary between self and other is overly blurred. From a feminist perspective, it is not surprising that this is the model of care we have inherited, for caring has usually been regarded as women's work, and traditional norms for women have stressed a denial of self. Feminist reflection, acutely aware of the limitations of these norms, precisely invites us to develop a healthier and more robust conception of proper caring (for further discussion, see Carse and Nelson 1996).

In another important instance, that which is associated with the private or domestic sphere is given short shrift in moral theory. Relations in the private sphere, such as parent-child relations, are marked by intimacies and dependencies, appropriate kinds of partiality, and positive but unchosen obligations that cannot be modelled as "contracts between equals." Furthermore, few would imagine that deliberations about how to handle such relations could be settled by some list of codified rules—wisdom here requires skills of discernment and judgment, not the internalization of set principles. But traditional moral theory tends to concentrate on moral questions that adjudicate relations between equal and self-sufficient strangers, to stress impartiality, to acknowledge obligations beyond duties of non-interference only when they are incurred by voluntary contract, and to emphasize a search for algorithmic moral principles or "policies" that one could apply to any situation to derive right action (Walker 1992a, Baier 1987).

This tendency to subsume all moral questions under a public "juridical" model tends, for one thing, to restrict the issues that will be acknowledged as important to those cast in terms of rights. "The" moral question about abortion, for instance, is often automatically cast as a battle between maternal and fetal rights, to the exclusion of, say, difficult and nuanced questions about whether and what distinctly maternal responsibilities might accompany pregnancy. And it often does violence to our considered sensibilities about the morality of relations involving dependencies and involuntary positive obligations. For instance, in considering what it is to respect patient autonomy, many seem to feel forced into a narrow consumer–provider model of the issue, in which the alternative to simply informing and then carrying out the patient's wishes must be regarded as paternalism. While such a model may be appropriate to, say, business relations between self-sufficient equals, it seems highly impoverished as a model for relations marked by the unequal vulnerabilities inherent in physician–patient relations. In these sorts of relations, all of the rich moral possibilities lie in between the two poles of merely providing information, on the one hand, and wresting the decision from the patient, on the other. For example, a proper moral stance might involve proactively helping a patient to sift through options, or proactively fostering the patient's independence by, say, discussing sensitive questions outside the presence of overly interfering family members.

Finally, when ethical approaches more characteristic of the private sphere do make it onto the radar screen, there is still a tendency to segregate these approaches from those we take to the public sphere. That is, in stark contrast to the tendency to subsume the morality of intimates into the morality of strangers, rarely do we ask how the moral lessons garnered from reflecting on private relations might shed light on moral issues that arise outside of the purely domestic context. To give just one example, patients often feel a deep sense of abandonment when their surgeons do not personally display a caring attitude toward them: the caring they may receive from other health care professionals, welcome as it may be, seems unable to compensate for this loss. This phenomenon will seem less puzzling if, borrowing a concept from the private realm, we realize that surgery involves a special kind of *intimacy*, as the surgeon dips into the patient's body. Seen under this guise, the patient's need becomes more understandable—and the surgeon's nontransferable duty to care clearer—for reflection on more familiar, domestic intimacies, such as those involved in sexual interactions, reminds us that intimacy followed by a vacuum of care can constitute a kind of abandonment.

In summary, then, reflection in feminist theory is important to bioethics in at least two distinct ways. First, it can reveal androcentric reasoning present in analyses of substantive bioethical issues—reasoning that can bias not only which policies are adopted, but what gets counted as an important question or persuasive argument. Second, it can help bioethicists to rethink the very conceptual tools used in bioethics—specifically, helping to identify where assumptions about gender have distorted the concepts commonly invoked in moral theory and, in doing so, clearing the way for the development of what might best be called "feminist-inspired" moral theory.

Notes

1. For excellent discussions of this theme in the history of science, see Russett (1989), Fausto-Sterling (1992, Chapter 4), and Rosenberg (1976, Chapter 2).
2. For extensive analysis of issues relating to public policy, see the essays in Institute of Medicine (1994, vol. 1).

3. Portions of this and the next few paragraphs are taken from my article, "Seeing and Caring: The Role of Affect in Feminist Moral Epistemology" (Little 1995).

References

Baier, Annette. 1987. The Need for More than Justice. In *Science, Morality and Feminist Theory*, ed. Marsha Hanen and Kai Nielsen, pp. 41-56. Calgary: University of Calgary Press.

Beauvoir, Simone de. 1952. *The Second Sex.* New York: Alfred A. Knopf.

Bem, Sandra L. 1993. *The Lenses of Gender.* New Haven and London: Yale University Press.

Bird, Chloe E. 1994. Women's Representation as Subjects in Clinical Studies: A Pilot Study of Research Published in JAMA in 1990 and 1992. In *Women and Health Research: Ethical and Legal Issues of Including Women in Clinical Studies,* vol. 2, Institute of Medicine, pp. 151–173. Washington, DC: National Academy Press.

Blackstone, William. [1765–1769] 1979. *Commentaries on the Laws of England.* Chicago: University of Chicago Press.

Bordo, Susan. 1986. The Cartesian Masculinization of Thought. *Signs* 11: 439–56.

Broverman, Inge K., Broverman, Donald M., Clarkson, Frank E., et al. 1970. Sex-Role Stereotypes and Clinical Judgments of Mental Health. *Journal of Consulting and Clinical Psychology* 34 (1): 1–7.

Carse, Alisa L., and Nelson, Hilde Lindemann. 1996. Rehabilitating Care. *Kennedy Institute of Ethics Journal* 6: 19–35.

Cotton, Paul. 1990. Examples Abound of Gaps in Medical Knowledge Because of Groups Excluded from Scientific Study. *Journal of the American Medical Association* 263: 1051, 1055.

———. 1993. FDA Lifts Ban on Women in Early Drug Tests. *Journal of the American Medical Association* 269: 2067.

Daniels, Cynthia. 1993. *At Women's Expense: State Power and the Politics of Fetal Rights.* Cambridge and London: Harvard University Press.

DeBruin, Debra A. 1994. Justice and the Inclusion of Women in Clinical Studies: An Argument for Further Reform. *Kennedy Institute of Ethics Journal* 4: 117–46.

Faden, Ruth; Kass, N.; and McGraw, D. In press. Women as Vessels and Vectors: Lessons from the HIV Epidemic. In *Feminism and Bioethics: Beyond Reproduction,* ed. Susan Wolf. New York: Oxford University Press.

Fausto-Sterling, Anne. 1992. *Myths of Gender: Biological Theories About Women and Men.* New York: HarperCollins.

GAO. U.S. General Accounting Office. 1990. *National Institutes of Health: Problems in Instituting Policy on Women in Study Populations.*

Gatens, Moira. 1991. *Feminism and Philosophy.* Bloomington: Indiana University Press.

Hamilton, Jean, and Parry, Barbara. 1983. Sex-Related Differences in Clinical Drug Response: Implications for Women's Health. *JAMWA* 38(5): 126–32.

Institute of Medicine: Committee on the Ethical and Legal Issues Relating to the Inclusion of Women in Clinical Trials. 1994. *Women and Health Research,* vols. 1 and 2. Washington, DC: National Academy Press.

Jaggar, Alison. 1989. Love and Knowledge: Emotion in Feminist Epistemology. In *Women, Knowledge, and Reality,* ed. Ann Garry and Marilyn Pearsall, pp. 129–55. Boston: Unwin Hyman.

Kant, Immanuel. 1960. *Observations on the Feeling of the Beautiful and Sublime,* Section Three (Of the Distinction of the Beautiful and Sublime in the Interrelations of the Two Sexes). Berkeley: University of California Press.

Laurence, Leslie, and Weinhouse, Beth. 1994. *Outrageous Practices: The Alarming Truth about how Medicine Mistreats Women.* New York: Fawcett Columbine.

Little, Margaret Olivia. 1995. Seeing and Caring: The Role of Affect in Feminist Moral Epistemology. *Hypatia* 10(3): 117–137.

Lloyd, Genevieve. 1983. Reason, Gender, and Morality in the History of Philosophy. *Social Research* 50: 490–513.

———. 1984. *The Man of Reason: Male and Female in Western Philosophy.* London: Methuem.

Lugones, Maria. 1987. Playfulness, World-Traveling, and Loving Perception. *Hypatia* 2(2): 3–19.

MacKinnon, Catharine A. 1987. *Feminism Unmodified: Discourses on Life and Law.* Cambridge and London: Harvard University Press.

Merton, Vanessa. 1994. Impact of Current Federal Regulations on the Inclusion of Female Subjects in Clinical Studies. In *Women and Health Research: Ethical and Legal Issues of Including Women in Clinical Studies,* vol. 2, Institute of Medicine, pp. 65–83. Washington, DC: National Academy Press.

Minow, Martha. 1990. *Making All the Difference: Inclusion, Exclusion, and American Law.* Ithaca and London: Cornell University Press.

Okin, Susan Miller. 1979. *Women in Western Political Thought.* Princeton: Princeton University Press.

Pateman, Carole. 1989. *The Disorder of Women.* Stanford: Stanford University Press.

Rosenberg, Charles. 1976. *No Other Gods: On Science and American Social Thought.* Baltimore: Johns Hopkins University Press.

Rothman, Barbara Katz. 1982. *In Labor: Women and Power in the Birthplace.* New York: Norton.

Rousseau, Emile. 1979. *Emile, or On Education.* New York: Basic Books.

Russett, Cynthia E. 1989. *Sexual Science: The Victorian Construction of Womanhood.* Cambridge and London: Harvard University Press.

Smith-Rosenberg, Caroll. 1972. The Hysterical Woman: Sex Roles in 19th Century America. *Social Research* 39: 652–78.

Tuana, Nancy. 1992. *Woman and the History of Philosophy.* New York: Paragon House.

Walker, Margaret Urban. 1992a. Feminism, Ethics, and the Question of Theory. *Hypatia* 7(3): 23–38.

———. 1992b. Moral Understandings: Alternative Epistemology for a Feminist Ethics. In *Explorations in Feminist Ethics,* ed. Eve Browning Cole and Susan Coultrap-McQuinn, pp. 165–75. Bloomington: Indiana University Press.

Chapter 2 PLURALISM AND MULTICULTURALISM

The Effect of Values and Culture on Life-Support Decisions

Jill Klessig

Many challenges to the physician–patient relationship occur in the period around a patient's death. Even in the best of circumstances, discussing starting and stopping life support is emotionally demanding. Poor communication between the physician and the patient or the patient's family can turn this situation into a nightmare. The psychological damage cannot be undone and may cloud the last memories the family has of the patient. Similarly, the physician will always carry the knowledge that the situation might have been handled better.

Instances of poor communication can occur if the cultural values of the health care professional and the patient are different, and each is unaware of the reasons underlying the other's behavior or viewpoint. This frequently leads to frustration, anger, and stereotyping. The problem is especially important when life-support measures are being discussed, as cultural patterns have great strength and influence in the period around a death.[1] It is unacceptable for a health professional to be ignorant or insensitive to the cultural beliefs of a dying patient....

It is not ethnicity per se but the social experiences of different groups that help shape particular cultural organization and value systems. These systems undergo constant, although sometimes slow, change as the social experiences of groups vary. Furthermore, all cultures are composed of individuals and, thus, intracultural variation can be as great as, or sometimes even greater than, intercultural variation.

I present this discussion to help physicians understand why patients might react in the way described, especially when such behavior is different from the physicians' expectations. I do *not* imply that any single member of an ethnic group will respond in the specific way or for the particular reasons mentioned here. To assume that a patient will react in a particular way can be as detrimental to the physician–patient relationship as ignoring the fact that differences exist among patients. Patients should always be treated as individuals first and members of a cultural group or groups second.

Religion is referred to here for several reasons. Religion is often important in shaping values and the moral fiber of societies and thus can help explain differing views toward death. In addition, often even persons who are not active in any religion revert to their religious roots when faced with death.[2]

The patients surveyed here were of low socioeconomic status, a class that frequently retains overt indications of traditional cultural values longer than higher socioeconomic classes.[3] The behaviors surrounding death are among the most resistant to change of any cultural or subcultural pattern.[4] Thus, in times of crisis, patients may return to cultural and religious traditions regardless of their socioeconomic status.

IRANIANS

Case Example

The patient, a 17-year-old Iranian girl, had a long history of diabetes mellitus with numerous episodes of ketoacidosis. On the day of admission, she was found unconscious. When the paramedics arrived she was asystolic, but a cardiac rhythm was restored en route to the emergency department. She was admitted to the intensive care unit (ICU) on full ventilatory support. On evaluation she was found to be brain dead. The family was informed of the diagnosis and the fact that legally she was dead. They objected to removing the ventilator and insisted on many unnecessary medical procedures. They remained in the ICU most of the time, interfering with the care of other patients. The physicians felt that the family was being unreasonable and inappropriate. On the second day of admission when the family was not present, life support was stopped. When the patient's parents found out what had happened, they became irate and refused to leave the ICU. The attending physician talked to them for a few minutes, became irritated, and left. The resident left in tears when the family told her that she had "murdered" the patient.

Discussion

Iranian patients are usually opposed to stopping life support in any situation. There appears to be little difference in the responses of the Muslims and the Christians in the study group, thus indicating that the trend was based in culture, not religion. Because, however, religious values have a tremendous influence on societal norms, and the predominant moral code of Iran is based on Islamic traditions, those will be discussed.

Life and death are viewed as controlled by God.[5, 6] All persons are entrusted with their body, and it is their moral duty to seek medical help when needed. The right to die is not recognized.[7]

Because only God can decide when someone will die and all are mandated to seek medical attention, life support is viewed as an obligation, not an option. Although stopping supportive measures is thought to be "playing God," starting these measures is not; instituting life support is an appropriate use of the "gift" of medical technology that has been given to humanity. Thus, to argue with Iranian patients or their families that to start therapy is also interfering with the will of God carries little moral validity.

The opposition to stopping life support holds true even if a patient is in considerable pain. Long-term suffering presents an opportunity to show courage and faith in God,[8] and taking a life to relieve suffering is forbidden.[6] Individual duress is acceptable if it obviates the societal duress of going against moral standards.[5]

Of note, these rules do not necessarily hold in the case of a defective newborn. Some people believe that evil spirits entered the child, and it is no longer human.[9] In these cases it might be permissible to withhold support, including nutrition.

Initiating a discussion of the issues of life support might anger a patient or family. This is based on the conviction that to tell a patient that there is no hope may hasten the dying process and is thus considered inappropriate and insensitive.[10] Given the necessity of obtaining informed consent in the United States, however, some form of dialogue about the terminal nature of a patient's disease is usually necessary. The manner in which such discussion is initiated is important. In Iranian culture it is rude to go directly to the point.[10] The physician should approach the subject slowly, first engaging in small talk. The family dynamics should also be investigated. If a patient is female, she may be under the guardianship of a male family member.[11] The patient's autonomy may not be honored if her decision is not in agreement with her husband's or father's.

In general, the concept of options and patient autonomy is foreign to traditional Iranian culture.[10] Patients are not used to being asked to make choices and may delay doing so. The health care team may become impatient with the patient or family because they "cannot make up their minds" when, in fact, the patient is expecting the physician to make the decisions regarding care.

Other factors can affect decisions about supportive measures in Iranian patients:

- The family's definition of death needs to be considered. In the case discussed here, the family felt that their daughter was still alive because she had a heartbeat and her skin was warm. Thus, to them, removing the ventilator was tantamount to murder.
- In Iran and in many other Middle Eastern countries, the family is expected to be demanding.[10] This shows concern for their family member. This is why the patient's family in this case stayed in the ICU and was so insistent on a wide range of medical care. Not to have done so would have indicated that they did not care about their daughter. Although physicians often become frustrated with this demanding behavior, to understand the reasons behind it may help alleviate some of the friction it causes.
- If a decision is made to stop life support in a Muslim patient, certain customs should be observed. The family should be allowed to stay in the room and recite the Koran (Qur'an) so that these are the last words the patient hears.[2, 11] In addition, family members should be allowed to move the bed so that the patient is facing Mecca when he or she dies. Finally, when a Muslim dies, a non-Muslim is not supposed to touch the body, so gloves should be worn.[12, 13]

KOREAN AMERICANS

Case Example

The patient, a 54-year-old Korean man, was admitted to the hospital with idiopathic pulmonary fibrosis. His condition deteriorated rapidly, and it was clear that death would occur within the next week. His physicians wanted to issue a do-not-resuscitate order, but his family disagreed, insisting that everything be done to keep him alive until arrangements could be made to fly him to Korea. The house staff thought that the family was unreasonable about the patient's prognosis and was causing him undue suffering. The family did not understand why the physicians were being so insensitive.

Discussion

There is little in the medical literature about Koreans and their views toward ethical issues in medicine, especially life support. The following factors are important, however: First, most Koreans are religious, with Buddhism and Protestantism exerting the greatest influence.[14–16] Many Koreans interpret stopping life support as interfering with God's will, although starting such measures is not. There is also still a strong Taoist influence in Korea, which places a great value on longevity.[14]

Another, perhaps more important, issue is that of filial piety, or loyalty to one's parents. In Korea as in many Asian countries, elders are to be respected and cared for.[14, 15, 17, 18] Children, especially the oldest son, owe their life to their parents. They are responsible for the parents and must preserve their lives at all cost. To agree to stopping life support, even if this is a parent's desire, may dishonor the family member in the eyes of relatives or the community. How people's actions are viewed by others is important.[19]

In addition to respect for elders, there is also a traditional concept of obedience to the male head of the family. This tradition has been shown to be still present in Korean-American families,[20 (p115)] and physicians may find that the father or husband makes life-support decisions about all family members.

Traditional values dictate that a patient die at home.[18] Thus, in this case example, the patient's family was aware of the terminal nature of his illness but wanted to keep him alive long enough to get him back to Korea. The fact that he would die en route was not important to them; the action was more important and preserved their honor.

CHINESE AMERICANS

Case Example

The patient, a 69-year-old Chinese-American woman, was admitted with complete right hemi-paresis and aphasia due to a stroke. She had a history of several previous infarcts, with a resulting dementia. A feeding tube was placed, but the patient repeatedly pulled it out. The family was asked to consent to a gastrostomy tube for feeding. They refused and, in addition, asked that all intravenous hydration be discontinued. Because of a question the patient's son had asked about the cost of nursing homes, the intern was certain that the family wanted the patient to die so they would not have to spend their potential inheritance on her care. The intern wanted to get a court order for the gastrostomy tube.

Discussion

Literature about traditional Chinese culture provides some explanations for the bipolar trend—both to stop life support and to believe strongly that all measures should be continued. For centuries the moral outlook of China has been shaped by Confucianism, Taoism, Buddhism, and, more recently, Marxism. This has led to an ethical perspective that is strongly virtue oriented.[21, 22] What is valued is not life itself but living in an ideal way. Taoism advocates nonaction and allowing things to be, and Buddhism emphasizes the transitoriness of life.[23] ("Death is only the vanishing of the human body, the true body exists forever."[24 (p13)]) These viewpoints, combined with the concept of *Ren* (benevolence, kindheartedness, humaneness),[25] lead many patients or their families to the belief that nature should be allowed to take its course, especially when a patient is suffering. Chinese philosophy has long included the right to choose death,[26] and there is evidence that most Chinese approve of passive euthanasia.[27]

In addition, each person is seen as part of the whole community, and individual actions must always take into consideration the effects on society.[22, 28] Thus, economic factors become an issue.[29] If life support is a financial burden on the family, the patient or family is likely to request that it be stopped.[30] An explanation for this view can be found in the teaching of Buddha: The principles of justice and compassion are central.[31] Justice requires an appropriate distribution of health care resources. Compassion encompasses justice. Thus, a patient who decides to forgo life-support measures so the family does not suffer, either emotionally or financially, is performing an act of compassion, which is highly valued.

Opposed to this is a traditional Chinese view that life should be valued and preserved at all costs and that physicians should do their best to save lives.[27, 30] This is partially based on the first Buddhist precept that prohibits killing, even when a person is suffering from a painful and incurable disease.[30] There is also the concern that to stop life support is to interfere with a person's *karma*—the idea that suffering is the result of some past deed and if the karma is not "worked out" in this life, the patient will be forced to suffer again in the next life.[31] Yet another factor involved is the concept of filial piety,[25, 27, 30, 32] discussed earlier.

ORTHODOX AND NON-ORTHODOX JEWS

Case Example

The patient, a 34-year-old man with alcoholic liver disease, was· admitted with his tenth episode of massive hematemesis over the past six months. During his previous admission 14 days before, the patient received 110 units of fresh frozen plasma and 68 units of red cells. On admission the patient had alcohol on his breath. After 24 hours he was still requiring constant transfusions. The attending physician decided to stop all blood products. On hearing this, the Jewish intern caring for the patient vehemently argued that such action was wrong and then left the ICU extremely upset.

Discussion

When raising the issue of life support with Jewish patients, identifying which sect they are associated with is essential. There is a great dichotomy between the views of Orthodox and non-Orthodox Jews. Both views are discussed here.

Traditional Orthodox teachings are firmly in favor of continuing life support. An Orthodox patient may become upset at a health care team for even bringing up the subject of stopping life-support measures. Reasons for this can be found in Orthodox teachings that take a strong prolife stance. Life is sacred and is to be preserved whenever possible.[33–35] Thus, it is mandatory to maintain one's health[35] and to seek health care when needed.[34] In addition, the traditional interpretation of the Bible says that physicians are mandated to save life when able[34, 35] and definitely should not assist a patient's death. (Someone who even closes the eyes of a dying person while the soul is departing is classified as a murderer.[36]) So strong is the requirement to preserve life that the risk of a loss of life supercedes most laws of the Sabbath.[34] Every life is of infinite worth, and even one moment of life is to be valued as if it were a month or a year. The sanctity of life is more important than its quality. Furthermore, physicians cannot make a judgment about another person's quality of life because life may have meaning under all conditions, even when the suffering is immense.[37] Thus, conservative interpretations of Jewish moral standards command that patients seek life-support measures and compel physicians to provide them. Although autonomy is valued, wishes that do not comply with these moral standards are not to be honored.[33]

On discussing his feelings, the intern in this case indicated that he was Orthodox and that he believed that not giving blood to this patient was wrong. This is an important case example because it shows how conflicts due to differences in values do not always come from patients. Physicians, too, carry value systems that relate to their past experiences, upbringing, and ethnic identity. Health care professionals need to be aware of their own biases when dealing with these potentially difficult situations.

The views explored here are not necessarily held by non-Orthodox Jews. Possible reasons for this include that Judaism does not glorify suffering by assigning it the redeeming features that

other faiths do. No one is required to withstand intractable pain to preserve life.[38] Judaism is committed to use all available resources to alleviate suffering to every extent possible.[39] Thus, pain should be treated. Prolonging the dying process is also prohibited.[34] Exactly what constitutes this dying process is unclear, but traditionally a person who is dying (a *goses*) is one who will not live more than 72 hours.[35] In this situation, it is permissible to stop life support because it is only prolonging the dying process. Another reason for being against life-prolonging measures is that Jews do not have the same belief in an afterlife or reincarnation that other faiths do. There is the feeling that "when it's over, it's over," and there is no point in prolonging futile care.

AFRICAN AMERICANS

Case Example

The patient, a 32-year-old African-American man, was admitted after receiving a stab wound to the heart. He had a cardiac arrest in the emergency department, suffering severe brain damage. A month later the patient had no notable return of cognitive function, although he was responsive to pain. He had continuous fevers, though no source of infection was found. The ICU team wished to issue a do-not-resuscitate order, stop antibiotic therapy, and transfer him to the general medical ward. The patient's wife disagreed and threatened to sue the hospital if these plans were carried out.

Discussion

An exploration of the views that African Americans hold toward do-not-resuscitate orders and life support is especially important because of the higher prevalence in the African-American community (than in the general population) of conditions likely to result in the need for a discussion of such issues. Overall, African Americans have higher incidences of cancer, accidents, the acquired immunodeficiency syndrome, hypertension, diabetes mellitus, and low-birth-weight babies[40–47]; they also have less access to needed primary health care.[48]

As is the case with all groups, African Americans cannot be lumped together, as past experiences, religion, and politics are extremely varied. Because of centuries of slavery and racism, their experiences in the United States are dissimilar from all other groups. Patients who recently arrived in the United States from Africa cannot be included in this group, as they have different experiences and medical belief systems.

Although the literature is sparse, there is some support for the finding that African-American patients are more likely to want life-support measures to be continued. Port and co-workers found fewer deaths due to the termination of dialysis in African-American patients than in whites.[49]

Several factors may influence decisions about life-support options. First, African Americans tend to be more religious and more devout than whites.[50] Many patients said that they would continue all measures until the end because it "is wrong" to stop and miracles are always possible. Patients said that they would feel enormous guilt about stopping support. This relates to both strong religious convictions and the observation that, in general, African Americans highly value their elders, long life (regardless of suffering), and the will to survive.[51–54] A physician's statement that the situation is hopeless may not be adequate: only God knows for sure. This may represent a distrust of the medical community rather than strictly religious conviction.

In addition, there are still problems with racism in the medical establishment. It has been shown that African-American patients receive less intense care[55] and are more likely to be negatively stereotyped than other patients.[56] These issues, combined with the perception of some African-American patients that their hospital stay was too short and the care less than satisfactory,[57] may lead to concerns that life support was stopped prematurely because of the patient's race.

FILIPINO AMERICANS

Case Example

The patient, a 44-year-old Filipino woman with metastatic breast cancer, was admitted with shortness of breath. On admission the house staff discussed the possibility of a do-not-resuscitate order with her. She agreed. Later, while the attending physician was examining the patient with her family in the room, he again brought up the subject of a do-not-resuscitate order. This time she denied that it was what she wanted. On leaving the room, the attending physician expressed displeasure with the resident who had initiated the order without "the patient's consent."

Discussion

The Republic of the Philippines is a diverse nation comprising more than 7,000 islands and with a culture that has been influenced by many countries and religions.[58] Compounding this diversity is the fact that there have been several different waves of immigration to the United States from the Philippines, with each group having unique experiences and backgrounds that would influence their belief systems. Despite this variety, most Filipino patients are apparently opposed to stopping life support.

Many of the Filipinos who have immigrated to the United States are Catholic[59] and believe that patients or physicians should not interfere with God's plan. The Catholic Church abhors "suicide" for any reason,[60] and it is morally wrong to encourage death with any action or omission. Thus, religious conviction is a major reason for continuing life support. Respect for elders is also important, as with Korean and Chinese patients.

The Filipino family greatly influences patients' decisions about health care.[58] Harmony is valued, and personal needs are subjugated to keeping group harmony. Thus, in this case, the patient actually did want the do-not-resuscitate order to be written and did not want life-support measures started. Her family objected, however, and because outright disagreement was to be avoided, she changed her mind.

The perceived cause of a patient's illness can also be a factor in decisions about supportive care. For example, for some Filipinos, illness may be attributed to a punishment from God,[57] and thus it would not be appropriate to interfere.

Others believe that people die because they have offended or are possessed by a spirit, a belief that is common throughout Southeast Asia.[61, 62] Patients or families may be reluctant to stop life support before the causative agent has been addressed. For example, the brother of a patient thought that she became ill because she swept dirt on a spirit who was walking by, thus offending the spirit. He believed that if the patient apologized enough she would get better, so stopping the ventilator was not appropriate.

MEXICAN AMERICANS

Case Example

The patient, a 43-year-old Mexican-American woman, was admitted with known metastatic breast cancer. On admission she said she wanted no heroic measures done. Over the next 24 hours her condition rapidly deteriorated, and she became comatose with imminent respiratory arrest. The issue of a do-not-resuscitate order was discussed with the patient's children. They were aware of her wishes but insisted that she be intubated, at least until their father was able to come from Mexico.

Discussion

Mexicans have a rich heritage, with their present culture influenced by indigenous native traditions as well as customs and beliefs imported from Spain and Africa. Mexican Americans have had these traditions modified further by the dominant American culture. This has led to a unique and diversified culture that only partially resembles those of other Spanish-speaking countries. Although Mexican Americans are the largest group of Latino patients,[7] a substantial number of persons come from other Hispanic countries. The following comments should not be assumed to relate to these other groups.

Mexican Americans' beliefs about illness causation are important in determining their views about life support. Health is a gift from God, and ill health, including accidents, may be due to a punishment from God or the saints. The suffering incurred is part of God's plan and should not be interfered with. Conversely, a patient may believe that the illness is caused by evil spirits or the Devil[67–70] and that a *curandero* (healer) may be able to cure the patient, even when Western medical practices have failed.

Other issues are equally important when discussing life support with Mexican-American patients. First, there is always hope the patient may get better, so to stop life support may cause the Mexican-American family great feelings of guilt. In addition, Mexican Americans believe that enduring sickness is a sign of strength.[70] Some studies suggest that Mexican Americans may have more fear of dying than other ethnic groups.[50] Last, more than 85% of Mexican American are Catholic[50] and against anything that hastens death.[71 (p282)]

When a patient is terminally ill, the family is involved in all aspects of decision making. The well-being of the family is valued over that of individual members. Traditionally the father or husband is the head of the household,[72, 73] and he should make or agree with all decisions. The wife's input is usually influential, however, even when it is not highly visible.

When discussing life support, physicians need to be aware of the concept of courtesy as it pertains to Mexican-American patients. Directly contradicting a physician is considered rude or disrespectful.[67, 72] Thus, a physician may think that a patient and the patient's family are in agreement with the plan of action when in fact they are strongly opposed to it. There is also still a strong tendency toward paternalism,[74] and physicians may be expected to make life-support decisions for their patients.

SUMMARY

The frustration that health care professionals experience when treating patients from different ethnic backgrounds can be mitigated by exploring the cultural foundation of the behavior in question. Variants of the factors discussed in this article occur in diverse cultures, although their degree of influence may vary. In addition, people who have identical reactions when confronted with the subject of stopping life support may have entirely different reasons for their behavior. Thus, when discussing do-not-resuscitate orders with patients from any culture, it is best to explore the following issues:

- What do they think about the sanctity of life?
- What is their definition of death?
- What is their religious background, and how active are they currently?
- What do they believe are the causal agents in illness, and how do these relate to the dying process?
- What is the patient's social support system?
- Who makes decisions about matters of importance in the family?

Health care professionals should remember that many patients have immigrated from countries where as much as three fourths of the population does not have access to basic health needs, such as clean drinking water. They have never before faced "high-tech" health care and do not have a clear concept of the implications or consequences of initiating life support. Finally, the concept of patient autonomy that is so highly valued in Western culture, and is the basis of many life-support decisions, is not as important in other cultures.

When faced with life-and-death decisions, all patients draw on a lifetime of experiences for strength and guidance in making decisions. Patients' societal traditions affect their interpretation of past experiences but are not the only factors involved. Each patient must be seen as a person who has a unique belief system, with ethnic background only a part, albeit an important part, of the equation. By discussing life-support issues in a culturally sensitive way, a physician can turn a potentially exasperating experience into an enriching one, with understanding and respect, if not agreement.

Notes

1. Counts D: The good death and Kaliai: Preparation for death in West New Britain, *In* Kalish R (Ed): *Death and Dying: Views From Many Cultures.* Farmingdale, NY, Baywood, 1980, pp 39–46.

2. Walker C: Attitudes to death and bereavement among cultural minority groups. *Nurs Times* 1982; 78:2106–2109.

3. Harwood A: *Ethnicity and Medical Care.* Cambridge, Mass, Harvard University Press, 1981.

4. Moore J: The death culture of Mexico and Mexican-Americans. *Omega* 1970; 1:271–291.

5. Sachedina AA: Islamic views on organ transplantation. *Transplant Proc* 1988; 20(suppl 1):1084–1088.

6. Hathout H: Islamic basis for biomedical ethics, *In Transcultural Dimensions of Medical Ethics, Symposium Proceedings*. Washington, DC, Fidia Research Foundation, 1990, pp 25–26.

7. Andrews M, Hanson P: Religious beliefs: Implications for nursing practice, *In* Boyle JS, Andrews M (Eds): *Transcultural Concepts in Nursing Care*. Glenview, Ill, Scott, Foresman, 1989, pp 357–417.

8. Al-Mutawa M: Health care ethics in Kuwait. *Hastings Cent Rep* 1989; 19:S11–12.

9. Shiloh A: The interaction between the Middle Eastern and Western systems of medicine. *Soc Sci Med* 1968; 2:235–248.

10. Meleis I, Jonsen R: Ethical crises and cultural differences. *West 1 Med* 1983; 138:889–893.

11. Henley A: *Asian Patients in Hospital and at Home*. London, Great Britain, King Edward's Hospital Fund, 1979 [distributor Pitman Medical].

12. Black J: Broaden your mind about death and bereavement in certain ethnic groups in Britain. *Br Med 1* 1987; 295:536–539.

13. McAvoy B, Donaldson L: *Health Care for Asians*. Cambridge, Great Britain, Oxford University Press, 1990.

14. Korean Overseas Information Service: *A Handbook of Korea*. Seoul, Korea, Samkhwai Printing, 1990.

15. Pang KY: The practice of traditional Korean medicine in Washington, DC. *Soc Sci Med* 1989; 28:875–884.

16. *Religions*. Seoul, Korea, Korean Overseas Information Service, 1983.

17. Pang KY: *Hwabyung:* The construction of a Korean popular illness among Korean elderly immigrant women in the United States. *Cult Med Psychiatry* 1990; 14:495–512.

18. *Customs and Traditions*. Seoul, Korea, Korean Overseas Information Service, 1982.

19. Chung HJ: Understanding the Oriental maternity patient. *Nurs Clin North Am* 1977; 12:67–75.

20. Yu EY, Phillips E, Yan ES: *Koreans in Los Angeles: Prospects and Promises*. Los Angeles, Calif, Koryo Research Institute, 1982.

21. Qiu RZ: *Medical Ethics and Chinese Culture. Transcultural Dimensions of Medical Ethics, Symposium Proceedings*. Washington, DC, Fidia Research Foundation, 1990.

22. Fox RC, Swazey JP: Medical morality is not bioethics—Medical ethics in China and the United States. *Perspect Biol Med* 1984; 27:336–360.

23. Chen-Louie T: Nursing care of Chinese American patients, *In* Orque M, Block B, Monrroy LSA (Eds): *Ethnic Nursing Care: A Multicultural Approach*. St Louis, Mo, CV Mosby, 1983.

24. *The Teachings of Buddha*. Tokyo, Japan, Dosaido Printing, 1966.

25. Ren-Zong Q (Qiu RZ]: Medicine—The art of humaneness: On the ethics of traditional Chinese medicine. *J Med Philos* 1988; 13:277–300.

26. Xu TM: China: Moral puzzles. *Hastings Cent Rep* 1990; 20:24–25.

27. Pu SD: Euthanasia in China: A report. *J Med Philos* 1988; 16:131–138.

28. Qiu RZ: Economics and medical decision-making: A Chinese perspective. *Sem Perinatol* 1987; 11:262–263.

29. Fox S: China: Diary of a barefoot bioethicist. *Hastings Cent Rep* 1984; 14:18–20.

30. Qiu RZ: Morality in flux: Medical ethics dilemmas in the People's Republic of China. *Kennedy Inst Ethics J* 1991; 1:16–27.

31. Ratanakul P: Bioethics in Thailand: The struggle for Buddhist solutions. *J Med Philos* 1988; 13:301–312.

32. Qiu RZ: 'No feeding tubes for me!' (Commentary). *Hastings Cent Rep* 1987; 17:523–26.

33. Steinberg A: Bioethics: Secular philosophy, Jewish law and modern medicine. *Isr J Med Sci* 1989; 25:404–409.

34. Rosner F: The physician-patient relationship: Responsibilities and limitations, *In* Meier L (Ed): *Jewish Values in Health and Medicine*. Lanham, Md, University Press of America, 1991, pp 95–110.

35. Perlin E: Jewish medical ethics and the care of the elderly. *Pharos* 1990; 53:2–5.

36. The Talmud. Shabbat 151b.

37. Frankl VE: The meaning of suffering, *In* Meier L (Ed): *Jewish Values in Bioethics*. New York, NY, Human Sciences Press. 1986, pp 117–123.

38. Bleich D: Care of the terminally ill, *In* Meier L (Ed): *Jewish Values in Health and Medicine*. Lanham, Md, University Press of America, 1991, pp 141–161.

39. Glick SM: *A View from Sinai—A Jewish Perspective on Biomedical Ethics*. Symposium Proceedings: Transcultural Dimensions of Medical

    Ethics. Washington, DC, Fidia Research Foundation, 1990, pp 19–21.

40. AMA Council on Ethical and Judicial Affairs: Black-white disparities in health care. *Conn Med* 1990; 54:625–628.

41. Joseph S: AIDS in the black community: Public health implications. *J Natl Med Assoc* 1988; 80:1173–1178.

42. Johnson C: Meeting the health care needs of our nation's black elderly. *J Natl Med Assoc* 1990; 82:823–827.

43. Evans T: Being black in America is hazardous to your health. *J Natl Med Assoc 1988*; 80:253–255.

44. Barber J: Black Americans in crisis. *J Natl Med Assoc* 1990; 82:664–665.

45. Dowling P, Fisher M: Maternal factors and low birthweight infants: A comparison of blacks with Mexican-Americans. *J Fam Pract* 1987; 25:153–158.

46. Miller W, Cooper R: Rising lung cancer death rates among black men: The importance of occupation and social class. *J Natl Med Assoc* 1982; 74:253–258.

47. Raju T, Hager S: The dilemma of less than 500 grams birth: Epidemiologic considerations. *Am J Perinatol* 1986; 3:327–331.

48. Hayward RA, Shapiro MF, Freeman HE, Corey CR: Inequities in health services among insured Americans—Do working-age adults have less access to medical care than the elderly? *N Engl J Med* 1988; 318:1507–1512.

49. Port FK, Wolfe RA, Hawthorne VM, Ferguson CW: Discontinuation of dialysis therapy as a cause of death. *Am J Nephrol* 1989; 9:145–149.

50. Kalish R, Reynolds DK: *Death and Ethnicity: A Psychocultural Study*. Los Angeles, Calif, University of Southern California Press, 1976, pp 200–221.

51. Lundgren L: Hospice: Concept and implementation in the black community. *J Commun Health Nurs* 1986; 3:137–144.

52. Spector R: *Cultural Diversity in Health and Illness*. New York, NY, Appleton-Century-Crofts, 1979.

53. Swanson WC, Harter CL: How do elderly blacks cope in New Orleans? *Aging Human Dev* 1971; 2:210–216.

54. Koenig R, Goldner N, Kresojevich R, Lockwood G: Ideas about illness of elderly black and white in an urban hospital. *Aging Hum Dev* 1971; (2):217–225.

55. Yergan J, Flood AB, LoGerfo JP, Diehr P: Relationship between patient race and the intensity of hospital services. *Med Care* 1987; 25:592–603.

56. Johnson SM, Kurtz ME, Tomlinson T, Howe KR: Students' stereotypes of patients as barriers to

clinical decision-making. *J Med Educ* 1986; 61(pt 1):727–735.

57. Blendon RJ, Aiken LH, Freeman HE, Corey CR: Access to medical care for black and white Americans—A matter of continuing concern. *JAMA* 1989; 261:278–281.

58. Orque M: Nursing care of Filipino American patients. *In* Orque M, Block B. Monrroy LSA (Eds): *Ethnic Nursing Care: A Multicultural Approach.* St Louis, Mo, CV Mosby, 1983, pp 149–182.

59. Anderson JN: Health and illness in Philipino immigrants. *West J Med* 1983; 139:811–819 [7–15].

60. Veith I: Changing concepts of health care: An historian's view. *West J Med* 1980; 133:532–538.

61. Sharp PT: Ghosts, witches, sickness and death: The traditional interpretation of injury and disease in a rural area of Papua New Guinea. *Papua New Guinea Med J* 1982; 25:108–115.

62. Orque M: Nursing care of South Vietnamese patients, *In* Orque M, Block B. Monrroy LSA (Eds): *Ethnic Nursing Care: A Multicultural Approach.* St Louis, Mo, CV Mosby, 1983, pp 245–269.

63. Maduro R: *Curanderismo* and Latino views of disease and curing. *West J Med* 1983; 139:868–874 [64–70].

64. Scheper-Hughes N, Stewart D: *Curanderismo* in Taos County, New Mexico—A possible case of anthropological romanticism? *West J Med* 1983; 139:875–884 [71–80].

65. Cockerham WC: *Medical Sociology.* Englewood Cliffs, NJ, Prentice-Hall, 1982.

66. Spector R: *Cultural Diversity in Health and Illness.* East Norwalk, Conn, Appleton & Lange, 1991.

67. Kuipers J: Mexican Americans, *In* Giger J, Davidhizar R (Eds): *Transcultural Nursing: Assessment and Intervention.* St Louis, Mo, Mosby Year Book, 1991, pp 185–202.

68. Gonzales HH: Health care needs of the Mexican American, *In Ethnicity and Health Care.* New York, NY, National League for Nursing, 1976, pp 21–28.

69. Dorsey PR, Jackson HQ: Cultural health traditions: The Latino/Chicano perspective, *In* Branch M, Paxton P (Eds): *Providing Safe Nursing Care for Ethnic People of Color.* New York, NY, Appleton-Century-Crofts, 1976, pp 41–80.

70. Schur C, Bernstein A, Berk M: The importance of distinguishing Hispanic subpopulations in the use of medical care. *Med Care* 1987; 25:627–641.

71. Dubois MJ: The dying human in Christian philosophy, *In* de Vries A, Carmi A (Eds): *The Dying Human.* Ramat Gan, Tel Aviv, Israel, Turtledove Publishing, 1979, pp 275–285.

72. Murillo N: The Mexican American family, *In* Martinez RA (Ed): *Hispanic Culture and Health Care.* St Louis, Mo, CV Mosby, 1978, pp 3–18.

73. Monrroy LSA: Nursing care of Raza/Latina patients, *In* Orque M, Block B, Monrroy LSA (Eds): *Ethnic Nursing Care: A Multicultural Approach.* St Louis, Mo, CV Mosby, 1983, pp 7115–148.

74. Escobar A: Human dying has changed. *Bull Pan Am Health Organ* 1990; 24:446–453.

The Impact of Culture on the Patient–Surgeon Relationship

Carolyn Ells and Donna A. Caniano

Practicing surgery in a multicultural setting poses numerous ethical challenges. Informed choice processes can be frustrated by cultural practices that locate decision-making authority in someone or some group (for example, family, brother, uncle, paternal grandmother) other than the patient, even when the patient has the capacity to make choices about treatment. Differences in meaning systems associated with the patient's culture and life experiences can frustrate disclosure and understanding of the relevant information on which the patient is to make an informed decision to choose or refuse an operation. This can be exacerbated in the presence of language differences and when translation is needed. In some cases, information from the surgeon is screened and altered by a family translator before it reaches the patient, because, for instance, cultural values hold that it would be wrong to frighten the patient. Sometimes cultural norms can prevent the patient from telling her family translator intimate details of her medical concerns, so a different story is told, leaving the surgeon with an inaccurate account of the medical problem to be solved. In many cultures, patients are not told the truth about cancer diagnoses or terminal prognoses. Surgeons can be asked not to disclose such information to patients or even to lie to patients, sometimes even to patients who directly ask about their diagnosis or prognosis.

Surgical procedures considered standard of care by the surgeon are sometimes refused on the basis of values and beliefs not shared by the surgical profession. Alternatively, surgical procedures are sometimes requested that violate the surgeon's standard of care. Not abiding by standard-of-care recommendations can result in consequences that the medical profession and the dominant culture have difficulty accepting. These and other cultural components of patient–surgeon relationships can challenge the values and standards on which the surgeon feels obliged to practice good patient care. Further, they can affect the success of the patient–surgeon relationship and the health outcomes for the patient. For these reasons, surgeons must attend to the cultural components of the patient–surgeon relationship and find ways to respond to them in an ethically and medically responsible manner.

This article tackles the issue, for surgeons, of "operating" with cultural sensitivity. We address this problem first by stepping back to review the nature of culture and why culture is important at all. Then, through case examples and discussion, we address several of the ethical challenges that surgeons can experience when they and their patients come from different cultures.

For ease of discussion, we assume a United States context in which surgeons belong to the dominant American culture that accepts most "Western" values and norms. The patients in our discussion belong to a nondominant culture within American society. Although many surgeons in the United States belong to, or share membership with, nondominant cultures, in their capacity as surgeons, surgeons are expected to

abide by the expectations of a medical profession imbued with the values of the dominant culture. Hence, the dominant culture always comes to bear on encounters with patients.

Although our case examples draw attention to the cultural traditions of at least some Japanese Americans, Hmong immigrants, and refugees from Somalia, it is important to realize that culture is not something unique only to people coming from "exotic" locales. American culture, with its particular beliefs, feelings, and behaviors, poses its own ethical challenges for American surgeons. An alternate set of case examples could well tackle issues related to operating on children and adolescents with trisomy-21 to make their faces look more "normal," cochlear implant surgery, and operating on intergender infants to make them appear male or female.

WHAT IS CULTURE, AND WHY IS CULTURE IMPORTANT?

"Culture" is the common and accepted way of thinking, feeling, and acting for a group of people.[1] As such, it involves the full range of common and accepted beliefs, values, attitudes, patterns of meanings, and behaviors held by a group of people.

Culture is important because it is culture that enables people to navigate and make sense of their world through shared sets of meanings and patterns of behavior. Individuals, and those they encounter in their cultural group, see and move through the world in roughly the same ways. A common social heritage builds solidarity among the group, helping to ensure continuity of group life. And when problems occur, culture is an "adaptive mechanism" that provides ready-made solutions to those problems[1] or tools to address them.

Aspects of culture are learned, shared, and perpetuated by members of the culture. Yet aspects of the culture such as how the group cares for its ill, the attitude it has toward women, or the value placed on certain rituals might change over time. The fluid nature of culture means that not all members of a culture share all of the beliefs, values, and patterns of behavior typical of that culture, so making predictions about any one person's beliefs, values, feelings, and so on based on general tendencies of the culture is highly problematic. General assumptions can create negative stereotypes and obscure the tremendous variability within cultures and the need to approach each person as a unique individual.[2]

Because culture is so broad in scope, political borders, religious traditions, or physical characteristics cannot in themselves constitute a culture. Immigrants, for example, frequently find ways to preserve their culture in adopted countries. Despite a shared faith, Native American Roman Catholics have meaning systems and patterns of behavior quite distinct from those of Roman Catholics in Ireland. People with the same skin color living in the United States might identify themselves culturally as Americans, African Americans, Caribbean, deaf, Jewish, or by some other cultural designation. Individuals or groups might blend the typical ways of thinking, feeling, and acting of two or more cultures. Indeed, terms such as "African American," "Native American," and "Japanese American" seem to suggest blended cultural traditions.

Despite tremendous cultural diversity within the United States, there are typical ways of thinking, feeling, and acting that together are distinctly "American." These include valuing freedom, individuality, industriousness, and ambition, values immortalized in the "American Dream." Being American is about life, liberty, and the pursuit of happiness. It is about rituals for Memorial Day weekend, Thanksgiving, family life, certain social etiquettes. It is about Disney, Hollywood, technology, driving a car, motherhood, and apple pie.

Understanding culture is important for surgeons. Health outcomes and professional values are just some of what can be at stake when patient and surgeon are from different cultures. More important than simply providing an explanation about *how* a people behave, culture provides reasons for *why* people of that culture tend to behave as they do. Understanding this how and why can

be immensely valuable in the development and ongoing nurturance of the patient–surgeon relationship. Culture, as the major context of people's lives, can help to identify underlying problems and can provide information (including information about beliefs, values, and preferences) needed to resolve those problems. But when two cultures meet, it is not just the patient's culture that the surgeon must be concerned with. The surgeon's own culture must also be understood. In fact, when relating to anyone from another culture, one must seek to understand one's own culture, the other's culture, and the interaction between the two. Although these tasks are as important for patients as they are for surgeons, we will focus on the perspective of the surgeon.

Patient 1

An elderly Japanese man with advanced pancreatic cancer is referred to a surgical oncologist to assess whether palliative surgery could relieve some of his pain and inability to eat. With the patient's daughter-in-law remaining at the patient's bedside, the patient's son first wishes to speak with the surgeon alone. The son explains that his father does not know that he has cancer and should not be told about the diagnosis. His father immigrated to the United States 35 years ago with his son and daughter-in-law, joining numerous other relatives who came many years earlier. The family continues to live according to Japanese cultural values and beliefs. Consistent with those values, a person should never be told the diagnosis of cancer, because it will be heard as a death sentence and will cause tremendous suffering. Likewise, a terminal prognosis should not be disclosed either. This situation is of immediate concern for the surgeon, who believes that disclosing this information is necessary for the patient to make an informed choice about whether to proceed with palliative surgery. Perhaps, knowing that time was short, the patient would not want to go through the ordeal of an operation. The surgeon is also aware that many people do not put their personal affairs in order until after learning of a terminal prognosis. For this reason also, the surgeon believes that respect for the father requires telling the truth. As the surgeon explains all of this to the son, the son becomes very distressed and pleads with the surgeon to conceal the truth from his father and to proceed with the operation if it will help relieve some of the suffering, imploring the surgeon to respect his father by respecting his father's cultural tradition.

Patient 2

A 60-year-old woman is being evaluated by the general surgical service of a large metropolitan hospital for chronic cholecystitis. She and her extended family are Hmong Vietnamese immigrants who have lived in the United States for many years. She speaks little English and resides in a large community of Hmong immigrants. The patient has had recurrent episodes of abdominal pain, fever, and vomiting secondary to cholelithiasis. The surgical consultant advises a laparoscopic cholecystectomy. The patient, through a family translator, refuses the operation. She informs the surgeon that her pain has a spiritual cause and that an operation will not help the spiritual imbalance in her body.

Patient 3

A gynecologist meets with a 12-year-old girl and her mother. Both are refugees from Somalia and have lived in the United States for 3 years. They ask for a genital "cutting" for the daughter in the tradition of their culture. The mother proudly explains that, because she cares so much for her daughter's well-being, she has decided to allow anesthesia and pain relief during the operation, because a pain-free operation will not diminish the cultural value of the genital cutting. The ritual procedure will mark a major transition for the daughter, as she moves from childhood into womanhood, and it will protect her future marriage potential. The gynecologist knows that all forms of genital cutting are not accepted in Western culture and in Western medicine. In fact, it is often characterized as mutilation and is illegal in most states. As the gynecologist explains that performing such operations is highly problematic in the United States, the mother and daughter start to cry. The mother

begs the gynecologist to try to understand. There are other, more serious, kinds of harms to be considered. If her daughter is to become a woman, to be a normal person, and to marry and have an honorable future, this operation is needed. But if all else fails, could the gynecologist provide the necessary pain relief and sterile conditions so that a traditional practitioner could perform the operation?

BEING SENSITIVE TO CULTURE

Each of these cases shows a meeting of different cultural beliefs, values, and ways of doing things. They invite us to ask: What does it mean to respect culture? What are the limits of respecting culture? In each case, answering these questions requires understanding the patient's culture, the surgeon's culture, and how those two cultures interact. In terms of limits, the surgeon must consider the limits of respecting each particular cultural tradition and the limits of respecting aspects of the cultural tradition of surgery. Within such limits, whenever possible, ways to honor all relevant, important values should be sought.

Understanding patients' cultures will involve understanding how and why patients act as they do. Communication is the most important tool for this. In addition to (an all-too-often scant) social history, surgeons need to inquire about the things that matter to their patients: what values, goals, and rituals are important to them and which take priority for them. By keeping in mind that any value, goal, or pattern of behavior can look nonsensical out of context, a surgeon will remember to seek out the context that makes sense of what patients claim to be important. Their culture is that context. For instance, claiming the importance of drinking some wine that is the blood of someone who lived and died 2,000 years ago might seem nonsensical without understanding the religious tradition that grounds that claim. Similarly, lying to a perfectly competent man about his cancer and calling that respect for the man might seem nonsensical without understanding the role of filial duty within the man's culture, the cultural emphasis on interdependence over individual autonomy, and the lie as a means to honor a cultural value of providing hope.

Not only should surgeons inquire about broader cultural aspects of patients' lives, but they must make it safe for patients to share this information, some of which will be private and personal, going right to the heart of a patient's identity and core values. In each instance, the patient should experience the surgeon's inquiries as genuine interest, with the patient's own well-being as the goal, as opposed to idle curiosity or seeking to criticize. The surgeon should be seen as wanting to create a therapeutic relationship that will enable the patient and the surgeon (and perhaps others) to work together to make good decisions about the patient's care. Although probing to understand patients' values, goals, and ways of doing things is appropriate, challenging the patient's culture is not. The surgeon should avoid negative remarks about the culture and actions or statements that intimidate, scare, or make the patient more vulnerable. Because of the inherent power imbalance that exists between patient and surgeon, the responsibility for creating good therapeutic relationships rests with the surgeon.[3] Accordingly, the surgeon should make reasonable efforts to create a therapeutic environment that encourages patients to share cultural aspects of their lives that bear on decisions and actions affecting health.

Surgeons might want to supplement their inquiry about culture by discussion with other knowledgeable persons, taking advantage of presentations about culture locally or at professional meetings, or by other personal research. Care must be taken not to breach patient confidentiality during these learning expeditions. In some cases, cultural brokers or community elders are used to help the patient and the surgeon to understand each other's culture and develop a good therapeutic relationship. Although using such liaisons can be very useful, surgeons might understandably resist this option because it requires bringing a third party, who is neither family nor part of the health care team,

into the therapeutic relationship. Yet the desire to keep outsiders from the therapeutic relationship can be a feature of the culture of surgery that the surgeon can forgo in favor of potential benefits, especially if the patient gives permission to include such third parties.

Over time, learning from many interactions with patients from different cultures, surgeons can build a substantial knowledge base about cultures present in their community and strategies for interaction when they meet patients from different cultures. Although this will help surgeons to work well with cultural differences in their practices, care must be taken not to make assumptions about any particular patient's cultural commitments. Generalizations about culture and signals of cultural membership can serve as triggers for further inquiry but should not be misinterpreted as the "truth" about any particular patient. For example, no assumption should be made about whether any particular Native American embraces or rejects the cultural aspirations of other Native Americans, or for that matter the aspirations of the dominant American culture.

Understanding one's own culture will be easier than understanding others' cultures. After all, we have first-person experience about how and why we behave as we do. But in many situations, it can take some effort to acknowledge and reflect on one's own ways of thinking, feeling, and acting. Often aspects of one's own culture seem natural and "right" simply because they are so established in one's experience and one is not called on to question or reflect on them, but when confronted with any ethical question or problem, one's cultural perspective must be acknowledged, including one's cultural biases toward certain actions and reasons for action over others. For each of us, our culture is the lens through which we experience the world. We cannot step out of it into some neutral position, so the notion of physicians as "morally neutral" is nonsensical. The "neutral" surgeon cannot really be neutral, although she or he can try to be fair.

For surgeons, understanding one's own culture also means understanding the culture of surgery. The typical ways that surgeons think, feel, and act must be understood and taken into account. Looking to professional commitments, codes of ethics, and policies will help in understanding the culture of surgery, for they set a standard of behavior and provide reasons for why surgeons do the things they do and what they stand for.[4] Although surgery has tended to be set slightly apart from medicine, it does share the basic assumptions of that tradition. The interests and well-being of patients take priority. Informed choice is valued. Anthropologists point to several tenacious assumptions in Western medicine that other cultures do not necessarily share: "nature" is distinct from the "supernatural"; nature is autonomous from human consciousness; nature is separate from culture, morality, and society; knowledge is produced by manipulation within a scientific program; each person is a free agent; the individual comes before and can choose his or her society and culture; relationships are external to the self; society is a potential enemy of freedom; the moral agent stands back from social roles to assess and pass moral judgment from a purely abstract point of view.[5]

There is a distance between patients and surgeons that is different from other kinds of medical practice. Drapes around the surgical site can reduce the patient to a technical problem.[6] In addition, although in some cases longterm patient–surgeon relationships exist, more often the surgeon is involved only for a short period when particular technical skills are needed. There is an air of pragmatism about surgeons: If it might work, do it. If it didn't work, try again. Communication might happen before and after an operation, but what surgeons *do* is the operation itself, and time pressures revolve around that.

Understanding the interaction between the different cultures of patient and surgeon involves understanding where there are consistencies and inconsistencies between each other's beliefs, values, feelings, patterns of behavior, and so on. Where there are inconsistencies pertinent to the therapeutic relationship or potential health outcomes, creative strategies might be needed to develop compromises acceptable to all. Respect for persons (i.e., patients) is often a mutually shared value, but cultural disagreements can still arise over what actions actually do constitute respect for a particular patient. Understanding how features of different cultures interact will also involve understanding the limits to compromise available to each culture. Through discussion of the case examples, we explore the interaction of different cultures further.

DISCUSSION OF CASES

In patient 1's case, the surgeon must decide how to handle a plea from the patient's son to conceal the truth about a cancer diagnosis and terminal prognosis. Note that the surgeon has not only been asked to hide the truth, she has inherited a situation in which the patient has already been deceived or possibly lied to outright. The surgeon is asked to begin a therapeutic relationship with a patient as a co-conspirator in a situation that she finds morally problematic. How she handles the situation will have ramifications for the patient, the patient's family, and the relationships that other health care professionals have with the patient.

The patient's son explains that "cancer" is heard in the Japanese cultural tradition as a death sentence and will cause the patient tremendous suffering. Likewise, a terminal prognosis causes tremendous suffering if disclosed to the patient. This cultural reaction is prevalent among numerous cultural groups including Italians, Greeks, Korean Americans, Mexican Americans, Sephardic Jews, Spanish, French, Eastern Europeans, Moroccans, and Japanese.[7, 8] For instance, in a study by Blackhall and colleagues,[8] it was discovered that Korean Americans and Mexican Americans were less likely than European Americans and African Americans to believe that patients should be told about a cancer diagnosis or a terminal prognosis. But the preferences about truth telling are not uniform within any of these cultural groups, although some tendencies among cultural groups can be identified. This means that membership in a cultural group cannot in itself guarantee that any particular person within the group affirms the value of with-holding the truth or telling the truth.

What is the surgeon's duty? The surgeon has a duty to offer truthful information to the patient that might aid the patient in making responsible decisions about treatment. The patient has a right to know such information, but the patient does not have a duty to be informed. The surgeon is not obliged to force information on the patient that the physician thinks is relevant but that the patient does not want to receive.[7, 9, 10] Although honesty is an important value that typically contributes to good therapeutic relationships and respect for patient autonomy, patients can waive their need for some disclosures of information: "Skip the gory details, doc. My mind is made up to have the operation." Waiving some disclosures of information does not shift the responsibility for choices made. The patient continues to have responsibility for his or her choices.[9] Key to ethical withholding of relevant information is that from the patient's perspective the physician is willing to make further disclosures at any time the patient asks: "I've changed my mind, doc. Tell me more about what's going on with my stomach."

The larger value to keep in mind is that priority is given to serving the overall best interests of the patient, *as defined by the patient* (within acceptable parameters of surgical practice). Where the surgeon has much expertise to contribute to assessments of a patient's interests related to physical and psychologic health, the patient is typically in the best position to determine his or her overall best interests, because these also include spiritual, cultural, and other interests as well. Hence the patient should be able to articulate general principles about disclosures and truth telling expected from surgeons: "I want to know everything" or "Talk to my son; he will handle it."

To guide physicians about ethical approaches to telling and withholding truth, the Italian Medical Association developed the Italian Deontology Code.[11] The code provides some latitude to physicians with regard to making judgments about whether it is appropriate, on the patient's cultural grounds, to with-

hold some information. Any information withheld from the patient is to be communicated to the family, but the code indicates that a patient's will is to be honored and a patient's questions are to be answered. Within an American culture context, where respect for autonomy is very highly valued, there is a slightly higher ethical standard. Physicians (and surgeons) should not simply guess what patients want or abide by family wishes with the caveat that they will tell the truth if asked. Rather, physicians (and surgeons) should solicit from their patients information about what level of disclosure patients desire and expect. And in any case, as with the Italian Code, any disclosures withheld should always be shared with the patient on the patient's request. For example, statements such as "Never tell me that I have cancer" should not be honored if the patient later asks, "Do I have cancer, doc?" The default assumption should be that patients are inquisitive and want detailed information about their condition.

To what extent does the culture speak for the patient? Because of the diversity within cultures, it is always important to clarify how much the patient wants to know.[7, 9, 10] In the case considered here, the patient's family lives according to traditional Japanese cultural values and beliefs. But has the patient himself affirmed that way of life? Perhaps the patient goes along with the family on most matters, but when the stakes are high or are personal, he would prefer something different. Perhaps, after 35 years in the United States, he does in fact personally support honesty and personal autonomy about such matters and feels that cancer and terminal prognoses are not as harmful to know about or talk about as others in his culture tend to believe.

How the surgeon initiates such conversations matters. Bluntly asking the patient if he wants to know the truth about his diagnosis and how much time he has left would likely be heard as "You have cancer and little time remaining." The same might be true for bluntly telling the patient that the operation will not proceed until these matters are discussed openly and thoroughly. Either approach would be disrespectful of the patient. A less direct approach is needed to learn more about the patient's cultural commitments. For instance, the surgeon might speak privately with the patient about family involvement in decision making, explaining that the family would like the surgeon to share information with them about the patient's condition and that the family is willing to accept some of the burden of decision making on behalf of the patient. The surgeon would assure the patient that the extent to which the family is involved depends solely on the patient's wishes and that the surgeon is seeking guidance from the patient on this matter. Taking cues from the patient's responses, the surgeon might need to probe further. For instance, if the patient acknowledges a preference for allowing the family to make at least some decisions on the patient's behalf without first consulting the patient, the surgeon might ask: "Is there anything specific that you would definitely want to know about or decide for yourself? Is there anything specific that you definitely want your family to handle without you? Are there some things that are very important to you that your family or I should know about?" In some situations, the patient might be inclined to give specific directions about disclosures: "Never tell me I have cancer. We don't do that in my family." In other situations, the patient might name particular values or goals that are to guide disclosures: "Handling this the Japanese way is important to me. My family will tell you how." Any time a patient waives his or her right to information or decision making, the surgeon must ensure that the patient understands that the patient is free to receive more information or take over decision making at any time in the future.

Although affirming this approach to truth telling in therapeutic relationships, Vicki Michel raises several difficulties that surgeons might encounter.[10] For instance, families might object to approaching patients to discuss how disclosures and decision making are to be addressed. In addition, even if raising the issue with the patient is acceptable to the family, conducting such conversations privately without the family present might be viewed as disrespectful to the cultural context of patients' lives. Yet the private conversation is usually needed for the surgeon to minimize the risk that the patient is being coerced or manipulated by family members.

Would it matter if the surgeon cannot accept the son's or the patient's wishes about withholding the truth and allowing the patient to make a less than fully informed choice about palliative surgery? Should the surgeon "resign" from the case and arrange for another surgeon to consult? A patient transferred to another surgeon's service is likely to experience that transfer as abandonment and punishment for not abiding by the wishes of the surgeon, someone whose preferences are relevant but do not have priority. Here it is best for the surgeon to strike a compromise. The surgeon can reaffirm the value she and her profession hold for developing a therapeutic relationship that gives priority to the overall best interests of the patient (as the patient defines those interests). With those patient-centered interests as a guide, the values of truth telling and informed choice can be honored by ascertaining and abiding by the patient's preferences on these matters and by always being ready to provide more information and decision-making support when the patient requests more. When the patient designates someone or some people to receive more information about the patient's condition or to participate in health care decision making, the surgeon honors both the patient's values and the surgeon's values by providing those people with the information and support they need. In the case considered here, if the patient indicates that discussions and decisions about diagnosis, prognosis, and operation should be handled largely by his family, then the surgeon should support that request by ensuring that the family is informed and enabled to make informed decisions on the patient's behalf. Discussions with the patient should be considerate of the limits set by the patient.

Note that the solution reached here is not a culture-specific solution. The solution is the same for any situation where one is asked to withhold the truth or lie to a patient. Although the situation might arise more often with patients from some cultural groups over others, surgeons should be prepared for it to arise in any patient encounter.

In patient 2's case, a Hmong woman refuses a laparoscopic cholecystectomy, believing that the proposed operation will not help the spiritual imbalance that causes her pain. Refusal of operation is common in the Hmong culture. There are taboos against it and other basic tools of Western medicine, such as blood tests, spinal taps, and anesthesia. For a Hmong person, these taboos are often viewed as guardians of one's identity, one's very soul.[12] But for surgeons and other health care providers, these taboos complicate the way they provide care and can put surgeons in a position of providing suboptimal care.

This case highlights how inextricably linked religion and medicine can be. When Anne Fadiman[12] was researching the tensions between the Hmong culture and the culture of Western medicine, she came to realize that, in the Hmong culture, "Medicine *was* religion. Religion was society. Society was medicine."[12] A bodily complaint is at the same time a complaint about one's spiritual life and a complaint about one's social relationship. A medical intervention intervenes on the body, the soul, the society, and perhaps even the whole universe. Hence, the patient and her Hmong community will understand a problem to be solved, and its solution, more broadly than many surgeons practicing Western medicine will understand it.

Decisions to break a taboo are not made easily in the Hmong culture and can involve a hierarchy of leadership within the Hmong community. Wives might need to ask husbands, who might need to ask elder brothers, who might need to ask clan leaders, who might need to ask more important clan leaders in other communities.[12] The most respectful and efficient approach surgeons can take might be to first clarify the extent to which the patient embraces her Hmong culture and then, consistent with that, involve those in the Hmong community who have an "official" role in mediating health care decisions. Doing so, the surgeon works with, rather than against, Hmong practices. Being careful to stay within

legal parameters, the surgeon will want to ensure that the patient with capacity (or the patient's surrogate) has veto power over any decisions made on his or her behalf by the community. Working with the culture might be easier with respect to who is involved with decision making than with the actual decisions the Hmong make. For instance, surgeons will understandably resist a choice for animal sacrifice instead of a recommended operation.

Part of what a surgeon will find challenging is grappling with the different explanations Western medicine and the Hmong culture give for the cause of illness. In the case considered here, the surgeon identifies cholelithiasis as the cause of the woman's recurrent episodes of abdominal pain, fever, and vomiting and concludes that a cholecystecomy is the most efficient and effective treatment. The patient identifies a spiritual cause and accordingly does not recognize the proposed operation as resolving the fundamental spiritual imbalance. Underlying the different causes of illness are vastly different concepts available to the surgeon and the Hmong patient with which they can discuss what each believes is going on. For instance, except for the heart, in the Hmong culture there are no concepts for internal organs.[12] Providing a simple explanation about "gallstones" and how they can interfere with the function of the gallbladder and cause certain symptoms to appear might not communicate much to a patient who does not grasp the more basic idea of internal organs. For their part, surgeons typically lack concepts that ground Hmong spiritual understandings.

Further confounding these challenges to understanding and communication is the need to use a translator. If a translator for a Hmong patient is available at all, it is usually, as in the case presented here, a family translator who has some understanding of English but typically is not fluent. Medical concepts, terms, and explanations need to be first understood by the translator and then communicated using Hmong concepts, terms, and meaning systems to the patient. When the translator indicates a patient's refusal of treatment that, from the surgeon's perspective, seems to be the best course of action, the surgeon will want to be certain that the patient's refusal of treatment is genuine, informed, and voluntary. If she has doubts, the surgeon might want to take extra steps to secure the services of a non-family translator who is more familiar with Hmong and Western cultures and the culture of Western medicine.

To help bridge the cultural divide between patients and surgeons of different cultures, "eight questions" developed by Arthur Kleinman and colleagues[13] might help. In cross-cultural therapeutic interactions, they suggest that physicians ask their patients: 1) What do you think has caused your problem? 2) Why do you think it started when it did? 3) What do you think your sickness does to you? How does it work? 4) How severe is your sickness? Will it have a short or long course? 5) What kind of treatment do you think you should receive? 6) What are the most important results you hope to receive from this treatment? 7) What are the chief problems your sickness has caused for you? 8) What do you fear most about your sickness?[13] The patient's answers to these questions will provide valuable insight into the patient's understandings, beliefs, values, and preferences. They also help to guide what happens next. Importantly, the questions are framed in such a way as to assume some authority and capacity on the part of patients to contribute to naming the problem and finding an acceptable solution. Patients might need to hear such appreciation for their point of view to enter into a successful therapeutic relationship with their surgeons.

Patients and surgeons must find ways to work together to achieve therapeutic goals. For instance, with the answers to the "eight questions" as a basis of understanding, the surgeon could work with the Hmong patient in "merging" the concept of a spiritual cause of illness with a bodily cause and determining how the operation could assist in recovery without violating the spiritual aspect of the illness. For example, part of the spiritual imbalance might be able to be viewed as, or as resulting in, an imbalance in the body brought on by, or manifested in, gallstones. The proposed operation might then be viewed as one of several means that, taken together, redress the spiritual cause. Alternatively, the operation might be able to be understood as valuable to produce symptom relief that would then enable the patient to better address the spiritual aspect of the illness.

Working with Hmong patients might entail reassessing usual health care practices, as in the case of a young Hmong child for whom the health care team decided to accept the possible loss of the child's lung by not insisting on an operation to clear a hemothorax in hopes that the family would continue to bring the child for life-sustaining dialysis.[14] Other features of that case included allowing a traditional Hmong shaman to come to the hospital to provide alternative treatment, discharging the patient home for healing rituals, and taking x-rays of the patient's lungs to determine the shaman's success at treatment. Yet the limits of compromise were carefully assessed by the health care team and articulated to the family: if dialysis were refused, Children's Protective Services would be notified. Because insistence on abiding solely by Western cultural values and traditions has been disastrous for the care of Hmong people, because respect for persons and autonomy demands patient-centered approaches, and because the patient defines the interests that ground therapeutic goals, surgeons and the institutions within which they work should be accepting of some compromises that do not put at risk other patients and staff, place burdensome demands on resources, or violate core professional or institutional values.

In the case of patient 3, the surgeon is asked by the mother to perform an operation that cuts the daughter's genitals in keeping with the family's cultural tradition. The genital "cutting" has important cultural meaning and is viewed by the mother (and presumably the daughter) as integral to the daughter's future acceptance and well-being within their cultural group. Pain associated with the procedure is viewed by the mother as a harm to be avoided, but avoiding pain and other potential harms appears to be secondary to the cultural value of undergoing genital cutting. The daughter's wishes and feelings about the operation are not clear in the case, but she cries when the surgeon begins to reject the request. Her tears may be a sign that her wishes and feelings are the same as her mother's, but alternatively they might be a sign that she fears a worse consequence: that the operation will be performed by a traditional practitioner without any pain relief or sterile conditions. The daughter's wishes and feelings will need to be explored.

A key issue in this case is different and competing notions of well-being and harm. The mother, who presumably is trying to ensure her daughter's well-being, understands that well-being in terms of her daughter's potential to flourish within the culture. Her assessment of cultural flourishing might not be unrealistic. She might be correct that, within the culture, measures of normalcy, privileges of adulthood, and potential for marriage within the cultural group (and with that a secure future) are major components of a good life that depend on the ritual genital cutting. Perhaps they even depend on undergoing the operation at this young age. On the mother's assessment, the potential harms of the operation, though considerable, are not as pronounced overall as the harms resulting from not having the operation. But the mother does want to minimize harms by involving the surgeon.

The surgeon would define well-being and rank potential harms differently. Physical harms that can include pain, bleeding, irreversible loss of the clitoris and labia, chronic infection, painful sexual intercourse and menstruation, infertility, difficult childbirth, and death are of great concern to Western surgeons.[15] Psychologic harms are also a concern. In addition, to have a good life in the dominant Western culture does not require genital cutting. Marriage potential (beyond this family's cultural group) and potential to care for oneself and one's family would likely be improved without the operation. As a systemic practice, genital cutting contributes to women's oppression around the world, in violation of the human rights standards

integral to Western culture. Precisely because of these harms and a notion of well-being that entails minimizing such harms, the operation is not accepted in the surgeon's Western culture. In fact, the whole range of such surgeries—from less invasive ritual cutting to full excision of the genitals—is emphatically rejected by Western culture. Note, for example, how public outrage squashed plans in Seattle to design a medically safe clitoridectomy.[15]

It is important to realize that women, particularly educated women, from African countries (including Somalia) where ritual genital procedures occur have spoken out against this custom because of its physical and psychologic harms and, very importantly, its contribution to the subjection of women. In discussions with the patient and her mother, the surgeon might wish to raise this point. If this information is new to the mother and daughter, it might prompt them to reevaluate their request for the procedure to know that support can be found within their culture to forgo this practice. In any case, discussion about this point and how cultural expectations and opportunities might change for the mother and daughter in America will help to determine what aspects of the culture the mother and daughter are firmly committed to.

The problem of the gynecologist's participation might appear easily solved by turning to the law. In the United States, the 1996 Federal Prohibition of Female Genital Mutilation Act prohibits the operation for anyone less than 18 years of age. (The same prohibition is made in the Canadian Criminal Code, section 268.) Because surgeons are obliged to comply with the law, and the law prohibits the operation on a minor, the gynecologist should not perform the operation. But still, there are questions about how the gynecologist should proceed. Should she provide pain relief and sterile conditions while a traditional practitioner performs the operation? Would it be the lesser of two evils if the gynecologist performed the operation in violation of the law? Should the mother be reported as suspected of child abuse? Should the gynecologist recommend that the daughter wait until she is 18 and then reconsider her desire to have the operation? After all, once she has lived in the United States for a number of years, the daughter (and mother) might come to have a different view of what practices will contribute to, or harm, well-being.

The age criterion stipulated in the law implies that the law is prepared to accept the operation for women 18 years of age and older. Presumably, conditions such as the woman making an informed choice to have the operation apply. Although genital cutting, like other risky behavior, might fall within the scope of informed choice, it is a separate issue whether genital cutting falls within the scope of professional practice of surgeons. That is, even if an adult woman has the mental capacity to make a choice about the operation, has adequate understanding about what that involves, is in a position to make a voluntary choice and does choose genital cutting, professional standards can still say: "No, this is not something surgeons do. It violates the mandate of surgical practice."

If the mandate of surgical practice is construed, as it often seems to be, as that which contributes to physical health, genital cutting for cultural purposes does not fit within that scope. Analogously, male circumcision solely for religious purposes is the role of the rabbi, not the surgeon. Yet the mandate of operation might seem to be elusive. Palliative surgery does not promote health so much as alleviate suffering, but that suffering does have physical causes. Using surgical means to achieve psychologic health, with no physiologic benefit, is sometimes controversial as in the case of amputating healthy limbs of people who identify themselves as amputees and are tormented by having limbs they believe they shouldn't have.[16] But at least some operations that do not have physiologic benefit are accepted within surgical practice, for example, breast reconstruction (which potentially has a psychologic benefit to help patients cope with the loss of a breast after mastectomy) and face lift (which might have neither physiologic nor psychologic benefits but might improve the marketability of someone in an acting profession). Accordingly, what seems to determine whether a particular practice is acceptable for surgeons turns on the cultural values of those surgeons and the American cultural community. Those values say "no" to genital cutting procedures.

Traditionally, in cultures where girls and women's genitals are cut in ritual ways, it is not surgeons who do this, but surgeons have special knowledge and skills and access to pain relief and sterile conditions. Hence involving surgeons in the ritual would reduce (but not eliminate) the potential harm to people undergoing the procedure. With important professional values that give priority to the interests and well-being of patients and to promoting the good and avoiding harm, surgeons might wonder whether they have a professional duty to assist, but given the illegal nature of the operation, advocacy to change dangerous cultural practices might be the best service that surgeons can justifiably participate in.

Although in the cases of patients 1 and 2, the operation proposed is consistent with the standard of care, in patient 3 the operation requested is meant to serve some end that is contrary to the standard of care. It is tempting to characterize the cases of patients 1 and 2 as involving operations that further "medical" ends while viewing the case of patient 3 as involving an operation that furthers a "cultural" end. To some extent this is correct, for reducing suffering (e.g., by palliative surgery) and improving health (e.g., by cholecystectomy) are central values of Western medicine, and the reasons given to perform a genital "cutting" do not fall under the usual mandate of Western medicine. But the surgeries in cases 1 and 2 also further "cultural" ends: the beliefs, values, and ways of doing things of the dominant Western culture and the culture of medicine. So in all three cases the distinction is between the dominant Western culture (including its culture of medicine) and incompatible beliefs, values, and ways of doing things of a nondominant culture.

CONCLUSIONS

The impact of culture on the patient–surgeon relationship can be profound. When different cultures meet, different ways of thinking, feeling, and acting come together. Some aspects of culture will be similar or the same, but many will differ. Almost inevitably, some important values will conflict, be prioritized differently, or require different—even contradictory—responses. For surgeons, attending to such cultural differences will be critical to the success of the therapeutic relationship because differences can alter expectations, understandings, and communication.

Several strategies will help surgeons in cross-cultural clinical situations. Some of these strategies include: listening and asking questions about the patient's and family's values, setting aside sufficient time to deal with a patient whose culture is different, and asking for help from other health care professionals in communicating with the patient and family. These might often be quite difficult for the busy surgeon to manage. There is also a need for health care organizations located where there are major populations whose cultural values might "challenge" the Western medical system to establish mechanisms for communication, such as through the use of community elders, education of a core of health care staff, and translation of patient teaching aids.

Notes

1. Brown C. *Understanding other cultures*. Englewood Cliffs, NJ: Prentice-Hall; 1963:1–35.
2. Koenig B, Gates-Williams J. Understanding cultural differences in care for dying patients. *West J Med* 1995; 163:244–249.
3. Canadian Healthcare Association, Canadian Medical Association, Canadian Nurses Association, and Catholic Health Association of Canada. Joint statement on preventing and resolving ethical conflicts involving health care providers and persons receiving care. *Can Med Assoc J* 1999; 160:1757–1764.
4. American College of Surgeons. Fellowship pledge and principles of patient care. In: Brody BA, McCullough LB, Rothstein MA, Bokinski MA, eds. *Medical ethics: codes, opinions, and statements*. Washington, DC: The Bureau of National Affairs; 2000:995–996.
5. Gordon DR. Tenacious assumptions in Western medicine. In: Lock M, Gordon D, eds. *Biomedicine examined*. Dordrecht, The Netherlands: Kluwer Academic Publishers; 1988:19–56.
6. Kirmayer LJ. Mind and body as metaphors. Hidden values in biomedicine. In: Lock M, Gordon D, eds. *Biomedicine examined*. Dordrecht, The Netherlands: Kluwer Academic Publishers; 1988:57–93.
7. Freedman B. Offering truth. *Arch Intern Med* 1993; 153:572–576.
8. Blackhall LJ, Murphy ST, Frank G, et al. Ethnicity and attitudes toward patient autonomy. *JAMA* 1995; 274:820–825.
9. Freedman B. A moral theory of informed consent. *Hastings Cent Rep* 1975; 5:32–39.
10. Michel V. Factoring ethnic and racial differences into bioethics decision making. *Generations* 1994; Winter:23–26.
11. Surbone A. Truth telling to the patient. *JAMA* 1992; 268:1661–1662.
12. Fadiman A. *The spirit catches you and you fall down*. New York: Farrar, Straus and Giroux; 1997:1–100.
13. Kleinman A, Eisenberg L, Good B. Culture, illness and care: clinical lessons from anthropologic and cross-cultural research. *Ann Intern Med* 1978; 88:251–258.
14. Wells R. Making room for alternatives. *Hastings Cent Rep* 2000; 30:26–27 [case study commentary].
15. Li X. Tolerating the intolerable: the case of female genital mutilation. *Philos Public Policy Q* 2001; 21:2–8.
16. Elliot C. A new way to be mad. *Atlantic Monthly* 2000; 286:72–84.

Truth Telling to the Patient

Antonella Surbone

And you shall know the truth, and the truth shall make you free. (John 8:32)

When I started writing this letter last year, I was practicing medical oncology in the United States. My work, based on providing thorough information to every patient, was that of an expert in a particular field as well as an educator. By explaining diagnosis, prognosis, and treatment options to the patient, I was creating the basis for freedom: freedom not only from symptoms and disease, but also freedom to make informed choices. At the same time, I grew to believe that truth telling goes far beyond providing mere information. Truth is not just the opposite of a lie, not just the sum of correct statements, but a reciprocal state in the patient-physician relationship. This relationship is established on the basis of mutual responsibilities. In such a context, information should never become a way of delegating the entire burden of medical decisions to the patient, thus limiting medical responsibilities. Truth should expand rather than limit professional responsibilities.

THE ITALIAN DEONTOLOGY CODE AND WITHHOLDING TRUTH

While reflecting on my responsibility to provide patients with information, which is an ethical duty of American physicians,[1] I often thought of the different approaches used in my country of origin, Italy, where patients are not always informed of their diagnosis and prognosis. In medical school at the University of Turin in the late 1970s, I learned the Italian Deontology Code, written by the Italian Medical Association, which included the following statement: "A serious or lethal prognosis can be hidden from the patient, but not from the family."[2]

During my first year of oncology fellowship in Italy in 1983, a middle-aged businessman was told he had gastritis, when dying of cachexia from end-stage carcinoma; a young, divorced housewife was told she had arthritis while receiving palliative radiation therapy for chemotherapy-resistant metastatic breast cancer; and a college student was told he had drug-induced hepatitis, but he was indeed progressing toward liver failure from widespread hepatic involvement with lymphoma. In each case the patient's family or only one family member was informed of the true diagnosis and prognosis. A ritual started, composed of sotto voce conversations between the physician and family members outside the patient's room: "Doctor, don't speak too loud" or "Doctor, tell me how much time is left for my husband, because I have to prepare." In each case, the patients knew or at least strongly suspected the truth, but they were part of a generally accepted farce of deception that prevented open discussion about the truth and how to act on it. Consequences of such deception varied from the unresolved financial problems left at the businessman's death, to the stressful, secret, and unsuccessful attempt of the dying single mother to find a way to provide for the future of her four children.

In 1986, an Italian public television survey of a sample population representative of the entire nation showed that Italians were more or less equally divided in their preferences for truth telling in medicine. A 1991 study of 1171 breast cancer patients and their physicians and surgeons in general hospitals in Italy evaluated the frequency of disclosure of the diagnosis of operable breast cancer.[3] Only 47% of these patients reported having been told that they had cancer, and 25% of their physicians stated they had not been given accurate information. After reading the results of this study, I asked myself, from an assimilated American perspective, how could such women not participate in the decision to undergo mastectomy or breast-conserving surgery, especially in those cases where we predict the outcomes to be equivalent?[4]

Later in 1991, I accepted my present position as vice-chairman in the oncology department of Santa Chiara Hospital in Pisa, Italy. The situation in the Italian medical world is rapidly evolving, with malpractice lawsuits increasing and the public skepticism of physicians on the rise.[5, 6] It is in this reality that bioethical issues, including patients' rights to information, are the subject of frequent discussions among physicians.

The Deontology Code was revised in 1989 and it now reads as follows:

> The physician has the duty to provide the patient—according to his cultural level and abilities to understand—the most serene information about the diagnosis, the prognosis and the therapeutic perspectives and their consequences; in the awareness of the limits of medical knowledge, in the respect of the person's rights, to foster the best compliance to the therapeutic proposals. Each question asked by the patient has to be accepted and answered clearly. The physician might evaluate, specifically in relationship with the patient's reactions, the opportunity not to reveal to the patient or to mitigate a serious or lethal prognosis. In this case it will have to be communicated to the family. In any event, the patient's will, freely expressed, should represent for the physician [an] element to which he will inspire his behavior.[7]

With regard to informed consent and participation in clinical studies, the Code states "experimentation is subordinated to the consent of the subject which has to be—if possible—freely expressed in writing."[8] In each of these statements the possibility of truth withholding still exists, and I think this can only be understood by considering the Italian cultural background.

I must first stress that I believe that ethics is inevitably connected to cultural values and, therefore, varies in different societies. This requires an implicit understanding of the dichotomy between believing in absolute values and respecting the pluralism of different cultures. This is to say, as difficult as it may sound for someone only used to one culture, that both the Italian and the American ways are ethical in their context.

AUTONOMIA E ISOLAMENTO

First, the Italian culture is strongly bound to the Greek and Latin approaches to medicine. "To benefit, at least not to harm," wrote Hippocrates. Benefit is the priority in the patient–physician relationship. In a recent public debate in Rome among physicians and journalists on truth telling, even those stating that information is the basis for the contract between patient and physician stressed that the first aim of such a contract is not information, but what is good for the patient.[9] In bioethics, practical directions derive from a balance between the two principles of beneficence and autonomy. While the concept of beneficence is quite similarly perceived in Italy and in the United States, autonomy is certainly viewed in different ways.

In the Italian culture, autonomy *(autonomia)* is often synonymous for isolation *(isolamento)*. The Italian patient is frequently viewed as being unable to learn enough to make appropriate autonomous health care decisions. Autonomy thus would easily become isolation for a person overwhelmed by complicated and frightening information that does not develop into knowledge. If information does not create knowledge, it does not create a positive autonomy. Protecting the ill family member from painful information is seen as essential for keeping the family together and not allowing the ill member to suffer alone. In addition, many Italians find it difficult to openly confront sickness and death.

Today, many Americans usually demand and are given information that enables them to make decisions either autonomously or with a physician's advice about their health care. Ancient Greek philosophers disputed the possibility of effectively communicating knowledge. Contemporary Italian attitudes perpetuate the belief that patients will never acquire enough knowledge to enable them to fully and appropriately participate in their care. As a result, the Italian physician remains a powerful, distant figure exercising unilateral decisions on the basis of knowledge that is assumed incommunicable.[10] "It is difficult to remain Imperator in the presence of a physician," said the Roman Emperor Hadrian in the second century,[11] and this seems to hold true even today.

TRUTH AND THE THERAPEUTIC RELATIONSHIP

We should never forget that the ill person, because of the nature of disease itself, is in a "uniquely dependent state."[12] The Italian Deontology Code thus allows physicians to use their experience and expertise to understand each patient and to establish how much information the patient can accept and process and in what manner the information is best conveyed. Any connection between patient and physician should be therapeutic. I firmly believe that truth is essential for a therapeutic relationship,[13] but I have to acknowledge that the Italian society is not prepared for the American way.

On the other hand, the Italian medical scene is rapidly changing, and physicians are now confronted with medicolegal issues that did not exist a few years ago. Although strongly believing in the truth, I am concerned that Italian physicians may communicate vast amounts of complicated information to unprepared patients only out of fear of litigation. Should this happen, it probably will not give rise to real truth telling and may result in exhaustive lists of information that will not improve the patient–physician relationship.

The Italian bioethical situation regarding truth telling to patients is often compared with the US situation a few decades ago.[14] I believe Italians should not borrow the American way, but they should learn from Americans and try to

find a better Italian way. I already see signs of this happening. There are now courses in bioethics at the universities of Florence and Rome, updates on bioethics in some regions of Italy,[15] medical meetings on truth telling[16] and communicating with patients,[17] and a project to establish a database for national and international bioethical issues.[18] From the patients' side, a spontaneous organization called "Tribunale per i Diritti del Malato" (Court for the Patient's Rights) now exists.[19]

For now, when dealing with my patients, I try to tell them the complete truth. But there are times when this is not so easy. For example, when faced with a family repeatedly asking me not to use the word "cancer," I rely on nonverbal communication to establish a truthful and therapeutic relationship with the patient. In all instances, I make an effort to listen to the patients and to respect their need for information. Since I believe the suffering person knows the truth, I think the only way to respect both Italian ethical principles and the patient's autonomy and dignity is to let the patient know that there are no barriers to communication and to the truth.

I hope all my Italian patients will soon ask me for the truth, and I hope I will never give information just for medicolegal reasons. Moreover, I hope I will contribute—together with my colleagues—to a positive change in our society.

Notes

1. Ad Hoc Committee on Medical Ethics. American College of Physicians Ethics Manual, I: history of medical ethics, the physician and the patient, the physician's relationship to other physicians, the physician and society. *Ann Intern Med.* 1984; 101:129–137.

2. Federazione Nazionale degli Ordini dei Medici Chirurghi e degli Odontoiatri. *Guida all'Esercizio Professionale per i Medici-Chirurghi a degli Odontoiatri.* Turin, Italy: Edizioni Medico Scientifiche; 1987:66–67.

3. Mosconi P, Meyerowitz BE, Liberati MC, et al. Disclosure of breast cancer diagnosis: patient and physician reports. *Ann Oncol.* 1991; 2:273–280.

4. Treatment of early-stage breast cancer. *JAMA*. 1991; 265:391–395. NIH Consensus Conference.

5. Sabbioni MEE. Speech is silver, silence is gold? *Ann Oncol*. 1991; 2:234.

6. Boeri S. Medici e no. *Panorama*. 1992; 1349:38–42.

7. Codice Deontologico 1989: informazione a consenso del paziente, art 39. In: Ordine dei Medici, ed. *Annuario dell'Ordine dei Medici della Provincia di Torino*. Turin, Italy: Ordine dei Medici; 1990:27.

8. Codice Deontologico 1989: sperimentazione, art 49. In: Ordine dei Medici, ed. *Annuario dell'Ordine dei Medici della Provincia di Torino*. Turin, Italy: Ordine dei Medici; 1990:28.

9. Il Medico d'Italia. Informazione al malato: come, quando e perché. Organo Ufficiale della Federazione Nazionale degli Ordini dei Medici Chirurghi e degli Odontoiatri. 1991; 41:1–2.

10. Zittoun R. Patient information and participation. In: Holland JC, Zittoun R, eds. *Psychosocial Aspects of Oncology*. Berlin, Germany: Springer-Verlag; 1990:27–44.

11. Yourcenar M. *Memoires d'Hadrien suivi de Carnets de notes de memoires d'Hadrien*. Paris, France: Gallimard; 1974.

12. Pellegrino ED. Altruism, self-interest, and medical ethics. *JAMA*. 1987; 258: 1939–1940.

13. Suchman AL, Matthews DA. What makes the patient-doctor relationship therapeutic? exploring the connexional dimension of medical care. *Ann Intern Med*. 1988; 108:125–130.

14. Novack DH, Plumer R, Smith RL, et al. Changes in physicians' attitudes toward telling the cancer patient. *JAMA*. 1979; 241:897–900.

15. Corso di formazione sulle tematiche bioetiche connesse al trattamento sanitario. Unitá Sanitaria Locale 12. Pisa, Italy. January-February 1992.

16. Il Medico d'Italia. Come informare il paziente grave. *Organo Ufficiale della Federazione Nazionale degli Ordini dei Medici Chirurghi e degli Odontoiatri*. 1992; 30:17.

17. Il Medico d'Italia. Come costruire e migliorare il rapporto medico-paziente. *Organo Ufficiale della Federazione Nazionale degli Ordini dei Medici Chirurghi e degli 0dontoiatri*. 1992; 26:16.

18. Il Medico d'Italia. Al via una banca dati sulla bioetica. *Organo Ufficiale della Federazione Nazionale degli Ordini dei Medici Chirurghi e degli Odontoiatri*. 1992; 40:4.

19. Tribunale per i Diritti del Malato. Sezione di Pisa, Ospedale Santa Chiara. Carta dei diritti del cittadino malato. Pisa, Italy, 1984.

Bioethics for Clinicians: Aboriginal Cultures

Jonathan H. Ellerby, John McKenzie, Stanley McKay, Gilbert J. Gariepy, and Joseph M. Kaufert

Mr. F, a 70-year-old Aboriginal elder who speaks only Ojibway, is admitted to a tertiary care hospital for diagnostic investigation of possible prostate cancer. Initially, only a female interpreter is available, and she has difficulty translating the physician's references to the penis while obtaining consent for cystoscopy. When asked to tell Mr. F that the procedure would aid in cancer diagnosis, she refuses to directly translate the concept of cancer and, instead, uses the word for "growth." The patient responds that he does not fully understand the diagnostic test but trusts the interpreter and the urologist and agrees to sign the

consent form. During cystoscopy both his son and a male interpreter are present to translate.

Following the biopsy and other diagnostic tests, Mr. F, his son, the male interpreter and the urologist meet. Addressing the son and the interpreter, the urologist explains that Mr. F has advanced cancer spreading to bone. When asked by the son about treatment, the urologist replies that any attempted curative treatment would probably cause more risk and discomfort than would pain relief and other palliative measures. The interpreter begins to translate the urologist's summary, but his explanation of the diagnosis is interrupted by the son, who says that he will communicate directly with his father. He states that the interpreter should not have used the Ojibway word *manitoc*, which denotes cancer through the cultural metaphor of "being eaten from within," and that direct reference to cancer and his father's terminal prognosis will promote fear and pain. He adds that his father has given him responsibility to interpret and to act as his proxy decision-maker.

The son further opposes the physician's attempt to communicate the prognosis directly to Mr. F, stating that direct references to death and dying may "bring death closer." The urologist argues that Mr. F needs to understand his diagnosis to give informed consent for treatment. The son replies that he will not lie to his father but that he needs time to communicate with his father through a more gradual and indirect process. The physician and son finally agree that the son will involve other family members over the next 48 hours.

The physician and family arrange to meet again in 2 days and, in the meantime, to hold a "sharing circle" (see Appendix 1 for definition) in which patient, family members and caregivers will discuss palliative care and answer Mr. F.'s questions.

WHAT IS ABORIGINAL BIOETHICS?

Although philosophies and practices analogous to bioethics do exist in Aboriginal cultures, the concept of "bioethics" is not generally differentiated from the ethical values and frameworks for decision-making that are applied in all dimensions of living. Accordingly, we will address ethical values that may be held by Aboriginal people rather than a formal, codified system of Aboriginal bioethics.

A recent review of the literature revealed that little has been published on the subject of Aboriginal health ethics.[1] In the scope of cultural bioethics, Aboriginal systems are unique in their respect for the visions and beliefs of the individual and concomitant respect for the community.[2] Aboriginal values are frequently dis-

counted by Western colonial culture. Primarily rooted in the context of oral history and culture, Aboriginal ethics are best understood as a process and not as the correct interpretation of a unified code.[1, 3] In their approach to ethical decision-making, Aboriginal cultures differ from religious and cultural groups that draw on Scripture and textual foundations for their ethical beliefs and practices. Despite these challenges, common themes and the diversity within Aboriginal ethics may be highlighted. Research conducted with Aboriginal elders[4] provides the basis for identifying widely held values in Aboriginal frameworks for decision-making.

Themes in Approaches to Communication and Caregiving

Some essential qualities of ethical approaches to communication and caregiving involving Aboriginal peoples are summarized in Table 1. Although these ethical values are important to understand and apply, examining specific applications of ethical care in detail is not as useful as developing a more generalized understanding of how to approach ethical decision-making with Aboriginal people in actual clinical settings. Aboriginal ethical decisions are often situational and highly dependent on individual values and on the context of the family and community.

In general, Aboriginal ethical values include the concepts of holism, pluralism, autonomy, community- or family-based decision-making, and the maintenance of quality of life rather than the exclusive pursuit of a cure. Most Aboriginal belief systems also emphasize achieving balance and wellness within all domains of human life (mental, physical, emotional and spiritual).

Aboriginal North American cultures share some ethical practices, such as the need to respect the integrity of the human body after death.[1, 2] Spirituality and cultural understandings of death, loss and the existence of Spirit Beings often play a role in the bioethical decisions of Aboriginal patients and families.[1] Acceptance is a common, deeply rooted aspect of Aboriginal relationships to death and the passage of time during illness.[11–16] Maintaining

Table 1

Essential qualities of ethical approaches to communications and caregiving involving Aboriginal people

Respect the individual: Individual experience and beliefs are viewed to be as valid and important as tradition or cultural norms.[1] Although closely bound to family and community in identity, individuals are recognized has having authority over their own health and "healing journey." When communicating with an Aboriginal person, it is important to show respect, especially for the aged and those with high status such as elders.

Practise conscious communication: Try to listen well and note responses, not only in speech but also, if possible, in body language. Emotional control is common among Aboriginal people and it may be difficult for non-Aboriginal people to "read" intonation and body language.

Use interpreters: Use an interpreter if there is any doubt as to fluency and understanding in English or French. Interpreters often assist in explaining and advocating for the patient.[5]

Involve the family: Often Aboriginal families will wish to be present during decision-making. Family members can be helpful in understanding the patient's beliefs and wishes. Patients may not strongly differentiate their own best interest from that of their family. Because of the individuality of values, however, family members may not always be suitable as interpreters. "Immediate family" can include many extended relations and may be very large and thus should be affirmed.[6]

Recognize alternative approaches to truth-telling: Aboriginal people may believe that speaking of a future illness or consequence will bring it to pass. Family members may not wish "bad news" to be communicated directly.[7, 8] Freedman's notion of "offering truth" may be helpful.[9] Mystery is an acceptable frame of reference for many Aboriginal people, and uncertainty in prognosis or disease progression is often easily accepted by Aboriginal people in contrast to non-Aboriginal people. Beneficence must be weighed carefully against the expressed wishes of Aboriginal patients and their families.

Practise noninterference: A patient's decisions should be based on a comprehensive reporting of options and be respected except for reasons of misunderstanding. Some decisions will be based on cultural knowledge or personal identity, and it will not be possible to reconcile these with medical knowledge. Also, many Aboriginal people accept medical advice without question as a sign of trust and respect for people in the role of "healer." It is important not to abuse this non-challenging trust when presented. Rational persuasion may be experienced as coercion by Aboriginal people.[10]

Allow for Aboriginal medicine: Aboriginal patients may desire the involvement of Aboriginal elders, healers, medicine people, or priests in their treatment. These practitioners are understood to be vital to the overall integrated health of a person and should be respected and honoured whenever possible. Sharing circles, smudging (using herbal-based incense) and traditional herbal remedies may be aspects of cultural medical treatments.*

*SEE APPENDIX 1 FOR DEFINITIONS OF SHARING CIRCLES AND SMUDGING.

quality of life is commonly seen as paramount to extending life. Simultaneously, life is to be preserved and should be pursued whenever meaningful quality can be maintained. Affirming the dignity of life is essential.[10]

Some Aboriginal people have a problem with advanced technology, and it is important to acknowledge this in treatment. Problems arise when a cultural heritage of nature-based medicine encounters biomedical treatment emphasizing technological interventions. Health care institutions such as urban teaching hospitals may be associated with a "culture of colonization" emphasizing technological solutions. There are diverse perspectives in Aboriginal communities regarding the use of technologically advanced and aggressive treatments such as transplantation, dialysis, and mechanical ventilation. However, many Aboriginal people, particularly the young, may be open to and desirous of using the full range of medical technologies available.

Barriers

Ethical care of Aboriginal peoples may include the current emphasis in bioethics on the moral context of individual relationships in clinical interactions. However, this approach does not fully engage the broader structural context of barriers that impede access to care or interfere with healing processes. Barriers include language problems, lack of cultural competence among health care providers, problems of transportation and communication in service delivery to remote communities, and institutional discrimination.

Applications of the bioethical principles of autonomy, beneficence and justice in contemporary relationships must recognize the historical context of power relationships between Aboriginal people and providers of health and social services. The dominant emphasis on respect for individual autonomy in bioethics may need to incorporate Aboriginal values emphasizing noninterference. The Aboriginal psychiatrist, Clare Brant,[10] observed:

> The ethic of non-interference is a behavioural norm of North America Native

tribes that promotes positive interpersonal relations by discouraging coercion of any kind, be it physical, verbal or psychological.

Approaches to guaranteeing autonomy in communication involving consent and truth-telling must accommodate this value of avoiding coercion. Direct, unmediated communication of "bad news" involving terminal prognosis or risks of impending death may violate some individual's and community's values. Cultural and spiritual traditions, including those of Navajo people in the United States and Dene people in Canada, assert that speaking explicitly about terminal illness and death may hasten death.[7, 8] Some families may therefore ask to be present to mediate communication of bad news and support the family. One potential way of recognizing alternative approaches to truth-telling in consent may resemble Freedman's concept of "offering truth."[9] This framework avoids "imposing truth" by allowing the person to define the level and explicitness of the information they require to interpret care options.

Emphasis on guaranteeing informed consent and minimizing risks to individuals in the decision-making process may be unduly influenced by historical relationships that discount Aboriginal values, which emphasize protection of the family and the community. In making consent decisions, Aboriginal patients and their families may balance the risks and benefits to the individual with interests of the family and community. For example, a patient may defer to the wisdom of an elder or healer or elect to use a proxy decision-maker from the family in signing consent agreements or advance directives.[8]

In ethical decision-making, power differences may be accentuated with language barriers among patients who are monolingual speakers of Aboriginal languages or who have limited fluency in English or French. In these situations ethical communication should involve the use of trained Aboriginal health interpreters who have competence in both biomedical terminology and Aboriginal concepts of health and healing.

Diversity and Pluralism

Diversity and pluralism are essential dimensions of Aboriginal ethics. Aboriginal ethics emphasize a pluralistic perspective that accepts that a wide spectrum of values and perspectives may be held by family members. In allowing for the expression of a plural spectrum of values, autonomy among individual family members is emphasized and respected. Aboriginal cultures and communities are diverse, and therefore it is difficult to develop generalizations about values or decision-making practices. Across Canada and within individual provinces and territories, there is a wide spectrum of cultural and language groups, and variations between individual Aboriginal communities and regional organizations. For example, Manitoba is home to Cree, Ojibway (Annishinabe), Metis, Inuit, Dene and Dakota people. Despite some shared beliefs, each cultural group must be treated with respect and an understanding of inherent diversity.

In considering the diversity of beliefs among Aboriginal people, one needs to recognize the impact of Christianity on Aboriginal communities. In many communities and families the introduction of Christianity increased the diversity of values influencing ethical decision-making. In some cases, the result has been division and animosity between family and community members who hold traditional Aboriginal values and those who assert Christian values.

WHY ARE ETHICS FOR ABORIGINAL PEOPLE IMPORTANT?

Population

The population of Aboriginal people who may benefit from culturally appropriate ethical decision-making is growing. There are alternative ways to define the Aboriginal population of Canada. Data from the 1996 Census indicated that about 800,000 people identified themselves with one or more Aboriginal groups (North American Indian, Métis, or Inuit).[17] The population includes about 41,000 who identified themselves as Inuit and about 210,000 as Métis.

Approximately 44% of Aboriginal people live in urban areas.[18] Of the more than 550,000 respondents who identified themselves as "North American Indian," about 60% indicated that they were a member of a First Nation or Band or had treaty status as defined by the Indian Act of Canada.[17] The ongoing transfer of control over health services to individual First Nations or Bands will mean that mandates to apply Aboriginal values in ethical decision-making will be emphasized in primary and tertiary health programs.

Access to Care

The importance of understanding Aboriginal perspectives on health ethics is often linked with differences in health status and utilization of health services. Lower health status and barriers to medical care access are engaged within the ethical context of distributive justice and equality. Research documenting the disproportionate burden of morbidity and mortality and high levels of health service utilization among Aboriginal people is often cited in medical literature. However, some Aboriginal health policy-makers have recently emphasized that epidemiological comparisons do not express the importance of individual and community historical relationships or contemporary experiences of racism in residential schools, social welfare programs, or the health care system.[19] In addition, there are many culturally distinct practices among Aboriginal people that necessitate a unique ethic of care.

Equitable access to high-quality health services is a central focus for both rural and urban Aboriginal people. Because of the centrality of family in Aboriginal people's experience of illness and treatment, and restrictions in the access of friends and family members, Aboriginal patients often feel isolated when in hospital.

Aboriginal approaches to decision-making commonly involve members of the extended family, and offering opportunities for family involvement should be considered a prerequisite of providing ethical and culturally appropriate services.[8]

HOW SHOULD I APPROACH THE PRACTICE OF ETHICS FOR ABORIGINAL PEOPLE?

To understand Aboriginal health ethics in clinical practice, several fundamental dimensions need to be recognized. Health care providers must recognize the risks of applying stereotyped values and spiritual beliefs, as well as the futility of attempting to develop generalized ethical formulas for communicating with Aboriginal patients. Plural belief systems and variation among individuals preclude the direct application of knowledge in reconciling Aboriginal beliefs with biomedical and bioethical criteria.

Aboriginal bioethics can best be viewed as an interpersonal process. Immediate and clearly defined approaches should not be expected. Aboriginal bioethical positions are largely situational; adopting a case-specific approach is therefore important. Health care providers working with Aboriginal people must first try to acknowledge the importance of autonomy, the centrality of family to health and identity, the diversity in beliefs and practices among Aboriginal people, and the value of developing and maintaining personal and emotionally sincere relationships with patients. Provider ethics emphasizing the maintenance of professional distance may contravene the Aboriginal affirmation of the power of human relationships in the healing process. Trust is paramount.

Health care providers might consider adopting the role of learner, allowing Aboriginal elders and each patient to lead in the articulation of the ethical principles guiding care. Not only is the process of family consultation critical in making decisions about acute and emergency care, but it is also an important dimension of day-to-day primary care. Health care providers should recognize that biomedical values may not always be reconcilable with Aboriginal values, despite improved communication methods or increased cross-cultural awareness.

If health care providers ignore differences related to Aboriginal culture, they will not be able to understand the wide spectrum of beliefs and attitudes that Aboriginal people draw on in making ethical decisions. Thus, although certain values such as respect for dignity, noninterference, sharing and the importance of family and community are widespread, other beliefs such as those about truth-telling may differ, even among members of the same family. Health care providers cannot take Aboriginal beliefs for granted and need to explore these carefully with each person. As well as respecting beliefs, health care providers need to respect the decisions of patients and families who request involvement of Aboriginal healers, elders, and medicine people in their care (Table 1).

THE FUTURE OF ETHICS AND ABORIGINAL PEOPLE

Aboriginal cultures can be identified as premodern in the sense that there is no separation between the self and the universe, between self, family and community or between mind, body and spirit. Thus, healing is not possible without spirituality, nor without relationships to family and community, and to the cosmos. Restoring these values and beliefs can balance biomedical treatments and lead to healing of the person as well as cure of disease.

Recent Western history has emphasized scientific and technological advances at the expense of, and exclusion of, spirituality. The consequences of this have been traumatic for many traditional Aboriginal people. When in need of health care, many Aboriginal people view health care institutions as dehumanizing: they experience mind-body separation and separation from family and community, and they are asked to participate in ethical decision-making guided by biomedical values.

The postmodern paradigm, which questions the existence of universal norms, scientific truth and "superior" cultures, presents an interesting challenge to modern medicine and its claims of exclusive efficacy in achieving cure. The current popularity of alternative healing methods, such as Aboriginal medicine, and the thirst for spiritual values are but a few indications of a postmodern culture that is more inclusive and holistic and thus more akin to traditional Aboriginal culture.

Aboriginal ethics is an important area of study because of its potential to make exceptional contributions to more generalized understandings of bioethical practice in increasingly diverse clinical and sociocultural environments. The emphasis in Aboriginal ethics on pluralism, diversity and the maintenance of a high level of respect for individuality challenges Western biomedical paradigms to become more responsive and dynamic in their approach to ethical decision-making. By incorporating a model of ethics that acknowledges pluralism and cultural context, medicine has the opportunity to develop models of ethics and care that are relevant to the cross-cultural treatment of the whole person.[20]

Considering the unique perspectives and experiences of Aboriginal people and the need for a dynamic, responsive framework for cross-cultural ethical decision-making, the Aboriginal population is clearly not the only cultural or religious group that is diverse and has a variety of beliefs and practices. By learning to respond to the nature of Aboriginal ethics, Western health care practitioners will become more responsive to the dynamics of culture in ethical decision-making for members of many ethnocultural communities.

THE CASE

The young female interpreter, out of respect for Mr. F's age, sex, and status, cannot discuss the urological procedure with him directly. However, by adhering to Ojibway beliefs, she does use a generalized term to refer to cancer and thus avoids contravening the belief that "speaking the future may bring it to pass." Although the male interpreter is able to use anatomic language without disrespect, Mr. F's son feels that explicit truth-telling about cancer is against traditional practice. In giving his son permission to be his interpreter and to be a proxy decision-maker, Mr. F is not undermining his own personal autonomy and instead is demonstrating shared family and communal responsi-

bility in decision-making. This is in contrast to the usual Western view of autonomy as conceding supremacy to the individual rather than to anyone else in making decisions. Only recently has the importance of relationships, especially as propounded in feminist ethics, been given a place in bioethics. It is worrisome for some that a cognitively competent individual is not being involved in making decisions about his future. Mr. F has, however, delegated responsibility to his son, even though non-Aboriginal patients more commonly accord such delegation to the medical team.

Given the principle of noninterference among Aboriginal people, the father's values and beliefs may differ considerably from those of his family. An important task of the interpreter and caregivers is to determine whether such differences are present. Aboriginal language interpreters are thus necessary not just for translation but to bring cultural awareness and sensitivity to interactions between patients, family members and health care providers. If differences in values are present, the physician may need to "offer truth" to ensure that Mr. F's views are respected. For example, Mr. F might be asked, "Are you the sort of person who likes to know all available information, or are you happy for your son to make decisions for you?" In this case it is reasonable that the father is not immediately told about his prognosis, since curative treatment is not being recommended. By being given extra time and a cultural medical treatment (i.e., a sharing circle in which caregivers, family, and the patient participate), Mr. F achieves "balance" between his diagnosis, the biomedical view, and his spiritual beliefs in a culturally appropriate manner. Following the sharing circle and a family meeting, the son, the urologist, and the interpreter meet with Mr. F, his wife, and two of his other children.

After this process of family consultation and gradual and prolonged truth-telling by the family, Mr. F understands his diagnosis and the implications of metastatic cancer. Together with his family, he consents to palliative care, including pain control and palliative radiation.

Notes

1. Gariepy GJ. *End of life issues in Aboriginal North America* [occasional paper]. Winnipeg: University of Manitoba; 1999.

2. Hultkrantz A. *Native religions of North America: the power of visions and fertility.* San Francisco: Harper Collins; 1987.

3. Ong WJ. *Orality and literacy.* New York: Methune; 1982. p. 57, 86, 145.

4. Ellerby JH. *Working with Aboriginal elders: understanding Aboriginal elders and healers and the cultural conflicts involved in their work in health care agencies and institutions.* Winnipeg: Earth Concepts and Biomedical Communications; 1999. p. 1–54.

5. Kaufert J, Koolage W. Role conflict among culture brokers: the experience of Native Canadian medical interpreters. *Soc Sci Med* 1984; 18(3):383–6.

6. Preston RJ, Preston S. Death and grieving among northern forest hunters: an East Cree example. In: *Coping with the final tragedy: cultural variations in dying and grieving.* Amityville (NY): Baywood; 1991. p. 135–56.

7. Carrese JA, Rhodes LA. Western bioethics on the Navajo reservation: Benefit or harm? *JAMA* 1995; 274:826–9.

8. Kaufert JM, Putsch RW, Lavallée M. End-of-life decision making among Aboriginal Canadians: interpretation, mediation, and discord in the communication of "bad news." *J Palliat Care* 1999; 15:31–8.

9. Freedman B. Offering truth: one ethical approach to the uninformed cancer patient. *Arch Intern Med* 1993; 153:572–6.

10. Brant CC. Native ethics and rules of behaviour. *Can J Psychiatry* 1990; 35:534–9.

11. Deloria V. Thinking in time and space. In: *God is red: a Native view of religion.* Golden (CO): Fulcrum Publishing; 1993. p. 62–77.

12. Deloria V. Death and religion. In: *God is red: a Native view of religion.* Golden (CO): Fulcrum Publishing; 1993. p. 165–84.

13. Hultkrantz A. North American Indian religion in a circumpolar perspective. In: Houins P, editor. *North American Indian studies: European contributions.* Gottingen: Hovens; 1981. p. 11–28.

14. Hultkrantz A. Health, religion and medicine in Native North American traditions. In: Sullivan LE, editor. *Healing and restoring: health and medicine in the world's religious traditions.* London: Macmillan; 1989. p. 327–58.

15. Hultkrantz A. *Shamanic healing and ritual drama: health and medicine in Native North American religious traditions.* New York: Crossroad; 1992. p. 15–6.

16. Hultkrantz A. *Shamanic healing and ritual drama: health and medicine in Native North American religious traditions.* New York: Crossroad; 1992. p. 164–8.

17. Population by Aboriginal group. In: *1996 Census.* Ottawa: Statistics Canada. Available: www.statcan.ca/english/Pgdb/People/Population/demo39a.htm (accessed 2000 Aug 29).

18. Royal Commission on Aboriginal Peoples. *Gathering strength.* Ottawa: The Commission; 1996.

19. O'Neil J, Reading J, Leader A. Changing the relations of surveillance: the development of a discourse of resistance in Aboriginal epidemiology. *Hum Organ* 1998; 57(2):230–7.

20. Dacher E. Towards a post-modern medicine. *J Altern Complement Med* 1996; 2(4):531–7.

21. Pohl A. *Building international awareness on Aboriginal issues.* Toronto: Citizens for Public Justice; 2000. p. 28–32.

Related Web sites

Aboriginal healing and wellness links (Turtle Island Native Network): www.turtleisland.org

Association of American Indian Physicians: www.aaip.com

Health Canada First Nations and Inuit Health Programs: www.hc-sc.gc.ca/msb/fnihp

Indian Health Service, US Department of Health and Human Services: www.ihs.gov

APPENDIX 1: GLOSSARY*

Aboriginal peoples: Groups or nations who were originally living in North America before European exploration.

Elder: Spiritual and community leader recognized by the Aboriginal community. Elders are cultural experts with special knowledge of community ethical values; some are also counselors and healers.

First Nations: Aboriginal societies that existed in Canada before Europeans arrived. Some Aboriginal people, including Inuit, do not see themselves as members of First Nations.

Inuit: A circumpolar Aboriginal people living in Canada, Greenland, Alaska, and Siberia.

Métis: A distinct and independent people whose ancestors were both of Aboriginal and European heritage and who currently do not have defined status within federal legislation.

Registered Indians: Aboriginal people who are registered under the Indian Act of Canada.

Sharing circle: An Aboriginal process in which each person has an opportunity to speak in turn. It is used for seeking consensus in decision-making, resolving conflicts between participants, and building community trust.

Smudging: A cleansing ceremony using the smoke from plant medicine.

Treaty Indians: Aboriginal people who are registered under the Indian Act of Canada and can prove descent from a band that signed a treaty.

---

*Aboriginal categories based on definitions proposed in *Building International Awareness on Aboriginal Issues*[21] and definitions on the Statistics Canada Web site.[17]

Deafness, Culture, and Choice

Neil Levy

There has been a great deal of discussion during the past few years of the potential biotechnology offers to us to choose to have only perfect babies, and of the implications that might have, for instance, for the disabled. What few people foresaw is that these same technologies could be deliberately used to ensure that children would be born with (what most people see as) disabilities. That this is a real possibility, and not merely the thought experiment of a philosopher, is brought home to us by the decision of an American lesbian couple to select a deaf sperm donor in order to maximise the chances that their children, Jehanne and Gauvin, would be deaf like them.[1] Their choice has sparked controversy, not only among medical ethicists, but in the opinion pages of newspapers across the world. Ought parents be permitted to make such choices?

If the parents of Jehanne and Gauvin have done anything wrong, it must consist in violating their child's right to an open future—limiting its future potential for choice.[2] But what does it mean to respect this right?

From the moment a child is born, her parents are making choices for her, which will powerfully shape her future. They will decide what kind of education she will have, what religious experiences, from among what group she can select friends. Thereby, they profoundly mould the person she will be and the life she will have.

When this activity is carried out within certain, ill-defined, limits, it is in no way objectionable. It is not merely a contingent fact about human beings that they must be educated in one way or another, and that this education will forever shape their future selves. It is, also, a profound metaphysical fact that freedom is necessarily constrained. If we did not bring values and expectations to our choices, we would have no basis upon which to make them. Thus, what is seen from one angle as the limiting of a child's future choices is, from another angle, the constitutive condition of her having choices at all. Only from within a certain, necessarily unchosen, framework can the child begin to make something of what she has been made.

Whether a parent's decisive choices on behalf of her child amount to an infringement of her right to an open future is, therefore, difficult to determine. We have no way of marking a precise boundary, within which such choices are the necessary preconditions of the child's own decisions, and beyond which too many options are foreclosed. All we can do is try to make some sort of judgment.

Does choosing deafness overstep this imprecise boundary? Deaf activists often argue that deafness is not a disability. Instead, it is the constitutive condition of access to a rich and valuable culture. For this reason, they might claim, choosing deafness falls well within the bounds of the permissible; it is a choice which opens up as many and as valuable options as it closes down. They cannot deny that, on average, the deaf do much worse than the hearing on a range of significant indicators of quality of life: unemployment, education levels, income, and so on. But they argue that this is a consequence of discrimination against them, overt and covert, and not of deafness itself. If society were structured to allow for the full participation of the deaf, they maintain, the negative effects of deafness would be entirely eliminated. In this sense, deafness is strictly analogous to blackness; blacks, too, do worse, on average, than their white peers, but this is an artefact of discrimination, not a consequence of skin colour.

If all the disadvantages which stem from deafness were traceable to discrimination, or even if they could all be eliminated by thoughtful planning, in the manner in which we can eliminate some of the disadvantages suffered by the wheelchair-bound by designing buildings with ramps, then this claim would be vindicated. And indeed, there is a great deal we can do to eliminate such disadvantages. We can caption television broadcasts, we can provide sign interpreters, and so forth. The internet has revolutionised the lives of many of the deaf, making communication, via email, as easy for them as it has been for most of us ever since the invention of the telephone. Though much has been done, however, and a great deal more could be achieved, we can

expect the deaf always to be at some disadvantage. We are, in many ways, a logocentric culture—one which is centred around the voice. The deaf will always be cut off from the buzz of conversation, always restricted to a narrower range of jobs, always slightly alienated from the mainstream of political, social, and cultural life. Deaf culture may have its compensations, but they cannot entirely make up for this estrangement.

Choosing deafness is, therefore, choosing a real (though not an especially severe) limitation, To that extent, deaf children have their future somewhat narrowed. Moreover, there is a sense in which this narrowing is uncompensated. For the children of the deaf, access to deaf culture is not the compensation they receive for their disability, it is their birthright. Culture, like language, is normally passed on without effort. Any baby, hearing or deaf, will pick up sign language and speak it as a first language, so long as it is exposed to it regularly. Thus, this couple did not need to make any special effort to ensure that their children would share their culture. A hearing child will pick up sign and a spoken language, just as the children of immigrants typically learn the language of their parents and the language of their adopted homeland. The hearing child of deaf parents might be said to have a maximally open future, since she participates, as a full member and not merely an onlooker, in two cultures.

The desire of parents to have their children share their culture is perfectly reasonable. It enhances empathy on both sides, enabling parents to assist their children in negotiating the road to adulthood that much more surely, and potentially increasing the satisfactions upon both sides. But deaf parents do not need to choose to exclude their children from the hearing world in order to include them in theirs; both are open to them. Though these parents might be guilty of restricting the range of their children's options to some extent, however, we ought not to be too hasty in condemning them. We ought to remember the extent to which they, like many other deaf people, felt isolated and alone as children, cut off not only from their schoolmates but also from their own family. They fear a similar fate for their children; that a nearly insuperable barrier will divide mother and child. In reality, their fear is misplaced. But it is comprehensible. Given this fact, and given the fact that the disadvantages which their children will suffer are likely to be relatively mild, we ought to react to them with compassion and understanding, not condemnation.

References

1. Mundy L. A world of their own. *Washington Post* 2002 Mar 31: W22.
2. On this right see Feinberg J. The child's right to an open future. In: Aiken W, LaFollette H, eds. *Whose child? Children's rights, parental authority, and state power.* Totowa, NJ: Littlefield, 1980: 124–53.

B. (R.) v. Children's Aid Society of Metropolitan Toronto, [1995] 1 S.C.R. 315

Summary prepared by Martina Munden

Sheena B was born prematurely. She had many ailments in the first few weeks of her life and received many treatments. Her parents, who were Jehovah's Witnesses, consented to all the treatments that were provided in those first few weeks, but requested, for religious reasons, that blood transfusions not be given. As Sheena B's condition deteriorated, the physicians believed that her life was in danger and that she might require a blood transfusion to treat potentially life-threatening congestive heart failure. The Court awarded the Children's Aid Society a 72-hour wardship of Sheena B in order that certain medical procedures, including a blood transfusion, could be administered to her. This order was based on the evidence of the physicians that a transfusion might be necessary and that the treatment would not be for experimental purposes. This order was later extended for 21 days. Sheena B was given a blood transfusion as part of an operation that she underwent. Although the wardship order was subsequently terminated and the child was returned to her parents, the parents appealed the court's decision. Ultimately, this case was heard by the Supreme Court of Canada.

The parents argued that the right to choose medical treatment for their infant was a liberty interest protected by s. 7 of the *Charter* and that the infringement of that interest did not conform to the principles of fundamental justice. The parents attacked the general procedure under the *Child Welfare Act*, and in particular, the specific way in which it was carried out in their case. The parents also argued that the *Act* deprived them of the right to refuse medical treatment for their child on religious grounds and thus violated their freedom of religion guaranteed under s. 2(a) of the *Charter*.

The majority of the Supreme Court of Canada held that in accordance with s. 7, the liberty interest of a parent includes the right to nurture a child, to care for its development, and to make decisions in fundamental matters such as medical care. It held that under s. 7, there is a protected sphere of parental decision-making and that "parental liberty" under s. 7 ensures that state intervention will be subject to *Charter* scrutiny for compliance with the "principles of fundamental justice." This finding recognized that there is a link between parental responsibilities and the correlative rights to exercise them, especially against the intrusion of the state into family relationships. The privileged role parents exercise in the upbringing of their children translates into a protected sphere of parental decision-making which is rooted in the presumption that parents should make important decisions affecting their children and that state intervention when it is considered necessary to safeguard the child's autonomy or health must be justified. The majority decision held that parental decision-making must receive the protection of the *Charter* in order for state interference to be properly monitored by the courts and to be permitted only when it conforms to the values underlying the *Charter*.

Although the SCC held that the liberty right under s. 7 encompasses parental decision-making for their children, upon reviewing the procedures contained in the *Child Welfare Act*, it concluded that those procedures were in accordance with the principles of fundamental justice. It also held that the application of the procedures in the present case was in compliance with the principles of fundamental justice.

With respect to whether the *Child Welfare Act* infringed the parents' freedom of religion, the majority decision held that the purpose of the *Act* was not directed at limiting the freedom of Jehovah's Witnesses to choose medical treatment for their children, including the freedom to refuse a blood transfusion on religious grounds. However, it found that the effects of the legislation denied the parents the right to choose medical treatment for their infant according to their religious beliefs. The majority decision held that the right of parents to rear their children according to their religious beliefs, including that of choosing medical and other treatments, was a fundamental aspect of freedom of religion. It held that the legislative scheme implemented by the *Act*, which culminated in a wardship order depriving the parents of the custody of their child, denied them the right to choose medical treatment for their infant according to their religious beliefs.

The SCC then explored whether the infringement was justified under s. 1 of the *Charter*. In holding that the restrictions imposed on parental rights were justified, the SCC noted that the state interest in protecting children at risk was a pressing and substantial concern, thus meeting the first requirement of a s. 1 analysis. It also held that the means chosen in overriding the parents' s. 2(a) *Charter* right were reasonable and demonstrably justified, noting that the process contemplated by the Act was carefully crafted, adaptable to a myriad of different situations, and far from arbitrary.

Although the majority decision of the SCC dismissed the appeal finding that the principles of fundamental justice had been complied with, its finding that the liberty interest covered by s. 7 of the *Charter* includes "parental liberty" is a significant one. Following this decision, decisions regarding parental rights to make decisions for medical care should proceed from the point that parental rights must be considered and state intervention must be justified, rather than proceeding from the perspective that parental decision-making regarding medical treatment is not a liberty right that parents can expect protection for under s. 7 of the *Charter*.

Chapter 3 HEALTH CARE IN CANADA

Sustaining Medicare: The Commission on the Future of Health Care in Canada

Ray Romanow

The heart of the Commission's mandate was to make recommendations "to ensure the long-term sustainability of a universally accessible, publicly funded health system." The rationale behind this mandate was quite simple. For a number of years now, Canadians have been told by some of their governments and a number of health policy experts that the system popularly known as medicare is no longer "sustainable."

At the same time, the Commission's extensive consultations with Canadians and its comprehensive research program clearly indicate that Canadians *want* the system to be sustainable, not only for themselves but for future generations of Canadians. They want it to change, and to change in some very fundamental and important ways. But they also want it to endure and, indeed, to thrive.

Is it possible to reconcile these two perspectives? The place to start is with a clear understanding of what makes a system sustainable and what needs to be done to ensure that Canada's health care system is sustainable in the future.

WHAT IS SUSTAINABILITY?

In some ways, the word "sustainability" both illuminates and obscures the debate. It is a word that is immediately understandable and yet open to multiple interpretations and misinterpretations. Moreover, much of the recent debate on health care has focused on one aspect only—namely costs. People conclude that the system is not sustainable because it costs too much money, it takes too large a proportion of governments' budgets, or it is an impediment to lowering taxes. There are others who argue that the problem with the system is the way it is organized and the inefficiencies that result. Reorganize the system, they argue, and there is more than enough money to meet our needs. Still other voices have argued that the only problem with the system is the lack of money provided in recent years. Restore and increase the financial resources, they argue, and all will be well.

In the Commission's view, this narrow focus on money is inadequate and does not help inform the debates or enable an overall assessment of whether or not Canada's health care system is sustainable.

Instead, the Commission takes the view that:

> Sustainability means ensuring that sufficient resources are available over the long term to provide timely access to quality services that address Canadians' evolving health needs.

For many years, health policy experts have focused on three essential dimensions that are each key to sustaining the health care system:

- **Services**—A more comprehensive range of necessary health care services must be available to meet Canadians' health needs. The services must be of a high quality and accessible on a timely basis. This aspect of sustainability involves looking at the changing ways health care services are delivered, whether they are accessible for Canadians, and whether they are efficiently and effectively delivered.

- **Needs**—The health care system must meet Canadians' needs and produce positive outcomes not only for individual Canadians but also for the population as a whole. This dimension examines how Canada's health care outcomes measure up to other countries, identifying disparities in the health of different Canadians and looking at trends in health.

- **Resources**—This includes not only financial resources but also the required health care providers and the physical resources (facilities, equipment, technology, research, and data) that are needed to provide the range of services offered.

There is no "invisible hand" that silently and unobtrusively keeps these elements in balance. Decisions about providing adequate resources imply that there is political support by governments and by Canadians to continue supporting the system through public funds and public oversight. Maintaining the balance is, in fact, a deliberate act of will on the part of society and, thus, it is the overall governance of the system at all levels that ultimately decides how these elements are balanced.

Governance involves the political, social and economic choices that Canadians, their governments, and those in the health care system make concerning how the system continues to balance the health services, health needs, and resources that make up the system.

The following sections of this chapter address the complex and thorny issue of sustainability from those three essential dimensions—services, needs and resources—and looks at the changing way the health care system has been governed. What this review shows is that the system continues to do many things well. At the same time, there are a number of things it can and must improve. The system is neither unsustainable nor unfixable, but action is required to maintain the right balance between the services that are provided, their effectiveness in meeting the needs of Canadians, and the resources that we, as Canadians, are prepared to dedicate to sustain the system in the future.

Ultimately, the question of whether and how the system is sustained comes down to choices by those who govern the health care system— by providers, by governments, by administrators and by Canadians themselves.

HEALTH AND HEALTH CARE SERVICES

Canada's health care system provides a range of services, some of which are covered by the *Canada Health Act* and the well-known five principles, some that are covered by provinces and territories, and some that are provided through the private sector. In large part, provinces and territories are responsible for organizing and delivering health care services to people across the country. Since medicare was first established, there have been considerable changes in both the scope of health care services provided in Canada and the different ways they are organized and delivered from relatively large regional health authorities to small clinics or doctors' offices.

Services offered in our health care system can be differentiated by their complexity and intensity: the more or less specialized nature of interventions to maintain or restore health and the number of qualified health personnel needed to see the interventions through.

At one end of the spectrum are a wide variety of services that are covered by the public health care system: public health programs aimed at the prevention of illness such as the immunization of children; visits to family physicians, pediatricians, or gynecologists; diagnostic tests; and day surgery. Moving across the spectrum, we find the complex and intense care that requires the increasing use of advanced technology as well as highly trained specialists and large support teams. In addition, long-term or continuing care is typically provided in nursing homes or other specialized residential settings for people who require ongoing medical attention and support but who do not need to be treated in hospitals. Palliative care is provided to people who are dying and is available in hospitals, hospices, and, to a growing extent, at home. Home care is an increasingly important component of health care that can allow people to avoid hospitalization or recover at home following a shorter hospital stay. At any point along the spectrum, people can and frequently do receive prescription drugs.

The key question in terms of sustainability is whether this vast continuum of services provided in Canada's health care system meets the needs of Canadians, is accessible, and can be adapted in the future to meet the changing needs of Canadians.

Health Care and the Canadian Constitution

The Canadian constitution does not address health and health care as a single subject nor does it explicitly allocate responsibility to one order of government or another. Both provincial and federal governments have varying degrees of jurisdiction over different aspects of the health care system (Braën 2002; Leeson 2002). However, through a number of court cases and legal interpretations, it is now well accepted that the provinces have primary jurisdiction over the organization and delivery of health care services in Canada. In contrast, Yukon, Nunavut, and the Northwest Territories do not have formal constitutional powers over health care, although they have assumed these responsibilities in recent years.

As Justice Estey of the Supreme Court of Canada pointed out in *Schneider v. The Queen:* "Health is not a subject specifically dealt with in the *Constitution Act* either in 1867 or by way of subsequent amendment. It is by the Constitution not assigned either to the federal or provincial legislative authority" (quoted in Gibson 1996, 1). In Peter Hogg's (1997, 485) words, "health is an 'amorphous topic' which is distributed to the federal Parliament or the provincial Legislatures depending on the purpose and effect of the particular health measure in issue." The reason for

this is that the concept of health care is a modern one with assumptions and meanings that could not have been predicted by the constitution. A simple analogy to "health and health care" would be "the environment," another contemporary concept foreign to 19th century thinking and, therefore, absent from the original constitutional division of powers.

While the provinces have primary responsibility for health care delivery, the federal government has constitutional authority and responsibility in a number of very specialized aspects of health care (e.g., the approval and regulation of prescription drugs) and in critical areas of publicly funded health care, including the protection and promotion of health. The federal government also is responsible for providing health services to specific groups of Canadians, including First Nations and Inuit peoples as well as members and veterans of the Armed Forces and members of the Royal Canadian Mounted Police.

Perhaps the most visible federal role in health care comes through its transfer of funds to the provinces through what is called the "federal spending power." This often-controversial power is not specifically identified in the constitution but rests on court decisions that have upheld the federal government's right to spend money in areas of provincial jurisdiction.

The spending power can be used to provide direct payments to individuals (such as Family Allowances in the past or the current Millennium Scholarships), to other third parties such as universities (e.g., the Canada Research Chairs), or to the provinces for such things as post-secondary education, social services or health care. Such transfers to the provinces often come with "conditions" on how the money is supposed to be spent.

The spending power has been contested by some provinces, which argue that health care is exclusively a provincial jurisdiction, that the "conditions" imposed by the federal government distort their own spending priorities, and that Ottawa's fiscal powers should be curtailed. In spite of these objections, various legal cases have consistently upheld the constitutionality of the federal spending power and, more specifically, the right to provide conditional funding to the provinces (Braën 2002).

Medicare and Beyond

Most Canadians give little thought to the constitutional division of powers over health care. When they think of medicare, they think, first and foremost, of the services that the system provides. However, there are many misconceptions about what medicare is and what it is not—and some of those misconceptions may stem from the complex relationship that has developed between the federal and provincial–territorial governments for funding and organizing the system.

In 1957, the federal government, under the *Hospital Insurance and Diagnostic Services Act* (HIDSA), agreed to reimburse provinces for a portion of the cost of providing hospital insurance to their residents. Some provinces had already created hospital insurance programs by this point and the others were encouraged to do so by the offer of partial federal funding. In the late 1960s and early 1970s, following the report of Justice Emmett Hall's Royal Commission on Health Services (1964) and building on the model introduced in Saskatchewan, the federal government again used its spending power to encourage provinces to expand hospitalization insurance to include basic physician services as well. They agreed to cover a portion of the cost of those expanded services under the *Medical Care Act* of 1966. This expanded the program that became known to the public as medicare. The result is complete coverage for all necessary hospital and physician services through a publicly funded "single-payer" insurance system. As a result, no Canadian has to pay for those services at the time he or she uses them.

In 1984, the *Medical Care Act* and HIDSA were replaced by the *Canada Health Act* (CHA), which enumerated the five principles that have, in recent years, come to define the Canadian health care system: public administration, universality, accessibility, portability, and compre-

hensiveness. These principles have also become the conditions that the federal government has placed on its transfer of funds to the provinces. The provinces must ensure that their health insurance programs meets the conditions set out in the *Canada Health Act* in order to receive their full share of federal funding, and they must report annually to the federal government on how they meet the conditions of the CHA. In 2001/02, CHA services amounted to almost $44 billion or 42.4% of total (public and private) health expenditures.

The federal government's role in relation to hospital and physician services covered under the *Canada Health Act* primarily involves transferring funds to the provinces and ensuring that the conditions of the Act are met. *Canada Health Act* services are insured and administered by the provinces and territories, and delivered through a variety of organizations such as regional health authorities, hospitals, physician practices, and health clinics. As discussed in more detail later in this chapter, the relative size of the federal transfer compared to the provincial cost of delivering health services has become a dominant and disruptive theme of contemporary intergovernmental relations in Canada.

In addition to hospital and physician services, provinces and territories provide a range of additional health care services including prescription drug plans, home care, continuing care, and long-term care. The nature and scope of these services vary considerably depending on the individual provincial and territorial plan. In addition, some provinces provide coverage for services such as rehabilitation, physiotherapy, or chiropractic care while others do not. Unlike the single-payer system for hospital and physician services, provincial coverage for prescription drugs and various other health services such as home care does not necessarily cover the full costs. Instead, provincial plans supplement, to varying degrees, private insurance and private payment. These services amounted to almost $26 billion, which was 25.2% of total health care expenditures in Canada in 2001/02. Moreover, public coverage for these other health care services is generally accompanied by co-payments, deductibles, and means testing and is, therefore, not the type of fully insured coverage we have come to expect for *Canada Health Act* services.

The private sector also plays a role in Canada's health care system. Private health care services are those that we either pay for directly ourselves or are covered through private insurance plans or employee benefit plans. For example, the vast majority of dental services in Canada are paid for through employer-provided insurance coverage or by individuals directly. Private services amounted to just over $33 billion in 2001/02, which was 32.4% of total health care expenditures.

There is also a small area of overlap between public and private health care services. This overlap includes two areas: services provided under workers' compensation programs for injuries sustained on the job, and tax subsidies to encourage the private sector to provide supplementary insurance (largely for prescription drugs and dental services not covered in provincial and territorial plans). Individuals also receive tax deductions if their medical expenses are more than 3% of their income. In 1994, these tax breaks were estimated to be worth about $2.5 billion (Smythe 2001). They have grown rapidly since that time and likely are worth closer to $4 billion today, including roughly $3 billion given up by governments for not taxing private health premiums paid by employers and a further $1 billion for the tax credits for individual health costs as well as various disability allowances. These tax subsidies are not typically included in estimates of public spending on health care.

The health care system has expanded considerably to respond to the changing nature of health care and medical science, the wishes of Canadians in different provinces and territories, and the availability of resources within any particular province. There are only minor differences between provinces in terms of the *Canada Health Act* services that are covered. For example, some provinces cover annual eye exams while some do not. Beyond these serv-

ices, all provinces provide some level of home care services, some form of public prescription drug insurance for vulnerable populations, and some range of continuing or long-term care.

There are also similarities in the way provinces have chosen to organize the delivery of health care services. The most prominent trend in recent years has been regionalization. Provinces have created regional health authorities with responsibility for organizing, delivering, and co-ordinating public health programs, hospital services, community care, and long-term or continuing care services within a particular region of the province. The province of Quebec led this move in the 1970s, but today every province has created health regions, although in Ontario these regions have only a consultative role.

Private For-Profit Service Delivery: The Debate

One of the most contentious issues facing Canadians is the extent to which the private sector should be involved in delivering health care services. Currently, provincial and territorial governments provide coverage for a range of services and those services can be delivered in any number of ways. Almost all Canadian hospitals are not-for-profit institutions and, in most provinces, are operated by regional health authorities. Most physician services are delivered by what are effectively owner-operated small businesses ranging from single-physician practices to multi-provider clinics that may include a range of health care providers. Large for-profit corporations deliver a narrower range of services including laboratory services and continuing and long-term care.

In the face of continuing pressures on the health care system, some argue that more private for-profit service delivery ought to be introduced in order to bring more resources, choice, and competition into the Canadian health care system and to improve its efficiency and effectiveness. Others argue as strongly that the private sector should be completely excluded from health care delivery, suggesting that private for-profit delivery runs counter to Canadians' values, is inequitable, and is less cost-effective than public delivery in the long run.

To try to make sense of this debate, it is important to distinguish between two types of services: direct health care services such as medical, diagnostic, and surgical care; and ancillary services such as food preparation, cleaning, and maintenance. An increasing proportion of ancillary services provided in Canada's not-for-profit hospitals are now contracted out to for-profit corporations. Canadians seem to find this role for private sector companies acceptable and some studies suggest that these enterprises achieve economies of scale (McFarlane and Prado 2002). Ancillary services are relatively easy to judge in terms of quality—the laundry is either clean or it is not, the cafeteria food is either good or it is not. Consequently, it is relatively easy to judge whether the company is providing the service as promised. Also, there is a greater likelihood that there are competitors in the same business to whom hospitals can turn for laundry or food services if their current contractor is unsatisfactory.

In terms of direct health care services, the precise number of for-profit facilities delivering direct health care services is unknown. One estimate in 1998 (Deber et al.) suggested that there were 300 private for-profit clinics in Canada delivering many diagnostic and therapeutic services formerly provided in hospitals, including abortions, endoscopies, physiotherapy, new reproductive technologies, and laser eye surgeries. In addition, there are a growing number of small private for-profit hospitals or stand-alone clinics in some provinces providing more complex surgeries, some requiring overnight stays. These facilities vary considerably in terms of the number of services they offer and their ownership structure. Furthermore, some provinces have expressed an interest in contracting out an increasing number of surgical services to private for-profit hospitals and clinics in the hope of realizing efficiencies.

Unlike ancillary services, direct health care services are very complex and it is difficult to assess their quality without considerable expertise. Indeed, the effects of poorly provided service may not be apparent until some time after the service has been delivered, as in the event of a post-operative complication. This is what most clearly distinguishes direct health care services from ancillary services—a poorly prepared cafeteria meal may be unpleasant, but poor quality surgery is another matter altogether. It is also unlikely that there would be a significant number of competitors able to offer health care services if a given for-profit provider is unsatisfactory. There simply is not a significant surplus of health care administrators or providers waiting in the wings to take over service delivery in a hospital. Thus, if services are of poor quality, it is going to be much harder to find a replacement once public facilities have stopped providing the services—the capacity that existed in the public system will have been lost.

Some suggest that private for-profit delivery is more efficient than not-for-profit delivery (Gratzer 1999 and 2002). Given that most of the private facilities currently operating and being planned focus only on providing a limited range of services, there are some important concerns that must be addressed in terms of how these facilities interact with the more comprehensive public system. In effect, these facilities "cream-off" those services that can be easily and more inexpensively provided on a volume basis, such as cataract surgery or hernia repair. This leaves the public system to provide the more complicated and expensive services from which it is more difficult to control cost per case. But if something goes wrong with a patient after discharge from a private facility—as a result, for example, of a post-operative infection or medical error—then the patient will likely have to be returned to a public hospital for treatment insofar as private facilities generally do not have the capacity to treat individuals on an intensive care basis. Thus, the public system becomes liable for the care triggered by a poor quality outcome within a private facility, yet under current arrangements there is no way for the public system to recover those costs from the private facility. In other words, the public system is required to provide a "back-up" to the private facilities to ensure quality care.

Proponents of for-profit care may insist that the quality of care is not an issue, but there is evidence from the United States to suggest that the non-profit sector tends to have better quality outcomes than the for-profit sector in such things as nursing home care (Harrington 2001; Marmor et al. 1987) and managed care organizations and hospitals (Kleinke 2001; Gray 1999). More recently, a comprehensive analysis of the various studies that compare not-for-profit and for-profit delivery of services concluded that for-profit hospitals had a significant increase in the risk of death and also tended to employ less highly skilled individuals than did non-profit facilities (Devereaux et al. 2002).

For those reasons, the Commission believes a line should be drawn between ancillary and direct health care services and that direct health care services should be delivered in public and not-for-profit health care facilities.

There are, however, several grey areas around the issue of private for-profit delivery. First, diagnostic services have expanded considerably in the past few years and, in many cases, these services are provided in private facilities under contracts with regional health authorities or provincial governments. Much of this involves relatively routine procedures such as laboratory tests and x-rays that can be done with little delay or wait on the part of the patient. But there appears to be a growing reliance on the private provision of more advanced and expensive diagnostics such as MRIs (magnetic resonance imaging), for which the waiting times in the public system can be frustratingly long because of what appears to be an under-investment in such technology within the public system. The growth of private advanced diagnostic facilities has permitted individuals to purchase faster service by paying for these services out of their own pocket and using the test results to "jump the queue" back into the public system for treatment. While this is not currently a common occurrence, Canadians made it clear to the Commission that they are deeply concerned

about the prospect of this becoming routine (Commission 2002a).

Medicare rests on the principle that an individual's financial resources should not determine access to services. In the Commission's view, governments have a responsibility to guarantee that the public system has sufficient resources to ensure appropriate access to advanced technology. Increased investment within the public system for new diagnostic technology can remove the temptation to "game" the system by individuals and health care providers through the private purchase of diagnostic tests that could allow them to jump the queue.

The second grey area is services provided to workers' compensation clients with job-related injuries and illnesses. Because of the belief that it is important to get these people back to work quickly, these clients get preferential treatment in accessing diagnostic and other health care services over those whose illness or injury is not work related or who may not be formally employed. As suggested in Chapter 2, this current exception under the *Canada Health Act* should be reconsidered.

The third grey area is contracting out of surgical services. In some cases, regional health authorities have contracted with private for-profit facilities that provide specific surgeries such as cataract and some day surgeries. Again, there is no clear evidence that this practice is more efficient or less costly than providing the services in an adequately resourced not-for-profit facility.

Services and Sustainability

Services are the first element in our definition of sustainability. The previous information suggests that there are complex, and sometimes confusing, relationships between the federal, provincial, and territorial governments. Much has changed since medicare was first introduced. The range of services is growing and changing with new advances in medicine and, as a result, the biggest growth in services is outside of hospital and physician services. Subsequent chapters will show that there is tremendous growth in home care and that prescription drugs have become the fastest growing part of the health care system. Canadians also are only too well aware of the fact that services are not always available on a timely basis. In areas like diagnostic services and some surgeries, people sometimes wait too long for access to the services they need. People in rural and remote communities also have problems in accessing services. In spite of what appears to be almost overwhelming support for primary health care, only limited progress has been made in extending primary health care across the country. All of these issues apply in every province and territory. The conclusion, then, on services and sustainability is that more needs to be done to ensure timely access to quality services. The answer, however, is not to look to the private sector for solutions. Instead, governments should seek the best solutions within the public system and ensure that adequate resources are available and services are accessible to all.

The Commission is strongly of the view that a properly funded public system can continue to provide the high quality services to which Canadians have become accustomed. Rather than subsidize private facilities with public dollars, governments should choose to ensure that the public system has sufficient capacity and is universally accessible. In addition, as discussed in Chapter 11, any decisions about expanding private for-profit delivery could have implications under international trade agreements that need to be considered in advance....

Needs and Sustainability

The second key dimension of assessing sustainability is needs, namely, Does the health care system adequately meet Canadians' needs? The answer is a qualified yes. Canada's health outcomes compare favourably with other countries and evidence suggests that we are doing a good job of addressing factors that affect the overall health of Canadians. There are, however, areas where there is room for improvement. And there are serious disparities in both access to health care and health outcomes in some parts of Canada. Clearly, more needs to be done to reduce these disparities and also to address a

number of factors that affect Canadians' health such as tobacco use, obesity, and inactivity. These factors are addressed specifically in Chapter 5 of this report. The other conclusion is that aging is not the ominous threat to future sustainability of our system that some would suggest. Aging will challenge and add costs to our health care system, but those costs can be managed, particularly if we begin to prepare and make adjustments to anticipate the impact of an aging population.

RESOURCES IN THE SYSTEM: THE CASE OF FUNDING

As was noted at the outset of this chapter, the third major component of the definition of sustainability relates to the availability of necessary resources. The health care system needs a variety of resources in order to deliver services and meet the health care needs of the population. That includes not only financial resources but also human and physical resources such as equipment, facilities, and technology. Chapter 3 deals with the information resources that are needed to allow providers, governments, and citizens to make informed decisions about the system generally and about their own personal care. Chapter 4 deals with the supply, distribution and changing role of health care providers. Chapter 6 deals with the availability and accessibility of equipment and facilities. All of these are essential for an efficient and effective health care system.

However, the primary focus of much of the debate about sustainability has been about money. Questions about the increasing costs of health care, who pays for what aspects of the health care system, and whether we will be able to afford the health care system in the future have played a significant part in the debates about medicare's sustainability. The debate has centered on whether there is too little public money in the system, whether there should be different ways of raising those public funds and whether the system as we know it is "affordable" any longer. Because other chapters do not deal with these issues in detail, the remainder of this chapter addresses the fiscal questions directly, beginning with how Canada's funding for health care compares with other countries, whether other options for funding should be considered, and the relative shares paid by different governments.

Canada's Reliance on Taxes

Canadians pay, directly or indirectly, for every aspect of our health care system through a combination of taxes, payments to government, private insurance premiums, and direct out-of-pocket fees of varying types and amounts. Some have suggested that Canada relies too heavily on taxation to support its health care system.

… 71% of the total funding for Canada's health care comes from taxation. In countries such as Germany, Japan, France, and the Netherlands, the majority of funding for health care comes from social insurance premiums in the form of employment payroll taxes. In most developed countries (other than those that rely heavily on social insurance), between 70 and 80% of total health care is funded through the taxation system (Mossialos et al. 2002)…. [I]t is hard to conclude that Canada depends too heavily on taxes to support health care.

Use of Private Insurance and Out-of-pocket Payments

One area where Canada differs from most OECD countries is in co-payments and user fees. While Canada relies almost entirely on taxes to fund hospital and physician services, co-payments and user fees for these services are common in most OECD countries. At the same time, Canada relies more heavily on private insurance and out-of-pocket payments for health care services that are not covered by the *Canada Health Act*.

… Dental services, for example, are almost entirely funded (94%) through private insurance and direct fees in Canada but are often part of public coverage in many Western European countries.

In comparison with selected countries, only Japan and Australia have higher levels of out-of-pocket expenditures than Canada while in the United Kingdom, Sweden, the Netherlands, Germany, and France all have substantially lower levels of out-of-pocket payments. This is because the fees charged in those countries are low and represent a relatively small proportion of the real cost of the services provided. Canadians, however, pay relatively high co-payments and deductibles for prescription drugs and health services outside the CHA and this results in Canada having a higher percentage of out-of-pocket payments than other countries.

Even though the co-payments and deductibles are high, the percentage of out-of-pocket payments in Canada accounts for a relatively small percentage of the total costs of health care services and is lower than the OECD average. Canada, like most of the wealthier OECD countries including the United States, relies primarily on funding provided through governments or through insurers. In high-income countries, what we call "third-party" payments (i.e., payments made by governments or insurers) make up between 80 and 90% of health expenditures (OECD 2002). In less wealthy OECD countries, however, there tends to be a much higher reliance on out-of-pocket payments.

The Balance between Public and Private Funding of Health Care

There is some debate in Canada about the appropriate balance between public and private funding for health care. Recently, a number of Canadian providers, scholars, and journalists argued in favour of a greater private role in funding Canadian health care on the assumption that Canadian health care spending is overly weighted to the public side (Gratzer 2002). However, a comparison with other industrialized countries shows that Canada is hardly an exception in terms of the public share of total health expenditures. The United Kingdom, Sweden, Germany, France, Japan, and Australia all have larger public health care sectors than Canada, while the Netherlands' public share is slightly lower than Canada's…. What is truly noteworthy is the extent to which these countries' public health care expenditures resemble each other.

While most wealthy countries rely heavily on public funding for health care, private insurance plays a significant role in funding health care in the United States. Private insurance in the United States is supported by tax breaks known as "tax expenditure subsidies." These subsidies exist, but to a much lesser extent, in all the comparison countries. Since these subsidies are not generally included when public health care expenditures are tallied, they are difficult to trace and are therefore referred to as "covert" expenditures (Mossialos and Dixon 2002). In fact, tax subsidies play an enormous role in providing health care coverage in the United States. When these tax breaks are taken into account, the public share of health care spending in the United States increases to nearly 60% of its total health care spending (Woolhandler and Himmelstein 2002). This changes the common perception that the United States has a predominantly private system of health care.

Even without including tax subsidies, the extraordinarily high level of total health care spending in the United States translates into far more spending per capita than in Canada and the other OECD countries. This has been described as tantamount to paying for national health insurance and, in return, getting a fragmented system with significant gaps in coverage—the worst of both worlds. While the United States' "health care system is usually portrayed as largely private," a more apt description is "[p]ublic money, private control" (Woolhandler and Himmelstein 2002, 22). Indeed, the larger the public share of health care financing beyond tax expenditure subsidies, the more total health expenditures are capable of being controlled. In contrast, the larger the private share of health care financing, the more difficult it is to control health care expenditures (Majnoni d'Intignano 2001).

Alternative Funding Sources

In recent years, a number of suggestions have been made that Canada should consider alternative ways of paying for health care services. These proposals may be a reaction to the fact that people see costs increasing, are worried about sustainability, and question whether we should change the current funding system to look for additional sources of revenue. Undeniably, each of these proposals has some potential to raise additional money to fund the health care system. But some pose problems in terms of the impact they would have on access and equity. A number of the most common proposals are critically examined below.

User Fees and Out-of-pocket Co-payments. User fees are definitely a "hot button" issue for many Canadians. While many are opposed to user fees because they discourage poorer people from accessing health care services, others see user fees as a necessary way of either raising additional funds for health care or curbing abuse of the health care system. Interestingly, during the Citizens' Dialogue sessions held by the Commission, the interest in user fees was not aimed at raising more revenue for the system but at curbing what some participants felt was abuse and unnecessary use of the system (Commission 2002a).

There is overwhelming evidence that direct charges such as user fees put the heaviest burden on the poor and impede their access to necessary health care. This is the case even when low-income exemptions are in place. The result may be higher costs in the long run because people delay treatment until their condition gets worse. In addition, user fees and payments also involve significant administrative costs that directly reduce the modest amount of revenue generated from the fees (Evans 2002a; Evans et al. 1993; Barer et al. 1993, 1979; CES 2001).

One of the key features of the *Canada Health Act* was its effective ban on user fees for hospital and physician services. Given what we know about the impact of even relatively low user fees, the Commission feels that this was the right decision then and remains the right decision today.

Medical Savings Accounts. Perhaps no recent suggestion for raising additional revenue has attracted as much attention as medical savings accounts, in part because they seem to address some of the criticisms of user fees. Medical savings accounts (MSAs) can be designed in a number of different ways but the fundamental concept is that individuals are allotted a yearly health care allowance and they can use it to "purchase" health care services (Gratzer 2002, 1999; Migué 2002; Ramsay 2002). If they have funds left in their MSA allowance at the end of the year, depending on how the plan is designed, they may be able to keep the funds or save them for future years when their health care costs may be higher.

MSAs are intended to provide patients with more control and to inject market forces into the organization and delivery of health care services. They provide patients with an incentive to "shop" for the best services and best prices, and to avoid unnecessary treatments, particularly if they get to keep any surplus in their account at the end of the year. If the costs of health care services people use in a year are higher than their yearly allowance, they would be required to pay all or a portion of the additional costs, depending on how the plan was designed. Most MSA proposals discussed in Canada involve a so-called "corridor" where people pay some of the cost of health care expenses above their annual allowance up to a certain point before catastrophic coverage funded entirely by government would cover any remaining costs (Mazankowski 2001).

Because medical savings account approaches are relatively new, we know very little about their effects and the literature to date is contradictory. MSAs have been implemented on a small scale in the United States, on an experimental basis in several cities in China, in South Africa where they constitute half of the private for-profit health insurance market, and on a nationwide basis in Singapore. It is difficult, however, to compare these experiences to the Canadian situation. With the exception of China, these countries have predominantly private financing and private delivery of health care services. This means people in those countries may have a much greater opportunity to "shop around" for health care services. Singapore's experience shows that hospitals tend not to compete on the basis of price for necessary services, but aggressively market expensive add-ons, some of which are of questionable value.

The limited evidence available suggests that medical savings accounts have a number of shortcomings that have been understated or ignored by their proponents (Maynard and Dixon 2002; Shortt 2002; Hurley 2000, 2002; Barr 2001). Overall, MSAs are based on the assumption that the use of necessary health care services is highly discretionary, when this is almost invariably not the case.

MSAs are unlikely to effectively control overall spending on health care (Forget et al. 2002). Most health care costs are incurred by a small proportion of people who have very high health care needs and they will continue to spend a lot regardless of whether or not they have an MSA. Under some designs, costs could actually increase because governments would not only provide the initial allowance but also continue to pay for catastrophic insurance to protect people against very high costs. If people were allowed to keep the money left in their MSA at the end of the year, this money would be lost to the health care system and would have to be made up through other means.

MSAs may compromise equity in access to health care services. If individuals are required to pay once they have used all of their MSA allowance, it could cause hardships for people with lower incomes or higher health care needs due to chronic or life-threatening conditions. This is precisely the reason why Canada's medicare system was introduced—to avoid a situation where wealthy people could get access to all the health care services they needed and poor people could not.

Tax-based Co-payments, Tax Credits, and Deductibles. A number of recent articles have focused on the use of the tax system as a way of increasing private payment in the health care system (Aba et al. 2002; Aba and Mintz 2002; Reuber and Poschmann 2002). The simplest way of doing this would be to include publicly provided health care services as a taxable benefit on individuals' annual income tax returns (Kent 2000). People would get something like a T4-H showing the cost of the health services they received in a year. This amount would be added to their taxable income and they would pay additional taxes to cover a portion of the cost of the health services they received.

On the positive side, this approach would raise additional revenues. People would know the costs of the services they received, and any additional taxes would be based on their ability to pay. On the other hand, the approach could potentially bankrupt people who had chronic health conditions or who suffered a catastrophic illness or injury. To address this concern, the amount of the co-payment or additional taxes a person paid could be capped at a certain percentage of his or her income and very low-income people could be exempt (Aba and Mintz 2002).

Even with these conditions, there are concerns with this approach. Fundamentally, it means that if people are sick or injured, they will be taxed more and pay more for health care. This is counter to the basic premise in Canada's health care system that access should be determined only by need and not by ability to pay. As in the case of MSAs or user fees, it may result in people not using needed health care services, a phenomenon that has been seen in a number of European systems (CES 2001). It also raises the question of whether middle- and higher-income earners, who currently pay the bulk of the costs of a universal health care system, will eventually become dissatisfied when they also have to pay even more at tax time based on their use of the health care system.

Public–Private Partnerships. While different options like user fees, taxable benefits, or medical savings accounts are designed to provide more private payments for health services, other approaches such as public–private partnerships (P3s) are being considered as a way of supporting capital projects. P3s involve a number of different options including long-term outsourcing contracts, joint ventures, strategic partnerships, or private financing models. In the United Kingdom, under private financing initiatives (PFI), private sector firms are awarded long-term contracts to design, build, finance, and operate hospitals.

While P3s may be a useful means of bringing the innovation of the private sector to bear, they are not without their critics. In many cases, governments find P3s attractive because the private sector company assumes the heavy capital costs of a project and governments are only required to pay "rental fees" over the longer term. Unfortunately, while P3s may cost governments and taxpayers less in the short term, these arrangements often cost more in the longer term (Sussex 2001). The rental costs charged to governments must be high enough to allow the private sector partner to recoup its costs and make a profit for its shareholders. The cost of borrowing is often higher for the private sector than for governments. And P3s often have higher administration costs. Critics also suggest that the quality of private for-profit run facilities can be lower than publicly run facilities and that, in some cases, these arrangements have resulted in beds being closed and staff being reduced (Pollack et al. 2001). This is not to say that P3s are without a place (for example in the case of health information systems), but they are no panacea and their use and value need to be carefully considered.

Should Canada Consider Alternative Funding Schemes? Each of the alternative options outlined above would raise more money for the health care system or free up money for governments to spend on other priorities such as lowering taxes or paying down debt. However, many of the options also compromise the principles and values on which Canadians built the health care system. Some of the options would simply shift the burden of health expenditures from the public purse to individuals and would ultimately undermine the equity that currently exists in both funding and access to needed health care services.

Through the Commission's consultations, Canadians indicated that they were willing to pay more in taxes to sustain the health care system, but only if changes are made to improve the current system. Consistent with this view, some have suggested a dedicated tax for health care. This could take a number of different forms. At one end of the spectrum is what public finance experts call a hypothecated tax—a single-purpose tax that is formally separated from all other revenue streams in a special fund similar to the Canada or the Quebec Pension Plans. At the other end of the spectrum, a health tax or premium could be established, but the money flows into the general revenue funds of governments. Both may satisfy the public's desire to ensure some degree of transparency and accountability but they provide less than perfect solutions in other respects.

In the case of the hypothecated tax, the amount collected could only be used for health care purposes, irrespective of shifting needs. This might be fine in normal years, but if any government needed to suddenly shift resources from health care to another priority in the face of an unexpected crisis, it would be prevented from doing so. In contrast to health care, pensions are a relatively small part of government expenditures so the impact of having dedicated taxes for pensions is not as great.

In the case of a notionally earmarked tax, given the sheer size of the health care system, it would be almost impossible to raise the necessary funding for health care through a single, dedicated tax. In fact, a number of provinces that once had sales taxes that were, in principle, earmarked for health and education have since dropped this type of labeling. At the same time, that is not to say that earmarked taxes could not be used to fund a portion of the health care bill (Senate 2002). During the Commission's Citizens' Dialogue, the idea of a dedicated tax was strongly supported by many Canadians because it would provide assurance that additional taxes paid by Canadians would, in fact, go to health care rather than other programs and services. It also is a way of improving transparency and accountability for the additional funds raised from taxpayers. Given this, it would be useful for governments to consider notionally earmarked taxes for health in the future.

Based on evidence both in Canada and internationally, progressive taxation continues to be the most effective way to fund health care in Canada. From what the Commission heard from Canadians through the Citizens' Dialogue and other consultations, the large majority of Canadians do not want to see any change in the single-payer insurance principle for core hospital and physician services. There also continues to be a strong consensus among Canadians that "ability to pay" should not be the predominant factor in how we fund key aspects of our health care system. Canadians want necessary hospital and physician services to be fully funded through our taxes. This may be because our tax-funded, universal health care system provides a kind of "double solidarity." It provides equity of funding between the "haves" and the "have-nots" in our society and it also provides equity between the healthy and the sick.

Future Sustainability. In many respects, the critical issue is not so much whether Canada's health care system is financially sustainable today but whether it will be sustainable in the future, given current trends and increasing costs. Making projections about future costs and financial sustainability may sound easy, but it is more than a simple accounting calculation. Forecasts of public revenues have to take into account the potential growth of the economy combined with interest payments on debt or long-term financial commitments as a result of past decisions. Forecasts depend on how various cost factors are assessed including the evolving needs and expectations of people served by particular programs. The projections also need to consider competing demands for spending on other programs or on tax reductions. In many cases, political assessments and value judgements of the relative merits of spending more in one area and less in another are very difficult to factor into projections for future spending.

That being said, it is important to look at the issue of future financial sustainability by examining Canada's spending on health care compared to other countries as well as the trends within Canada, both in terms of provincial–territorial funding and federal funding. It also is important to consider the role of the health care sector in Canada's economy, not just as a driver of costs but also as a significant contributor to economic growth.

Comparisons with Other Countries. If we look back to 1970, total and public health care costs have increased in Canada as a percentage of Gross Domestic Product (GDP). At the time medicare was introduced, Canada spent about 7% of GDP on total health care costs. Thirty years later, Canadian health care costs take up about 9.1% of our GDP. On the public side, Canada was spending approximately 5% of GDP on health in 1970 and by 2000 this had grown to 6.5% (see Appendix E).

In terms of current comparisons with specific OECD and G7 countries, Canada's spending on health care on both a per capita basis and as a percentage of GDP is slightly higher than the OECD average but very comparable to the G7 average....

Looking at comparisons with the United States ... Canadian spending closely tracked American spending until the early 1970s when the addition of physicians' services to single-payer insurance plans broke the pattern. Since that time, the long-term trend in health care costs in Canada has been more in line with trends in European countries while the United States has moved further away from the OECD average.

Canada's proximity to the United States is both an opportunity and a challenge. The exposure of Canadian scientists, researchers, patients, and health care providers to American medical and scientific innovations, American research organizations, and high-end health care facilities (such as the Mayo Clinic) raises expectations of what can be done in Canada. While all OECD countries face increasing health care costs, Canada's pressures will always be more intense because of our relationship with, and proximity to, the United States.

Health Care Spending Trends in Canada. Like all other OECD countries, Canada's spending on health care is increasing. But to address the question of sustainability, it is important to break down the various components of the health care system to see where the costs are increasing the most. The cost of hospital and physician services has grown at a much slower rate than other health care services and programs covered by the provinces and territories.... Both private and provincial government per capita spending on non-CHA services has grown considerably in recent years while per capita spending on hospital and physician services is currently no higher than it was in 1991 when it reached a peak of $1,265 per person. On a national basis, hospital and physician services now constitute about 63% of total provincial–territorial health care spending compared to 77% in 1975.... Thus the overall increase in provincial per capita health care spending—which rose 15.6% between 1991 and 2001—reflects the fact that the cost of non-CHA services is rising faster than CHA services (CIHI 2002) and is illustrative of the way in which the use of health care services is changing.

Prescription drugs provide the most graphic example of the shift in the various components of spending within the health care budget. In 1975, prescription drug costs made up a relatively stable share of about 6% of health care spending. But by the mid-1980s, that share had begun a steady climb and, by 2001, the share had doubled to 12% (CIHI 2002). The rapid escalation of drug costs has added over half a percentage point to the share of Canada's national income (GDP) that is spent on health care.

There also have been significant increases in other components of provincial and territorial spending on health care since 1975, including public spending on:

- Home care services, which has increased from $26 million in 1975 to approximately $2.7 billion in 2001 (CIHI 2001a; HC 2002d);
- Other institutions such as nursing homes, which has grown from $800 million in 1975 to $6.8 billion in 2001 (CIHI 2002); and
- Non-physician professional health care services, which has increased from $120 million in 1975 to $800 million by 2001.

This does not mean, therefore, that we can simply target growing costs in key areas—such as prescription drugs and home care, as the culprits in increasing health care costs. Expanding use of prescription drugs and home care has reduced the reliance on more expensive hospital care and are part of changing trends in how health care services are delivered. These changing trends and the connections between various components of the health care system need to be considered as part of any analysis of the future costs of the system.

Federal and Provincial–Territorial Shares of Health Care Spending. As noted earlier in this chapter, federal, provincial, and territorial governments share responsibility for funding health care. This partnership has changed over time as has the benchmark for determining the appropriate contribution of each order of government. In the last decade or more, defining that balance in terms of funding has been the subject of considerable acrimony and debate. Provinces accuse the federal government of no longer shouldering its traditional share of the rising costs of health care while the federal government counters by saying provinces have chosen to finance tax cuts over health care.

Since medicare began, there have been three major regimes through which the federal government has provided funds to the provinces for health care. The first federal transfer regime for health began in 1957 with the *Hospital Insurance and Diagnostic Services Act.* The formula for federal funding involved matching the costs of providing hospital insurance in the provinces on a per capita basis (half of which was based on their individual costs and the other half on the national average). A similar cost-sharing arrangement was introduced (but calculated solely on the basis of the per capita share of the national average) in 1966 with the passage of the *Medical Care Act* that extended federal contributions to physician services in the provinces. These funding arrangements were based on 50/50 cost sharing for eligible provincial hospital and physician services, not all provincial

health expenditures. The federal share in the final year of this cost-sharing regime for total physician and hospital services was close to 47%, which can easily be assumed to be close to 50% of eligible services.

These early pieces of legislation provided the dedicated funding for hospital and physician services that were necessary to put medicare in place. Under the original design, however, the financial cost of medical and hospital insurance posed significant problems for the federal, provincial, and territorial governments. For the federal government, a primary concern was that relevant spending decisions were being made in the provinces and the federal government could not control the level of transfers to the provinces under shared-cost arrangements.

Provincial and territorial governments also sought an increased degree of autonomy with regard to the disbursement of federal funds. Funding was confined to hospital and physician services at a time when provincial health systems were expanding beyond this narrow set of services, and health services that were not eligible for federal funding under the original cost-sharing arrangements were taking up an increasing share of provincial and territorial health care spending.

To address these concerns, a new block transfer mechanism for funding both health and post-secondary education was negotiated and introduced in 1977. This second transfer regime, known as Established Programs Financing (EPF), effectively broke the link between actual expenditures for hospital and physician services made by provinces and territories and the level of federal transfers for health. From this point on, increases in federal funding were based on a formula in which transfers increased in relation to growth in the economy (measured as per capita Gross National Product) rather than based on actual provincial and territorial expenditures for hospital and physician services. The importance of this change was that after EPF, provincial expenditures on health that exceeded the rate of economic growth and population change were borne exclusively by provincial governments, thus providing the federal government with the predictability it sought in terms of its own expenditures. At the same time, EPF provided provinces with increased flexibility because federal funds were no longer exclusively designed to support hospital and physician services. In addition, under the new arrangements, the way in which transfers were delivered was changed. In the first year of the agreement, provinces would receive a cash transfer equal to one-half of the total value and the remainder would come in the form of tax points: the federal government reduced its percentage of personal and corporate income taxes to give room to the provinces to increase their own taxes. After 1977, the cash portion would increase according to the escalator formula, while the tax points would increase in accordance with growth in the provincial economy as reflected in increased tax revenues collected. Since a tax point yields less revenue in low-income than in high-income provinces, the value of the tax points were to be equalized to the national average.

These arrangements served the short-term needs of both orders of government, but there were significant and unforeseen consequences to the new formula. Some provinces used this new flexibility to allow physicians and hospitals to extra-bill or charge user fees to patients as a means of offsetting increased health care costs and demands for increases in professional fees paid to doctors. But what this did was shift a larger portion of those increasing costs to those who most needed health care services—the poor and the sick. In response, Justice Emmett Hall (1980) conducted a review of health services in Canada and reported to then federal Minister of Health, Monique Bégin. The result was the creation of the *Canada Health Act* introduced by Bégin in 1984. It enumerated the five principles we know today and also allowed the federal government to withhold a portion of cash transfers to provinces that allowed extra-billing or user fees.

… [T]he CHA was, in the years immediately following its passage, an effective means for the federal government to discourage the use of

extra-billing or user fees. By initially reducing transfers to those provinces that allowed extra-billing but then restoring the funding once provinces eliminated such charges, the federal government succeeded in rolling back such practices. However, the federal government has proven to be reluctant to impose penalties related to other provincial practices that could be seen to be in violation of the five principles of the Act, but which did not involve user fees or extra-billing. Thus, while the CHA was very successful in changing provincial behaviour in the narrow sense of eliminating user fees and extra-billing, it was less successful as a general guarantor of medicare as a whole.

Another consequence of EPF became apparent in 1982 when the federal government unilaterally changed the formula for its contribution. The total EPF transfer was now calculated for each province on the basis of the per capita entitlement in the base year, escalated by nominal GNP and population growth. The cash portion of the transfer was calculated as the difference between the value of the tax points and the total provincial entitlement. In addition, the federal government unilaterally reduced the value of the escalator formula, first in 1986 and again in 1989. In 1991, EPF entitlements were frozen at their 1989/90 levels. At the same time, the notional value of the tax points continued to grow as a proportion of the total entitlement relative to the cash portion. In one estimate, federal cash transfers for health were anticipated to completely disappear for all provinces by 2010 (Smith 1995). By their very nature, tax point transfers are essentially unconditional since there is no mechanism whereby the federal government could withhold transfers in the event a province or territory failed to comply with the conditions attached to federal dollars.

In 1995, the third federal transfer regime was introduced in the form of the Canada Health and Social Transfer (CHST). The CHST has been a contentious program since it was introduced. In addition to health care and post-secondary education that were part of EPF, social assistance and social services were added to the new omnibus

CHST transfer. Like EPF before it, only a portion of the CHST is intended for health care and involves a mix of cash and the tax points. The combination of funding three major social programs through a single block transfer, in addition to the complexities of the cash and tax portions of the arrangements, make estimating the value of the federal contribution to health care extremely obscure to even the most informed.

Historically, there has been a powerful and direct relationship between increasing health care spending and the overall growth in the economy, with costs for health care services increasing slightly more than increases in the nation's wealth. This was captured under both the original cost-sharing arrangements. As health expenditures at the provincial and territorial level increased so too did the federal contribution. What the original cost-sharing arrangements lacked, however, was an incentive for cost-containment as the relationship between federal transfers and provincial and territorial expenditures was open-ended. EPF made the correlation between economic growth and health services spending more direct by linking federal transfers to growth in GNP. The escalator under EPF had the effect of restraining the growth of health care expenditures to a level comparable to growth in the economy.

… Since the 1960s, health expenditures have consistently grown at a higher rate than growth in the economy. The very high ratio of health spending to economic growth in the 1960s reflects the early stages of medicare as the system was being constructed. However, the ratio moderated over time as the system matured. The relationship over the entire period averages out to roughly 1.25, meaning that for every 10% increase in GDP our health services expenditures have increased by 12.5%. This suggests that even the escalator formula for EPF with its direct link to growth in the economy was not sufficient to keep pace with health care costs. This became exacerbated by unilateral federal reductions in the escalator and finally with the freeze on EPF increases.

Under the CHST, there is no mechanism for providing for natural increases in health care spending in the calculation of federal transfers. Increases in CHST transfers are at the discretion of the federal government. Since its inception there have been two increases, one in 1999 and another in September 2000. The absence of an escalator formula for increases in federal contributions to provincial and territorial health expenditures means that there is no link between the growth in either health expenditures or the growth in the economy. This results in provinces making regular demands for increases in the transfer and has contributed to the highly politicized and acrimonious nature of the debate over health care funding in recent years.

This is the historical context in which the current debate over appropriate levels of funding has taken place. Looking at the impact of these various shifts in funding arrangements over time, the relative share between the federal and provincial governments has become increasingly obscure. In part, the complexities of the arrangements themselves have largely contributed to this confusion.

Health Care Spending as a Share of Provincial Budgets. As a result of growing costs, provincial governments have, in recent years, warned both their residents and the federal government that health care spending is "crowding out" other spending and policy priorities such as education, infrastructure, debt reduction, and tax cuts. Except for a short period in the early to mid-1990s, real provincial and territorial spending on health care has been climbing…. Adjusting for inflation, per capita provincial and territorial spending on health care rose from an average of $1,200 per person in 1975 to almost $2,100 per person in 2001 (CIHI 2001b).

… [H]ealth care spending is taking up an increasing share of total provincial and territorial spending on programs. In 1999/2000, health spending accounted for 35.4% of provincial and territorial program spending compared to 28% in 1974 to 1978. There are a number of reasons why health care spending is taking up an increasing share of governments' budgets and the reasons vary among provinces and territories. However, three reasons are common to all provinces:

- The impact of cost-cutting in the early 1990s compromised public confidence in the system and created the need to reinvest in recent years (Tuohy 2002);
- The growing cost of prescription drugs, home care, and other health care expenses is constantly driving up provincial spending on health care even though hospital and physician care may be growing at a more acceptable rate (Evans 2002b); and
- The cost of recent large increases in health care provider remuneration following years of restraint in the 1990s.

However, not all commentators accept the provinces' arguments that their current expenditure patterns are unsustainable. Boychuk (2002) argues that provincial health expenditures relative to GDP are the same now as a decade ago and that recent increases are a result of unleashing the "pent-up demand" created by the expenditure cuts of the mid-1990s. The system is only unsustainable, he argues, if we accept that:

- Spending will increase even faster than is necessary to deal with an aging population and the increase in the cost of current services; or
- There is a consensus that the tax burden on Canadians is itself unsustainable and must be lowered.

The perception that there is a fiscal crisis in health care is as important as the reality, however, since the perception undermines the public's confidence in the system regardless of whether steps are taken to contain costs.

These issues are important ones for the provinces and territories. Shouldering the lion's share of risk for growing health care costs, they face far greater anxiety about their ability to fund health care in the future. Furthermore, both federal and provincial governments now are politically committed to a policy of phased-in tax reductions. These tax cuts are estimated to be worth $40 billion in total in 2001/02 (Yalnizyan 2002)—one half from the federal government and one half from the provinces. In comparison to these tax cuts, federal health funding increased by $2.8 billion while provincial spending on health care increased by $4.8 billion in the same year….

Health as a Major Contributor to the Economy. Discussions about health care are most often focused on costs while, in fact, health care is also a major contributor to Canada's economy and economies around the world.

According to American economist William Nordhaus, the "medical revolution over the last century appears to qualify, at least from an economic point of view, for Samuel Johnson's accolade as 'the greatest benefit to mankind'" (2002, 38). This increase in economic value comes from numerous directions including improvements in:

- Basic knowledge from the germ theory of disease at the beginning of the 20th century to the more recent DNA revolution;
- Public health capital and infrastructure;
- Diagnostic tools and processes;
- Logistics in terms of obtaining critical care (e.g., emergency response);
- Treatment technologies and protocols including pharmaceuticals.

In the early 1990s, rising health care costs were seen in many countries as an obstacle to balancing budgets and cutting taxes. This created the view that health care costs were a threat to future national competitiveness. But based on Nordhaus' calculations, it appears that health care spending contributed at least as much to the American economy as spending on all other consumption expenditures combined. Canadian economist Tom Courchene (2001) has made a similar argument about viewing health care expenditures as a dynamic investment in the economy rather than simply as consumption.

Health care investments not only lead to longer and more productive working lives on an individual basis; properly targeted public health care investments can also provide countries with a competitive advantage. According to the Canadian Council of Chief Executives' submission to the Commission (2002, 2), "Canada's business leaders have been strong supporters of Canada's universally accessible public health care system" because it provides a "significant advantage in attracting the people and investment that companies need to stay competitive." Indeed, the "big three" automakers (Ford, General Motors, and Daimler-Chrysler) recently signed joint letters with their largest union, the Canadian Autoworkers, expressing support for Canada's publicly funded health care system and noting that it provides an important competitive advantage to the Canadian auto and auto-parts industries relative to their American counterparts. In short, it is more economical for the employers to pay taxes in support of medicare than to be forced to buy private health insurance for their workers.

It is also true that health care is what economists call a superior good in that, as individuals, we tend to spend progressively more on health care than other goods and services as our incomes go up. Based on a series of international studies summarized by Gerdtham and Jönsson (2000), higher income is the single most important factor determining higher levels of health spending in all countries. Indeed, the more economically developed the country, the more pronounced the effect (Scheiber and Maeda 1997). According to Reinhardt et al. (2002, 171), per capita GDP is without doubt "the most powerful explanatory variable for international differences in health spending."

Resources and Sustainability

What conclusions can we draw about resources and sustainability? Canada's spending on health care is comparable with other OECD countries although we spend considerably less per capita than the United States. All OECD countries are facing increasing health care costs and experience suggests that the wealthier the country, the more it spends on health care. Some suggest that Canada relies too heavily on taxation, and yet, comparisons show that we are not much different from other countries. A look at various alternative ways of funding health care shows that each option raises a number of problems and many would simply shift the burden of funding from governments to individual Canadians. At the same time, there are serious problems in the balance between federal and provincial–territorial funding for health care, and health care is taking up an increasing proportion of provincial budgets. Later chapters of this report address specific ways in which steps can be taken to control rising costs, especially for prescription drugs. But the reality is that health care costs are likely to continue to increase and choices have to be made about how those costs will be managed. Overwhelmingly, Canadians told the Commission that they are prepared to pay more for health care to ensure the system's sustainability, provided the system is prepared to change to meet their needs and expectations.

References

Aba, S., W.D. Goodman, and J. M. Mintz, 2002. *Funding Public Provision of Private Health: The Case for a Copayment Contribution through the Tax System.* C.D. Howe Institute Commentary 163. Toronto, C.D. Howe Institute.

Aba, S., and J. Mintz. 2002. Should Public Health Care Benefits Be Included as Part of Taxable Income? Paper presented at the Roundtable on Financing Options for the Commission on the Future of Health Care in Canada. May 24, C.D. Howe Institute, Toronto.

Barer, M., V. Bhatia, G.L. Stoddart, and R.G. Evans. 1993. *The Remarkable Tenacity of User Charges: A Concise History of the Participation, Positions, and Rationales of Canadian Interest Groups in the Debate over "Direct Patient Participation" in Health Care Financing.* Vancouver, Centre for Health Services and Policy Research, University of British Columbia.

Barer, M., R.G. Evans, C. Hertzman, and J. Lomas. 1979. Controlling Health Care Costs by Direct Charges to Patients: Snare or Delusion? Toronto, Ontario Economic Council, Occasional Paper No. 10.

Barr, M.S. 2001. Medical Savings Accounts in Singapore: A Critical Inquiry. *Journal of Health Politics, Policy and Law* 26(4), 709–726.

Boychuk, G.W. 2002. The Changing Political and Economic Environment of Health Care in Canada. Discussion Paper prepared for the Commission on the Future of Health Care in Canada.

Braën, A. 2002. Health and the Distribution of Powers in Canada. Discussion Paper prepared for the Commission on the Future of Health Care in Canada.

Canada. 1964. *Royal Commission on Health Services, Volumes 1 and 2.* [Emmet M. Hall, Chair]. Ottawa, Royal Commission on Health Services.

Canada. Senate. 2002. *The Health of Canadians – The Federal Role. Final Report on the State of the Health Care System in Canada. Volume Six: Recommendations for Reform.* [M.J.L. Kirby, Chair]. Ottawa, Standing Senate Committee on Social Affairs, Science and Technology.

Canadian Council of Chief Executives. 2002. Written submission to the Commission on the Future of Health Care in Canada, entitled "Shared Enterprise: Sustaining and Improving Health Care for Canadians."

CES (Collége des Économistes de la Santé). 2001. Utilisation Fees Imposed to Public Health Care System Users in Europe. Proceedings of the Workshop on November 29 organised for the Commission on the Future of Health Care in Canada. Paris, Collége des Économistes de la Santé.

CIHI (Canadian Institute for Health Information). 2002. Unpublished statistical data compiled by the Canadian Institute for Health Information for the Commission on the Future of Health Care in Canada.

———. 2001a. *Home Care Estimates in National Health Expenditures. Feasibility Study.* Ottawa, Canadian Institute for Health Information.

———. 2001b. *National Health Expenditures Trends, 1975–2001.* Ottawa, Canadian Institute for Health Information.

Commission. 2002a. *Report on Citizens' Dialogue on the Future of Health Care in Canada.* Prepared for the Commission on the Future of Health Care in Canada by J. Maxwell, K. Jackson, and B. Legowski (Canadian Policy Research Networks), S. Rosell and D. Yankelovich (Viewpoint Learning), in collaboration with P.-G. Forest and L. Lozowchuk (Commission on the Future of Health Care in Canada). Saskatoon, Commission on the Future of Health Care in Canada.

Courchene, T. 2001. *A State of Minds: Toward a Human Capital Future for Canadians.* Montreal, Institute for Research on Public Policy.

Deber, R. 2002. Delivering Health Care Services: Public, Not-for-Profit, or Private? Discussion Paper prepared for the Commission on the Future of Health Care in Canada.

Devereaux, P.J., P.T.L. Choi, C. Lacchetti, B. Weaver, H.J. Schünemann, T. Haines, J.N. Lavis, B.J.B. Grant, D.R.S. Haslam, M. Bhandari, T. Sullivan, D.J. Cook, S.D. Walter, M. Meade, H. Khan, N. Bhatnagar, and G.H. Guyatt. 2002. A Systematic Review and Meta-Analysis of Studies Comparing Mortality Rates of Private For-Profit Hospitals and Private Not-For-Profit Hospitals. *CMAJ* 166(11), 1399–1406.

Evans, R.G. 2002a. Financing Health Care: Taxation and the Alternatives. In *Funding Health Care: Options for Europe.* Edited by E. Mossialos, A. Dixon, and J. Figueras. Buckingham, Open University Press, 31–58.

———. 2002b. Raising the Money: Options, Consequences and Objectives for Financing Health Care in Canada. Discussion Paper prepared for the Commission on the Future of Health Care in Canada.

Evans, R.G., M.L. Barer, G.I. Stoddart, and V. Bhatia. 1993. *It's Not for the Money, It's the Principle: Why User Charges for Some Services and Not Others?* Vancouver, Centre for Health Services and Policy Research, University of British Columbia.

Forget, E.L., R. Deber, and L.L. Roos. 2002. Medical Savings Accounts: Will They Reduce Costs? *CMAJ* 167(2), 143–147.

Gibson, D. 1996. The Canada Health Act and the Constitution. *Health Law Journal* 4, 1–33.

Gratzer, D. Ed. 2002. *Better Medicine: Reforming Canadian Health Care.* Toronto, ECW Press.

Gratzer, D. 1999. *Code Blue: Reviving Canada's Health Care System.* Toronto, ECW Press.

Gray, B.H. 1999. *The Empirical Literature Comparing For-Profit and Nonprofit Hospitals, Managed Care Organizations and Nursing Homes: Updating the Institute of Medicine Study*. Washington, DC, Coalition for Nonprofit Healthcare.

Harrington, C. 2001. Residential Nursing Facilities in the United States. *BMJ* 323, 507–510.

Hall. 1964. See Canada. 1964.

HC (Health Canada). 2001. *Health Expenditures in Canada by Age and Sex, 1980–81 to 2000–01. Statistical Annex*. Ottawa, Health Canada.

Hogg, P. 1997. *Constitutional Law of Canada: Fourth Edition*. Scarborough, ON: Carswell.

Hurley, J. 2002. Medical Savings Accounts Will Not Advance Canadian Health Care Objectives. *CMAJ* 167(2), 152–153.

———. 2000. Medical Savings Accounts: Approach With Caution. *Journal of Health Services Research and Policy* 5(3), 130–132.

Kent, T. 2000. *What Should Be Done about Medicare?* Ottawa, Caledon Institute of Public Policy.

Kleinke, J.D. 2001. *Oxymorons: The Myth of a U.S. Health Care System*. San Francisco: Jossey-Bass.

Leeson, H. 2002. Constitutional Jurisdiction Over Health and Health Care Services in Canada. Discussion Paper prepared for the Commission on the Future of Health Care in Canada.

Majnoni d'Itignano, B. 2001. *Santé et économie en Europe*. Paris, Presses Universitaires de France.

Marmor, T.R. M. Schlesinger, and R.W. Smithey. 1987. Nonprofit Organizations and Healthcare. In *The Nonprofit Sector: A Research Handbook*. Edited by W.W. Powell, New Haven, Yale University Press, 1–35.

Maynard, A., and A. Dixon. 2002. Private Health Insurance and Medical Savings Accounts: Theory and Experience. In *Funding Health Care: Options for Europe*. Edited by E. Mossialos, A. Dixon, J. Figueras, and J. Kutzin. Buckingham, Open University Press, 109–127.

Mazankowski, D. 2001. [Alberta 2001.] *A Framework for Reform. Report of the Premier's Advisory Council on Health*. D. Mazankowski, Chair. Edmonton, Premier's Advisory Council on Health.

McFarlane, L., and C. Prado. 2002. *The Best-Laid Plans: Health Care's Problems and Prospects*. Montreal, McGill-Queen's University Press.

Migué, Jean-Luc. 2002. Funding and Production of Health Services: Outlook and Potential Solutions. Discussion Paper prepared for the Commission on the Future of Health Care in Canada.

Mossialos, E., and A. Dixon. 2002. Funding Health Care: An Introduction. In *Funding Health Care: Options for Europe*. Edited by E. Mossialos, A. Dixon, J. Figueras, and J. Kutzin. Buckingham, Open University Press, 1–30.

Mossialos, E., A. Dixon, J. Figueras, and J. Kutzin, eds. 2002. *Funding Health Care: Options for Europe*. Buckingham, Open University Press.

Nordhaus, E. 2002. The Health of Nations: The Contribution of Improved Health to Living Standards. Cambridge, National Bureau of Economic Research, Working Paper 8818.

OECD (Organisation for Economic Co-operation and Development). 2002. *OECD Health Data 2002b. A Comparative Analysis of 30 Countries*. Paris, Organisation for Economic Co-operation and Development.

Pollack, A., J. Shaoul, D. Rowland, and S. Player. 2001. Public Services and the Private Sector: A Response to the IPPR. London, Catalyst, Working Paper.

Ramsay, C. 2002. A Framework for Determining the Extent of Public Financing of Programs and Services. Discussion Paper prepared for the Commission on the Future of Health Care in Canada.

Reinhardt, U.E., P.S. Hussey, and G. F. Anderson. 2002. Cross-National Comparisons of Health Systems Using OECD Data, 1999. *Health Affairs* 21(3), 169–181.

Reuber, G.L., and F. Poschmann, 2002. Increasing Patient Incentives to Improve the Financial Stability of the Health Care System. Paper presented May 24 at the Roundtable on Financing Options for the Commission on the Future of Health Care in Canada. C.D. Howe Institute.

Scheiber, G., and A. Maeda. 1997. A Curmudgeon's Guide to Financing Health Care in Developing Countries. In Innovation in Health Care Financing, Edited by G.J. Schieber. Washington, DC, World Bank, World Bank Discussion Paper No. 365, 1–38.

Senate. 2002. See Canada. Senate. 2002.

Shortt, S.E.D. 2002. Medical Savings Accounts in Publicly Funded Health Care Systems: Enthusiasm Versus Evidence. *CMAJ* 167(2), 159–162.

Smith, Miriam. 1995. "Retrenching the Sacred Trust: Medicate and Canadian Federalism." In *New Trends in Canadian Federalism*. Edited by F. Rocher and M. Smith. Peterborough: Broadview Press.

Smythe, J.G. 2001. Tax Subsidization of Employer-Provided Health Care Insurance in Canada: Incidence Analysis. Edmonton, Department of Economics, University of Alberta, Working Paper.

Sussex, J. 2001. *The Economics of the Private Finance Initiative in the NHS*. London, The Office of Health Economics.

Tuohy, C.H. 2002. The Costs of Constraint and Prospects for Health Care Reform in Canada. *Health Affairs* 21(3), 32–46.

Woolhandler, S., and D.U. Himmelstein. 2002. Paying for National Health Insurance – and Not Getting It. *Health Affairs* 21(4), 88–98.

Yalnizyan, A. 2002. Paying for Keeps: How the Feds Can Save Medicare. Canadian Centre for Policy Alternatives Monograph.

Ethics, Economics, and Public Financing of Health Care

Jeremiah Hurley

INTRODUCTION

Is there an ethical rationale for publicly financed health insurance? It would seem there is a variety of (sophisticated, complex, and sometimes mutually incompatible) arguments rooted in different ethical frameworks. However, because public financing is a particular institutional arrangement that is valued not intrinsically but only to the extent that it contributes to achieving a higher end, a wide variety of such arguments share a common structure.[1] Although these arguments differ considerably in detail, they share a structure built on four logically related propositions regarding: (1) the ultimate purpose of a human life or human society; (2) the role of health and its distribution in society in advancing this ultimate purpose; (3) the role of access to or utilisation of health care in maintaining or improving the desired level and distribution of health among members of society; and (4) the role of public financing in ensuring the ethically justified access to and util-

isation of health care by members of society. Because the dominant concern of modern economic analysis is the consequences of alternative institutional arrangements of economic activity, economic reasoning has much to contribute to the development of such ethical arguments. Indeed, economic analysis is a necessary ingredient since the rationale for public financing rests at least in part on demonstrating that the ethically required access to and utilisation of health care cannot be achieved through a system of solely private financing. Equity arguments alone are not sufficient: if markets function well a system of public subsidies for the purchase of private insurance could deal with equity concerns. Rather, full public financing for health care requires demonstrating that, even in the presence of appropriate subsidies, private financing through insurance markets fails to promote the requisite access to or utilisation of health care. Economic reasoning is crucial to any ethical argument that proceeds in this fashion.

The paper is organised around the four propositions listed above, focusing on propositions (3) and (4) where economics offers the greatest potential contributions. To help make matters more concrete, I illustrate key points with reference to ethical analysis of public financing within three specific ethical frameworks: (1) classical utilitarianism; (2) extra-welfarism, particularly as developed in the health sector[2, 3]; and (3) Rawlsian-style contractarianism.[4, 5] I choose these because they are commonly used in health sector analysis, they represent broad approaches to social ethics for which there are numerous particular refinements, they differ in their focus for valuation and in the decision rules used to rank institutional arrangements, and they derive from very different philosophical and ethical traditions. Space constraints mean that I can give each only the most cursory treatment; their use is meant purely to illustrate points, not to develop the fundamental argument.

THE STRUCTURE OF ETHICAL ARGUMENTS REGARDING PUBLIC FINANCING OF HEALTH CARE

The Purpose of Life, Ultimate Ends, and a Just Society

The purpose of life has of course been a central question in moral and political philosophy for thousands of years and a question to which philosophers have provided a wide range of answers. All theories of justice and the "good" society are based (implicitly or explicitly) on such an ultimate end, and within any such theory the characteristics of a just society are those that foster the posited ultimate end. For Bentham, Mill, and classical utilitarians the ultimate human end was happiness and the good society maximised happiness among its members. Extra-welfarists, in contrast, eschew utility in favour of more objective outcomes such as functionings and capabilities and the good society allocates resources to foster these among its members.[6, 8] For Rawls the ultimate end was "the satisfaction of [a person's] rational desire" in the form of a rational plan of life,[9] and in a good society devia-

tions from equality of basic primary goods can be justified only to the extent that they improve the lot of the least advantaged member of society.[4]

Health

Health is ethically good to the extent that it contributes to the realisation of the ultimate end sought—happiness, capabilities and functionings, fulfilment of a rational life plan, etc. Among the various "goods" that contribute to the ultimate end, health is often accorded special ethical significance because it is necessary to achieving most intermediate and ultimate ends; ill health and injury are unpredictable and largely beyond the control of an individual (most of those who fall ill have done nothing knowingly to deserve or cause the ill health); and ill health represents a time of considerable vulnerability and dependency on others, giving society's response to those who suffer illness and injury particular ethical salience.

But simply arguing that health is ethically important is not enough. A crucial question is: what does an ethical analysis demand about the just level and distribution of health in society? Maximising the level of health in society is unlikely to be ethically justified given that health is only one contributor to an ultimate end and that health cannot be directly redistributed among members of society (though of course it can be indirectly redistributed via the allocation of health-influencing resources). Welfarist reasoning cannot identify the just distribution of health a priori because the just distribution depends on the structure and distribution of preferences in society with respect to health and other things. The just level and distribution of health is the one that maximises average utility among members of society. If one assumes diminishing marginal utility, then utilitarianism would have a bias toward more equal distributions of health (up to the point where the additions to utility from this are offset by reductions in utility from transferring additional resources from other activities to health). From an extra-welfarist health perspective, Culyer and Wagstaff argue that the only ethically defensible distribution of health is an equal distribution, subject to some side constraints such as the imperative not to deliberately reduce one person's health status to equalise health levels.[10, 11] Rawls did not include health or health care in his set of primary goods, but more recently he has explored how health might be integrated into his framework.[12] Rawls's difference principle would permit a deviation from an equal distribution of health if it improved the health and well-being of the least advantaged member of society; it is silent on the characteristics of the distribution above this minimum level. (See Williams and Cookson[13] for an analysis within an economic framework of the demands of a wide variety of equity criteria with respect to the distribution of health among members of society.)

Access to and Utilisation of Health Care

Health care, which is generally defined to include those goods, services, and activities the primary purpose of which is the maintenance or improvement of health,[14] is one of a complex array of factors that determine health.[15] Health care as such is not intrinsically ethically valuable; it is ethically valuable because it contributes to health. From this it follows directly that the ethically justified distribution of access to and utilisation of needed health care is the one which generates the desired level and distribution of health.

This conclusion rests on two controversial, often confusing concepts—access and need—central to many discussions of ethics and health care. Economic reasoning has contributed in recent years to clarifying access, need, and competing definitions of these concepts (see, for example Culyer and Wagstaff, Mooney, Le Grand, Pereira, and Wagstaff and Van Doorslaer[10, 16–20]) even if it may not have generated greater consensus. Economics identifies access with the concept of feasible choice sets.[10, 18, 22] A person's feasible choice set includes all those things it is possible for them to obtain or accomplish given their resources and constraints beyond their control. Therefore, access is greater in situation B compared to situation A if the feasible choice set under B is larger

than (and fully encompasses) the feasible choice set in A. Two individuals have equal access if they have identical feasible choice sets. Empirically measuring access remains a tremendous challenge, but this analytic approach provides considerable insight into the implications for resource allocation of calls for differing types of access.

It is not access to or utilisation of health care services *as such* that is ethically justified, but access to or utilisation of *needed* health care services. The notion of need is highly contested,[21, 23, 28] but economists generally favour instrumentalist conceptions of need: a need exists when there is a good, activity, or service that is effective (and some would add cost-effective[23]) in attaining an ethically legitimate end for a person. The question of effectiveness is in large part technical; the question of what constitutes an ethically legitimate end is in large part social, political, and moral. Unlike most areas of economics, for which goods are assumed to contribute directly to welfare, the technical production relationship between health care and health allows for a more precise use of the concept of need than is possible even in other areas where needs talk is prevalent (for example, housing, food, education). This production relationship means that a health care need is very specific— one needs a specific health care service that has been shown to be effective for the particular health problem, for which there are often few substitutes. Unlike most goods, health care itself is often a "bad" that causes considerable short-term pain and suffering, but which is consumed only because of its expected health benefits. This provides a sounder basis for third-party judgments of need, especially need in relation to socially defined objectives.

The fact that the primary purpose for consuming health care is to improve health and that there is a basis for third-party judgments of need (as opposed to mere wants) generates good-specific distributional concerns about health care. Welfarist frameworks model this through utility interdependences that generate good-specific caring externalities associated with health status and the consumption of needed health care.[29, 30] That is, person A's utility depends in part on person B's health status and, by implication, her consumption of needed health care; where access itself is the focus of concern, person A's utility depends in part on person B's access to health care (though person B may choose not to consume even needed care).

Welfarists seldom investigate the underlying source of such utility interdependence (for example, the view that health care is a right, notions of solidarity with other members of society, etc), but regardless of that, such externalities imply that within welfarist frameworks broad access to and utilisation of needed health care may be ethically justified. As ever, the preferred distribution depends on the precise nature of preferences and utility interdependences, but a priori such externalities give rise to distributional concerns not associated with most goods and services. Culyer and Wagstaff's health-oriented extra-welfarism calls for access to and utilisation of health care services that generate an equal distribution of health. This will call for broad access to health care services for all members of society, though they specifically note that the ethically justified distribution is unlikely to coincide with allocation according to need and equal access to health care.[10] A Rawlsian demand for a minimal level of health for all in society would also demand a minimal level of access to or utilisation of needed health care services by all in society.

What is noteworthy is that each of these frameworks calls, to some extent, for utilisation of health care to be associated with need and health status, not simply ability to pay, and that this fact demands broad (but not necessarily equal) access to needed health care services by all members of society.

The Role of Public Financing

The last link in the chain of reasoning is the demonstration that public financing of health care is either necessary to generate the ethically justified distribution of access and utilisation or that it does this better than other financing arrangements. This requires examining the properties of alternative private market and public

financing arrangements. In the discussion I distinguish four configurations of financing with increasing reliance on public financing: (1) fully private financing through private insurance purchases and direct payments by patients to providers; (2) public subsidies to support the purchase of insurance in private markets, and/or public insurance for certain population subgroups (for example, as in the US); (3) single-source, universal, first-dollar (free of charge) publicly financed insurance, with a parallel private insurance sector offering coverage for the same services insured by the public sector (for example, as is the case in the UK); and (4) single-source, universal, first-dollar publicly financed insurance with no parallel private insurance sector (for example, as is the case for physician and hospital services in Canada).

INSURANCE, INSURANCE MARKETS, AND FINANCING HEALTH CARE

Unpredictability in the need for health care and the high costs of health care (which can exceed an amount that even many forward-looking, prudent members of society could afford) generate an important role for insurance in health care financing. Insurance pools individuals' financial risks associated with health care, reducing the total amount of risk in society and allowing those who fall ill to obtain the care they need. From an ethical perspective, it is interesting to note that, unlike most goods and services, the production of insurance is by definition a collective activity: it is literally impossible for a single individual to "produce" insurance (except in the very limited sense of pooling risk over time through saving). One can produce insurance only by joining together with others (even if through market-based, voluntary transactions) to form a risk pool.

A system of private insurance markets alone (even one that is well-functioning by economic criteria discussed below) could not provide the broad access called for by the analysis in the previous section. Markets allocate goods and services on the basis of a person's ability and willingness to pay. Low-income members of society would be unable to afford health care insurance policies. This is particularly so given the well-established inverse relationship between socioeconomic status and health status, which would make premiums in a private market highest on average for those with the fewest economic resources (and the most need). From an economic perspective, however, this is simply a problem of the distribution of income. If health care insurance markets are otherwise well-functioning, all that may be required to address this problem is a system of public subsidies to allow the purchase of health care insurance by all members of society.

A role for public financing beyond a system of subsidies for private insurance depends on how well a system of private health care insurance markets functions, or, in economic language, the extent to which markets fail to allocate resources efficiently. Economics defines a situation to be efficient if one beneficial activity cannot be increased without decreasing some other beneficial activity.[31] The ethical force of this concept of efficiency within a consequentialist line of reasoning is clear: to tolerate an inefficient allocation of resources is to forgo an opportunity to provide benefit (however one wants to measure this) to one person or group without decreasing benefit to anyone else.

Within this broad concept, economists distinguish three types of efficiency. Technical efficiency requires that we not waste physical or human resources when producing goods and services. Cost-effectiveness efficiency integrates the relative costs of resources, and requires that we use the least-cost combination of inputs to produce goods and services. And allocative efficiency integrates a consideration of the value of goods and services to members of society. It asks whether society is producing the "right" amount of each good and service and distributing those goods and services in accord with the "value" individuals place on them. The "right" mix and distribution of goods depends, of course, on how value to an individual is assessed (utility, health, other notions of wellbeing) and on the decision-

criterion by which different allocations are ranked, (for example, a maximisation criterion, a Pareto criterion, a Rawlsian maxmin criterion).

ECONOMIES OF SCALE

Private health care insurance markets suffer from two sources of technical inefficiency that can be mitigated or avoided through public financing. The fixed costs to a private insurer of providing insurance (for example, the cost of determining risk-rated premiums), which are the same whether the insurer sells 100 policies or 100 million policies, generate economies of scale in insurance provision that make it impossible in many settings to sustain competitive markets for insurance if firms are to operate at technically efficient sizes.[32] In addition, systems of private insurance with multiple insurance organisations are technically inefficient because they require a host of administrative costs absent from public insurance programmes (for example, rate-setting, marketing, claims administration). Estimates suggest, for example, that administrative costs within the private, multi-payer US system account for 19–24% of health care spending while they account for only 8–11% in Canada's publicly financed system.[33]

Allocative inefficiency in private insurance markets that arises from informational asymmetries between sellers and purchasers of insurance further supports the argument that public financing is necessary to achieve broad access to health care. In private insurance markets that form risk pools by voluntary enrolment, informational asymmetries between insurance providers and insurance purchasers can cause risk selection. Risk selection arises when insurers selectively enroll low-risk individuals (cream-skimming) or when high-risk individuals selectively seek out more generous insurance (adverse selection). Risk selection, and adverse selection in particular, can make it impossible to sustain private insurance markets. As a consequence, even people who are willing and able to purchase insurance at a price that reflects their risk status are unable to do so because the dynamic of adverse selection makes it impossible to sustain an insurance market. Although risk-adjusted premiums can reduce such risk selection, it is not possible to risk-adjust premiums accurately enough to eliminate risk selection. Universal, publicly financed insurance that covers all residents of a jurisdiction completely avoids risk selection.

Asymmetry of information between patients and health care providers furnishes an additional rationale for public financing and for first-dollar coverage with no patient cost-sharing. Individuals are frequently unable to identify what is wrong with them and, once diagnosed, what health care services they need to resolve their health problem. A primary reason for seeing a health professional is precisely to obtain such information. This informational asymmetry gives health care providers tremendous market power and can generate inefficiency-inducing supply-side moral hazard (higher prices, increased use of marginally beneficial services). Moral hazard plagues both privately and publicly financed insurance systems, but public insurers within single-payer systems of finance may have more effective policy levers and the countervailing power required to control better the various forms of supply-side moral hazard.[32, 34]

Patient-provider informational asymmetry also suggests that patient cost-sharing will be inefficient by leading to non-optimal health care consumption. The fact that patients often cannot distinguish between necessary and unnecessary care, that cost-sharing discriminates on the basis of ability to pay, and that those with low income, on average, have greater needs for care, means that cost-sharing leads to a reduction in both necessary and unnecessary care, with potentially important adverse health effects.[35]

KEY MESSAGES

The key messages of such efficiency analyses are that: (1) it will likely be more costly to produce insurance through private markets than through a public, single-payer system; (2) a system of private insurance markets will be incomplete, leaving members of society with either no insurance or less-than-complete insurance (for reasons other than ability to pay) while public insurance can provide universal coverage; (3) the usual prescription of cost-sharing within insurance systems is not supported in the health care sector. Taken together, they imply that a system of publicly financed insurance is more likely to provide the broad access to and utilisation of health financing demanded by the utilitarian, extra-welfarist and Rawlsian frameworks than is a system of private insurance markets. Indeed, these efficiency arguments, when combined with equity considerations provide a strong rationale for universal, mandatory, first-dollar public insurance for health care. A few qualifications to this general conclusion are required.

Within the utilitarian calculus, the benefits of such a programme of public financing, which provides the same amount of insurance to all members of society, would have to be weighed against a welfare cost that arises in a world of heterogeneous risk attitudes and preferences for insurance. A system of public financing that provides everyone with the same level of insurance forces some to consume more insurance than they desire and others less insurance than they desire. The size of this welfare loss depends on the extent of heterogeneity relative to the welfare cost of imperfect market arrangements. The universal programme may still be justified, but technically it becomes an empirical matter.

Secondly, given the correlation between health and other markers of socioeconomic status (for example, income, education, control, etc.), the "least advantaged" member of society is likely to be one of those most disadvantaged under private insurance markets and most helped by a system of public financing. Hence, the rationale for public financing is likely to be quite strong within a Rawlsian framework. Similarly, given that within the extra-welfarist framework health can only be equalised by improving the health of those with low health status (recall the side constraint on not lowering the health of anyone), the rationale for public financing is again likely to be quite strong within health-oriented extra-welfarism.

Thirdly, although significant public financing may be a necessary condition for achieving the access and utilisation sought by the different frameworks, the funding, organisation, and delivery of services will have an important impact on realising the full vision.

Lastly, the patterns of income redistribution associated with public finance through progressive systems of taxation advance broader social objectives, an aspect not considered above.[32, 34] Private insurance with risk-rated premiums does not embody any *ex ante* redistribution of income (though of course, *ex post*, it redistributes from the well to the sick in the insurance pool). In contrast, public financing embodies both *ex ante* redistribution from the wealthy (and generally healthy) to the poor (who generally have lower health status) as well as *ex post* redistribution from the healthy to the sick.

Public Financing with No Parallel Private Finance

The vast majority of countries with universal publicly financed systems of health care insurance allow a parallel private insurance sector in which individuals can purchase private insurance for publicly insured services. The benefits of such insurance to its beneficiaries may include a wider range of treatment choices, the ability to jump a public queue, and so forth. Advocates also argue that such private insurance helps improve access to the public sector by lessening the demands placed on it. Is there an ethical rationale, however, for going beyond the provision of universal public finance by prohibiting such parallel private insurance, as is done in Canada for medically necessary physician and hospital services?

Restricting private insurance this way might follow directly from certain ethical approaches that demand equal access to health care or equal maximum possible consumption of health care by all members of society (for example, perhaps some solidarity-based approaches). It would not, however, follow directly from any of the three ethical frameworks considered in this paper or many other approaches framed within the four

propositions identified above. But within a wide range of consequentialist approaches, such a restriction might derive indirectly from the operation of parallel systems of finance. That is, it is an empirical question whether a system of financing that prohibits private insurance for publicly insured services better advances the access and utilisation patterns ethically demanded. Evidence suggests that this is at least plausible.

Parallel systems of private finance can drain resources from the public system, erode public support for the public system, lead to longer waiting times in the public sector, and make it harder to provide all members with timely access to high-quality services.[36] Parallel private insurance is in general associated with an expansion of resources devoted to health care, though these additional resources are often used for services that generate smaller health gains (otherwise, they would have been given greater priority within the public system).

These dynamics imply that a parallel private insurance sector is not, as is commonly suggested, simply an add-on to a publicly financed system. Rather, complex interaction occurs that affects the viability of the publicly financed system, which leads to cross-subsidies (most often from public to private), and which may draw scarce resources into the health sector that are allocated in ways not consistent with the ethically justified patterns of access and utilisation.

Once again, this potential empirical justification is perhaps most tentative within a utilitarian framework, as the benefits of such a restriction on parallel private insurance must be weighed against its cost in the form of frustrated preferences among those who would prefer to purchase such insurance. The rationale is perhaps strongest within the extra-welfarist approach that calls for an equal distribution of health and which strongly de-emphasises utility effects in the valuation process. Given that on average it is those who are of low income and poor health status who are hurt most by the dynamics of parallel systems of finance, such a restriction may well also be supported within a Rawlsian framework.

CONCLUSIONS

My hope is that this short paper has documented at least two contributions of economic reasoning to the development of ethical arguments regarding public financing of health care. First, that economic methods have helped to clarify concepts such as access and need, which are central to discussions of ethically justified allocations of health care resources. And second, that economic analysis, which has demonstrated both analytically and empirically that private insurance markets suffer a number of both equity- and efficiency-relevant deficiencies, has a central role to play within a wide range of ethical approaches in identifying the ethically justified institutional arrangements for financing health care. Both of these points exemplify a broader cross-fertilisation between ethics and economics that has emerged in recent years (see, for example, Sen, Hausman and McPherson, and Broome[6, 37, 39] among others) which promises to advance both disciplines.

Notes

1. Health care financing refers to the raising of revenue from individuals in society to support the provision of health care services. *Public* financing refers to raising the revenues through the public tax system. Financing should be distinguished from delivery. Delivery refers to the actual provision of health care services. There is no logical relationship between the nature (i.e., public or private) of financing and the nature (i.e., public or private) of the delivery system: public financing can be (and often is) combined with the delivery of health care services by private organisations (not-for-profit, not-only-for-profit, and for-profit organisations).

2. Culyer AJ. The normative economics of health care finance and provision. *Oxford Review of Economic Policy* 1989; 5:34–58.

3. Culyer AJ. Commodities, characteristics of commodities, characteristics of people, utilities and quality of life. In: Baldwin S, Godfrey C, Propper C, eds. *Quality of life: perspectives and policies.* London: Routledge, 1990: 9–27.

4. Rawls J. *A theory of justice.* Oxford: Oxford University Press, 1971.

5. Wolff RP. *Understanding Rawls.* Princeton: Princeton University Press, 1977.

6. Sen A. *On ethics and economics.* Oxford: Blackwell, 1987.

7. Sen A. *The standard of living.* Cambridge: Cambridge University Press, 1987.

8. Sen A. *Commodities and capabilities.* Oxford: Oxford University Press, 1999.

9. See reference 4: 92.

10. Culyer AJ, Wagstaff A. Equity and equality in health and health care. *Journal of Health Economics* 1993; 2:431–57.

11. Culyer AJ. *Equality of what in health policy? Conflicts between the contenders.* York: University of York Centre for Health Economics, 1995. Discussion paper 142.

12. Rawls J. *Political liberalism.* New York: Columbia University Press, 1993.

13. Williams A, Cookson R. Equity in health. In: Culyer AJ, Newhouse JP, eds. *Handbook of health economics.* Amsterdam: North-Holland, 2000: 1863–910.

14. Health care is sometimes consumed for reasons other than improving health, such as a diagnostic test that provides information valued by the patient even if it will not alter treatment decisions or health. This definition holds true for a large portion of health care consumption.

15. Evans RG, Barer M, Marmor T. *Why are some people healthy and others not?* New York: DeGrutyer, 1994.

16. Mooney G. Equity in health care: confronting the confusion. *Effective Health Care* 1983; 1:179–85.

17. Mooney G. *Key issues in health economics.* New York: Harvester Wheatsheaf, 1994.

18. LeGrand J. *Equity and choice.* London: HarperCollins Academic, 1991.

19. Pereira J. What does equity in health mean? *Journal of Social Policy* 1993; 21:19–48.

20. Wagstaff A, Van Doorslaer E. Equity in health care finance and delivery. In: Culyer AJ, Newhouse JP, eds. *Handbook of health economics.* Amsterdam: North-Holland, 2000: 1803–62.

21. Williams A. Need—an economic exegesis. In: Culyer AJ, Wright KG, eds. *Economic aspects of health.* London: Martin Robertson, 1978: 32–45.

22. Olsen EO, Rogers DL. The welfare economics of equal access. *Journal of Public Economics* 1991; 45:91–105.

23. Culyer AJ. Need—is a consensus possible? *Journal of Medical Ethics* 1998; 24:77–80.

24. Robertson A. Critical reflections on the politics of need: implications for public health. *Social Science and Medicine* 1998; 47: 1419–30.

25. Braybrooke D. *Meeting needs.* Princeton: Princeton University Press, 1987.

26. Barry B. *Political argument.* London: Routledge, 1965.

27. Thomson G. *Needs.* London: Routledge and Kegan Paul, 1987.

28. Springborg P. *The problem of human needs and the critique of civilization.* London: George Allen and Unwin, 1991.

29. Culyer AJ, Simpson H. Externality models and health: a Ruckblick over the last twenty years. *Economic Record* 1980; 56:22230.

30. Evans RG, Wolfson AD. *Faith, hope and charity: health care in the utility function.* Vancouver, BC: University of British Columbia, 1980. Discussion paper 20–46.

31. Nicholson W. Efficiency and welfare. *Intermediate microeconomics and its application.* New York: Dryden Press, 1983: 541–69, at 542.

32. Evans RG. *Strained mercy: the economics of Canadian health care.* Toronto: Butterworths, 1984.

33. Woolhandler S, Himmelstein D. The deteriorating efficiency of the US health care system. *New England Journal of Medicine* 1991; 324:1253–8.

34. Evans RG. The welfare economics of public health insurance: theory and Canadian practice. In: Soderstrom L, ed. *Social insurance.* Amsterdam: North Holland, 1983: 71–103.

35. Stoddart GL, Barer M, Evans RG. *User charges, snares and delusions: another look at the literature.* Toronto: Premier's Council on Health, Well-being and Social Justice, 1994.

36. MacDonald P, Shortt S, Sanmartin C, Barer M, Lewis S, Sheps S. *Waiting lists and waiting times for heatlh care in Canada: more management!! More money??* Ottawa: Health Canada, 1998.

37. Hausman D, McPherson MS. *Economic analysis and moral philosophy.* New York: Cambridge University Press, 1996.

38. Broome J. *Weighing goods.* Oxford: Basil Blackwell, 1991.

39. Broome J. *Ethics out of economics.* Cambridge: Cambridge University Press, 1999.

The Many Meanings of Deinsuring a Health Service: The Case of in Vitro Fertilization in Ontario

Mita Giacomini, Jeremiah Hurley, and Greg Stoddart

INTRODUCTION

Background

"Priority-setting" and "resource allocation" have become bywords for health system reform. Health insurance programs around the world—public and private—are reviewing both their processes for making coverage decisions and covered services themselves, to fashion more affordable and acceptable packages of basic service. Policy analysts have described a number of principles to guide systematic decisions about the priority and coverage eligibility of individual services (Crawshaw et al., 1990; Eddy, 1991; GCCHC, 1992; OTA, 1992; Ham, 1993; Deber et al., 1994; Klein, 1994; CMA, 1995; Wilson et al., 1995 and DCE [Danish Council of Ethics], 1997). Most approaches emphasize traditional technology assessment criteria of effectiveness and efficiency, mediated by community values (e.g., ethical principles, participatory structures, population and individual preferences, etc.) (Klein, 1993; Tymstra and Andela, 1993; Goold, 1996; Lenaghan et al., 1996; Richardson and Waddington, 1996; Lomas and Stronks et al., 1997). Health policy makers often expect (or at least hope) that explicit and principle-based deinsurance exercises will achieve multiple health system goals: lower spending and improved health by eliminating payment for—and practice of—dubiously effective or unnecessary medical care. Stricter coverage criteria also potentially create stronger incentives for new technologies to "prove themselves" via rigorous scientific evaluation.

Alongside these policy initiatives, critiques and case studies of actual priority setting processes are also beginning to appear. In practice, political or organizational imperatives have compromised technocratic, principle-based approaches—sometimes to the demise of the priority-setting process altogether (e.g., Redmayne and Klein, 1993; Campbell, 1995; Cooper, 1995; Ham, 1995; Blumstein, 1997; Chinitz and Israili, 1997). Early reports suggest that decisions can be strongly influenced by stakeholders' varying interpretations of "what is at stake" in the coverage of a given technology (e.g., Redmayne and Klein, 1993; Giacomini, 1999). To date there has been little research documenting stakeholder responses to actual deinsurance decisions made through explicit priority-setting processes.

This paper reports experience from the case of deinsuring in vitro fertilization (IVF) in the Canadian province of Ontario. It extends the current literature by analyzing not only the reasoning that went into the deinsurance decision, but also the impact of the decision in terms of stakeholders' understanding of the essential "meaning" of the policy and the part these meanings play in their initial responses to the policy.

The findings illustrate the complexity of implementing deinsurance and tracing its effects. This case suggests that priority-setting decisions based on incomplete information, inconsistently applied principles, and too little attention to health system dynamics (perhaps the current norm in "real world" priority-setting) can have the perverse effect of undermining progress toward improving health, reducing expenditures, and evaluating services rigorously. Although some of the findings are specific to IVF or Ontario, we believe many of the same types of effects can be expected for other procedures in other jurisdictions. This analysis offers several lessons for improving the process,

the credibility, and the health effects of other priority-setting exercises. First, individual services are embedded within systems of service. Removing even "inefficient" or "ineffective" service can affect remaining services and costs in the system, potentially in ways that offset anticipated gains. Second, criteria-based priority-setting can lose its legitimacy through the failure to articulate key criteria (e.g., "medical necessity") or through selective, rather than systematic, application of criteria across services. Finally, even scientific "evidence-based" decisions can lead to confusion and dissent among stakeholders affected by a deinsurance policy. Different stakeholders hold often incompatible views on what evidence is relevant and what types or "levels" of evidence are credible. Relegating a still-experimental service to the commercial sector (rather than to research settings) through deinsurance can send especially confusing messages about both effectiveness as a coverage criterion and the value of evaluation evidence.

METHODS

Our case study of deinsuring IVF focused on two research questions: (1) what was the nature of the IVF deinsurance policy and the scope of stakeholders' interests in the policy? and (2) what meanings have various stakeholders attributed to deinsurance and what have been their initial responses based on these interpretations? The approach was guided by a conceptual framework (Giacomini et al., 1996a; Giacomini et al., 1996b) derived from the growing body of literature addressing the social dimensions of financial incentives (e.g., Whyte et al., 1955; Kerr, 1975; Backoff and Mitnick, 1981; Kohn, 1993a, 1993b; Stone, 1997). This "communication model" of financial incentives characterizes funding structures as means of communicating complex policy objectives, rather than as mechanistic reward-penalty systems. This view supports a qualitative, interpretive approach to the empirical investigation of financial incentives. The case study methods implied by the communication model of financial incentives

(Giacomini and Goldsmith, 1996) have been applied to other recent cases of health care funding changes (see, e.g., Hurley et al., 1997a, 1997b; Lomas and Rachlis, 1997; Giacomini and Peters, 1998). In the analysis, we characterize stakeholders' interpretations of the deinsurance policy and identify common themes regarding what deinsurance can mean to those expected to respond to the policy.

Several sources of data were used. We conducted a qualitative content analysis of documents concerning IVF in Ontario, the deinsurance decision and reactions to it (e.g., policy documents and bulletins, unpublished research reports, news media; academic editorials, letters to the editor and published scholarly analyses; stakeholders' press releases, position statements, briefs submitted to policy makers, and orientation materials; clinic patient education materials). We conducted 21 semi-structured interviews with individuals representing public and private clinic providers, members of the provincial Joint Review Panel that recommended deinsuring IVF, an Ontario consumer advocacy organization for the infertile, the federal Royal Commission on New Reproductive Technologies, IVF evaluation researchers, the Ontario Ministry of Health, and the Ontario Medical Association. Interviews explored the perceived meaning of the deinsurance policy, its early consequences, and its likely implications. Follow-up interviews were conducted as necessary to clarify and triangulate key findings. We also conducted a telephone survey of the 12 Ontario IVF clinics (five public, seven private) in 1996 regarding utilization patterns, fees, and research involvement before and since deinsurance. Eight clinics responded (four public, four private), three did not respond after several attempts, and one refused to participate in the survey. Of the responding clinics, most were only able to give partial information on utilization trends before and since deinsurance (which, although disappointing, was not surprising as there are currently no provincial or federal standards for maintaining utilization and outcome data or for making them publicly available).

Analysis involved identifying key themes of policy interpretation and elucidating both sub-themes and conceptual relationships between these categories.

THE POLICY AND THE POLICY MAKING PROCESS

In February of 1994, the Ontario Ministry of Health announced that, on the recommendation of an ad hoc review committee, physician payment for IVF for indications other than completely blocked fallopian tubes would be removed from the Ontario Health Insurance Plan (OHIP) Schedule of Benefits. The Ministry of Health described the policy in a press release on 17 Feb 1994 (MoH, 1994a):

> The services that will be removed from OHIP coverage [include, among 7 others] ... in vitro fertilization, except for complete fallopian tube blockage, for a maximum of three cycles ... Doctors may continue to provide these treatments, but will charge patients for them, using the Ontario Medical Association's fee schedule as a guide.

The deinsurance initiative began in the summer of 1993 when a "Joint Review Panel" of the Ontario Ministry of Health and the Ontario Medical Association (hereafter, "the Panel") convened to review a set of services proposed for deinsuring to meet a $20 million total physician expenditure reduction by "removing services [from the physician fee schedule] that were not medically necessary..." (MoH, 1994a). The impetus was cost control in the physician sector; deinsuring IVF was expected to save $4.4 million per year in physician billings (Pringle, 1995). However, the Ministry's later explanations (and rationalizations) of the decision noted several other policy objectives including the application of "medical necessity" as a criterion for coverage, the implementation of recommendations of a Royal Commission concerned with the appropriate use of new reproductive technologies, and the consideration of scientific evidence and professional opinion in coverage decision-making. The Ministry argued that, "IVF is expensive, it is not medically necessary and the medical community is split on its effectiveness" (Brooks, 1994, p. 970) and that the policy "agree[d] with a recently released federal government report [i.e., the Royal Commission on New Reproductive Technologies] that recommended IVF should not be publicly funded except for fallopian tube blockage" (MoH, 1994a, p.1).

The decision-making process unfolded as follows. The Panel was chaired by the Dean of Nursing at the University of Toronto; members included two representatives from the Ontario Medical Association, two representatives of the Ministry of Health, and two public representatives. The Panel deliberated for three months, soliciting limited public input through one day of hearings in Toronto and through voluntary written submissions and letters. The Panel began with a list of nineteen services for possible deinsurance—eight services proposed by the Ontario Medical Association and eleven proposed by the Ministry of Health (see Table 1). These services were selected by "[taking] into account the earlier public reaction and the experience in other provinces" (Pringle, 1995, p. 3). Notwithstanding its mandate to save $20 million, the first principle of the Panel's process was: "do not take costing into account in decision-making" (neither did the Panel address the related issue of cost-effectiveness). The other two principles were, "seek gender and age equity" and, "do not consider whether Ontario Medical Association or Ministry of Health is source of item" (Pringle, 1995). Despite the brief opportunity for public consultation, the Chair maintains that, "public input [was] enormously influential in persuading the panel what not to delist" (Pringle, 1995). The volume of testimony in support of not deinsuring IVF was second only to that supporting the annual health exam.

The Panel relied on information formulated concurrently by the federal Royal Commission on New Reproductive Technologies (hereafter, "the Royal Commission"), which issued its final

report on November 15, 1993. The Royal Commission reviewed the social, ethical, and medical implications of many new reproductive technologies, including IVF and eventually published the following recommendations regarding IVF specifically:

> 128. IVF for bilateral fallopian tube blockage be an insured service under provincial medical programs within the regulatory framework recommended by the Royal Commission on New Reproductive Technologies.

> 129. The province of Ontario discontinue coverage of IVF for indications other than bilateral fallopian tube blockage and that the resources be reallocated to fund clinical trials of unproven but promising techniques (RCNRT, 1993b, p. 564).

The regulatory framework referenced in the first recommendation includes elements such as the funding and oversight of basic and clinical research, compulsory licensing and reporting requirements for all providers, practice guidelines regarding appropriate assessment and referral for IVF, and confining unproven drugs and procedures to practice under research protocols with human subject protections (as opposed to allowing unproven services to be available in the private market) (RCNRT, 1993b). The Royal Commission's two recommendations, together with its regulatory framework, comprised a policy package designed to be adopted in whole to stem privatization and increasingly inappropriate use of IVF. However, the only portion of these recommendations implemented in Ontario was the deinsurance of IVF for non-blocked tubes. Ontario deinsurance policy deviated from the Royal Commission's recommendations insofar as it did not reallocate resources to fund clinical trials.

Neither federal nor provincial agencies implemented the Royal Commission's broader regulatory framework to contain the effects of IVF deinsurance or otherwise control the use of new reproductive technologies. In July of 1995,

Table 1

Final recommendations concerning services for deinsurance (Sources: MoH, 1994a and Pringle, 1995)

	Who Suggested	*Estimated annual physician billings ($m)*
Recommended deinsuring:		
In vitro fertilization for conditions other than complete fallopian tube blockage	MoH	4.4
Reversal of sterilization	MoH	1.5
Routine newborn, ritual, or cosmetic circumcision	MoH	1.0
Removal of tattoos (except resulting from abuse)	MoH	0.1
Repair of torn earlobes (except from acute trauma)	MoH	0.2
Removal of acne pimples	MoH	2.0
Injection of simple varicose veins	MoH	2.5
Removal of certain benign skin lesions	MoH	5.9
Recommended NOT deinsuring:		
Annual health examinations (but do plan to phase out, replace with age/risk periodic health examinations)	OMA	40
General anesthesia for uninsured dental procedures	MoH	1.8
Otoplasty to correct outstanding ears	MoH	0.5
Removal of port wine stains on the face and neck	MoH	0.3
Travel assessments/immunization clinics	OMA	0.25
Insertion of testicular prosthesis	OMA	0.05
Insertion of penile prosthesis for impotence	OMA	0.22
Intracorporeal injection for impotence	OMA	0.22
Uvulopalatopharyngoplasty (for snoring and sleep apnea)	OMA	0.22
Excision of calcaneal spurs (heel spurs)	OMA	0.057
No recommendation:		
Weight loss clinics	OMA	1.6

the federal Health Minister called a voluntary moratorium on a selected set of nine particularly controversial reproductive technologies, some associated with IVF (e.g., egg-selling, sperm-selling, surrogacy contracting, and embryo selection by sex). Some IVF providers publicly defied the moratorium (see, e.g., Canadian Press, 1995). In 1996, the federal parliament failed to pass legislation criminalizing the nine practices and proposing a "management regime" for regulating reproductive technology (e.g., Dickens, 1996; McTeer, 1996).

Members of the Panel have mixed opinions about the value of their work. The Chair has described the list of candidate services as a "haphazard" and "bizarre," commenting that, "… this exercise in delisting was a failure as a process for rationally determining what medical procedures should and should not be publicly insured … working from a haphazard collection of procedures is no place to start this kind of process" (Pringle, 1995, p. 8). She also felt the hurried schedule allowed neither systematic analysis nor thorough public consultation. The Chair and the two consumer representatives issued a public statement cautioning that the Panel had not been able to consider the systemic implications of its deinsurance policy (MoH, 1994a):

> The [Panel] process … was regarded as a piecemeal approach to a systemic problem. Questions about the meaning of delisting, the ultimate results in terms of costs to individuals, effects on the health status of the population, practice changes by physicians, risks of a two-tiered system, etc. have still not been answered and are likely to recur. The relationship of this process to any reform of the health care system was a cause of much concern.

Panel members objected to the ultimate policy goal of saving $20 million in physician billings and favored instead non-budgetary principles such as medical necessity and equity for screening the services. They characterized the cost-saving goal as, "arbitrary, unrelated to 'medical necessity', [and] a cause for doubt as to the sincerity of the review process" (McInnes, 1994).

At first glance, Ontario's act of deinsuring IVF—i.e., removing the service from insured benefits—seems relatively straightforward. However, the deinsurance policy is neither simple nor clear to those involved with IVF services. First, deinsurance applies only to particular *uses* of the service. Public payment for IVF now depends upon diagnosis (Table 2): Ontario women with blocked tubes have coverage for all infertility treatments; Ontario women without blocked tubes have coverage for infertility treatments other than IVF (such as intrauterine insemination, donor insemination, and tubal surgery). Second, deinsurance added one more barrier to a number of existent barriers to IVF access. Patient selection criteria varied between clinics (Ikonomidis and Lowy, 1994; Ikonomidis and Dickens, 1995). Those undergoing publicly-insured IVF faced considerable out-of-pocket costs; privately-paid drugs and ancillary services typically totaled several thousand dollars. The Joint Panel, noting these extra costs to public IVF, deemed IVF an "inequitable technology" geared to wealthier OHIP beneficiaries and so less appropriate for public subsidy (Panel member interview). Importantly, IVF was already available on a private pay basis in the province. Individuals able to pay a higher premium, unwilling to wait several months for treatment, failing public clinic selection criteria, or wishing to attempt a fourth or fifth try have always had the option of seeking care at a private clinic for an additional cost of about $3250–7200 per cycle.

Table 2

Diagnosis and procedure contingencies for public insurance, before and after IVF deinsurance

Diagnosis	*Services Covered by OHIP*	
	IVF	*Non-IVF treatments*
Totally blocked fallopian tubes	Before deinsurance: yes;	After deinsurance: yes
	Before deinsurance: yes;	After deinsurance: yes
Other infertility diagnoses	Before deinsurance: yes;	After deinsurance: NO
	Before deinsurance: yes;	After deinsurance: yes

Third, "IVF" per se was not listed in the OHIP Schedule of Benefits as a discrete service with a discrete billing code and fee attached to it. Rather, IVF involves a complex set of procedures including diagnostics, surgery, laboratory interventions and drugs. Many have distinct billing codes that may be used in contexts other than an IVF regimen. A list of the typical elements in the IVF process appears in Table 3

(RCNRT, 1993b). The deinsurance policy withdrew public payment for two procedures crucial to the treatment regime (oocyte retrieval and embryo transfer) and implicitly deinsured the remaining elements by reemphasizing standing policy that, "… any service provided by a physician, laboratory or hospital that supports an uninsured service is not an insured benefit" (MoH, 1994b, p. 4).

Table 3

Services comprising the "IVF service"

Description[a]	Generic type of service
Diagnosis (f)	Exam
	Diagnostic lab procedure
Diagnosis (m)	Diagnostic lab procedure
Ovulation induction (f)	Fertility drugs
	Diagnostic procedures (bloodwork, ultrasound)
Semen analysis (m)	Diagnostic lab procedure
Egg retrieval (f)	Diagnostic lab
	Operative procedure Z718: "laparosopy for oocyte retrieval"[b]
Sperm wash	Lab procedure
Egg fertilization	Lab procedure
Embryo transfer (f)	Operative procedure Z585[b]: "hysteroscopy with embryo transfer"[c]
Implantation determination (f)	Diagnostic lab procedure
	Ultrasound
Emergency procedures[d]	Hospital procedures
	Hospital stay

[a] KEY: M = MALE PARTNER OF COUPLE; F = FEMALE PARTNER OF COUPLE. SOURCES: PATIENT SERVICES ADAPTED FROM DESCRIPTION OF IVF PROCESS DESCRIBED BY THE RCNRT (1993); DELISTING POLICY FROM MINISTRY OF HEALTH BULLETIN 4265.

[b] THESE ARE THE TWO EXPLICITLY "DELISTED" PROCEDURES.

[c] HYSTEROSCOPY MAY NOW BE REPLACED BY CATHETER IMPLANTATION (PROVIDER INTERVIEW); THE MOH BULLETIN REFERS ONLY TO HYSTEROSCOPY.

[d] ALL OTHER PROCEDURES ARE DELISTED IMPLICITLY ACCORDING TO THE FOLLOWING POLICY "… ANY SERVICE PROVIDED BY A PHYSICIAN, LABORATORY OR HOSPITAL THAT SUPPORTS AN UNINSURED SERVICE IS NOT AN INSURED BENEFIT. THEREFORE, NO CLAIMS TO THE MINISTRY SHOULD BE MADE FOR ANY INITIAL CONSULTATIONS, FOLLOW-UP ASSESSMENTS, COUNSELLING, DIAGNOSTIC INVESTIGATIONS (E.G., ULTRASOUND, LABORATORY TESTS), PREOPERATIVE LABORATORY WORK/ASSESSMENTS WHICH ARE IN SUPPORT OF AN UNINSURED SERVICE SUCH AS … UNINSURED IVF …" (MINISTRY OF HEALTH, BULLETIN 4265, "CHANGES TO MINISTRY OF HEALTH SCHEDULE OF BENEFITS OF OCTOBER 1ST, 1992". 8 MARCH 1994 [DISTRIBUTED TO PHYSICIANS, HOSPITALS, CLINICS AND LABORATORIES] P. 4).

Providers have remained confused about how exactly to carve "IVF other than for completely blocked fallopian tubes" out of publicly-supported infertility treatment regimens. Ambiguity remains about both the services covered (or not) and valid diagnostic indications; some providers may capitalize on this ambiguity to "game" the system on the behalf of some patients (interviews with providers, consumer advocate). Compliance is not directly monitored or enforced. The deinsurance policy applies only to physician billings and IVF remains substantially publicly subsidized through global operating budgets to university and hospital-based clinics. Some independent clinics also receive public research grants which subsidize salaries for laboratory and clinical personnel (Table 4).

WHAT MESSAGES DID IVF DEINSURANCE SEND?

IVF deinsurance sent a variety of policy messages to stakeholders interested in IVF. Interpretations of the policy message focus around three broad themes: (1) imperatives for demonstrating health service *effectiveness*, (2) the meaning of *medical necessity* (and related concepts) as principles guiding health service coverage and, (3) intentional or unintentional effects on health service *market dynamics*, including supply and demand side responses, delineation between public and private health service sectors, and effects on health expenditures.

The Effectiveness Imperative

To some, the deinsurance policy exemplifies "evidence-based decision making" guided by the principle of clinical effectiveness. To others, it represents the capricious use of evidence to rationalize deinsuring an expensive service. The Panel justified its decision to deinsure IVF on the grounds that there was no decisive evidence of the service's effectiveness for conditions other than blocked tubes.

IVF has been difficult to evaluate using rigorous randomized controlled trials (Goeree et al., 1993; Solimon et al., 1993). The two only two such reports published by 1993 (and indeed, up to the present time) both came from a trial conducted in Ontario public IVF clinics prior to deinsurance (Jarrell et al., 1993; Solimon et al., 1993). The trial, apparently the only one of its kind, aimed to assess the effectiveness of IVF to normal care while waiting for IVF (during which time other infertility treatment may or may not be pursued[1]). Results showed a statistically significant benefit for individuals with blocked tubes. Effectiveness for other conditions was inconclusive due to too few study subjects; a positive but statistically insignificant effect was found for endometriosis (Solimon et al., 1993).

Table 4

Diagnosis, site of care, and possible sources of payment for IVF, before and after IVF deinsurance

Infertility diagnosis	*Site of care*	
	Public clinic	*Private clinic*
Blocked fallopian tubes	Before deinsurance: public insurance	Before deinsurance: patient/public insurance
	After deinsurance: public insurance	After deinsurance: patient/public insurance
Other diagnoses	Before deinsurance: public insurance	Before deinsurance: patient/public insurance
	After deinsurance: patient	After deinsurance: patient

Clinical trials notwithstanding, IVF advocates and skeptics disagree over what constitutes good evidence. These disagreements hinge on issues such as what specific function of IVF should be evaluated (e.g., producing pregnancies or babies, diagnosis or treatment, mental health or physical health) and what evaluation designs (e.g., controlled trials, descriptive statistics, individual case reports, anecdote) are credible. Altogether, the policy sends unclear messages regarding the importance of evidence-based coverage, evidence-based clinical practice, and evaluation research to generate evidence.

Different stakeholders apply different standards of scientific evidence to the question, "does IVF work?" Policy makers questioning the value of IVF (i.e., the Panel, the Royal Commission, consulting clinical epidemiologists) applied the most stringent standard of clinical evaluation (randomized, controlled clinical trial findings) and found evidence of IVF's effectiveness lacking except in the case of blocked tubes. IVF for other diagnoses, such as endometriosis, was not demonstrated to be ineffective, rather, the study was inconclusive due to limitations of the research design. This lack of evidence translated into the Ontario Health Minister's statement to the press (explaining IVF deinsurance) that "test tube babies" remain "experimental" (Papp, 1994).

In contrast to the dearth of controlled trials of IVF's essential effectiveness, the scientific literature abounds with case series as well as controlled trials comparing different techniques of IVF to each other. Many IVF advocates find credible "evidence" of effectiveness in stories of personal success and the reports of uncontrolled clinical trials and cases. Cases (rather than populations) have always provided the primary data for developing and practicing IVF. The procedure involves a great deal of direct observation of—and participation in—the conception process. Because of this direct experience by both providers and patients, IVF participants are often unwilling to allow that anyone in the experimental group of an IVF trial could get pregnant by any means other than IVF.

Even more contentious than the question of legitimate study design is the question, "if it works well, how well is 'well enough' to justify public payment?" While policy makers and clinical epidemiologists seek a substantially increased probability of live births from IVF, many consumers and providers seek mere "possibilities." They speak in terms of being given "chances," "miracles," and so forth, not in terms of statistical likelihoods and rational optimization. For example, a newsletter for allied professionals in Ontario infertility clinics describes the gratification of achieving "a miracle" against the odds calculated by evaluative science: "… somehow we made it work when 'statistics and research' said it would not be possible" (OFSN, 1992).

Policy makers and evaluation researchers also differ from providers and consumers with regard to what they believe to be the salient benefit of IVF. Clinical research has evaluated IVF as a treatment technology to produce pregnancies or live births. But some providers argue that IVF produces important benefits even when it fails to produce a baby. For example, IVF also functions in some cases as a diagnostic technology. It offers clients and providers unique insight into the couple's reproductive function and when it fails, unique demonstration that "nothing can be done" for the couple's infertility (provider interviews). This additional diagnostic information and emotional closure can potentially benefit the woman's physical health by obviating further infertility interventions; it benefits couples' and individuals' emotional health by allowing them to "get on with their lives."

These differing views on what constitutes "evidence" create serious tensions for priority-setting exercises committed to principles of both "values" and "effectiveness." If coverage decisions are to reflect both scientific evidence and social values, policy makers will have to come to terms with the fact that the public, the profession, and policy analysts can value fundamentally different types of scientific evidence. The ethos of "chances," "hope," or "miracles" for individuals (which consumers tend to value) is inconsistent with the ethos of "clinically important effect sizes" or "statistically significant differences" for populations (which technology assessors value). It would be antithetical to the trend toward involving public values in coverage decisions to dismiss one basis as irrational or irrelevant.

Ironically, the "evidence based" coverage deinsurance decision may have weakened both incentives and means for investigators to test IVF's effectiveness through randomized trials. First, after deinsurance, providers face less, not more, pressure from payers to demonstrate the value of their service through randomized trials. The new "payer" (the private consumer) is in a weaker position to insist upon rigorous evaluation than the province and typically does not "believe in" the results of clinical evaluation to the degree that provincial policy makers or other health care administrators do.

Second, public clinic queues have provided the only ethical and practical source of control cases for controlled trials for assessing IVF's effectiveness. The new user fees have virtually eliminated these queues and consequently controlled trials. Although the Royal Commission had recommended that the province offset deinsurance with IVF research subsidies, this recommendation was not followed. Consequently, deinsurance halted Ontario's randomized trial, the first and, thus far, the last "in which IVF treatment is compared with no IVF treatment with respect to clinical pregnancy rates" (Jarrell et al., 1993 para 24; provider interview).

Medical Necessity

The Ministry portrayed "medical necessity" as a key criterion in its review of selected services and deinsurance of IVF (Gerard, 1993; Brooks, 1994; MoH, 1994a). Because "medical necessity" is the basis for coverage mandated by the 1984 Canada Health Act, this term has high currency in debates over which services belong in provincial health insurance plans. However, it remains a largely undefined and slippery concept for policy making purposes (e.g., Bergthold, 1995; Rachlis, 1995; Charles et al., 1997; Hurley et al., 1997a, 1997b).

The concept of medical necessity played an influential but highly ambivalent role in shaping both Ontario's deinsurance decision and stakeholders' interpretations of its meaning. The Panel's and Ministry's use of "medical necessity" to justify deinsuring IVF has been interpreted to mean several things: (1) that if a service is deemed not medically necessary, it means that the condition it treats is not a legitimate medical problem; (2) that the lack of a principled definition and ambiguity of the concept of "medical necessity" can be used capriciously to justify cutting health benefits for other reasons; or, (3) that "medical necessity" can be determined inductively by evidence of its coverage in other jurisdictions or its similarity with other provincially insured services (rather than deductively by the application of principles).

Because policy makers invoked the rationale of "medical necessity," some interpret IVF's deinsurance as a judgment about the legitimacy of *need* for IVF (apart from the merits of IVF itself). Consumers argue vehemently that infertility is a legitimate medical condition and IVF a legitimate treatment: "Infertility is a serious medical condition resulting in the abnormal function of the reproductive system and deserves treatment as does any other medical condition" (IAAC, 1994). Indeed, the Panel's consensus was that infertility is a medical need and infertility treatment legitimate medical care. The Panel declared in its submitted recommendation that, "In Ontario treatment of infertility is considered medically necessary and is, therefore, covered by OHIP" (MoH, 1994a). Announcing the final decision to deinsure IVF, the Ministry stated that the deinsured services generally were not "medically necessary," but in the same announcement affirmed that infertility treatments are considered "medically necessary." Nevertheless, the infertile felt that deinsuring IVF along with several cosmetic services reinforced a message that the service is frivolous— elective but not medically needed.

Consumer advocates protest that the idea of "medical necessity" is nowhere legislatively defined and implies no specific criteria or processes for deinsurance (IAAC, 1994; Tennant, 1994). They advocate an individualized determination of medical necessity: rather than applying the concept at a system-wide level to determine covered benefits, they argue that it should be applied at a clinical level in treatment decision making: "What is medically necessary for one person may not be medically necessary for another one" (Kennedy, 1995, p. A10). Similar conclusions have been reached by critics of deinsurance more generally (Klein, 1994; Rachlis, 1995; Charles et al., 1997; Hurley et al., 1997, 1997b). Although deinsurance made IVF coverage diagnosis-contingent, providers and consumers complain that coverage on the basis of tubal blockage still offers too little discretion for matching treatment regimens to specific individual needs (provider, consumer advocate interviews).

Deductive reasoning based on definitions, principles and algorithms is one way to apply the concept of "medical necessity." However, Ontario stakeholders also used two types of inductive analysis to argue for or against the medical necessity of IVF. First, they referred to IVF coverage policies in other jurisdictions. This strategy was used to legitimate both opposing claims: that IVF should be publicly funded and that it should not. The Panel noted the lack of IVF coverage in other Canadian provinces, who are all obligated by federal law to cover "medically necessary" services and considered this evidence that IVF is not medically necessary (Panel member interviews). Canada's federal Health Minister did not view the coverage of IVF in Ontario as evidence of its status as a "core" service to be covered by all provinces (Pole, 1995). Consumers advocates, on the other hand, argued that IVF's medical necessity is evident in its public coverage in countries outside Canada (e.g., some UK jurisdictions, Australia, The Netherlands, France) and its legislated inclusion in private insurance packages for several U.S. states (Redmayne and Klein, 1993; IAAC, 1995).

A second inductive critique considered whether services "like" IVF remained covered. Those who feel that deinsuring IVF was capricious compare IVF to other services to illustrate

that IVF has been unfairly "singled out" for deinsurance, while many covered services share similar characteristics of medical necessity (IAAC, 1994; Tennant, 1994). A submission to the Panel, for example, questioned: "… I wonder why IVF has been singled out and lumped together with such 'lifestyle' issues as tattoo removal and vasectomy reversal … if [not life-threatening] is the definition of medical necessity, then many, many procedures could be delisted … cataract surgery, for example, or hip replacement" (Tennant, 1994). Rhetoric arguing for public coverage compares IVF variously to joint replacement, optometry, psychoanalysis, or abortion with regard to its qualifying features for public coverage (e.g., its use to restore function rather than prolong life, its instrumental use in family planning) (Panel member interview; IAAC, 1994). This practice of inducing medical necessity criteria from examples, rather deducing it from abstract principles, has been found in policy arguments for service coverage since the inception of medicare in Canada (Charles et al., 1997).

Further complicating the issue of medical necessity is IVF's role as a reproductive health service. Deinsuring reproductive care is not new in Canada. An entire spectrum of reproductive services—low and high cost, low and high technology, for birth achievement as well as birth control—have been proposed for deinsurance in some provinces over the past decade. Nevertheless, the relationship of IVF to reproductive capacity and behaviour is indeed an important feature of the deinsurance "message" as understood by stakeholders.

The idea of "rights" coloured reactions to the IVF deinsurance policy. Some advocates of IVF argue that people have a right to reproduce. Symbolically, public funding affirms this privilege; withdrawing public support violates it. Infertility Awareness cited in its brief to the Panel the United Nations 1948 Universal Declaration of Human Rights, which "recognizes the right of everyone to have children" (IAAC, 1994). IVF advocates introduce the theme of rights to reproductive "choices" rather delicately with the suggestion that provinces who offer the choice of abortion should offer the symmetric choice of a full range of infertility interventions, e.g.: "The tax dollars of the infertile pay for reproductive health care for the fertile—they pay for maternity and sterilization and abortions" (Papp, 1994). The intention is not to question the coverage of abortion, but to invoke similar principles to cover IVF (IAAC, 1994). The Women's Health Bureau supported publicly insuring IVF under the rubric of women's reproductive services (Panel member interviews). Some providers agree that deinsuring IVF impinges reproductive rights and choices, or constitutes government interference in private family life (provider interviews; Gerard, 1993). Other providers clearly see access as less of a "right," for example when they refuse IVF to candidates they consider psychosocially unfit for treatment or parenthood (Ikonomidis and Lowy, 1994).

IVF coverage has been cast not only as a "right to reproduce" issue, but also a "right to health care" issue. Many involved in the IVF debate question whether it is essentially medical care, or foremost some other type of nonmedical social or personal service. Some insist that infertility care is essentially a medical service for a physical or even mental health problem (provider interview). Some see it as medical intervention for a non-"health" problem because IVF simply circumvents but does not remedy the underlying pathology that causes infertility (provider interview). Others have characterized IVF (along with other deinsured services) as more of a lifestyle choice or a luxury; in support of the deinsurance policy, the Ontario Medical Association president declared, "We've allowed the frills to creep in. Because we've not been willing to say no—until now" (Kennedy, 1993, p. A10). The Royal Commission, according to a well-articulated ethical framework based on an "ethic of care," argued that infertility treatment is a not a medically unnecessary luxury (RCNRT, 1993c).

Deinsurance and Market Dynamics

In Ontario, deinsuring IVF did not mean that it became unavailable. Rather, it became available only privately at market-determined fees. This introduced a new market dynamic to IVF provision in the province. Stakeholders express particular concerns about issues such as the fairness of a 100% user charge for a service popular among the infertile, the appropriateness of private enterprise by infertility care providers, and whether this instance of deinsurance portends more health care privatization in general.

Deinsuring IVF blurred further an already a fuzzy boundary between the public and private IVF sectors. "Public" IVF clinics in Ontario are those whose overhead costs are funded by the provincial health system through hospital operating budgets. "Private" IVF clinics (mostly for-profit and physician- or investor-owned) are those whose overhead costs are covered through private fees. Physicians in both public and private clinics have always been able to bill the public health insurance plan for covered services and to bill patients privately for services not covered by the public plan (e.g., cryopreservation and sperm assessment) as well as other costs (e.g., 'program development'). In addition, providers often work in both public and private clinics, so that clients assessed in the public clinics are sometimes offered the option of seeing (for a fee) the same physicians at a private clinic with a shorter wait and access to services not available in the public system (consumer advocate, provider interviews).

The intertwining of the public and private IVF sectors generates financial cross-subsidies in both directions. Public funds continue to subsidize many aspects of private IVF (e.g., Baird, 1995). These subsidies include public insurance for pregnancies and complications of private IVF, increased incidence of multiple births and low-birthweight babies with long-term disabilities, and the associated costs of social support. Public funds also support the medical centres that house IVF programs, provide access to patients, and train physicians who practice private IVF. In the other direction, private IVF fees generate extra revenue for publicly-funded hospitals, which is sometimes used to subsidize other non-IVF hospital services (provider interview).

Demand for IVF persists despite high out-of-pocket prices. Many view this demand as rooted in the unique psychology of the desire for children. Some view IVF-seekers' powerful yearning with compassion (RCNRT, 1993c), while others view it with more derision or skepticism (Panel member, provider interviews; Tennant, 1994). Many infertile individuals endure financial hardship and unknown medical risks—if not through IVF, then through any accessible treatment—for the slightest possibility of having a child. Anecdotes abound of people selling their houses or cars, depleting their savings, using credit cards, borrowing relatives' money, or moonlighting to fund the out-of-pocket costs of IVF (consumer advocate, provider interviews). As a consequence of the increasing personal expense of IVF, patients increasingly sell some of their eggs to finance each IVF cycle (Nisker 1995, 1996). In doing so, women decrease their own chances of conceiving through IVF and incur undetermined health risks. For these reasons, the Royal Commission declared egg-selling unethical.

Deinsuring IVF also encourages substitution among infertility treatments and clinics. Individuals unable to finance private IVF have turned to services still publicly insured, such as surgery or repeated cycles of intrauterine insemination (provider interview; IAAC, 1995). Because deinsurance has reduced the disparity in financial costs between the public and private sectors, it appears to have led to substitution of private clinic use for public clinic use. Although standard measures of utilization are not available, in the Toronto area (with several public as well as private clinics), after deinsurance the average wait in public clinics dropped from 36 months to 3 months in two and from 12 months to 0 in the third, while two private clinics report a 140% increase and a 4% decrease in demand.

Consumers, then, seem to have reacted largely as one would expect. Given inelastic demand, many go to great lengths to obtain IVF despite increased personal costs. Where this is not possible, they substitute lower-cost alternatives. Given the equalizing of public and private financial costs, they are preferentially using private clinics where the "time costs" in waiting have

traditionally been lower (and the quality of care or amenities are perceived by some to be higher).

Deinsurance also potentially affects the supply of IVF providers and services. While the number of public IVF clinics in Ontario remains unchanged at five, IVF capacity in the private sector did increase coincident with deinsurance. Private IVF clinics have attracted venture capital in recent years, especially for more technologically "advanced" services. The number of private clinics increased from 6 to 7 in 1994. Urban clinics have also added private "satellite" clinics in outlying areas to perform all services up to the stage of egg retrieval (after which the central IVF clinic takes over).

Competition among clinics appears to be increasing, although more in terms of quality than of price. The Ministry's deinsurance policy advised that clinics "use the OHIP fee schedule as a guide" for determining private IVF fees. But prices vary considerably. Public clinics' physician fees range threefold, from $1000 to $3200 (provider survey). Some clinics set prices to pursue objectives such as attracting patients for clinic-based research, matching local competitors, or increasing service volumes (provider interviews). Quality competition is based on "state-of-the-art" technology, staff with impressive clinical credentials or compassionate manner, or "beautiful facilities" (provider, consumer advocate interviews). Providers market their services with claims based on varying definitions of a "success rate," varying methods of calculating rates and little comparability across clinics (RCNRT, 1993a). Although consumer advocates try to educate consumers about these variations in outcome reporting and to pressure clinics to express rates in consistent terms, advertised IVF outcomes remain unstandardized. This is a major concern of those who have examined the IVF markets in Canada and the U.S. (e.g., RCNRT, 1993a; Neumann, 1997).[2]

Making IVF coverage conditional on diagnosis has introduced an incentive for strategic diagnostic and treatment behaviour. Some providers have contested the Ministry's anatomically-based definition of "totally blocked fallopian tubes," arguing for a broader, function-based definition (provider interview).[3] In addition to the incentive for "diagnostic creep" (Simborg, 1981), providers and patients are sometimes choosing less sensitive tests that do not as readily rule out totally blocked fallopian tubes, thereby preserving their entitlement to public funding for IVF (provider interview). Diagnosis-based strategic marketing in the IVF field is not new. While standardized infertility rates show little change over the past few decades, public awareness of infertility and its new "high tech" treatments has generated the perception of a growing infertility epidemic in North America (Scritchfield, 1989; RCNRT, 1993d). Some IVF clinics start IVF earlier in the infertility experience, before less invasive measures have been exhausted (provider interviews). More generally, the IVF industry is cultivating new markets of "infertile" people, e.g., post-menopausal women, fertile women postponing childbearing (the potentially infertile) (Medical Post, 1995) and even those seeking posthumous conception (e.g., Toronto Star, 1995).

Deinsurance was intended above all to control public spending for physician services. In the most immediate sense, the policy did save public money: it supported a contractual decrease of the provincial physician budget by $20 million. However, it remains unknown whether IVF- and infertility-related spending within Ontario's physician budget have changed, or by how much. Data necessary for evaluation (e.g., reliable utilization statistics on IVF and substitute and complementary services) remain uncollected and unavailable. The effect on costs cannot be calculated by simply subtracting the IVF physician fees from the provincial health care budget. Deinsuring physician payment associated with IVF affects the delivery and use of other health care services (e.g., rates of surgery and intrauterine insemination, commitments of specialists between public and private clinics, hospital investment in capital for IVF clinics, and cross-subsidization of other hospital programs with private IVF revenues). The ripple of utilization adjustments in turn affects health care

needs (e.g., due to complications from alternative procedures, multiple births).

Importantly, deinsurance was not the only policy tool available to control provincial expenditures for IVF and IVF-related needs and services. Infertility consumer advocates argued against IVF deinsurance on the grounds that larger cost savings might come from regulatory reforms to cut down on poor treatment practices, such as standard clinical guidelines for IVF and the accreditation of IVF providers (IAAC, 1994). Such regulation was also recommended by the Royal Commission but has not been implemented provincially or federally.

DISCUSSION

Deinsuring IVF was intended to support several policy goals: (1) To save the Ontario Health Insurance Plan $4.4 million through reduced physician billings for IVF; (2) To affirm that public payment be restricted to "medically necessary" care; (3) To apply scientific evidence of effectiveness as a criterion for the medical necessity of a service; and, (4) To take a first step toward applying the painstakingly formulated recommendations of the federal Royal Commission on New Reproductive Technologies.

To those who advocate evaluation-based coverage of health care technologies, it may seem that Ontario policy makers took a modest and constructive step by removing one service of dubious effectiveness and high cost from public insurance coverage. As it plays out, however, Ontario's deinsurance of IVF could inadvertently accomplish the opposite of what policy makers had hoped. It remains unclear whether public infertility- and IVF-related spending has gone up or down. "Medical necessity" was inconsistently defined and understood by stakeholders to refer to various service characteristics: experimental status, effectiveness, legitimacy of infertility as a medical indication, coverage status in other jurisdictions and as a Trojan horse for obscuring "real" decision criteria such as cost control. Rigorous evaluation of IVF's effectiveness has stalled and uses for unproven purposes have moved further into the private sector. Utilization of other underevaluated infertility interventions in the public sector may have increased as a result of deinsurance.

As a financial incentive tool, deinsurance does not necessarily create an incentive discouraging inappropriate services. Ontario's deinsurance of IVF conveyed ambiguous signals about "the right thing to do," as well as "how to do the right thing." This case suggests some generic lessons for other jurisdictions engaged in priority-setting and service deinsurance: (1) individual services interact with the rest of the system, (2) inconsistent use of coverage principles can undermine popular legitimacy of priority-setting principles and processes, (3) "evidence-based" decisions can founder on differing stakeholder perceptions of valuable types and topics of evidence, as well as the inconsistent message given by commercializing unacceptably ineffective (or unproven) care.

First, many services are inextricably connected to other parts of the health care system. For service priority-setting, it is seldom easy to define either "the" service in question, or "the" alternative to which it might be compared (Ham, 1993; Giacomini, 1999). IVF's purposes have been variously conceived (so to speak) by different stakeholders as: to produce a baby (any baby, a genetically related baby, or a healthy baby), or, barring a baby, to produce pregnancy, hope, diagnostic answers, or psychological relief. Alternatives to publicly-paid IVF, then, could be anything from other clinical interventions for achieving conception (e.g., tuboplasty, waiting, private IVF), other means of producing psychological relief (e.g., counseling), or other means of achieving parenthood (e.g., adoption, surrogacy). The purpose of and alternatives to IVF depend upon the goals of its users, its payers, and the economic and organizational context in which it is delivered.

As an item on a list of potentially deinsurable services, IVF appears deceptively discrete. In practice however it is better thought of as a component integrated into a system of services. Its removal has systemic effects on other serv-ices and on the care that particular populations receive. If IVF is less available, demand for its variously understood "alternatives" increases. Thus, a policy about the role of a given service is by implication also a policy about the role of its alternatives. The health effects and social costs of turning to alternatives such as tubal surgery, private IVF, surrogacy, adoption, or "giving up" remain poorly understood. The ad hoc deinsurance of a discrete service—according to a limited characterization of that service and a non-comparative understanding of its expense and effectiveness—guarantees neither lower spending nor improved outcomes in populations or individuals.

Second, the selective or incomplete application of assessment principles can undermine the popular legitimacy of health service priority-setting. Despite the Panel's public explanations of its process and its rationale for deinsuring IVF, stakeholders remain confused (and skeptical) about the true criteria and agenda driving the decision. Perceived criteria for the decision include clinical effectiveness (a criterion the Panel did use), the legitimacy of the need for infertility services (a criterion the Panel explicitly rejected) and coverage in other jurisdictions (an impetus for examining IVF, but not a criterion officially used by the Panel to judge it). The concept of medical necessity was used repeatedly to justify the decision, but left vaguely defined. Medical necessity and its various connotations (need, effectiveness, etc.) appear to have functioned more as post hoc rationalizations rather than as a priori rationales for withdrawing coverage. The highly selective application of the review process to only a few services appeared very unfair to consumers and providers who believe in the value of IVF, as well as to the Panel members doing the review. The net effect has been unclear understanding of how health services are valued, a general consensus that the service restrictions were primarily cost-reducing, and residual skepticism about priority-setting exercises.

This case suggests that the legitimacy of structured decision-making processes will rest not only on the integrity of the criteria and reasoning used in the algorithms (e.g., GCCHC, 1992; Deber et al., 1994). Legitimacy will also depend on how effectively the criteria are communicated to and agreed to be valid by stakeholders and on how consistently the criteria are applied across services. A seminal Dutch proposal for determining service coverage has suggested the four "screens" of: necessity, effectiveness, efficiency, and whether the service should be left to individual responsibility or provided out of a community commitment to solidarity (GCCHC, 1992). When applying this decision-making algorithm hypothetically to IVF, the authors conclude that, "… from the medical-professional viewpoint, in vitro fertilization would be necessary care, reasonably effective and, compared to alternatives, reasonably efficient," but that it fails on the basis of solidarity: "… a broad, not to mention compulsory, solidarity would not seem to be justified, so that in vitro fertilization will not be included in the basic package" (GCCHC, 1992, p. 88).

The Ontario case suggests that this type of rational priority-setting would not be so straightforward. Canadian stakeholders in 1994 did not agree readily on IVF's effectiveness status, or even on acceptable effectiveness parameters. Efficiency was all but disregarded: although cost was a central concern, cost-effectiveness principles and data played little role in the policy debate. Many remain unconvinced that infertility treatment is established as valid necessity, despite both the Royal Commission's and the Panel's explicit attempts to validate the needs of the infertile and to separate these from the issue of IVF payment. Finally, opinions diverge on a solidarity basis for IVF coverage and ideas about solidarity can be difficult to distinguish from ideas about rights as well as necessity.

IVF clearly represents many things to many people. These qualitative dimensions and stakeholders' strong opinions about which ones count, can confound standardized approaches to priority-setting. In jurisdictions outside of Canada, health system administrators have also diverged in their understanding of the essential,

defining qualities of IVF for the purpose of coverage decision-making. Redmayne and Klein (1993) investigated the widely varying reasoning behind the in vitro fertilization (IVF) coverage decisions of six UK purchasing authorities. Reasons for declining to cover IVF included: a belief that those in need of IVF are not "really ill"; local affluence and the ability to pay privately; high cost; reluctance to ration by volume to control costs; the argument that money could be spent on more reliably effective services (specifically, hip replacements); and a local opinion-leader's conviction that IVF is not effective. Reasons for deciding to cover IVF included: its inclusion in a larger package of infertility services; strong lobbying by a local provider or local pressure groups; concern about psychological and marital stress due to infertility; a commitment to "the family"; a sense of moral obligation given the coverage of other reproductive services such as contraception and abortion; a belief that the epidemiological need for IVF is limited (creating a natural limit to IVF spending); explicit limitation of the service to women/couples under 40 with no more than one child (again to limit spending); and a belief that the procedure is effective. The UK experience illustrates the multitude of criteria that decision makers have applied to deinsurance in general and to IVF in particular.

Beneath technologies, their purposes and their alternatives, lie constituent interests. In the policy world, selective divestment from certain health services readily translates into selective divestment from certain populations' needs. Because IVF deinsurance selectively deinsures only *some* infertile people for only *some* treatments, consumers have interpreted the policy to be divisive to the "community" in need. More generally, IVF privatization through deinsurance signals a movement away from the solidarity principles underlying social insurance (Stone, 1993).

Finally, even "evidence-based" coverage decisions can send mixed messages about the proper role of evidence as well as the proper role of yet-unproven or ineffective technologies. The Panel's reference to scientific evidence as justification for deinsuring IVF was, outwardly, a step toward rationalizing benefits through technology assessment. However, as stakeholders interpret the policy, the deinsurance of IVF does not herald more stringent evidentiary standards for health service coverage. Stakeholders disagree over key issues such as whether relevant evidence was used, whether services should be disqualified for a lack of evidence of effectiveness or only for proven ineffectiveness, whether clinical evidence applies at the level of provincial coverage decision-making vs. service-level clinical decision-making and whether it is appropriate to apply evidence standards to discrete services (e.g., IVF) rather than to programs of care (e.g., infertility treatment) for defined conditions. Deinsurance also seems unlikely to create incentives for more rigorous evaluation in the future. Individual infertile consumers seem less insistent on rigorous evaluation evidence than are collective payers such as insurance plans. Despite official announcements to the contrary, deinsurance did not send a clear message that IVF remains "experimental." Its dispatch to the private sector (rather than to research protocols and stringent ethical oversight) served to characterize it rather as an "elective."

Acknowledgements

We foremost thank the many anonymous informants interviewed for this project, for sharing their thoughts and time with us, as well as for critiquing work in progress. David Schneider, Laurie Goldsmith, and Susan West provided research assistance on the project. Cathy Charles, Jonathan Lomas, Laurie Goldsmith, the Polinomics Group at CHEPA, and two anonymous reviewers gave helpful suggestions on earlier drafts. This project was funded through a grant from National Health Research and Development Program, NHRDP Project Number 6606-5665-303. Our work was also supported by the collegial environment and resources of the Centre for Health Economics and Policy Analysis (CHEPA), which is funded in part through a grant from the Ontario Ministry of Health.

Notes

1. In the absence of a waiting list for IVF, it is difficult to convince individuals to participate in a controlled trial. Control group members are likely to seek IVF elsewhere or drop out of the study. With a queue, individuals can be randomized to "early" versus "late" treatment with IVF (by randomizing their position in the queue). Pregnancy rates in those still waiting can then be compared to rates in those who have received treatment.

2. There is tremendous variation in claims of effectiveness in marketing and information materials offered by North American IVF providers. "Success rates" may be calculated based on any number of populations and endpoints, the choice of which can dramatically alter "success rates" and confuse anyone trying to make unbiased comparisons of effectiveness.

3. An anatomically blocked tube has a physical obstruction that is evident even in the absence of an egg's passage through it. Functionally blocked tubes may not be anatomically obstructed but nevertheless be impassable by an egg. Anatomical blockage is a subset of functional blockage.

References

Backoff, R.W. and Mitnick, B.M., 1981. The systems approach, incentive relations and university management. In: Wilson, J. Editor, 1981. *New Directions for Higher Education: Management Science Applications to Academic Administration* 35. Jossey-Bass, San Francisco, 73–92.

Baird, P., 1995. Hidden costs of two-tier health system. *Toronto Star,* 29 Aug 1995, A17.

Bergthold, L.A., 1995. Medical necessity: do we need it? *Health Affairs* 14, 180–190.

Blumstein, J.F., 1997. The Oregon experiment: The role of cost-benefit analysis in the allocation of medicaid funds. *Social Science and Medicine* 45, 545–554.

Brooks, J., 1994. Infertility treatment targeted as Ontario delists services. *Canadian Medical Association Journal* 150, 970–972.

Campbell, A., 1995. Defining core health services: the New Zealand experience. *Bioethics* 9, 252–258.

Canadian Press, 1995. Fertility firms scornful of call for moratorium. *Toronto Star,* 28 July 1995, A8.

Charles, C., Lomas, J., Giacomini, M., Bhatia, V. and Vincent, V., 1997. The role of medical necessity in Canadian health policy: four meanings and... a funeral? *Milbank Quarterly* 75, 365–394.

Chinitz, D. and Israeli, A., 1997. Health reform and rationing in Israel. *Health Affairs* 16, 205–210.

CMA (Canadian Medical Association), 1995. Core and comprehensive health care services. *Canadian Medical Association Journal* 152, 740A–740B.

Cooper, M.H., 1995. Core services and the New Zealand health reforms. *British Medical Bulletin* 51, 799–807.

Crawshaw, R., Garland, M., Hines, B. and Anderson, B., 1990. Developing principles for prudent health care allocation: The continuing Oregon experiment. *Western Journal of Medicine* 152, 441–446.

(DCE) Danish Council of Ethics, 1997. Priority Setting in the Health Service. Available at website: http://www.etiskraad.dk/publikationer/eng002.htm.

Deber, R., Ross, E., Catz, M. (1994). Comprehensiveness in Health Care: Report to the Heal Action Lobby. Toronto: Department of Health Administration, University of Toronto.

Dickens, B., 1996. Do not criminalize new reproductive technologies. *Policy Options* 17(2), 11–14.

Eddy, D.M., 1991. What care is 'essential'? What services are 'basic'? *JAMA* 265, 782–788.

GCCHC (Government Committee on Choices in Health Care), 1992. *Choices in Health Care* Ministry of Welfare, Health and Social Affairs, Zoetermeer, the Netherlands.

Gerard, W., 1993. Test-tube babies: the high cost of conception. *Toronto Star,* 27 May 1993, F5–F7.

Giacomini, M., 1999. The 'which' hunt: assembling health technologies for assessment and rationing. Journal of Health Politics, Policy and Law 24(4), 715–758.

Giacomini, M. and Goldsmith, L., 1996. Case Study Methodology for Studying Financial Incentives in Context. McMaster University Centre for Health Economics and Policy Analysis, Working Paper 96-15.

Giacomini, M., Hurley, J., Lomas, J., Bhatia, V. and Goldsmith, L., 1996a. The many meanings of money: a health policy analysis framework for understanding financial incentives. McMaster University Centre for Health Economics and Policy Analysis, Working Paper 96-06.

Giacomini, M., Hurley, J. and Lomas, J., Bhatia, V. and Goldsmith, L., 1996b. The devil in the details: conclusions about how funding changes translate into financial incentives in the Canadian health system. Hamilton, Ontario: McMaster University Centre for Health Economics and Policy Analysis, Working Paper 96-14.

Giacomini, M. and Peters, M.A., 1998. Beyond 'financial incentives': what the funding structure for midwifery in Ontario means to the stakeholders. *Canadian Public Administration* 41(4), 553–586.

Goeree, R., Jarrell, J. and Labelle, R., 1993. Methodological challenges in evaluating a new and evolving technology: the case of in vitro fertilization. New reproductive technologies and the health care system: the case for evidence-based medicine. Ottawa: Canada Communications Group. (Royal Commission on New Reproductive Technologies research volume 11.)

Goold, S.D., 1996. Allocating health care: cost-utility analysis, informed democratic decision making, or the veil of ignorance? *Journal of Health Politics Policy and Law* 21, 69–98.

Ham, C., 1995. Synthesis: what can we learn from international experience? *British Medical Bulletin* 51, 819–830.

Ham, C., 1993. Priority setting in the NHS: reports from six districts. *British Medical Journal* 307, 435–438.

Hurley, J., Birch, S., Stoddart, G. and Torrance, G., 1997. Medical necessity, benefit and resource allocation in health care. *Journal of Health Services Research and Policy* 2, 223–230

Hurley, J., Lomas, J. and Goldsmith, L., 1997. Physician expenditure caps in Canada: a common property perspective. *Milbank Quarterly* 75(3), 343–364.

IAAC (Infertility Awareness Association of Canada), Toronto Chapter, 1994. Unpublished written submission to the Joint Review Panel, 10 Jan 1994.

IAAC (Infertility Awareness Association of Canada), Toronto Chapter, 1995. Orientation packet/organizational literature.

Ikonomidis, S. and Dickens, B., 1995. Ontario's decision to defund in vitro fertilization treatment except for women with bilateral fallopian tube damage. *Canadian Public Policy* 21 (3), 379–381.

Ikonomidis, S. and Lowy, F., 1994. Access to in vitro fertilization in Canada. *Journal of the Society of Obstetricians and Gynecologists of Canada* 16, 1831–1837.

Jarrell, J.F., Labelle, R., Goeree, R., Milner, R. and Collins, J., 1993. In vitro fertilization and embryo transfer: a randomized controlled trial. Online Journal of Current Clinical Trials. Document No. 73.

Kennedy, M., 1993. Surgery on medicare. *Hamilton Spectator,* 24 Aug 1993, A10.

Kennedy, M., 1995. Taking the pulse of medicare. *Hamilton Spectator,* 16 Sept 1995, A10.

Kerr, S., 1975. On the folly of rewarding A, while hoping for B. *Academy of Management Journal* 18(4), 769–783.

Klein, R., 1994. Can we restrict the health care menu? *Health Policy* 27, 103–112.

Klein, R., 1993. Dimensions of rationing: who should do what? *British Medical Journal* 307, 309–311.

Kohn, A., 1993a. Why incentive plans cannot work. *Harvard Business Review* (Sept/Oct): 54–63.

Kohn, A., 1993b. *Punished by Rewards: The Trouble with Gold Stars, Incentive Plans, A's, Praise and Other Bribes.* Houghton Mifflin Company, Boston.

Lenaghan, J., New, B. and Mitchell, E., 1996. Setting priorities: Is there a role for citizens' juries? *British Medical Journal* 312, 1591–1593.

Lomas, J., and Rachlis, M., 1997. Moving rocks: Block funding in P.E.I. as an incentive for cross-sectoral reallocations among human services. *Canadian Public Administration* 39(4), 581–600.

Lomas, J., 1997. Reluctant rationers: Public input to health care priorities. *Journal of Health Services Research and Policy* 2, 103–111.

McInnes, C., 1994. OHIP to stop paying for some in vitro, other procedures. *Globe and Mail,* 18 Feb 1994, A7.

McTeer, M.A., 1996. A regime to regulate reproductive technologies. *Policy Options* 17(2), 29–33.

Medical Post, 1995. Eggs stored from young women can be used later in life. *Medical Post,* November 1995.

MoH (Ontario Ministry of Health), 1994. Grier accepts Pringle report. (News release of 17 Feb 1994) 94/037.

MoH (Ontario Ministry of Health), 1994. Bulletin 4265, "Changes to Ministry of Health Schedule of Benefits of October 1st, 1992." 8 March 1994 [distributed to physicians, hospitals, clinics and laboratories].

Neumann, P.J., 1997. Should health insurance cover IVF? Issues and options. *Journal of Health Politics, Policy and Law* 22, 1215–1237.

Nisker, J., 1995. A user-friendly framework for exploration of ethical issues in reproductive medicine. *Assisted Reproduction Reviews* 5, 272–279.

Nisker, J., 1996. The use of IVF patients as oocyte 'donors': Unwise despite its apparent appeal. *Policy Options* 17(2), 25–29.

OFSN (Ontario Fertility Services Network), 1992. Ontario Fertility Services Network Newsletter, summer issue.

OTA (Office of Technology Assessment, Congress of the United States), 1992. *Evaluation of the Oregon Medicaid Proposal: Summary.* Office of Technology Assessment, Washington, DC.

Papp, L., 1994. Annual check-ups survive OHIP axe. *Toronto Star,* 18 Feb 1994, A1.

Pole, K., 1995. Feds won't lead quest to define medical necessity. *Medical Post,* 7 Feb 1995, 33.

Pringle, D., 1995. Deinsuring medical services: practical or perverse? Presentation to the Annual Meeting of the Canadian Health Economics Research Assiociation, Waterloo, Ontario, 25 Aug 1995.

Rachlis, M., 1995. Defining basic services and deinsuring the rest: the wrong diagnosis and the wrong prescription. *Canadian Medical Association Journal* 152, 1401–1405.

RCNRT (Royal Commission on New Reproductive Technologies), 1993. *Proceed With Care: Final Report of the Royal Commission on New Reproductive Technologies.* Ottawa: Minister of Government Services Canada.

RCNRT (Royal Commission on New Reproductive Technologies), 1993. Infertility treatments: in vitro fertilization. In: *Proceed With Care: Final*

Report of the Royal Commission on New Reproductive Technologies. Ottawa: Minister of Government Services Canada, 497–580.

RCNRT (Royal Commission on New Reproductive Technologies), 1993. What guided our deliberations: Ethical framework and guiding principles. In: *Proceed With Care: Final Report of the Royal Commission on New Reproductive Technologies.* Ottawa: Minister of Government Services Canada, 49–67.

RCNRT (Royal Commission on New Reproductive Technologies), 1993. Prevalence of infertility. In: *Proceed With Care: Final Report of the Royal Commission on New Reproductive Technologies.* Ottawa: Minister of Government Services Canada, 179–198.

Redmayne, S. and Klein, R., 1993. Rationing in practice: the case of in vitro fertilization. *British Medical Journal* 306, 1521–1524.

Richardson, R. and Waddington, C., 1996. Allocating resources: community involvement is not easy. *International Journal of Health Planning and Management* 11, 307–315.

Scritchfield, S.A., 1989. The social construction of infertility: from private matter to social concern. In: Best, J. Editor, 1989. *Images of Issues: Typifying Contemporary Social Problems.* Aldine de Gruyter, New York, 99–114.

Simborg, D., 1981. DRG Creep: a new hospital acquired disease. *New England Journal of Medicine* 304, 1602–1604.

Solimon, S., Daya, S., Collins, J. and Jarrell, J., 1993. A randomized trial of in vitro fertilization versus conventional treatment for infertility. *Fertility and Sterility* 59, 1239–1244.

Stone, D., 1993. The struggle for the soul of health insurance. *Journal of Health Politics Policy and Law* 18, 286–317.

Stone, D.A., 1997. Inducements. In: *Policy Paradox: The Art of Political Decision Making.* W.W. Norton and Co, New York, 263–281.

Stronks, K., Strijbis, A.-M., Wendte, J.F. and Gunning-Schepers, L.J., 1997. Who should decide? Qualitative analysis of panel data from public, patients, healthcare professionals and insurers on priorities in health care. *British Medical Journal* 315, 92–96.

Tennant, D., 1994. Firsthand Knowledge: A Consumer's View of Proposed Delisting of IVF. Unpublished written submission to the Joint Review Panel.

Toronto Star, 1995. Fathering babies from the grave: corpse's sperm can fertilize eggs but should it? *Toronto Star,* Dec. 1995.

Tymstra, T. and Andela, M., 1993. Opinions of Dutch physicians, nurses and citizens on health care policy, rationing and technology. *JAMA* 270, 2995–2999.

Whyte, W.F., Dalton, M., Roy, D. et al., 1955. On symbols and interaction. In: *Money and Motivation: An Analysis of Incentives in Industry* Harper and Brothers, New York, 241–249.

Wilson, R., Rowan, M.S. and Henderson, J., 1995. Core and comprehesive health care services: 1. Introduction to the Canadian Medical Association's decision-making framework. *Canadian Medical Association Journal* 152, 1063–1066.

Eldridge v. British Columbia (Attorney General), [1997] 3 S.C.R. 624

Summary prepared by Lisa Forman

Medical care in British Columbia is administered through the *Hospital Insurance Act*, which reimburses hospitals for the medically required services they provide to the public, and the *Medical and Health Care Services Act,* which funds medically required services provided by doctors and other health care practitioners. Neither program pays for sign language interpretation for the deaf.

Free medical interpreting services were provided until 1990 by a private non-profit agency, the Western Institute for the Deaf and Hard of Hearing, but were discontinued because of insufficient funding. The Institute's two requests of the Ministry of Health for funding were declined, on the basis that it would strain available resources and create a precedent to fund similar services for the non-English speaking immigrant community.

The appellants—Robin Eldridge and John and Linda Warren—were born deaf, and their preferred means of communication is sign language. They contended that the absence of interpreters impaired their ability to communicate with their doctors and health care providers, increasing the risk of misdiagnosis and ineffective treatment.

This case concerned the question of whether a provincial government's failure to provide funding for sign language interpreters for deaf persons when they receive medical services violates s. 15(1) of the *Canadian Charter of Rights and Freedoms*. The appellants argued that the failure to pay for interpreters infringed their right to equal benefit of the law without discrimination based on physical disability, in that the communication barrier between deaf persons and health care providers resulted in a lesser quality of medical services for deaf persons than for hearing persons.

The judgment of the Supreme Court of Canada was delivered by Justice La Forest. The SCC considered first whether this decision violated the appellant's equality rights under section 15(1) of the *Charter*, and if so, whether it was a reasonable limitation under s. 1.

The SCC recognized that as deaf persons, the appellants belong to an enumerated group under section 15(1)—the physically disabled. The SCC also found that there was no question that the distinction drawn between the appellants and others was based on a personal characteristic irrelevant to the functional values underlying the health care system—the promotion of health, the prevention and treatment of illness and disease, and the realization of those values through a publicly funded health care system.

The SCC considered that the only question in this case was whether the appellants had been afforded the "equal benefit" of the law without discrimination within the meaning of s. 15(1). Although the medicare system applies equally to deaf and hearing populations, the applicant's claim was one of "adverse effects" discrimination. A discriminatory purpose or intention is not a necessary condition of a s. 15(1) violation, and it is sufficient if the effect of the legislation is to deny someone the equal protection or benefit of the law. Adverse effects discrimination is especially relevant in the case of disability, as the government will rarely single out disabled persons for discriminatory treatment. More common are laws of general application that have a disparate impact on the disabled. In the present case, the adverse effects suffered by deaf persons stems from a failure to ensure that they benefit equally from a service offered to everyone.

The Court of Appeal had found that failing to provide medically related sign language interpretation was not discriminatory, because interpretation services were not "medically required" but were "ancillary services," which, like other non-medical services, are not publicly funded. Justice La Forest found this reasoning to seriously mischaracterize the practical reality of health care delivery, where effective communication is an integral part of the provision of medical services. When deaf patients cannot communicate effectively with their doctors without an interpreter, they could not be said to receive the same level of medical care as hearing persons. To do so they must bear the burden of paying for the means to communicate with their health care providers, despite the fact that the system is intended to make ability to pay irrelevant. Where necessary for effective communication, sign language interpretation should not be viewed as an "ancillary" service, but as the means whereby deaf persons receive the same quality of medical care as the hearing population.

The SCC found that to argue that governments should be entitled to provide benefits to the general population without ensuring that disadvantaged members of society have the resources to take full advantage of those benefits "bespeaks a thin and impoverished vision of s. 15(1)." The SCC found that the failure to provide sign language interpretation where necessary for effective communication constituted a prima facie violation of the s. 15(1) rights of deaf persons. This failure denies them the equal benefit of the law and discriminates against them in comparison with hearing persons.

The SCC then moved on to its considerations under s. 1 of the *Charter*. This section states that the *Charter* "guarantees the rights and freedoms set out in it subject only to such reasonable limits prescribed by law as can be demonstrably justified in a free and democratic society." Justice La Forest found the government had failed to demonstrate a reasonable basis to deny medical interpretation services for the deaf as a minimum impairment of their rights. The estimated cost of providing sign language interpretation for the whole of British Columbia was only $150,000, or approximately 0.0025 percent of the provincial health care budget at the time. The SCC found the refusal to expend this relatively insignificant sum could not constitute a minimum impairment of the appellants' constitutional rights.

The government argued that recognizing the appellants' claim would force governments to spend precious health care dollars accommodating myriad disadvantaged persons. However the SCC rejected this reasoning, in that the appellants' claim was not for a benefit that the government, in the exercise of its discretion to allocate resources to address various social problems, had chosen not to provide. Rather, they asked only for equal access to services available to all. The SCC found no evidence that this type of accommodation extended to other government services would unduly strain the fiscal resources of the state.

The SCC found clear evidence that deaf persons receive medical services inferior to the hearing population. Given the centrality of good health in the quality of life of all persons, this diminished the overall quality of their lives. The SCC found the government had not made a "reasonable accommodation" of the appellants' disability to the point of "undue hardship." The SCC allowed the appeal, granting a declaration that the failure was unconstitutional and directing the government of British Columbia to administer the relevant acts in a manner consistent with the requirements of s. 15(1) of the *Charter*.

Cameron v. Nova Scotia (Attorney General) (1999), 172 N.S.R. (2d) 227 (C.A.)

Summary prepared by Josephine Johnston

The appellants were a husband and wife who had been unable to conceive a child due to the husband's "severe male factor infertility" (reduced sperm count). In an effort to conceive a child they had both undergone surgery before they were referred by their physicians for intro cytoplasmic sperm injection (ICSI). ICSI is a specialized form of in vitro fertilization (IVF) in which a single sperm is injected into an egg and the resulting fertilized egg is transferred to the woman for implantation and gestation. ICSI is considered the treatment of choice for severe male factor infertility.

The appellants had undergone four cycles of ICSI (two in Toronto and two in Calgary) and the woman had received two frozen embryo transfers. None of the procedures had been successful and the appellants had incurred costs of approximately $40,000 for the treatments, drugs, travel, and lodging. They had been unable to recover any of these costs from Maritime Medical Care, Inc. (MMC) because MMC said that the services accessed were not considered insured services in Nova Scotia.

Among other remedies, the appellants sought recovery of their out-of-province fertility treatment costs, a declaration that they were entitled to coverage for any further treatment, and an order directing the Nova Scotia Minister of Health to establish a mechanism for payment for IVF and ICSI procedures.

After failing in the Nova Scotia Supreme Court, the appellants appealed to the Nova Scotia Court of Appeal. They claimed that IVF and ICSI were "insured services" under Nova Scotia's Health Services and Insurance Act and its subsequent Regulations. Specifically, they argued that the services they accessed in Toronto

and Calgary (and IVF generally) were "medically necessary" services and so ought to be covered under the Nova Scotia medical plan.

If the services were not insured services under Nova Scotia policy, then the appellants claimed that this policy was in breach of s. 15(1) of the *Canadian Charter of Rights and Freedoms*. In particular, the appellants claimed that the decision not to cover IVF and ICSI amounted to discrimination against the infertile under the *Charter*. They claimed that infertility is a disability and that the application of Nova Scotia's policy regarding IVF and ICSI has a disproportionate effect on them because, while "every aspect of having children" is covered by medicare, infertile persons can only access treatments at their own cost. They argued that such discrimination could not be justified in a free and democratic society (s. 1 of the *Charter*).

The three-member Court of Appeal dismissed the appellants' appeal, delivering two separate judgments. In the first judgment, Justice Chipman (with Justice Pugsley concurring), found that IVF and ICSI were not among the services and procedures listed in the Regulations to the Health Services and Insurance Act. They were also not "medically required" services despite the fact that they were the treatment of choice for cases of severe male infertility. Quoting the trial judge that "neither 'medically indicated' nor 'standard medical practice' equates to 'medically required'," Justice Chipman concluded that whether a service was "medically required" may well depend on economic constraints. Justice Chipman stated:

> In my opinion, the hospital and medical care available under the policy of the Act

is universal in that it applies to all residents of the Province without restriction. It is comprehensive, but by no means all-inclusive…. Of necessity, what is or is not medically required must be judged by those placed in charge of administration of the policy. The judgment requires an appreciation not only of medical procedures, but the availability of funds.

Establishing a breach of the *Charter* required that the appellants show that the law drew a distinction between them and other Canadians based on a personal characteristic, or that the law failed to take account of their already disadvantaged position in society due to a personal characteristic. They would then need to show that the differential treatment was based on a characteristic listed in s. 15 (for example, physical disability) and that the differential treatment discriminates in a manner that has the effect of perpetuating a stereotype or denigrating the individual.

Justice Chipman found that the province's policy regarding IVF and ICSI reinforced the disadvantage of the infertile and drew a distinction based on a personal characteristic. He also found that infertility was a physical disability within the meaning of s. 15 of the *Charter*. Finally, he accepted that the policy's differential treatment of the appellants was discriminatory because they are denied the services that may be the most significant to them.

However, Justice Chipman accepted the respondents' defence that any discrimination under s. 15 was justified by s. 1 of the *Charter*. In effect, the judge deferred to the policy-making authority of the Nova Scotia Government. He stated:

It is the administrators of the policy who have drawn the line that excludes IVF and ICSI from the category of insured services … they must be "accorded some flexibility" in apportioning social benefits among the vast number of competing

procedures and the conditions of patients that call for them…. We should not second guess them.

He concluded that the violation of the appellants' s. 15 rights was rationally connected to the aim of the Nova Scotia *Health Services and Insurance Act* and the policy developed under it. The exclusion of IVF and ICSI services was discriminatory, and unfortunate, but it was also justifiable enough to be saved by s. 1 of the *Charter*.

In a separate judgment, Justice Bateman agreed with Justice Chipman on the question of whether IVF and ICSI were insured services in Nova Scotia, and with the result he reached on the question of whether the Nova Scotia policy breached the *Charter*. However, she disagreed with Justice Chipman's analysis of the *Charter* issue. Principally, she found that the appellants were not disabled, and that the denial of funding for IVF and ICSI was not discriminatory.

Like the trial judge, Justice Bateman considered that the denial of IVF and ICSI services in Nova Scotia medical policy was a denial of funding for specific treatments, rather than a denial of equality under the law. She also found that the appellants were not "excluded from mainstream society" in the way necessary to establish disability under the *Charter*. All decisions not to fund treatments inevitably result in someone suffering disadvantage, she found. However, this disadvantage alone did not make each person disabled.

Justice Bateman also ruled that the Nova Scotia policy was not discriminatory because it did not "function by stereotype or otherwise to perpetuate the view by society that the infertile is less deserving of concern, respect or consideration than others." Rather, like Justice Chipman, she considered the policy to be an example of the inevitable consequences of administering health care. Having ruled that the policy was not discriminatory, Justice Bateman did not need to consider whether it was justifiable in a free and democratic society.

Auton (Guardian ad litem of) v. British Columbia (Attorney General), (2003), 220 D.L.R. (4th) 411 (B.C.C.A.)

Summary prepared by Lisa Shields

This case was brought on behalf of a group of British Columbia children with autism or autism spectrum disorder (ASD). Their parents brought a legal action against the provincial government seeking funding for treatment of their children's conditions and a declaration that the government's refusal to provide such treatment was a violation of ss. 7 and 15 of the *Canadian Charter of Rights and Freedoms*. Autism or ASD is a neurobehavioural syndrome that leads to behavioural impairments in social interaction and communication. Without appropriate therapy, almost all individuals with autism or ASD will lead a life of isolation and will eventually be institutionalized.

The parents sought coverage for a specific type of early, intensive behavioural therapy called the "Lovaas Autism Treatment." This method of therapy had been credited with increasing the independence and level of functioning of autistic children. The parents argued that the treatment provided their children with the greatest possible opportunities in life and consequently significantly contributed to the children's well-being. Each of the children involved had already shown notable improvements using the Lovaas method. Unfortunately the treatment was extremely expensive and consequently one of the parents was unable to continue.

Under its health care legislation, the British Columbia government provided for the medically necessary treatment of all citizens, regardless of their ability to pay for the treatment. The government nonetheless refused to fund the Lovaas Autism Treatment because of a concern that providing treatment for autism or ASD would lead to other similar demands for coverage, thereby placing too great a financial strain on the provincial health care system. The government also questioned the efficacy of the Lovaas Autism Treatment and argued that any treatment was futile given that there is no cure for autism or ASD.

The B.C. Court of Appeal (BCCA) agreed with the parents that some sort of early, intensive behavioral therapy was medically necessary for children with autism or ASD, but this treatment did not have to be the Lovaas Autism Treatment. The BCCA found that the province's failure to provide such treatment was a violation of the children's rights guaranteed in s. 15(1) of the *Canadian Charter of Rights and Freedoms* to be free from discrimination based on disability.

The British Columbia health care plan itself was not flawed as it provided that necessary medical treatment would be provided to all residents. Instead, the *Charter* violation rested in the government's own interpretation of the law as excluding treatment for autism or ASD. Necessary medical treatment was being provided to children who did not have autism or ASD. Therefore, the government's failure to provide necessary medical treatment for children with autism or ASD constituted discrimination based on a disability, contrary to s. 15(1) of the *Charter*.

Furthermore, the BCCA rejected the government's argument that the treatment was too expensive, finding instead that it was likely cheaper to provide the treatment than to pay for the life-long care that would be required without treatment. Although the BCCA recognized the government's financial constraints, it felt that treatment could be provided without financially destroying the health care system. It was more important that the province remedy its discriminatory practice against children with autism or ASD than that it limit its health care spending.

PART 2

Decision-Making in Therapeutic Settings

Chapter 4   RESOURCE ALLOCATION

The Prostitute, the Playboy, and the Poet: Rationing Schemes for Organ Transplantation

George J. Annas

In the public debate about the availability of heart and liver transplants, the issue of rationing on a massive scale has been credibly raised for the first time in United States medical care. In an era of scarce resources, the eventual arrival of such a discussion was, of course, inevitable.[1] Unless we decide to ban heart and liver transplantation, or make them available to everyone, some rationing scheme must be used to choose among potential transplant candidates. The debate has existed throughout the history of medical ethics. Traditionally it has been stated as a choice between saving one of two patients, both of whom require the immediate assistance of the only available physician to survive.

National attention was focused on decisions regarding the rationing of kidney dialysis machines when they were first used on a limited basis in the late 1960s. As one commentator described the debate within the medical profession:

> Shall machines or organs go to the sickest, or to the ones with most promise of recovery; on a first-come, first-served basis; to the most "valuable" patient (based on wealth, education, position, what?); to the one with the most dependents; to women and children first; to those who can pay; to whom? Or should lots be cast, impersonally and uncritically?[2]

In Seattle, Washington, an anonymous screening committee was set up to pick who among competing candidates would receive the life-saving technology. One lay member of the screening committee is quoted as saying:

> The choices were hard ... I remember voting against a young woman who was a known prostitute. I found I couldn't vote for her, rather than another candidate, a young wife and mother. I also voted against a young man who, until he learned he had renal failure, had been a ne'er do-well, a real playboy. He promised he would reform his character, go back to school, and so on, if only he were selected for treatment. But I felt I'd lived long enough to know that a person like that won't really do what he was promising at the time.[3]

When the biases and selection criteria of the committee were made public, there was a general negative reaction against this type of arbitrary device. Two experts reacted to the "numbing accounts of how close to the surface lie the prejudices and mindless cliches that pollute the committee's deliberations," by concluding that the committee was "measuring persons in accordance with its own middle-class values." The committee process, they noted, ruled out "creative nonconformists" and made the Pacific Northwest "no place for a Henry David Thoreau with bad kidneys."[4]

To avoid having to make such explicit, arbitrary, "social worth" determinations, the Congress, in 1972, enacted legislation that provided federal funds for virtually all kidney dialysis and kidney transplantation procedures in the United States.[5] This decision, however, simply served to postpone the time when identical decisions will have to be made about candidates for heart and liver transplantation in a society that does not provide sufficient financial and medical resources to provide all "suitable" candidates with the operation.

There are four major approaches to rationing scarce medical resources: the market approach; the selection committee approach; the lottery approach; and the "customary" approach.[1]

THE MARKET APPROACH

The market approach would provide an organ to everyone who could pay for it with their own funds or private insurance. It puts a very high value on individual rights, and a very low value on equality and fairness. It has properly been criticized on a number of bases, including that the transplant technologies have been developed and are supported with public funds, that medical resources used for transplantation will not be available for higher priority care, and that financial success alone is an insufficient justification for demanding a medical procedure. Most telling is its complete lack of concern for fairness and equity.[6]

A "bake sale" or charity approach that requires the less financially fortunate to make public appeals for funding is demeaning to the individuals involved, and to society as a whole. Rationing by financial ability says we do not believe in equality, but believe that a price can and should be placed on human life and that it should be paid by the individual whose life is at stake. Neither belief is tolerable in a society in which income is inequitably distributed.

THE SELECTION COMMITTEE PROCESS

The Seattle Selection Committee is a model of the committee process. Ethics Committees set up in some hospitals to decide whether or not certain handicapped newborn infants should be given medical care may represent another.[7] These committees have developed because it was seen as unworkable or unwise to explicitly set forth the criteria on which selection decisions would be made. But only two results are possible, as Professor Guido Calabrezi has pointed out: either a pattern of decision-making will develop or it will not. If a pattern does develop (e.g., in Seattle, the imposition of middle-class values), then it can be articulated and those decision "rules" codified and used directly, without resort to the committee. If a pattern does not develop, the committee is vulnerable to the charge that it is acting arbitrarily, or dishonestly, and therefore cannot be permitted to continue to make such important decisions.[1]

In the end, public designation of a committee to make selection decisions on vague criteria will fail because it too closely involves the state and all members of society in explicitly preferring specific individuals over others, and in devaluing the interests those others have in living. It thus directly undermines, as surely as the market system does, society's view of equality and the value of human life.

THE LOTTERY APPROACH

The lottery approach is the ultimate equalizer which puts equality ahead of every other value. This makes it extremely attractive, since all comers have an equal chance at selection regardless of race, color, creed, or financial status. On the other hand, it offends our notions of efficiency and fairness since it makes *no* distinctions among such things as the strength of the desires of the candidates, their potential survival, and their quality of life. In this sense it is a mindless method of trying to solve society's dilemma which is caused by its unwillingness or inability to spend enough resources to make a lottery unnecessary. By making this macro spending decision evident to all, it also undermines society's view of the pricelessness of human life. A first-come, first-served system is a type of natural lottery since referral to a transplant program is generally random in time. Nonetheless, higher income groups have quicker access to referral networks and thus have an inherent advantage over the poor in a strict first-come, first-served system.[8, 9]

THE CUSTOMARY APPROACH

Society has traditionally attempted to avoid explicitly recognizing that we are making a choice not to save individual lives because it is too expensive to do so. As long as such decisions are not explicitly acknowledged, they can be tolerated by society. For example, until recently there was said to be a general understanding among general practitioners in Britain that individuals over age 55 suffering from end-stage kidney disease not be referred for dialysis or transplant. In 1984, however, this unwritten practice became highly publicized, with figures that showed a rate of new cases of end-stage kidney disease treated in Britain at 40 per million (versus the US figure of 80 per million) resulting in 1500–3000 "unnecessary deaths" annually.[10] This has, predictably, led to movements to enlarge the National Health Service budget to expand dialysis services to meet this need, a more socially acceptable solution than permitting the now publicly recognized situation to continue.

In the US, the customary approach permits individual physicians to select their patients on the basis of medical criteria or clinical suitability. This, however, contains much hidden social worth criteria. For example, one criterion, common in the transplant literature, requires an individual to have sufficient family support for successful aftercare. This discriminates against individuals without families and those who have become alienated from their families. The criterion may be relevant, but it is hardly medical.

Similar observations can be made about medical criteria that include IQ, mental illness, criminal records, employment, indigency, alcoholism, drug addiction, or geographical location. Age is perhaps more difficult, since it may be impressionistically related to outcome. But it is not medically logical to assume that an individual who is 49 years old is necessarily a better medical candidate for a transplant than one who is 50 years old. Unless specific examination of the characteristics of older persons that make them less desirable candidates is undertaken, such a cut off is arbitrary, and thus devalues the lives of older citizens. The same can be said of blanket exclusions of alcoholics and drug addicts.

In short, the customary approach has one great advantage for society and one great disadvantage: it gives us the illusion that we do not have to make choices; but the cost is mass deception, and when this deception is uncovered, we must deal with it either by universal entitlement or by choosing another method of patient selection.

A COMBINATION OF APPROACHES

A socially acceptable approach must be fair, efficient, and reflective of important social values. The most important values at stake in organ transplantation are fairness itself, equity in the sense of equality, and the value of life. To promote efficiency, it is important that no one receive a transplant unless they want one and are likely to obtain significant benefit from it in the sense of years of life at a reasonable level of functioning.

Accordingly, it is appropriate for there to be an initial screening process that is based *exclusively* on medical criteria designed to measure the probability of a successful transplant, i.e., one in which the patient survives for at least a number of years and is rehabilitated. There is room in medical criteria for social worth judgments, but there is probably no way to avoid this completely. For example, it has been noted that "in many respects social and medical criteria are inextricably intertwined" and that therefore medical criteria might "exclude the poor and disadvantaged because health and socioeconomic status are highly interdependent."[11] Roger Evans gives an example. In the End Stage Renal Disease Program, "those of lower socioeconomic status are likely to have multiple comorbid health conditions such as diabetes, hepatitis, and hypertension" making them both less desirable candidates and more expensive to treat.[11]

To prevent the gulf between the haves and have nots from widening, we must make every reasonable attempt to develop medical criteria that are objective and independent of social worth categories. One minimal way to approach this is to require that medical screening be reviewed and approved by an ethics committee with significant public representation, filed with a public agency, and made readily available to the public for comment. In the event that more than one hospital in a state or region is offering a particular transplant service, it would be most fair and efficient for individual hospitals to perform the initial medical screening themselves (based on the uniform, objective criteria), but to have all subsequent non-medical selection done by a method approved by a single selection committee composed of representatives of all hospitals engaged in the particular transplant procedure, as well as significant representation of the public at large.

As this implies, after the medical screening is performed, there may be more acceptable candidates in the "pool" than there are organs or surgical teams to go around. Selection among waiting candidates will then be necessary. This situation occurs now in kidney transplantion, but since the organ matching is much more sophisticated than in hearts and livers (permitting much more precise matching of organ and recipient), and since dialysis permits individuals to wait almost indefinitely for an organ without risking death, the situations are not close enough to permit use of the same matching criteria. On the other hand, to the extent that organs are specifically tissue- and size-matched and fairly distributed to the best matched candidate, the organ

distribution system itself will resemble a natural lottery.

When a pool of acceptable candidates is developed, a decision about who gets the next available, suitable organ must be made. We must choose between using a conscious, value-laden, social worth selection criterion (including a committee to make the actual choice), or some type of random device. In view of the unacceptability and arbitrariness of social worth criteria being applied, implicitly or explicitly, by committee, this method is neither viable nor proper. On the other hand, strict adherence to a lottery might create a situation where an individual who has only a one-in-four chance of living five years with a transplant (but who could survive another six months without one) would get an organ before an individual who could survive as long or longer, but who will die within days or hours if he or she is not immediately transplanted. Accordingly, the most reasonable approach seems to be to allocate organs on a first-come, first-served basis to members of the pool but permit individuals to "jump" the queue if the second level selection committee believes they are in immediate danger of death (but still have a reasonable prospect for long-term survival with a transplant) and the person who would otherwise get the organ can survive long enough to be reasonably assured that he or she will be able to get another organ.

The first-come, first-served method of basic selection (after a medical screen) seems the preferred method because it most closely approximates the randomness of a straight lottery without the obviousness of making equity the only promoted value. Some unfairness is introduced by the fact that the more wealthy and medically astute will likely get into the pool first, and thus be ahead in line, but this advantage should decrease sharply as public awareness of the system grows. The possibility of unfairness is also inherent in permitting individuals to jump the queue, but some flexibility needs to be retained in the system to permit it to respond to reasonable contingencies.

We will have to face the fact that should the resources devoted to organ transplantation be limited (as they are now and are likely to be in the future), at some point it is likely that significant numbers of individuals will die in the pool, waiting for a transplant. Three things can be done to avoid this: 1) medical criteria can be made stricter, perhaps by adding a more rigorous notion of "quality" of life to longevity and prospects for rehabilitation; 2) resources devoted to transplantation and organ procurement can be increased; or 3) individuals can be persuaded not to attempt to join the pool.

Of these three options, only the third has the promise of both conserving resources and promoting autonomy. While most persons medically eligible for a transplant would probably want one, some would not—at least if they understood all that was involved, including the need for a lifetime commitment to daily immunosuppression medications, and periodic medical monitoring for rejection symptoms. Accordingly, it makes public policy sense to publicize the risks and side effects of transplantation, and to require careful explanations of the procedure be given to prospective patients *before* they undergo medical screening. It is likely that by the time patients come to the transplant center they have made up their minds and would do almost anything to get the transplant. Nonetheless, if there are patients who, when confronted with all the facts, would voluntarily elect not to proceed, we enhance both their own freedom and the efficiency and cost-effectiveness of the transplantation system by screening them out as early as possible.

CONCLUSION

Choices among patients that seem to condemn some to death and give others an opportunity to survive will always be tragic. Society has developed a number of mechanisms to make such decisions more acceptable by camouflaging them. In an era of scarce resources and conscious cost containment, such mechanisms will become public, and they will be usable only if they are fair and efficient. If they are not so perceived, we will shift from one mechanism to another in an effort to continue the illusion that tragic choices really don't have to be made, and that we can simultaneously move toward equity of access, quality of services, and cost containment without any challenges to our values. Along with the prostitute, the playboy, and the poet, we all need to be involved in the development of an access model to extreme and expensive medical technologies with which we can live.

Notes

1. Calabresi G, Bobbitt P: *Tragic Choices.* New York: Norton, 1978.
2. Fletcher J: Our shameful waste of human tissue. *In:* Cutler DR (ed): *The Religious Situation.* Boston: Beacon Press, 1969; 223–252.
3. Quoted in Fox R, Swazey J: *The Courage to Fail.* Chicago: Univ of Chicago Press, 1974; 232.
4. Sanders & Dukeminier: Medical advance and legal lag: hemodialysis and kidney transplantation. *UCLA L Rev* 1968; 15:357.
5. Rettig RA: The policy debate on patient care financing for victims of end stage renal disease. *Law & Contemporary Problems* 1976; 40:196.
6. President's Commission for the Study of Ethical Problems in Medicine: *Securing Access to Health Care.* US Govt Printing office, 1983; 25.
7. Annas GJ: Ethics committees on neonatal care: substantive protection or procedural diversion? *Am J Public Health* 1984; 74:843–845.
8. Bayer R: Justice and health care in an era of cost containment: allocating scarce medical resources. *Soc Responsibility* 1984; 9:37–52.
9. Annas GJ: Allocation of artificial hearts in the year 2002: *Minerva v National Health Agency. Am J Law Med* 1977; 3:59–76.
10. Commentary: UK's poor record in treatment of renal failure. *Lancet* July 7, 1984; 53.
11. Evans R: Health care technology and the inevitability of resource allocation and rationing decisions, Part II. *JAMA* 1983; 249:2208, 2217.

Air-Support Treatment: A Case Study in the Ethics of Allocating an Expensive Treatment

Benjamin Freedman, James Gilbert, and Lois A. Kaltsounakis

Charm ache with air ...

William Shakespeare, *Much Ado about Nothing*

A HOSPITAL UNDER PRESSURE

The first use of air-support treatment in the Jewish General Hospital (JGH) in Montreal gave notice of the sorts of issues—ethical, administrative, and personal—that would be associated with it thereafter. Mrs. S, a patient in her late sixties with advanced senile dementia of the Alzheimer's type, was being treated in orthopedics for a broken hip. In the course of a lengthy convalescence, she developed pressure sores that did not respond to ordinary nursing measures.

A grandson, acting as family spokesperson for Mrs. S, conducted his own investigation into treatment options and launched a successful pressure campaign resulting in the hospital's leasing, and then purchasing, an air-support bed. Surgery to cover Mrs. S's deepest pressure sores with skin grafts, allowing her removal from this expensive apparatus, was refused.

After many months on this bed without healing, the family was informed that Mrs. S would be removed from it so that another patient, in greater need and with greater prospects for improvement, might benefit from it. The family, a demanding group that had often, in the past, used arguments, community pressure, and threats of litigation to get its own way, informed the hospital that it would sue if Mrs. S was not continued on air-support treatment. Among the morals of this story: the hospital needs a rational policy in order to ethically allocate this particular resource.

THE INSTITUTIONAL CONTEXT

The Jewish General Hospital, in common with other hospitals in Canada (and especially Quebec), is a natural laboratory of institutional allocation of health-care resources. A 628-bed McGill University teaching hospital with a very elderly catchment population (of 195,000 patient-days provided last year, 55,000 were for long-term care), it operates within a tight global operating budget. For the year ending March 31, 1990, the JGH's budget was set by the provincial ministry of health at $102 million (in Canadian funds: all following dollar figures refer to Canadian costs unless otherwise noted). From that budget, whose distribution is the hospital's responsibility rather than the government's, all operational needs of the hospital must be satisfied; or in other words, each hospital service and amenity is in budgetary competition with all others. Success in operating within the budget is rewarded: the hospital is permitted to keep any surplus funds and has been given a further grant of around one million dollars as a *cout de système,* an adjustment on behalf of meeting advancing technology and serving an ever-more-needy population. And failure is punished: a deficit is met by a governmentally imposed freeze for the following year on construction, equipment purchase, and the funding of new programs. Given the already fierce competition among existing hospital services, new programs and expensive technologies such as air-support treatment need to be rigorously scrutinized before their introduction into the hospital.

THE AILMENT

As appealing as the prospect of lying in bed for extended periods of time may sometimes be, there are serious side effects to this activity. The only portions of skin on the human body capable of withstanding pressure over 40 mmHg for prolonged periods are the soles of the feet; normal capillary pressure elsewhere ranges from 25 to 35 mmHg. Lying in bed causes the weight to be distributed over other body surfaces with bony prominences (hip, coccyx, heels, and so on) unable to withstand prolonged pressure. With more pressure *on* the capillaries than *in* them, circulation slows, and blood flow is reduced or obstructed. Unless the external pressure is relieved, tissue damage results due to the lack of oxygen.

A dermal ulcer (in prior parlance, decubitus ulcer or pressure ulcer) is the end stage of damage to the skin and its underlying tissue. The risks of developing a dermal ulcer are much greater for seriously ill or debilitated patients because of their immobility that causes pressure on the capillaries, and because their condition (for example, dehydration) may itself contribute to having considerably reduced capillary pressure. It has been estimated that 3 to 5 percent of all patients admitted to hospitals will develop a dermal ulcer; estimated costs of treatment range from $5,000 to $35,000 (US) per ulcer.[1] Over the past year (April 1989 to March 1990) JGH had almost sixty patients who had either stage 3 or stage 4 dermal ulcers, making them priority candidates for the treatment discussed below.

THE THERAPY

As early as 1873, experiments were being conducted on ways to relieve pressure to prevent tissue damage.[2] Over the years, various materials such as moss, straw, feathers, sand, springs, rubber, plastic, foams, and plaster of paris have been used for pressure relief.

In 1961, John Scales started experiments to study the support of the body by temperature controlled air at pressures that would not cause undesirable physiological changes.[3] From this early work it became apparent that patient-support systems, based on the principle of air support but with the air contained and separated from the patient by a membrane permeable to water vapor, could be developed. The low air-loss bed system first came into use at Scales's institution in Stanmore, England, in March 1971.[4] Air-fluidized beds have been available since 1969. These beds contain ceramic beads covered by a closely woven polyester sheet. Warm, pressurized air is forced throughout the particulate mass in order to make the particles behave as a fluid. The patient "floats" on the bed without pressure on the bony prominences. These beds provide an ideal environment for prevention, as well as an excellent treatment for skin breakdown.[5] This therapy may also serve a useful role in the treatment of cancer patients (by providing pain relief) and patients with burns (by permitting skin regeneration). The disadvantage of this therapy, however, is its cost. Air-support therapies vary in technique and technology; purchase price of the beds ranges from $35,000 to $150,000. Maintenance contracts average $3,500 annually. The cost of replacement pillows is $4,142 every second year. The daily rental cost ranges from $65 to $150 depending on the type of bed, and some companies add an installation charge of $100.[6]

These figures put in perspective the issue of allocation posed by air-support beds. The beds are expensive in absolute terms to purchase and maintain, and further problems are posed when an unbudgeted rental is required. These equipment costs are borne by the hospital's budget for nursing, which represents just under half the global hospital budget. However, that nursing budget itself is dominated by personnel costs, which consume well over 85 percent of the total. The average cost per patient-day for the past year was $524, so that a rental at JGH adds 18 percent (based on $100 per day) to the expense of a day of care. Dolezal and his colleagues, estimating air-support therapy to add only 4 to 6 percent to the total hospital bill, state that "the additional expense is justifiable considering the safety of postoperative healing and the comfortable environment provided for these patients."[7] The constraints within which JGH operates do not allow them the latitude to justify costs in this fashion.

Because the JGH has only one air-support therapy bed that has many uses and an increasing patient demand, there is always a queue. In order to ethically decide the order of the queue, a sound policy of allocation of this particular resource is needed.

ETHICAL ALLOCATION I: PATIENT-CENTERED FACTORS

A justifiable scheme for the allocation of medical resources must involve two components. It must provide technically sound patient-centered decisions. That is, it must incorporate a realistic appraisal of the resource in relationship to the needs of the specific patient in question, to ensure that the resource is being used wisely and efficiently. The scheme must also be sensitive to the broad context within which the resource is to be provided. Patients' rights must be respected while the needs and interests of the institution and the population it serves are accommodated. Ethical reasoning is relevant to both of these dimensions of sound allocative policy.

When a patient is admitted to the hospital, a nurse does a skin and wound assessment within the first twenty-four hours. Preventive measures are implemented for patients identified as at risk for dermal ulcer development. Risk factors can be divided into environmental factors (for example, pressure, shear, and friction) and systemic factors (such as age, weight, mobility, nutritional status, moisture problems—incontinence and drainage—and predisposing diseases).

Generally, the greater the number of factors present, the greater the risk. All dermal ulcers are identified according to stage using criteria adapted from Shea.[8] Because tissue breaks down more readily in the presence of systemic risk factors, continued nursing assessment is critical. This initial assessment, along with the factors presented below, forms the basis of what therapy, if any, will be used on the patient.

Patients with ulcers at higher stages usually receive priority for air-support treatment.

A resource is wasted unless given to those who need and may benefit from it. Patients who are not bedfast do not need air support; they prevent and heal dermal ulcers by walking around. Likewise, bedfast patients who are not immobile can turn themselves to prevent and heal dermal ulcers. Because air-support therapy is the optimal treatment for and only for bedfast patients who cannot be positioned off their ulcers, it should be restricted to them.

It is obvious that to qualify for air-support therapy the patient must be able to benefit from it. One class of patients that does not qualify includes those that have the necessary ailments but have such poor nutritional (especially protein) intake that healing cannot take place.[9]

When we talk about a patient "benefiting" from a particular treatment, we usually require that the patient experience the benefit. This is always the case if the benefit received from a treatment is the reduction of pain. It is part of the logic of the word pain that it is experienced. (One cannot say "I am in pain yet I have no sensation of it.") What if the goal of the treatment is simply to heal a dermal ulcer? A patient whose mental status is so compromised that she could not experience the benefit of having her ulcer healed would, in a technical sense, still be benefiting from having the ulcer healed. But unexperienced benefit is of little value: were someone to open up a bank account in a man's name, without his knowing it, and deposit a million dollars in it, he would benefit from this. Even if it never came to his attention that he had this money, he would technically be a millionaire. It would, however, be a useless benefit if, unaware of the transaction, he never spent the money or at least had a chance to revel in the fact that he was so rich. Likewise for the patient who does not experience the benefit of a particular treatment. We therefore choose to exclude patients who cannot and will never experience the benefit of air-support therapy from this costly treatment.

In allocating this particular resource we are forced to address the issue of sometimes conflicting medical goals. Benefit from air-support therapy we have seen can fall into two analytically distinct categories: healing of the dermal ulcer and relief from pain or discomfort. These usually go together, but not always: a stage 4 ulcer causes such extensive neural damage that the patient experiences little or no pain or discomfort. For this patient, benefit from air-support therapy means nothing more than the healing of an ulcer. The reciprocal of this, the patient with an unresponsive ulcer who feels more comfortable on air support, was the case with Mrs. S.

There are many ways of relieving pain other than using air-support therapy. Therefore, policy must ordinarily assign relative priority to the goal of healing. The presence of intractable pain, however, can still be a decisive factor in determining allocation. If two patients are equally qualified for air-support therapy, yet only one of them is experiencing intractable pain that can be relieved by air support, then both reason and emotion dictate that this patient should receive the therapy.

A final principle: a patient that will probably die before the objective of air-support treatment can be realized should be excluded. The justification of this harsh principle follows from the same means-end rationality as has been applied to the nursing evaluation: there is no justification to instituting medical measures from which benefit will not be derived. However, in applying this principle, attention must be paid to the specific treatment goal for which air support is proposed. When air support is proposed as the appropriate comfort measure for a person with, for example, bone metastases, imminent death should not be an exclusion….

ETHICAL ALLOCATION II: ISSUES AND PRINCIPLES OF CONTEXT

The patient-centered level of consideration establishes that the resource may be justified vis-à-vis a particular patient. But without considering the context of the allocation, one could not conclude whether that would represent the best use of the resource, or whether another patient is entitled to the resource. The two-party, doctor–patient model of decisions, so common in medical ethics, is inadequate to this purpose of institutional allocative decisions.

The first issue needing to be addressed is whether any patient has a *right* to the scarce resource, or in other words, is any patient or group of patients *entitled* to air-support treatment? The fundamental importance of this question is expressed in the philosopher's maxim, "Rights are trumps." In our understanding of ethics and jurisprudence, satisfying a person's right takes precedence over all other claims.

We believe that no patient has a right, legal or moral, to receive air-support treatment. Legally, the ministry does not compel the hospital to make this treatment available to any person. While Canadians by law possess a positive right to "medically necessary treatment,"[10] considerable discretion in describing the boundaries of this concept is provided and necessary. "Medically necessary treatment" in practice extends well beyond the concept of "minimally decent health care," a concept appealed to by American theorists;[11] but it does not encompass a patient's right to optimal treatment, with no regard to cost.

These points, while valid legally and administratively, do not settle the ethical question: is a patient *morally* entitled to air-support treatment? We believe not, for any argument supporting such a right would need to surmount the following obstacle. Precisely because of the peremptory, powerful character of rights, a liberal social scheme must formulate them so that the rights of each are compatible with the right of all. Jurists say, for example, that one's right to freedom of action ends at the tip of someone else's nose—that is, at the point where the exercise of the right infringes the rights of another. The difficulty faced by claiming that a patient has a positive right to some treatment is that the right imposes a correlative duty upon the institution to pay for the satisfaction of that right.

Air-support therapy in our allocative scheme is in competition with all other forms of treatment. Patient candidates are in a zero-sum game with the medical needs of all other patients; one patient's gain is another's loss. With the possible exception of emergency services,[12] no medical treatment within the hospital possesses such a degree of need and urgency as to automatically trump all of its competitors—precisely the condition that would be described were we to say that a patient has a *right* to a particular treatment.

One other possibility, though, requires analysis. Although a patient is not entitled to an air bed paid for by the hospital, he or she may have another source of entitlement. An insurance policy might include this treatment within its coverage, in which case the patient is entitled to have the hospital rent a bed with its costs reimbursed by insurance. Some private health insurers in Canada, such as Blue Cross, have agreed to cover the costs of air-support therapy after case evaluation; similar coverage may be provided by governmental insurers that cover workers' and automobile accidents. This suggests a further criterion of exclusion: the hospital will not pay for air-support treatment on behalf of a person entitled to have it provided from any other source. These persons are to obtain the funding for the treatment from the other source, in effect removing them from the hospital queue.

We have denied that a patient has a right to air-support treatment funded by JGH. Rather, within our understanding, a patient may have a *claim* to that treatment. It is the job of ethics to assess how well grounded is the claim, relative to other claimants.

What if a person is a candidate for, but not yet eligible for, air support provided by the hospital, and he wishes to pay for it out of his own funds? Should he be permitted to buy his way out of the fate shared in common by other patients?

The question has somewhat more bite within the Canadian system, with its egalitarian commitment to the provision of health care, than within the United States. One great political advantage of a universal entitlement to health care is that all are in the same boat—the rich as well as the poor, the politically powerful as well as the disenfranchised—with the former group's self-interest effectively satisfying the latter's needs.

Nonetheless, we tend to favor this exemption. As argued above, there is no entitlement to air-support therapy *per se*; therefore, permitting a patient to buy his way off the queue does not violate universality as it is imperfectly realized at present. And, this exemption is compatible with such egalitarian views as those held by Rawls and his followers.[13] When a patient is allowed to buy his way off the queue, he is being treated in a way that satisfies Rawls's difference principle, allowing unequal treatment that will redound to the benefit of the least advantaged. In our context, the "least advantaged" person in question is the last person on the queue, and his or her situation is improved because one person ahead has left the line. For these reasons we conclude that one who prepares his own bed—or pays for it—can lie in it.

Even granted that a patient initially has no right to air-support treatment, does the fact that he or she is now in it ground an entitlement to continue? It is often the case that a person is not initially entitled to some good, but, once the good has been offered, the supplier is duty bound to continue. A person has no right to be seen by Dr. Zhivago, but once the doctor has begun to treat her (and perhaps even as soon as he has agreed to see her), a doctor–patient relationship has been established that generally justifies her expectation that it will continue. In general, one who undertakes to supply health care must continue. Does this principle apply to air-support therapy, creating a right to continue on behalf of patients beginning the therapy?

We have decided to the contrary. Just as the patient's rights are not violated when air-support treatment is withheld, so are they not violated when it is withdrawn. This view accords with the general consensus regarding life-support equipment, stated by the President's Commission for the Study of Ethical Problems in Medicine among others, that there is no decisive moral difference between withholding and withdrawing medical treatment.[14] (That there is no difference in principle is assured by the arbitrary way in which we "count" medical treatments. Is each drop in the IV, or each cycle on the respirator, to count as a separate initiation of treatment? In the case of air support, is the treatment reinstituted each time the patient is replaced on the bed after a bath, or after the pillows have been changed?)

Moreover, while there is no significant *moral* difference of principle between withholding and withdrawing a treatment, there are significant *practical* differences that suggest that, in general, the advantage lies with withdrawing rather than withholding the treatment in question. The reason is that a treatment's worth to a specific patient can often only be accurately assessed following a trial period of treatment.

The President's Commission suggested that those institutions that feel comfortable in withholding ventilation from patients, but have difficulty in withdrawing it, are prone to two sorts of errors. First, patients who had been put on ventilation, for whom it is no longer appropriate, continue treatment at a cost of anguish to the patient and at a financial cost to the institution. And second, for fear of being locked into maintaining a patient indefinitely on ventilation, institutions never institute a trial period in others who might in fact have a reversible condition. A regime that permits withholding treatment while prohibiting withdrawing it overtreats the first set of patients while undertreating the second, because it has no way of trying a treatment to see how it goes and deciding on that basis.

The same points apply to air-support therapy. We need to recognize that a treatment that has proven futile may be withdrawn, for the same reason that one that promises to be futile may be withheld. The point in fact applies with even greater force in our case, because of the scarcity of the resource and since the treatment period may be fairly lengthy.[15]

Because there are always several patients in the hospital who could benefit to some degree from air-support therapy, efficiency demands that the bed always be in use, assigned to the patient with the greatest need. In the past, however, the bed has sometimes been unused, for fear that the patient in the greatest need would linger on it indefinitely, locking out other patients whose improvement on air support

would be more rapid and assured. This situation should not recur in an institution that allocates the bed rationally, rather than by reference to a fallacious presumption of a right to continue.

One last consideration flows naturally from the above discussion. A bed treating two is more efficient than one helping a single patient, and so some allowance for the stage of the candidates' ulcers needs to be made in the evaluation process. In general, it would seem that priority should be given to Patient A—with stage 4 ulcers (that extend through skin and fat into muscle and/or bone)—*unless* it is the case that patients B and C, with stage 3 ulcers (extending through skin and fat only), could be prevented from progressing to stage 4 in the same treatment interval that it would have taken A to regress back to stage 3. While rationality seems to demand that we think about the intervention as secondary prevention as well as treatment, inherent prognostic uncertainties, as well as interstaff and interservice political realities, may make it difficult to incorporate this "soft" factor into evaluating priority access.

CONCLUSION

Our attempt to formulate an ethically justified approach to the allocation of air-support treatment presents a means for defining those persons who are eligible for the treatment (those who are "on the queue"), and a basis for considering the relative weight of claim to treatment on the bed of eligible persons.

As a contribution to practical ethics, proposed policy must be clearly useful as well as justified. We feel the deliberation that goes into constructing a policy is itself useful, in forcing the reexamination of preconceptions and the clarification of hospital practice. The points made about defining need and potential for benefit, for example, are nothing more than organized common sense. The same may be said, though, about good nursing or hospital administration; and, there is clearly merit in organizing common sense.

Within our deliberations, we tried first to identify and track the relevant points raised about who should have access to this bed, and then to formalize that within a policy. It is fair to ask, "What advantage is there in having such a policy? Isn't the proposed policy the same old considerations, dressed up so they will appear decent in public?" The objection ignores what may be the chief advantage a policy statement may offer. By definition, the allocation of scarce resources involves conflict, often expressed in interpersonal tension or intrapersonal ambivalence. In the heat of a situation, some principles of choice that had earlier been rejected become appealing once again; others, that had in a calmer moment proven fair, may be forgotten. It is then that a policy is most needed.[16]

The role of philosophy in formulating these sorts of policies is worthy of further thought. In this case, it was most useful playing a critical rather than constructive role, showing that some ideas such as the right of a patient to be treated on air support or the entitlement to continuing treatment were spurious. It might be pleasing to think that the cure for philosophy is more (and better) philosophy; less happy is the thought that the final cure for philosophy might be no philosophy at all.

Yet it seems to us that this criticism asks too much of philosophy. The yearning for constructive principles ultimately rests on the idea that there are right answers to the distribution of scarce resources that philosophy should discover or validate. This may be too much to hope for. Perhaps all that can be done is to eliminate the wrong responses, leaving discretionary choice within a range of equally justified, yet equally problematic answers.

Acknowledgments

The authors appreciate the assistance provided by Charles Kaplan, Director of Finance, Jewish General Hospital, and Patricia Rawlings, Quality Assurance Coordinator, JGH.

Notes

1. C. Van Ness and C.A. Sacramento, "The Implementation of a Quality Assurance Study and Program to Reduce the Incidence of Hospital Acquired Pressure Ulcers," *Journal of Enterosotomal Therapy* 16, no. 2 (1989): 61–64.

2. J. Scales, "Pressure Sore Prevention," *Care Science and Practice* 1 (June 1982): 9–17.

3. J.T. Scales, H.F. Lunn, PA. Leneid, *et al.,* "The Prevention and Treatment of Pressure Sores Using Air Support Systems," *Paraplegia* 12 (August 1974): 118–31.

4. Scales, "Pressure Sore Prevention."

5. Whether these beds would continue to play a necessary role even when optimal nursing care is provided is a matter of professional dispute. See B.L. Moody, J.E. Fanale, M. Thompson, *et al.,* "Impact of Staff Education on Pressure Sore Development in Elderly Hospitalized Patients," *Archives of Internal Medicine* 148 (October 1988): 2241–43.

6. Information on prices as of summer 1990 was provided by the sales office of Kinetic Concepts Inc., whose help is gratefully acknowledged.

7. R Dolezal, M. Cohen, and R. Schultz, "The Use of Clinitron Therapy Unit in the Immediate Postoperative Care of Pressure Ulcers," *Annals of Plastic Surgery* 14 (January 1985): 36.

8. J.D. Shea, "Pressure Sores: Classification and Management," *Clinical Orthopedics* 112 (1975): 89–100; R. Bennett, M.F. Bettantoni, and J. Ouslander, "Air Fluidized Bed Treatment of Nursing Home Patients with Pressure Sores," *Journal of the American Geriatrics Society* 37, no. 3 (1989): 235–42.

9. R.M. Allman, J. Walker, M. Hart, and C. Laprade, "Air-Fluidized Beds or Conventional Therapy for Pressure Sores: A Randomized Trial," *Annals of Internal Medicine* 107, no. 5 (1987): 641–48. For a contrary view see Bennett, Bettantoni, and Ouslander, "Air Fluidized Bed Treatment."

10. *Statutes of Canada,* "Medical Care Act."

11. See, for example, discussion in H.T. Engelhardt, Jr., *The Foundations of Bioethics* (New York: Oxford University Press, 1986), chap. 8.

12. Were the hospital in the position of a closed system, the sole supplier of service to members of the catchment area, presumably emergency services would definitely trump alternative hospital services. That condition is not present for JGH, which is, for example, permitted to impose an ambulance ban when its allocated emergency services are overloaded, resulting in patients being sent to other hospitals in the Montreal municipal community.

13. J. Rawls, *A Theory of Justice* (Cambridge, MA: Harvard University Press, 1971); R. Green, "Health Care Justice in Contract Theory

Perspective," in *Ethics and Health Policy,* ed. R. Veatch and R. Branson (Cambridge, MA: Ballinger, 1976); N. Daniels, "Health Care Needs and Distributive Justice," *Philosophy and Public Affairs* 10, no. 2 (1981): 146–79.

14. President's Commission for the Study of Ethical Problems in Medicine and Biomedical and Behavioral Research, *Decisions to Forgo Life-Sustaining Treatment* (Washington, DC: Government Printing Office, 1983); G. Povar, "Withdrawing and Withholding Therapy: Putting Ethics into Practice," *Journal of Clinical Ethics* 1 (Spring 1990): 50–56; J. Burden, B. Freedman, A. Gelb, "Ethical and Family Management Problems in the Intensive Care Unit—An Illustrative Case," *Canadian Journal of Anaesthesia* 34, no. 3 (1987–1988): 274–79.

15. Shea, "Pressure Sores."

16. B. Freedman, "The Last Bed in the ICU," in *Cases in Bioethics,* ed. C. Levine (New York: St. Martin's Press, 1989), 229–31.

Murray Menkes v. The General Manager, the Ontario Health Insurance Plan

Health Services and Review Board

SUMMARY

This is an appeal from a decision of the General Manager of the Ontario Health Insurance Plan ("OHIP") which denied the Appellant's request for full payment of the costs of a living donor renal transplant performed at the Mayo Clinic in Rochester, Minnesota.

BACKGROUND

The Appellant, Murray Menkes, was diagnosed with renal failure in October 1998. By February 1999, the Appellant required dialysis treatments three times per week. The Appellant's Nephrologist, Dr. Edward Cole, suggested kidney transplant. Dr. Cole is Director of the Nephrology Division and Director, Renal Transplantation at the Toronto General Hospital. The Appellant was placed on the transplant list for a cadaveric organ, but was informed that waiting times for organs could be lengthy (three to four years), since there are many more individuals awaiting transplant than there are suitable organs available from the donor pool.

Because of the shortage of cadaver donors, kidney transplant programs are increasingly tuning to living donor transplants, in which a kidney from a living donor—frequently a rela-

tive of the recipient—is transplanted into the recipient. During the course of the Appellant's dialysis treatments, the Appellant's live-in housekeeper came forward and offered to donate one of her kidneys to the Appellant. The housekeeper has been employed by the Appellant's family for a number of years and is described by the Appellant as being very much a part of his extremely close extended family. The Appellant apparently was extremely moved by his housekeeper's offer, but initially was reluctant to accept. He ultimately decided to explore the viability of this living-donor transplant option, however, when she continued to make her offer.

The Appellant and the housekeeper (hereafter referred to as "the donor") underwent a series of tests to determine whether she was a suitable match for purposes of the renal transplant. The work-ups showed that the donor was a good candidate, and they proceeded to move forward with the "living donor transplant." In addition to medical testing, the Appellant and the donor were also interviewed by the transplant program's social worker. Among other things, the social worker apparently questioned the donor about her motives in offering her kidney to the Appellant. Due to ethical concerns, including issues relating to voluntary consent and the potential for financial compensation for organ donation in these circumstances (employer–employee relationship), the donor apparently signed an agreement stating that she would not be compensated for the donation of her kidney, and confirming that she was offering to donate her kidney on her own initiative.

The Appellant testified that transplant surgery was scheduled for August of 1999, then postponed until early September 1999. Shortly before the scheduled surgery date, the hospital called the Appellant to inform him that it would not perform the transplant due to ethical concerns. The evidence also indicates that the ethical concerns related specifically to the employer–employee relationship that exists between the recipient and donor. Among other things, in the context of organ donation such a relationship gives rise to issues relating to the potential for compensation, as well as issues relating to the imbalance of power between recipient and donor. Unfortunately in this case there is very little evidence detailing the ethics review process, the guidelines, if any, that are used in such ethical reviews within the Toronto General Hospital or in Ontario transplant programs more broadly, or the specific reasons for the transplant program's decision in the Appellant's case.

According to the Appellant, the hospital arrived at its decision following review by an internal ethics review committee, as well as an ethics consultant from Chicago. A letter from Dr. Cole dated December 6, 2000 and submitted in support of this hearing described the decision-making process as follows:

> This man received a living donor transplant from an employee which was done at the Mayo Clinic in Rochester, Minnesota. He had come forward to me with this potential living donor and subsequently both donor and recipient had extensive workups at the Toronto General Hospital. A concern arose because the donor was an employee of the recipient. This was reviewed by several ethical consultants as well as mem-

bers of the Kidney Transplant Program at the Toronto General Hospital. In the end, it was felt that it would be impossible for the donor to freely give a kidney to her employer with no possibility of compensation. Accordingly, the Program declined to do the transplant.

Following the Toronto Hospital's refusal to perform the transplant, the Appellant asked his physicians if the operation could be performed elsewhere. He contacted a physician at St. Michael's Hospital who apparently said he would refuse to perform the transplant on the same grounds. Additional inquiries to transplant programs at the London Health Sciences Centre and a Vancouver hospital yielded a similar response.

The Appellant also explored both cadaveric and living donor transplant at three transplant programs in the United States, including Jackson Memorial, the University of Pittsburgh and the Mayo Clinic. In September 1999 the Appellant and donor traveled to Rochester Minnesota to attend the Mayo Clinic where they underwent medical testing and were interviewed by one of the hospital's social workers. The Appellant indicated that the nature of the recipient–donor relationship was raised by the hospital, but the Mayo Clinic ultimately was satisfied that the donor was acting on compassionate grounds and agreed to perform the transplant surgery. The living donor renal transplant surgery was performed at the Mayo Clinic in October 1999. The Appellant received additional out-patient and surgical services at the Mayo Clinic between November 1999 and April 2000. The surgery was successful, and Dr. Cole indicates that the Appellant has had an excellent result.

Dr. Cole completed a "Prior Approval Application for Full Payment of Insured Out-of-Country Health Services" on behalf of the Appellant. It appears that the prior approval application was signed by the Appellant in September 2000 (prior to the out-of-country treatment), but was not signed by Dr. Cole until December 2000. Dr. Cole completed the form to show a clinical diagnosis of "endstage renal disease requiring renal transplant." The proposed out-of-country treatment for which payment is requested is stated as renal transplant.

Dr. Cole completed both Part A of the Prior Approval Application (for services performed in Ontario) and Part 4B (for services not performed in Ontario). The first questions posed in Part 4A address the issue of delay. They ask:

> Is this service required out of Canada to avoid a delay in obtaining the service in Ontario that would:
>
> (a) result in death?
> (b) result in medically significant irreversible tissue damage?

Dr. Cole's responses to the questions posed in Part A indicate that the service is not required out of Canada to avoid a delay in obtaining the service in Ontario that would result in death. Dr. Cole did not answer "yes" or "no" to the question relating to tissue damage, however he has written the following in the lines below: "Living donor renal transplant would not be done here because of ethical concerns re: donor. Waiting time for cadaver transplant (3–4 yr) might well have increased morbidity."

In Part 4B Dr. Cole indicates that the treatment is generally accepted in Ontario as appropriate for a person in these medical circumstances, that the treatment is not considered experimental, and that it is not performed in Ontario by an identical or equivalent procedure.

Dr. David Cow, Medical Consultant with the Ministry of Health and Long Term Care, denied the Appellant's request for payment in a letter to Dr. Cole dated January 23, 2001. In denying the Appellant's request for full funding of the out-of-country health services Dr. Cow wrote, in part:

> … Review of available information indicates that while this particular transplant scenario is not considered ethical in Ontario, renal transplants are available at a number of centres in Ontario.
>
> In view of the preceding, I regret to inform you that this request for prior

approval of full payment for health services outside of Canada has been denied….

The Appellant appeals that decision….

ISSUES

The broad issue before the Board is whether the services for which the Appellant seeks full funding are insured services under the *Health Insurance Act*. To answer this question, the Board must determine whether the services in question meet the criteria and conditions for insured out-of-country medical services on a prior approval basis….

Specifically, in this appeal the Board must consider the following issues:

1. Are the services generally accepted in Ontario as appropriate for a person in the same medical circumstances as the Appellant?
2. Are the services not performed in Ontario?
3. If the services are performed in Ontario, would a delay in obtaining treatment in Ontario result in death or medically significant irreversible tissue damage?

REASONS

… The Board is of the view that in cases involving organ donation, in determining whether the transplant is generally accepted in Ontario as appropriate for a person in the same medical circumstances, the phrase "medical circumstances" encompasses both recipient and donor, and the relationship between them. As Dr. Fisher noted in response to a question from the Board, "there is no transplant without a donor." The Board is also of the view that the notion of "medical circumstances" also incorporates the "ethical" aspects of the particular transplant scenario at issue, since ethical review and ethical decision-making constitute an essential part of medical decision-making in relation to organ transplant. However, while ethical considerations are critical to the issue of general acceptance in this case, the Board's role is not to "re-decide" the underlying ethical issue, but rather to determine whether the treatment meets the criteria and conditions under the *Health Insurance Act.* In this case the Board must first determine whether there is sufficient evidence to support a finding that this particular transplant scenario is generally accepted in Ontario as appropriate....

The Prior Approval Application asks the referring physician to address the issue of general acceptance directly. The first question in Part 4B of the application asks, "is the treatment generally accepted in Ontario as appropriate for a person in these medical circumstances?" The completing physician, Dr. Cole, checked the box marked "yes" in response to this question. He also indicates that the treatment is performed in Ontario by an identical or equivalent procedure.

Taken alone, Dr. Cole's response to the first question on the prior approval application suggests that the treatment that the Appellant received at the Mayo clinic is generally accepted as appropriate in Ontario for a person in the same medical circumstances as the Appellant. However, there is other evidence suggesting that this is not the case and that Dr. Cole's response to the question of general acceptance relates to renal transplant generally, as opposed to the specific circumstances of this particular transplant scenario. In Part 4B of the Prior Approval Application Dr. Cole goes on to note that this living donor renal transplant would not be done in Ontario because of ethical concerns relating to the donor's relationship to the recipient. He notes further that two Toronto centres declined to do the transplant that was performed at the Mayo Clinic. The Appellant testified that transplant programs in London, Ontario and Vancouver, British Columbia also indicated that they would refuse to perform the surgery on ethical grounds.

The evidence in this case suggests that while renal transplantation is generally accepted as appropriate in the treatment of end-stage renal disease, this particular renal transplant scenario is not generally accepted in Ontario as appropriate on the basis of ethical considerations arising from the recipient–donor relationship.

The only evidence that would support a finding that this particular treatment scenario is generally accepted in Ontario as appropriate is Dr. Cole's affirmative response (provided by checking a box marked "yes") to the question posed on the prior approval application respecting general acceptance. Such a response can be persuasive in some cases. In this case, however, the evidence indicates that the Toronto Hospital refused to perform the transplant on ethical grounds following an internal ethics review. Two other transplant centres in Ontario indicated that they too would refuse to perform the surgery due to ethical concerns relating to the relationship between donor and recipient. Further inquiries to a Vancouver transplant centre received a similar response and, while not determinative on the issue of general acceptance in Ontario, suggest that the position taken by Ontario hospitals may be shared more broadly across Canada.

The materials filed by the Appellant also included several abstracts for journal articles relating to living donor transplantation obtained through a search of the National Library of Medicine's PubMed database. A number of these abstracts deal with the ethical issues surrounding living donor transplant, including transplants involving non-family or "altruistic" donors. However, while these abstracts do indicate the benefits of living donor transplantation for organ recipients, they also suggest that the ethical issues are complex, and further that there is no consensus with respect to the ethical issues surrounding non-family living donors. More significantly, the abstracts are for American and European journal articles and do not provide evidence of Ontario (or Canadian) ethical perspectives, or the general acceptance in Ontario of living donor transplants involving an employer–employee or other non-family relationship. The Board is therefore of the view that the abstracts do not provide support for a finding that this particular transplant scenario is generally accepted in Ontario as appropriate.

The Board also considered evidence relating to the substantial advantages of earlier transplant to the Appellant, as well as the potential advantages to the health care system. These benefits are discussed in some of the medical journal abstracts, as well as in a letter from Dr. Cole dated December 6, 2000. In that letter Dr. Cole wrote:

> … From the patient's point of view, I believe there is a substantial advantage in terms of the quality of his life and also how long he will live, since recent information indicates that patients survive longer with transplants than on dialysis, and that longer periods on dialysis have an adverse impact on survival following transplantation.
>
> Furthermore, there would be an advantage to our health care system of transplanting him sooner, since the long term costs associated with transplantation are far lower than those associated with dialysis.

Dr. Fisher conceded in his testimony that there may be substantial advantages associated with renal transplantation and that the medical literature indicates that renal transplantation is preferable to dialysis. However, while the Board accepts this evidence, we are of the view that this does not provide evidence to support the general acceptance of this particular transplant scenario, but rather speaks to the benefits and advantages of renal transplantation more generally….

In support of a finding that this transplant scenario is not generally accepted in Ontario we have a one-hundred percent refusal rate by Ontario transplant centres due to ethical concerns relating to the recipient–donor relationship. The Vancouver transplant program's refusal and the divergence of opinion on the ethical issues seen in the medical literature suggest that the Ontario perspective is not unique. After considering all of the evidence in this case, the Board is of the view that the evidence supports a finding that this particular living donor renal transplant scenario is not generally accepted in Ontario as appropriate due to ethical concerns relating to the relationship between recipient and donor….

OTHER ISSUES

The Board has found that this particular transplant scenario is not generally accepted in Ontario as appropriate. In light of this finding, it is not necessary for the Board to consider the remaining issues relating to availability in Ontario, or delay in obtaining treatment in Ontario….

Appeal dismissed….

The Ethics of Setting Limits on ICD Therapy

Barry Hoffmaster

"It is in high technology areas where we face the stark reality of patient need against scarce resources in life and death situations that we see rationing with all its sharp edges exposed."

David Mechanic[1]

One discussion of the legal and ethical implications of implantable cardioverter defibrillator (ICD) therapy begins by observing that "… the legal and ethical issues involved in most aspects of the development of the ICD have not been fundamentally different from those raised by many other therapies".[2] With respect to the issues inherent in discontinuing treatment, for example, ICD therapy does not seem fundamentally different.[3] But the advent of ICDs does pose questions about the allocation and rationing of scarce health care resources in a particularly stark and dramatic, even if not fundamentally different, manner. Why is that?

It is because of the collective features of ICDs. ICDs are generally safe. ICDs have been demonstrated to be effective, unlike, for example, "last chance" investigational chemotherapy. ICDs serve an important need, unlike some forms of cosmetic surgery, for instance. ICDs, it can be argued, are cost effective compared with alternative drug therapy. And ICDs are very expensive. Even if ICDs are cost effective compared with alternative treatments, cost effectiveness does not entail cost savings. A proliferation of the use of ICDs would impose a heavy financial burden on the health care system. The principal, and perhaps sole, deterrent to the widespread use of ICDs is, therefore, economic. Should a health care technology that has been demonstrated to be safe and effective in prolonging life be withheld from patients simply because it is too expensive? That is the moral question that ICDs force on us. With ICDs, the edges of rationing become razor sharp.

ALLOCATION AND RATIONING— CLARIFYING TERMS

Discussions of the health care crisis and whether it is necessary to ration health care services are hampered and confused by imprecise, inconsistent uses of the terms "rationing" and "allocation".[4] Historically, 'to ration' has meant "to distribute equitably," so a notion of fairness or justice has been intrinsic to the understanding of rationing.[5] Lately, however, "rationing" seems to have lost its essential association with equity and has acquired pejorative connotations, particularly in the United States, where access to health care depends largely on the ability to pay. To say that health care is rationed on an economic basis in the United States is to now connect rationing with explicit inequity. In the United States it has even been proposed that "rationing" be used to mean "societal toleration of inequitable access (eg, based on ability to pay) to services deemed necessary, as defined by reference to appropriate clinical guidelines".[6] In one influential setting, therefore, the meaning of "rationing" has shifted from being conceptually linked with equity to being conceptually linked with inequity.

Distinguishing between "allocation" and "rationing" is complicated, too, by the multiple hierarchical levels at which decisions about

health care resources are made. At the highest or "macro" level are decisions about what proportion of a society's total budget should be devoted to health care. The federal and provincial governments have to determine how much money to allocate to health care as opposed to, for example, education, welfare, and the environment. A provincial ministry of health or a regional health care authority then has to distribute the delegated proportion across the health care field—they must decide how much to devote to physicians' salaries, hospitals, drugs, diagnostic and therapeutic services, prevention, and long term and chronic care, for example. At the intermediate or "meso" level, hospitals, organizations providing community and home care, and other health care institutions then must distribute the fixed budget that they receive across their divisions, programs, and services. Finally, at the level of patient care, the "micro" level, health care professionals must make decisions about how extensive a series of diagnostic tests should be, how aggressively a condition should be treated or when rehabilitation should be discontinued, for instance. When such decisions are constrained by the limited availability of resources or are influenced by considerations of whether a particular use of a resource would be worthwhile, rationing occurs.

Once these various levels are recognized, "allocation" and "rationing" are often distinguished by drawing a line in the hierarchy. "Allocation" is used to refer to higher level decisions, decisions that constrain the availability of resources. 'Rationing' is used to refer to lower level decisions, decisions about the use of limited resources. Doing so is consistent with the original understanding of "rationing," according to which a "ration" means the amount of food, supplies, money, or whatever given to an individual. Here the term "rationing" will be restricted to decisions about which individual patients receive ICDs, and "allocation" will be used for all of the decisions higher in the hierarchy that determine how many ICDs are available for clinical use. This is purely a stipulative, terminological point that has no implications for the substantive moral issues associated with the allocation and rationing of health care services.

THE STATUS QUO

How are decisions about the allocation and rationing of ICDs currently made? Provinces allocate funds for ICDs differently, but there seems to be two general approaches. On the one hand, a provincial ministry of health may control how much money goes to an expensive technology such as ICDs by assigning annual quotas to hospitals. On the other hand, hospitals may receive global budgets from a province and then have to determine for themselves how much of that budget to expend on ICDs. In either event, doctors in a hospital subsequently have to decide which patients will receive the limited number of ICDs that is available.

Given that the supply of ICDs is restricted, doctors are forced to ration. They may try to avoid doing so by implanting ICDs in every patient who, in their clinical judgment, is likely to benefit. But that is simply rationing on the basis of "first come, first served." And what happens when the supply is exhausted? Patients who also may have benefited, perhaps to a greater extent, will not get ICDs. What if doctors appeal to the hospital administration and argue successfully for more ICDs? Then their patients will benefit, but other people in the hospital will suffer. The doctors may be shielded from the consequences of that allocation decision. Now they might not have to ration, but someone else will.

Moreover, doctors are going to be pushed inexorably to make harder and more contentious decisions. Consider the following vignettes (G Klein and C Simpson, personal communication):

Case 1: A 75-year-old man with a long history of coronary artery disease has suffered two myocardial infarctions (MIs). His left ventricular ejection fraction measures 10% by two-dimensional echocardiography, and he has New York Heart Association class IV heart failure. He had an in-hospital cardiac arrest (due to ventricular fibrillation) six months previously, was successfully resuscitated and started on amiodarone. He again presented with unstable ventricular tachycardia (VT) and was cardioverted by direct current shock in an emergency room.

This patient technically fulfills the criteria for an ICD, but he is very sick, with a prognosis of 50% mortality in one year. He most likely will die of some cause other than a ventricular arrhythmia. He has failed on amiodarone so he could be given an ICD. Is it worth it?

Case 2: An 86-year-old woman is resuscitated after cardiac arrest. She had an uncomplicated anterior wall MI four years ago, but otherwise she is in good health. Investigations demonstrate no reversible ischemia or other remediable cause for the cardiac arrest. She and her family have read about ICDs and have requested that one be implanted.

This patient technically fulfills the Anti-arrhythmics Versus Implantable Defibrillator (AVID) study criteria for an ICD (7), but should she get amiodarone first? She has requested an ICD. And what about her age? Is it worth it?

Case 3: A 52-year-old man had sustained VT on the second day after coronary artery bypass surgery, which required cardioversion because of hemodynamic instability. He had an MI six months previously, leaving a small apical scar. Despite this, left ventricular ejection fraction was virtually normal at 55%. A coronary angiogram performed after the VT episode confirmed that all grafts were widely patent. Serum potassium measured two hours before the VT episode was slightly low at 3.2 mmol/L.

This patient is immediately postoperative, a time at which arrhythmias are common but are usually self-correcting or self-limiting. His low potassium may be the cause of the VT, and if that problem were corrected, his risk may be reduced. In the AVID trial,[7] this class of patients benefited the least. Should he nevertheless receive an ICD?

One could argue that these are no more than clinical management problems. If an ICD is clinically indicated and is available, the patient should get it. Physicians should think about and act on only what is in the best interest of their patients.

In theory, that stance is clinically and morally attractive. In practice, though, as the gulf expands between the number of available ICDs and the number of patients who may benefit from or want ICDs, it becomes increasingly harder to sustain. The pressure on doctors to ask not just, "Will it help" but also, "Is it worth it?" can only mount.

How are decisions about the rationing of ICDs now made? Doctors will, of course, consult with colleagues about particularly troublesome cases, and on occasion they may even ask a hospital ethics committee for advice. But, for the most part, they make these bedside rationing decisions on their own.

That approach is unsatisfactory for at least two reasons. First, and perhaps surprisingly, doctors do not like being put in this position. One cardiologist has commented to the author that deciding whether a patient gets an ICD is the hardest thing he has to do in medicine. Second, having doctors ration ICDs is contrary to bioethics orthodoxy. Doctors should not be "gate-keepers" for society, because that role forces them to have divided loyalties. On the one hand, as personal physicians they have a fiduciary duty to their patients that requires them to act solely in the best interest of their patients. Respect for and adherence to that duty is the basis of the trust that patients repose in their physicians. On the other hand, as gatekeepers, they have an obligation to the society that funds health care to ensure that limited health care resources are used efficiently and optimally. When doctors wear their gatekeeper hat, they have to consider whether an ICD that might benefit their patient could benefit some other patient even more. They have to think about the pool of patients that may need ICDs, not just the patients for whom they are immediately responsible. And if the fiscal year is three-quarters over and there are only two of the annual quota of 40 ICDs left for the remaining three months, should their patient, for whom an ICD offers some real but modest benefit, get one? Patient advocate or gatekeeper—which should the physician be?

The status quo imposes divided loyalties on physicians and forces them to make decisions that they do not like and perhaps even resent. There are other difficulties, too. Because physicians' discretion to ration ICDs is unfettered, their clinical judgments are likely to be variable, which means potential inequities for patients. Even worse, that flexibility could be abused if decisions manifested arbitrariness, arrogance, or favouritism. Moreover, as long as rationing remains an exercise of physicians' clinical judgments, the need for and the existence of rationing will be hidden from the public. And if it were to become known that doctors are unilaterally making these kinds of rationing decisions, faith in the medical profession might erode.

THE SEARCH FOR AN ALTERNATIVE

So what should be done? The orthodox and familiar answer is that the discretion of physicians needs to be fettered. The eligibility conditions for an ICD need to be specified, and that can be accomplished by developing clinical practice guidelines. The argument for this position rests on four assumptions.[8]

The first assumption is that the courts will decline to make rationing decisions. That assumption is reasonable on practical and theoretical grounds. With respect to the former, judges likely would find rationing decisions as difficult and uncomfortable as physicians do and be eager to defer to the clinical judgments of doctors. With respect to the latter, Fuller[9] has argued that what he calls "polycentric" problems are inherently unsuited to adjudication, and allocative or distributive matters are paradigms of "polycentric" situations.

The second assumption is that, despite persistent calls for "society" to make allocation and rationing decisions, "society"—however that vague notion is understood—does not want to do so. Writing in the context of the National Health Service in Britain, Klein et al.[8] conclude:

> … the results of various surveys … agree on one point. This is that people believe that it is doctors not they, [National Health Service] managers or the government—who should be responsible for

deciding on priorities. There is, therefore, no strong case for arguing that the strategy of asking the public about priorities should be pursued more vigorously.

The third assumption is that rationing by denial is too crude and too inequitable. How, for example, would one decide *what* was to be denied? Would general categories of services be pitted against one another, such as acute care services against mental health services? Or would the competition be between specific kinds of treatment, heart transplantations compared with in vitro fertilization, for instance? Or would the decisions be about *to whom* services should be denied? Would the claims of the old be weighed against the claims of the young, for example?

The fourth assumption is that the vast majority of health care services benefit someone, in one way or another. Klein et al.[8] remark that "… most treatments do benefit *someone,* even if at a low level of probability …"

The result of these assumptions is that the kind of rationing that should be done is rationing by selection: "The real issue … is not so much which services or types of care should be on offer but which patients should be selected for what kinds of treatment and at what level of intensity".[8] Moreover, rationing in the "strict sense," that is, rationing "at the bedside" by doctors, is inevitable for clinical and moral reasons.

The clinical reasons are the uncertainty, complexity, and contingency that pervade the practice of medicine. These features are inevitable and ineliminable because they are inherent in the enterprise of applying general rules to specific patients in particular circumstances. Even if randomized clinical trials conclusively identified classes of patients for whom ICDs were clearly beneficial, trying to apply those results to the care of an idiosyncratic patient with a unique history and distinctive problems would require interpretation. The criteria used to select patients for randomized clinical trials are always limited, partial, and oriented to features that are objectively identifiable and quantifiable. Patients who fulfill all of these criteria could possess additional features that would make ICDs inappropriate or perhaps even harmful. Patients could possess some, but not all, of the features. Or patients could possess closely analogous features that would make it reasonable to extend the results of the clinical trial to them. Deciding how the care of a specific patient should be guided by the general norms of medicine, norms that are derived from medical school lectures, authoritative textbooks, personal experience, conversations with colleagues, or published research studies, always has and always will require clinical judgment.

The moral reasons are that the notions of equity and need are too abstract, too elusive and too elastic to be practically determinative. The formal definition of justice or equity is treating like cases alike, but that definition is useful only if there are precise substantive criteria for identifying relevant similarities and dissimilarities. And, while the notion of need is at the core of health care, its definitions are almost as numerous as those who work in and make use of the health care system.

The result of these clinical and moral realities is an inexorable process of "downward delegation" that culminates in clinical discretion. Decisions about the use of scarce health care resources are pushed from the top of the hierarchy, from policy-making levels in government offices and hospital administrations, to the bottom of the hierarchy, to the bedsides of patients. "Downward delegation" is not the product of doctors mobilizing to protect their turf but instead represents a reasonable way of responding to situations that are imposed on them:

> Once we accept the problematic nature of the concepts of equity and need—and the difficulties involved in trying to operationalize them—then the use of discretion at the point of service delivery becomes not a perversion of policy in the process of implementation but a rational response to the difficulty of devising decision-making rules that are sufficiently specific and robust to cope with

all contingencies. Just as the case for pushing responsibility from the national level to the local level rests on the argument that need can only be interpreted in context— taking account of specific circumstances—so the argument for pushing responsibility down from the local level to the service deliverers rests on the argument that only they can interpret the complexity of individual circumstances. Discretion, in short, is a function of ambiguity. And considerations of equity revolve primarily around the way in which that discretion is exercised: it becomes a process criterion, where the currency of evaluation is freedom from bias and the absence of arbitrariness in the allocatory judgements made.[8]

The ethical focus, in this view, shifts from substance to procedure. Given the rampant clinical and moral indeterminacy, it does not make sense to ask whether a particular rationing decision is right, because that would necessitate invoking general clinical and moral principles to try to justify the decision. Instead, one asks whether the decision was made in the right way, for example, by a procedure that is open, fair, and not tainted by favouritism or arbitrariness.

The principal advantages of a procedural alternative are that it promotes the consistency, and thus the fairness, of treatment; it makes rationing more visible; it reduces the burden on individual physicians; and it enhances the accountability of doctors and the medical profession. The main disadvantage is that it camouflages the responsibilities of politicians and civil servants to set priorities in health care. Rationing at the bedside occurs because there are too few resources to offer patients all the options that physicians believe might be clinically beneficial. But the amount of resources available is a result of decisions made higher up in the hierarchy, for example, by officials in the ministry of health who decide how to allocate a global health care budget, and by provincial and federal politicians who determine how large that health care budget

will be. Concentrating on bedside rationing deflects attention away from the allocation decisions that create the need to ration and, by so doing, tacitly endorses those allocation decisions:

> Rationing at the bedside occurs because health care resources are consumed by organizational, professional, and political arrangements that force rationing downstream. The real ethics of rationing should focus on these arrangements. For when moral philosophers or concerned individuals focus on how to ration fairly at the bedside or in a given situation, they in effect legitimate and support those who have set the budget or who benefit from institutional, budgetary, or professional arrangements that help produce the existing situation of scarcity.[10]

That is a serious and neglected moral concern.

The ethics of allocation and rationing is, then, ultimately about matters of institutional design— how to develop morally defensible structures and procedures for making these decisions. Are there any ethical guidelines that might govern this enterprise? Writing about the coverage of "last chance therapies" by health maintenance organizations in the United States, Daniels and Sabin[11] argue that the decision procedures for setting limits on health care services have to have four general features to be legitimate and fair:

- Limit-setting decisions and their rationales must be publicly accessible.
- A rationale must constitute a reasonable construal of how to meet the medical needs of a covered population under acceptable resource constraints.
- Mechanisms must exist for challenging and revisiting decisions and resolving disputes.
- There must be voluntary or public regulation of the process to insure that conditions 1 through 3 are met.

Public accessibility, review, and appeal mechanisms, and voluntary or public regulation are plausible components of any morally defensible decision-making procedure. What counts as a "reasonable construal" of how to meet needs under "acceptable resource constraints" and what resource constraints should be deemed "acceptable" leave much to be settled, however. Resolutions of these matters could vary considerably. How much difference should be accepted, and how much discretion may be ineliminable? Those remain worrisome questions.

TWO RESIDUAL PROBLEMS

Differential treatment: One assumption behind the regionalization of health care is that decisions about health care priorities are better made close to the populations being served, where need can be more accurately assessed and more appropriately evaluated in light of local contexts. The result, however, is that different local authorities make different decisions. Given a procedural approach to the allocation of health care resources, those variable decisions are legitimate if they have been made in the right way. Is the existence of such differential treatment morally palatable?

Daniels and Sabin[11] think that differential treatment may be more acceptable in a national health care system, such as that of the United Kingdom, than in a decentralized system, such as that of the United States:

> In the United Kingdom ... it might seem more troubling that Groucho did not get his transplant in London but Harpo got his in Manchester. Here ... there might be disagreements among meaningful political units, the districts, about what constituted the "best" procedure. If that is true, then there might be even more reason to tolerate variation than there is in the United States where people are grouped into insurance schemes, not meaningful political units that have ways of selecting their procedures in a democratic fashion.

That argument could, of course, be extended to Canada as long as local and regional health authorities qualified as "meaningful political units" and set their priorities "in a democratic fashion."

But as Daniels and Sabin[11] recognize, the issue remains tricky:

> In a national health care system, the political rationale for uniformity would have to show that differential treatment among districts was less acceptable than giving them autonomy to select their own procedures. If meaningful political units, like districts, felt strongly enough about their choices of procedures, the costs of uniformity might be too high. For the problem we are facing, then, it remains unclear how acceptable it would be for Harpo to get a last chance when Groucho does not.

Or how acceptable it would be for Harpo to get an ICD when Groucho does not. Certain meaningful political units in Canada—the provinces—undoubtedly would feel strongly about protecting their autonomy in health care. Regional or local health care authorities within a province may be more inclined to uniformity, if only because consistency with other jurisdictions could be cited as a reason for the tough choices they have to make. The conflict between autonomy and uniformity will not be easy to sort out.

Indications creep: The complexity, uncertainty, and contingency that dog clinical decision making will continually challenge the efficacy of practice guidelines and will persistently exert pressure to expand the indications for ICDs. Practice guidelines will never eliminate "grey zones" for the use of ICDs. But then consider this scenario (C Simpson, personal communication). A patient who had an ICD implanted for a "grey zone" indication lives out the lifespan of the device (five to seven years) without ever needing it. Should it be replaced? Many physicians may say no, but in practice the device is frequently replaced. Such patients are not common now, but if ICDs were to be put in patients who are less and less "ill," their numbers would increase.

As with any health care technology (witness transplantation), the more that ICDs are used, the more they will become used. The pressure to implant them in patients who are less sick and who may potentially benefit from them will be strong. And when it is a matter of life and death, that pressure is hard to resist. Who would want to trade places with physicians who have to look patients in the eye and tell them that they are not going to get something that could save their lives because it costs too much? Would the physicians who have to make clinical judgments about ICDs and about invoking ICD practice guidelines be able to withstand that pressure?

CONCLUSION

Despite these reservations, a procedurally oriented approach to the allocation and rationing of ICDs is the only escape from a morally untenable situation. It is simply not reasonable for doctors, for patients or for "society" to have decisions about the use of ICDs made through the unfettered discretion of physicians. The scope of their discretion needs to be restricted, and the manner in which their discretion is exercized needs to be constrained. That means that more responsibility for decisions about the use of ICDs needs to be pushed back up the decision-making hierarchy. There needs to be more explicit allocation and less implicit rationing.

How can that be accomplished? It can be done through institutional design, but institutional design that occurs systematically and comprehensively. In Ontario, for example, the Ontario Ministry of Health, the Cardiac Care Network of Ontario, hospitals, and individual units all would have to be involved. Matters of legitimacy and fairness would have to be identified within each institutional venue, and structures and processes that are morally defensible would have to be designed for each venue. Then those institutional approaches would have to be melded so that the overall system operated coherently, legitimately, and fairly. That, of course, is a tall order. But what is the alternative?

Acknowledgements

The author's work in this area was instigated by Dr George Klein and Dr Chris Simpson. The author is grateful for their encouragement, and their patient support and tutelage.

Notes

1. Mechanic D. *From Advocacy to Allocation: The Evolving American Health Care System*. New York: Free Press, 1986.
2. Anderson MH, Camm AJ. Legal and ethical aspects of driving and working in patients with an implantable cardioverter defibrillator. *Am Heart J* 1994; 127:1185–93.
3. Quill TE, Barold SS, Sussman BL. Discontinuing an implantable cardioverter defibrillator as a life-sustaining treatment. *Am J Cardiol* 1994; 74:205–7.
4. Hoffmaster CB, Wolf SM. *Allocation and Rationing of Resources in Long-Term and Chronic Care*. London: Westminster Institute for Ethics and Human Values, 1993.
5. *Merriam-Webster's Collegiate Dictionary*, 10th edn. Springfield: Merriam-Webster, 1993.
6. Hadorn, DC, RH Brook. The health care resource allocation debate. *JAMA* 1991; 266:3328–31.
7. A comparison of antiarrhythmic-drug therapy with implantable defibrillators in patients resuscitated from near-fatal ventricular arrhythmia. The Antiarrhythmics Versus Implantable Defibrillators (AVID) investigators. *N Engl J Med* 1997; 337:1576–83.
8. Klein R, Day P, Redmayne S. *Managing Scarcity*. Philadelphia: Open University Press, 1996.
9. Fuller LL. The forms and limits of adjudication. *Harv Law Rev* 1978; 92:353–409.
10. Light DW. The real ethics of rationing. *PennBioeth* 1998; 4:3–4.
11. Daniels N, Sabin JE. Last chance therapies and managed care. *Hastings Cen Rep* 1998; 28:27–41.

Rationing Fairly: Programmatic Considerations

Norman Daniels

Despite its necessity, rationing raises troublesome questions about fairness. We ration in situations in which losers, as well as winners, have plausible claims to have their needs met. When we knowingly and deliberately refrain from meeting some legitimate needs, we had better have justification for the distributive choices we make. Not surprisingly, health planners and legislaters appeal to bioethicists for help, asking what justice requires here. Can we help them? I think we are not ready to yet, and I will support this claim by noting four general rationing problems that we remain unsure how to solve, illustrating how they plague Oregon's rationing plan.

Before turning to the four problems, I want to make several preliminary remarks. First, philosophers (including me) have traditionally underestimated the importance of rationing, thinking of it as a peripheral, not central problem. Since we cannot afford, for example, to educate, treat medically, or protect legally people in all the ways their needs for these goods require or the accepted distributive principles seem to demand, rationing is clearly pervasive, not peripheral.

Rationing decisions share three key features. First, the goods we often must provide—legal services, health care, educational benefits—are not divisible without loss of benefit, unlike money. We thus cannot avoid unequal or "lumpy" distributions. Meeting the educational, health care or legal needs of some people, for example, will mean that the requirements of others will go unsatisfied. Second, when we ration, we deny benefits to some individuals who can plausibly claim they are owed them in principle. They can cite an accepted principle of distributive justice that governs their situation and should protect them. Third, the general distributive principles appealed to by claimants as well

as by rationers do not by themselves provide adequate reasons for choosing among claimants: they are too schematic. This point was driven home to me by the way in which my "fair equality of opportunity" account of just health care (Daniels 1985, 1988) fails to yield specific solutions to the rationing problems I shall survey. Finally, even the best work in the general theory of justice has not squarely faced the problems raised by the indeterminacy of distributive principles. Rawls (1971), for example, suggests that the problem of fleshing out the content of principles of distributive justice is ultimately procedural, falling to the legislature. Perhaps, but the claim that we must in general turn to a fair democratic procedure should not be an assumption, but the conclusion, either of a general argument or of a failed search for appropriate moral constraints on rationing. If however, there are substantive principles governing rationing, then the theory of justice is incomplete in a way we have not noticed. This point cuts across the debates between proponents of "local justice" (Walzer 1983; Elster 1992) and "global justice" (Rawls 1971; Gauthier 1986), and between liberalism and communitarianism (cf. Emanuel 1991; Daniels 1992).

FOUR UNSOLVED RATIONING PROBLEMS: ILLUSTRATIONS FROM OREGON

The Fair Chances

Before seeing how the fair chances/best outcomes problem arises in Oregon's macrorationing plan, consider its more familiar microrationing form: Which of several equally needy individuals should get a scarce resource, such as a heart transplant? Suppose, for example, that Alice and Betty are the same age, have waited on queue the same time, and that each will live only one week without a transplant. With the transplant, however, Alice is expected to live two years and Betty twenty. Who should get the transplant (cf. Kamm 1989)? Giving priority to producing best outcomes, a priority built into some point systems for awarding organs, would mean that Betty gets the organ and Alice dies (assuming persistent scarcity of organs, as Brock (1988) notes). But Alice might complain, "Why should I give up my only chance of survival—and two years of survival is not insignificant—just because Betty has a chance to longer? It is not fair that I have to give up everything that is valuable to me just so Betty can have more of what is valuable to her." Alice demands a lottery that gives her an equal chance with Betty.

Some people agree with Alice's complaint and agree with her demand for a lottery. Few would agree with her, however, if she had very little chance at survival; more would agree if her outcomes were only somewhat worse than Betty's. Still, at the level of intuitions, there is much disagreement about when and how much to favor best outcomes. Brock (1988), like Broome (1987) proposes breaking this deadlock by giving Alice and Betty chances proportional to the benefits they can get (e.g., by assigning Alice one side of a ten-sided die). Kamm (1989, 1993) notes that Brock's proposal must be amended once we allow differences in urgency or need among patients. She favors assigning multiplicative weights to the degree of need or urgency. Then, the neediest might end up with no chance to receive a transplant if their outcomes were very poor, but, compared to Brock's "proportional chances" proposal, they would have greater opportunity to get an organ if their outcomes were reasonably high.[1] Both Brock's and Kamm's suggestions seem ad hoc. That there is some force to each of Alice's and Betty's demands does not, as Brock would have it, mean the force is clearly equal; similarly, assigning weights to more factors, as Kamm does, seems to add an element of precision lacking in our intu-

itions about these cases. Our intuitions may fall short of giving us clear, orderly principles here.

We might try to break the deadlock at the level of intuitions by appealing to more theoretical considerations. For example, we might respond to Alice that she already has lost a "natural" lottery; she might have been the one with twenty years expected survival, but it turned out to be Betty instead. After the fact, however, Alice is unlikely to agree that there has already been a fair "natural" lottery, even assuming that there were no prior differences in access to care and so on. To undercut Alice's demand for a new lottery, we would have to persuade her that the proper perspective for everyone to adopt is *ex ante*, not *ex post* information about her condition (cf. Menzel 1989). But what should Alice know about herself *ex ante*? If Alice knows about her family history of heart disease, she might well not favor giving complete priority to best outcomes. Perhaps Alice should agree it is reasonable to adopt more radical *ex ante* position, one that denies her all information about herself, a thick "veil of ignorance." Controversy persists. Behind such a veil, some would argue that it would be irrational to forego the greater expected payoff that would result from giving priority to best outcomes.[2] Citing Rawls' adoption of a minimum strategy, Kamm (1993) argues against such "gambling" behind the veil. Alternatively, she appeals to Scanlon (1982): if Alice would "reasonably regret" losing to Betty, then she should not be held to a scheme that favors best outcomes. Unclear about our intuitions, we are also stymied by a controversy at the deepest theoretical levels.

The best outcomes problem arises in macrorationing as well. Consider HSS Secretary Louis Sullivan's (1992) recent refusal to grant a Medicaid waiver to Oregon's rationing plan. Sullivan's main criticism of the Oregon plan is that in preferring treatments that provide greater net benefits the plan discriminates against the disabled.[3] The clearest example of such discrimination would be this: Two groups of patients, both in need of a treatment that can give them a net benefit of a given magnitude; because one group has a disability, e.g., difficulty walking, that would not be affected by the treatment, we deny them the treatment. Neither Sullivan nor the NLC give an example, even hypothetical, of how this situation could arise in the Oregon scheme. The denial of coverage for aggressive treatment of very low birthweight (<500 gr) neonates, which they do cite as an example of discrimination, is not an appropriate example, because the denial is premised on the lack of benefit produced by aggressive treatment of such neonates.

Consider an example suggestive of the Oregon scheme. Suppose two treatments, T1 and T2, can benefit different groups of patients, G1 and G2 as follows. T1 preserves life for G1s (or provides some other major benefit), but it does not restore a particular function, such as walking, to G1s. T2 not only preserves life for G2s (or provides some other major benefit), but it also enables them to walk again. The Oregon Health Service Commission ranks T2 as a more important service than T1 because it produces a greater net benefit (I ignore the OTA [1991] argument that net benefit is not a major contributor to rank). Sullivan says that it is discriminatory to deny G1s T1, even though a single person would clearly consider relative benefit in deciding between T1 and T2.

The Sullivan/NLCMDD objection can, with charity, be interpreted as a version of Alice's complaint that favoring best outcomes denies her a fair chance at a benefit. Interpreted this way, the Sullivan/NLCMDD objection is that we cannot rule out giving G1s any chance at the benefit treatment would bring them simply because G2s would benefit more from the use of our limited resources. In effect, they seem to be saying we should give no weight to best outcomes. As I noted earlier, this extreme position does not seem to match our intuitions in the microrationing case. But neither does the alternative extreme position, that we must always give priority to better outcomes. The point is that a rationing approach that ranks services by net benefit, whether it turns out to be Oregon's scheme or simply Hadorn's (1991) alternative

proposal, thus carries with it unsolved moral issues. To justify ranking by net benefit we must be prepared to address those underlying issues.

The Priorities Problem

Oregon's (intended) methodology of ranking by net benefit also ignores the moral issues I group here as the priorities problem. Suppose that two treatment condition pairs give equal net benefits. (Remember, this [does] not generally mean they produce the same health outcomes, only the same net benefits). Then the OHSC should rank them equal in importance. But now suppose that people with C1 are more seriously impaired by their disease or disability than people with C2. Though T1 and T2 produce equivalent net gains in benefit, people with C2 will end up better off than people with C1, since they started out better off. Nothing in the method of ranking treatment/condition pairs by net benefit responds to this difference between C1s and C2s. Nevertheless, most of us would judge it more important to give services to C1s than it is to give them to C2s under these conditions. We feel at least some inclination to help those worse off than those better off. For example, if C1s after treatment were no better off than C2s before treatment, we are more strongly inclined to give priority to the worst off. Our concern to respect that priority might decline if the effect of treating C1s but not C2s is that C1s end up better off than C2s. How troubled we would be by this outcome might depend on how great the new inequality turned out to be, or on how significant the residual impairment of C2s was.

Suppose now that there is greater net benefit from giving T2 to C2s than there is from giving T1 to C1s. If C1s are sufficiently worse off to start with than T2s, and if C1s end up worse off or not significantly better off than C2s, then our concern about priorities may compel us to forego the greater net benefit that results from giving T2 to C2s. But how much priority we give to the worst off still remains unclear. If we can only give a very modest improvement to the worst off, but we must forego a very significant improvement to those initially better off, then we may overrule our concern for the worst off. Our intuitions do not pull us toward a strict priority for the worst off.

Just what the structure of our concern about priority is, however, remains unclear. The unsolved priorities problem not only affects a methodology that ranks by net benefit or by net QLY's. It affects cost/benefit and cost/effectiveness rankings, including Eddy's (1991a) "willingness to pay" methodology. So too does the aggregation problem, to which I briefly now turn.

The Aggregation Problem

In June of 1990, the Oregon Health Services Commission released a list of treatment/ condition pairs ranked by a cost/benefit calculation. Critics were quick to seize on rankings that seemed completely counter-intuitive. For example, as Hadorn noted (1991), toothcapping was ranked higher than appendectomy. The reason was simple: an appendectomy cost about $4,000, many times the cost of capping a tooth. Simply aggregating the net medical benefit of many capped teeth yielded a net benefit greater than that produced by one appendectomy.

Eddy (1991b) points out that our intuitions in these cases are largely based on comparing treatment/condition pairs for their importance on a one:one basis. One appendectomy is more important than one toothcapping because it saves a life rather than merely reduces pain and preserves dental function. But our intuitions are much less developed when it comes to making one:many comparisons (though we can establish indifference curves that capture trades we are willing to make; cf. Nord 1992). When does saving more lives through one technology mean we should forego saving fewer through another? The complex debate about whether "numbers count" has a bearing on rationing problems. How many legs should we be willing to forego saving in order to save one life? How many eyes? How many teeth? Can we aggregate *any* small benefits, or only those that are in some clear way significant, when we want to weigh theses benefits against clearly significant benefits (e.g., saving a life) to a few? Kamm (1987,

1993) argues persuasively that we should not favor saving one life and curing a sore throat over saving a different life, because curing a sore throat is not a "competitor" with saving a life. She also argues that benefits that someone is morally not required to sacrifice in order to save another's life also have significant standing and can be aggregated. If we are not required to sacrifice an arm in order to same someone's life, then we can aggregate arms saved and weigh them against lives saved. She suggests that our judgments about aggregation differ if we are in contexts where saving lives rather than inducing harms (positive vs. negative duties) are at issue.

Kamm shows that we are not straightforward aggregators of all benefits and that our moral views are both complex and difficult to explicate in terms of well-ordered principles. These views are not compatible with the straightforward aggregation (sum ranking) that is presupposed by the dominant methodologies derived from welfare economics. Yet we do permit, indeed require, some forms of aggregation. Our philosophical task is to specify which principles governing aggregation have the strongest justification. If it appears there is no plausible, principled account of aggregation, then we have strong reason to rely instead on fair procedures and an obligation to give any of them.

The Democracy Problem

When Sullivan rejected Oregon's application for a Medicaid waiver, he complained that the methodology for assessing net medical benefit drew on biased or discriminatory public attitudes toward disabilities. Adapting Kaplan's (Kaplan and Anderson 1990) "quality of well-being" scale for use in measuring the benefit of medical treatments, Oregon surveyed residents, asking them to judge on a scale of 0 (death) to 100 (perfect health) what the impact would be of having to live the rest of one's life with some physical or mental impairment or symptom; for example, wearing eyeglasses was rated 95 out of 100, for a weighting of –0.05. Many of these judgments seem downright bizarre, whether or not they reflect bias. For example, having to wear eyeglasses was rated slightly worse than the –0.046 weighting assigned to not being able to drive a car or use public transportation or the –0.049 assigned to having to stay at a hospital or nursing home. Other weightings clearly reflected cultural attitudes and possibly bias: having trouble with drugs or alcohol was given the second most negative weighting (–0.455) of all conditions, much worse than, for example, having a bad burn over large areas of your body (–0.372) or being so impaired that one needs help to eat or go to the bathroom (–0.106). Having to use a walker or wheelchair under your own control was weighted as much worse (–0.373) than having losses of consciousness from seizures, blackout or coma (–0.114).

Claiming that people who experience a disabling condition, like being unable to walk, tend to give less negative ratings to them than people who have experienced them, Sullivan argued Oregon was likely to underestimate the benefit of a treatment that left people with such disabilities. Excluding such treatments would thus be the result of public bias.[4] His complaint carries over to other methodologies, e.g., Eddy's (1991) willingness-to-pay approach and the use of QLY's in cost-effectiveness or cost-benefit analyses.

Sullivan's complaint raises an interesting question: Whose judgments about the effects of a condition should be used? Those who do not have a disabling condition may suffer from cultural biases, overestimating the impact of disability. But those who have the condition may rate it as less serious because they have modified their preferences, goals, and values in order to make a "healthy adjustment" to their condition. Their overall dissatisfaction—tapped by these methodologies—may not reflect the impact that would be captured by a measure more directly attuned to the range of capabilities they retain. Still, insisting on the more objective measure has a high political cost and may even seem paternalistic.

Sullivan simply assumes that we must give priority to the judgments made by those, experiencing the condition, but that is not so obvious. Clearly, there is something attractive about the idea, embedded in all these methodologies, of

assessing the relative impact of conditions on people by asking them what they think about the impact (cf. Menzel 1992). Should we give people what they actually want? Or should we give them what they should want, correcting for various defects in their judgment? What corrections to expressed preferences are plausible?

The democracy problem arises at another level in procedures that purport to be directly democratic. The Oregon plan called for the OHSC to respect "community values" in its ranking of services. Because prevention and family planning services were frequently discussed in community meetings, the OHSC assigned the categories including those services very high ranking. Consequently, in Oregon, vasectomies are ranked more important than hip replacements. Remember the priority and aggregation problems: it would seem more important to restore mobility to someone who cannot walk than to improve the convenience of birth control through vasectomy in several people. But, assuming that the Commissioners properly interpreted the wishes of Oregonians, that is not what Oregonians wanted the rankings to be. Should we treat this as error? Or must we abide by whatever the democratic process yields?

Thus far I have characterized the problem of democracy as a problem of error: a fair democratic process, or a methodology that rests in part on expressions of preferences, leads to judgments that deviate from either intuitive or theoretically based judgments about the relative importance of certain health outcomes or services. The problem is how much weight to give the intuitive or theoretically based judgments as opposed to the expressed preferences. The point should be put in another way as well. Should we in the end think of the democratic process as a matter of pure procedural justice? If so, then we have no way to correct the judgment made through that process, for what it determines to be fair is what counts as fair. Or should we really consider the democratic process as an impure and imperfect form of procedural justice? Then it is one that can be corrected by appeal to some prior notion of what constitutes a fair outcome of rationing. I suggest that we do not yet know the answer to this question, and we will not be able to answer it until we work harder at providing a theory of rationing.

CONCLUSION

I conclude with a plea against provincialism. The four problems I illustrated have their analogues in the rationing of goods other than health care. To flesh out a principle that says "people are equal before the law" will involve decisions about how to allocate legal services among all people who can make plausible claims to need them by citing that principle. Similarly, to give content to a principle that assures equal educational opportunity will involve decisions about resource allocation very much like those involved in rationing health care. Being provincial about health care rationing will prevent us from seeing the relationships among these rationing problems. Conversely, a rationing theory will have greater force if it derives from consideration of common types of problems that are independent of the kinds of goods whose distribution is in question. I am suggesting that exploring a theory of rationing in this way is a prolegomenon to serious work in "applied ethics."

Acknowledgement

This work was generously supported by the National Endowment for the Humanities (RH20917) and the National Library of Medicine (1R01LM05005). I also wish to thank Tufts University and Harvard's Program in Ethics and the Professions for Sabbatical support.

Notes

1. Kamm (1989, 1993) distinguishes urgency, that is, how imminent death would be without a transplant, from need. Need should, on her view, reflect how important living longer is to an individual; specifically, living longer may be more important to someone who has lived a short life than it is to someone who has lived a longer life, so there may be a decreasing marginal utility of living longer.

2. I have argued as such in a Battelle project on heart transplantation in the early 1980s; others have made similar arguments.

3. I am taking Sullivan's criticism at face value, though I suspect the rejection of the Medicaid waiver was motivated by political considerations, not incompatibility with the ADA (cf. Hadorn 1992; Capron 1992; Menzel 1992).

4. The OTA (1991) notes that men gave dysmenorrhea a greater negative weight than women. The effect of this weighting is that greater net benefit, and thus higher rank, accrues to treating dysmenorrhea if we include the judgments of men than if we counted only the judgments of women.

References

Brock, Dan. 1988. "Ethical Issues in Recipient Selection for Organ Transplantation." in D. Mathiey (ed.) *Organ Substitution Technology: Ethical, Legal, and Public Policy Issues*. Boulder: Westview. pp. 86–99.

Broome, John. 1987. "Fairness and the Random Distribution of Goods." (unpublished manuscript).

Capron, Alexander. 1992. "Oregon's Disability: Principles or Politics?" *Hasting Center Report* 22: 6 (November–December): 18–20.

Daniels, Norman. 1985. *Just Health Care*. Cambridge: Cambridge University Press.

Daniels, Norman. 1988. *Am I My Parents' Keeper? An Essay on Justice Between the Young and the Old*. New York: Oxford University Press.

Daniels, Norman. 1992. "Liberalism and Medical Ethics." *Hastings Center Report*. 22:6 (November–December): 41–3.

Eddy, D. 1991a. "Rationing by Patient Choice," *JAMA* 265:1 (January 2): 105–108.

Eddy, D. 1991b. "Oregon's Methods: Did Cost-Effectiveness Analysis Fail?" *JAMA* 266: 15 (October 16): 2135–41.

Elster, John. 1992. *Local Justice: How Institutions Allocate Scarce Goods and Necessary Burdens*. New York: Russel Sage.

Emanuel, Ezekial. 1991. *The Ends of Human Life: Medical Ethics in a Liberal Polity*. Cambridge, MA: Harvard University Press.

Gauthier, D. 1986. *Morals By Agreement*. Oxford: Oxford University Press.

Hadorn, David. 1992. "The Problem of Discrimination in Health Care Priority Setting." *JAMA* 268:11 (16 September): 1454–9.

Kamm, Frances. 1987. "Choosing Between People: Commonsense Morality and Doctors' Choices." *Bioethics* 1:255–271.

Kamm, Frances. 1989. "The Report of the US Task Force on Organ Transplantation: Criticisms and Alternatives." *Mount Sinai Journal of Medicine* 56:207–220.

Kamm, Frances. 1993. *Morality and Mortality, Vol. 1.* Oxford: Oxford University Press (in press).

Kaplan, R.M. Anderson, J.P. 1990. "The General Health Policy Model: An Integrated Approach." in B. Spilker (ed.) *Quality of Life Assessments in Clinical Trials.* New York: Raven Press.

Menzel, Paul. 1989. *Strong Medicine.* New York: Oxford University Press.

Menzel, Paul. 1992. Oregon's Denial: Disabilities and Quality of Life." *Hastings Center Report* 22:6 (November–December): 21–25.

National Legal Center for the Medically Dependent and Disabled. 1991. Letter to Representative Christopher H. Smith.

Nord, Eric. 1992. "The Relevance of Health State after Treatment in Prioritising Between Different Patients." *Journal of Medical Ethics.* (forthcoming).

Office of Technology Assessment. 1991. *Evaluation of the Oregon Medicaid Proposal.* U.S. Congress (final draft in press).

Oregon Health Services Commission. 1991. *Prioritization of Health Services: A Report to the Governor and Leguslature.*

Rawls, John. 1971. *A Theory of Justice* Cambridge, MA: Harvard University Press.

Scanlon, Thomas. 1982. "Contractualism and Utilitarianism." In Amartya Sen and Bernard Williams, eds. *Utilitarianism and Beyond*, pp. 103–28. Cambridge: Cambridge University Press.

Sullivan, Louis. 1992. Press Release (August 3, 1992). Health and Human Services Press Office.

Walzer, Michael. 1983. *Spheres of Justice.* New York: Basic.

Four Models of the Physician–Patient Relationship

Ezekiel J. Emanuel and Linda L. Emanuel

During the last two decades or so, there has been a struggle over the patient's role in medical decision making that is often characterized as a conflict between autonomy and health, between the values of the patient and the values of the physician. Seeking to curtail physician dominance, many have advocated an ideal of greater patient control.[1, 2] Others question this ideal because it fails to acknowledge the potentially imbalanced nature of this interaction when one party is sick and searching for security, and when judgments entail the interpretation of technical information.[3, 4] Still others are trying to delineate a more mutual relationship.[5, 6] This struggle shapes the expectations of physicians and patients as well as the ethical and legal standards for the physician's duties, informed consent, and medical malpractice. This struggle forces us to ask, What should be the ideal physician–patient relationship?

We shall outline four models of the physician–patient interaction, emphasizing the different understandings of (1) the goals of the physician–patient interaction, (2) the physician's obligations, (3) the role of patient values, and (4) the conception of patient autonomy. To elaborate the abstract description of these four models, we shall indicate the types of response the models might suggest in a clinical situation. Third, we shall also indicate how these models inform the current debate about the ideal physician–patient relationship. Finally, we shall evaluate these models and recommend one as the preferred model.

As outlined, the models are Weberian ideal types. They may not describe any particular physician–patient interactions but highlight, free from complicating details, different visions of the essential characteristics of the physician–patient interaction.[7] Consequently, they do not embody minimum ethical or legal standards, but rather constitute regulative ideals that are "higher than the law" but not "above the law."[8]

THE PATERNALISTIC MODEL

First is the *paternalistic* model, sometimes called the parental[9] or priestly[10] model. In this model, the physician–patient interaction ensures that patients receive the interventions that best promote their health and well-being. To this end, physicians use their skills to determine the patient's medical condition and his or her stage in the disease process and to identify the medical tests and treatments most likely to restore the patient's health or ameliorate pain. Then the physician presents the patient with selected information that will encourage the patient to consent to the intervention the physician considers best. At the extreme, the physician authoritatively informs the patient when the intervention will be initiated.

The paternalistic model assumes that there are shared objective criteria for determining what is best. Hence the physician can discern what is in the patient's best interest with limited patient participation. Ultimately, it is assumed that the patient will be thankful for decisions made by the physician even if he or she would not agree to them at the time.[11] In the tension between the patient's autonomy and well-being, between choice and health, the paternalistic physician's main emphasis is toward the latter.

In the paternalistic model, the physician acts as the patient's guardian, articulating and implementing what is best for the patient. As such, the physician has obligations, including that of placing the patient's interest above his or her own and soliciting the views of others when lacking adequate knowledge. The conception of patient autonomy is patient assent, either at the time or later, to the physician's determinations of what is best.

THE INFORMATIVE MODEL

Second is the *informative* model, sometimes called the scientific,[9] engineering,[10] or consumer model. In this model, the objective of the physician–patient interaction is for the physician to provide the patient with all relevant information, for the patient to select the medical interventions he or she wants, and for the physician to execute the selected interventions. To this end, the physician informs the patient of his or her disease state, the nature of possible diagnostic and therapeutic interventions, the nature and probability of risks and benefits associated with the interventions, and any uncertainties of knowledge. At the extreme, patients could come to know all medical information relevant to their disease and available interventions and select the interventions that best realize their values.

The informative model assumes a fairly clear distinction between facts and values. The patient's values are well defined and known; what the patient lacks is facts. It is the physician's obligation to provide all the available facts, and the patient's values then determine what treatments are to be given. There is no role for the physician's values, the physician's understanding of the patient's values, or his or her judgment of the worth of the patient's values. In the informative model, the physician is a purveyor of technical expertise, providing the patient with the means to exercise control. As technical experts, physicians have important obligations to provide truthful information, to maintain competence in their area of expertise, and to consult others when their knowledge or skills are lacking. The conception of patient autonomy is patient control over medical decision making.

THE INTERPRETIVE MODEL

The third model is the *interpretive* model. The aim of the physician–patient interaction is to elucidate the patient's values and what he or she actually wants, and to help the patient select the available medical interventions that realize these values. Like the informative physician, the interpretive physician provides the patient with information on the nature of the condition and the risks and benefits of possible interventions. Beyond this, however, the interpretive physician assists the patient in elucidating and articulating his or her values and in determining what medical interventions best realize the specified values, thus helping to interpret the patient's values for the patient.

According to the interpretive model, the patient's values are not necessarily fixed and known to the patient. They are often inchoate, and the patient may only partially understand them; they may conflict when applied to specific situations. Consequently, the physician working with the patient must elucidate and make coherent these values. To do this, the physician works with the patient to reconstruct the patient's goals and aspirations, commitments and character. At the extreme, the physician must conceive the patient's life as a narrative whole, and from this specify the patient's values and their priority.[12, 13] Then the physician determines which tests and treatments best realize these values. Importantly, the physician does not dictate to the patient; it is the patient who ultimately decides which values and course of action best fit who he or she is. Neither is the physician judging the patient's values; he or she helps the patient to understand and use them in the medical situation.

In the interpretive model, the physician is a counselor, analogous to a cabinet minister's advisory role to a head of state, supplying relevant information, helping to elucidate values and suggesting what medical interventions realize these values. Thus the physician's obligations include those enumerated in the informative model but also require engaging the patient in a joint process of understanding. Accordingly, the conception of autonomy is self-understanding; the patient comes to know more clearly who he or she is and how the various medical options bear on his or her identity.

THE DELIBERATIVE MODEL

Fourth is the *deliberative* model. The aim of the physician–patient interaction is to help the patient determine and choose the best health-related values that can be realized in the clinical situation. To this end, the physician must delineate information on the patient's clinical situation and then help elucidate the types of values embodied in the available options. The physician's objectives include suggesting why certain health-related values are more worthy and should be aspired to. At the extreme, the physician and patient engage in deliberation about what kind of health-related values the patient could and ultimately should pursue. The physician discusses only health-related values, that is, values that affect or are affected by the patient's disease and treatments; he or she recognizes that many elements of morality are unrelated to the patient's disease or treatment and beyond the scope of their professional relationship. Further, the physician aims at no more than moral persuasion; ultimately, coercion is avoided, and the patient must define his or her life and select the ordering of values to be espoused. By engaging in moral deliberation, the physician and patient judge the worthiness and importance of the health-related values.

In the deliberative model, the physician acts as a teacher or friend,[14] engaging the patient in dialogue on what course of action would be best. Not only does the physician indicate what the patient could do, but, knowing the patient and wishing what is best, the physician indicates what the patient should do, what decision regarding medical therapy would be admirable. The conception of patient autonomy is moral self-development; the patient is empowered not simply to follow unexamined preferences or examined values, but to consider, through dialogue, alternative health-related values, their worthiness, and their implications for treatment.

COMPARING THE FOUR MODELS

The Table compares the four models on essential points. Importantly, all models have a role for patient autonomy; a main factor that differentiates the models is their particular conceptions of patient autonomy. Therefore, no single model can be endorsed because it alone promotes patient autonomy. Instead the models must be compared and evaluated, at least in part, by evaluating the adequacy of their particular conceptions of patient autonomy.

The four models are not exhaustive. At a minimum there might be added a fifth: the *instrumental* model. In this model, the patient's values are irrelevant; the physician aims for some goal independent of the patient, such as the good of society or furtherance of scientific knowledge. The Tuskegee syphilis experiment[15–17] and the Willowbrook hepatitis study[18, 19] are examples of this model. As the moral condemnation of these cases reveals, this model is not an ideal but an aberration. Thus we have not elaborated it herein.

A CLINICAL CASE

To make tangible these abstract descriptions and to crystallize essential differences among the models, we will illustrate the responses they suggest in a clinical situation, that of a 43-year-old premenopausal woman who has recently discovered a breast mass. Surgery reveals a 3.5-cm ductal carcinoma with no lymph node involvement that is estrogen receptor positive. Chest roentgenogram, bone scan, and liver function tests reveal no evidence of metastatic disease. The patient was recently divorced and has gone back to work as a legal aide to support herself. What should the physician say to this patient?

	Informative	*Interpretive*	*Deliberative*	*Paternalistic*
Patient values	Defined, fixed, and known to the patient	Inchoate and conflicting, requiring elucidation	Open to development and revision through moral discussion	Objective and shared by physician and patient
Physician's obligation	Providing relevant factual information and implementing patient's selected intervention	Elucidating and interpreting relevant patient values as well as informing the patient and implementing the patient's selected intervention	Articulating and persuading the patient of the most admirable values as well as informing the patient and implementing the patient's selected intervention	Promoting the patient's well being independent of the patient's current preferences
Conception of patient's autonomy	Choice of, and control over, medical care	Self-understanding relevant to medical care	Moral self-development relevant to medical care	Assenting to objective values
Conception of physician's role	Competent technical expert	Counselor or adviser	Friend or teacher	Guardian

Comparing the Four Models

In the paternalistic model a physician might say, "There are two alternative therapies to protect against recurrence of cancer in your breast: mastectomy or radiation. We now know that the survival with lumpectomy combined with radiation therapy is equal to that with mastectomy. Because lumpectomy and radiation offers the best survival and the best cosmetic result, it is to be preferred. I have asked the radiation therapist to come and discuss radiation treatment with you. We also need to protect you against the spread of the cancer to other parts of your body. Even though the chance of recurrence is low, you are young, and we should not leave any therapeutic possibilities untried. Recent studies involving chemotherapy suggest improvements in survival without recurrence of breast cancer. Indeed, the National Cancer Institute recommends chemotherapy for women with your type of breast cancer. Chemotherapy has side effects. Nevertheless, a few months of hardship now are worth the potential added years of life without cancer."

In the informative model a physician might say, "With node-negative breast cancer there are two issues before you: local control and systemic control. For local control, the options are mastectomy or lumpectomy with or without radiation. From many studies we know that mastectomy and lumpectomy with radiation result in identical overall survival, about 80% 10-year survival. Lumpectomy without radiation results in a 30% to 40% chance of tumor recurrence in the breast. The second issue relates to systemic control. We know that chemotherapy prolongs survival for premenopausal women who have axillary nodes involved with tumor. The role for women with node-negative breast cancer is less clear. Individual studies suggest that chemotherapy is of no benefit in terms of improving overall survival, but a comprehensive review of all studies suggests that there is a survival benefit. Several years ago, the NCI suggested that for women like yourself, chemotherapy can have a positive therapeutic impact. Finally, let me inform you that there are clinical trials, for which you are eligible, to evaluate the benefits of chemotherapy for patients with node-negative breast cancer. I can enroll you in a study if you want. I will be happy to give you any further information you feel you need."

The interpretive physician might outline much of the same information as the informative physician, then engage in discussion to elucidate the patient's wishes, and conclude, "It sounds to me as if you have conflicting wishes. Understandably, you seem uncertain how to balance the demands required for receiving additional treatment, rejuvenating your personal affairs, and maintaining your psychological equilibrium. Let me try to express a perspective that fits your position. Fighting your cancer is important, but it must leave you with a healthy self-image and quality time outside the hospital. This view seems compatible with undergoing radiation therapy but not chemotherapy. A lumpectomy with radiation maximizes your chance of surviving while preserving your breast. Radiotherapy fights your breast cancer without disfigurement. Conversely, chemotherapy would prolong the duration of therapy by many months. Further, the benefits of chemotherapy in terms of survival are smaller and more controversial. Given the recent changes in your life, you have too many new preoccupations to undergo months of chemotherapy for a questionable benefit. Do I understand you? We can talk again in a few days."

The deliberative physician might begin by outlining the same factual information, engage in a conversation to elucidate the patient's values, but continue, "It seems clear that you should undergo radiation therapy. It offers maximal survival with minimal risk, disfigurement, and disruption of your life. The issue of chemotherapy is different, fraught with conflicting data. Balancing all the options, I think the best one for you is to enter a trial that is investigating the potential benefit of chemotherapy for women with node-negative breast cancer. First, it ensures that you receive excellent medical care. At this point, we do not know which therapy maximizes survival. In a clinical study the schedule of follow-up visits, tests, and decisions is specified by leading breast cancer experts to ensure that all the women receive care that is the best available anywhere. A second reason to participate in a trial is altruistic; it allows you to contribute something to women with breast cancer in the future who will face difficult choices. Over decades, thousands of women have participated in studies that inform our current treatment practices. Without those women, and the knowledge they made possible, we would probably still be giving you and all other women with breast cancer mastectomies. By enrolling in a trial you participate in a tradition in which women of one generation receive the highest standard of care available but also enhance the care of women in future generations because medicine has learned something about which interventions are better. I must tell you that I am not involved in the study; if you elect to enroll in this trial, you will initially see another breast cancer expert to plan your therapy. I have sought to explain our current knowledge and offer my recommendation so you can make the best possible decision."

Lacking the normal interchange with patients, these statements may seem contrived, even caricatures. Nevertheless, they highlight the essence of each model and suggest how the objectives and assumptions of each inform a physician's approach to his or her patients. Similar statements can be imagined for other clinical situations such as an obstetrician discussing prenatal testing or a cardiologist discussing cholesterol-reducing interventions.

THE CURRENT DEBATE AND THE FOUR MODELS

In recent decades there has been a call for greater patient autonomy or, as some have called it, "patient sovereignty,"[20] conceived as patient *choice* and *control* over medical decisions. This shift toward the informative model is embodied in the adoption of business terms for medicine, as when physicians are described as health care providers and patients as consumers. It can also be found in the propagation of patient rights statements,[21] in the promotion of living will laws, and in rules regarding human experimentation. For instance, the opening sentences of one law state: "The Rights of the Terminally Ill Act authorizes an adult person to *control* decisions regarding administration of life-sustaining treatment…. The Act merely provides one way by which a terminally-ill patient's *desires* regarding the use of life-sustaining procedures can be legally implemented" (emphasis added).[22] Indeed, living will laws do not require or encourage patients to discuss the issue of terminating care with their physicians before signing such documents. Similarly, decisions in "right-to-die" cases emphasize patient control over medical decisions. As one court put it:[23]

> The right to refuse medical treatment is basic and fundamental…. Its exercise requires no one's approval…. *[T]he controlling decision belongs to a competent informed patient….* It is not a medical decision for her physicians to make…. *It is a moral and philosophical decision that, being a competent adult, is [the patient's] alone.* (emphasis added)

Probably the most forceful endorsement of the informative model as the ideal inheres in informed consent standards. Prior to the 1970s, the standard for informed consent was "physician based."[24–26] Since 1972 and the *Canterbury* case, however, the emphasis has been on a "patient-oriented" standard of informed consent in which the physician has a "duty" to provide appropriate medical facts to empower the patient to use his or her values to determine what interventions should be implemented.[25–27]

> True consent to what happens to one's self is the informed exercise of a choice, and that entails an opportunity to evaluate knowledgeably the options available and the risks attendant upon each…. *[I]t is the prerogative of the patient, not the physician, to determine for himself the direction in which his interests seem to lie.* To enable the patient to chart his course understandably, some familiarity with the therapeutic alternatives and their hazards becomes essential.[27] (emphasis added)

SHARED DECISION MAKING

Despite its dominance, many have found the informative model "arid."[20] The President's Commission and others contend that the ideal relationship does not vest moral authority and medical decision-making power exclusively in the patient but must be a process of shared decision making constructed around "mutual participation and respect."[20, 28] The President's Commission argues that the physician's role is "to help the patient understand the medical situation and available courses of action, and the patient conveys his or her concerns and wishes."[20] Brock and Wartman[29] stress this fact-value "division of labor"—having the physician provide information while the patient makes value decisions—by describing "shared decision making" as a collaborative process

> in which both physicians and patients make active and essential contributions. Physicians bring their medical training, knowledge, and expertise—including an understanding of the available treatment alternatives—to the diagnosis and management of patients' condition. Patients bring knowledge of their own subjective aims and values, through which risks and benefits of various treatment options can be evaluated. With this approach,

selecting the best treatment for a particular patient requires the contribution of both parties.

Similarly, in discussing ideal medical decision making, Eddy[30] argues for this fact-value division of labor between the physician and patient as the ideal:

> It is important to separate the decision process into these two steps…. The first step is a question of facts. The anchor is empirical evidence…. [T]he second step is a question not of facts but of personal values or preferences. The thought process is not analytic but personal and subjective…. [I]t is the patient's preferences that should determine the decision…. Ideally, you and I [the physicians] are not in the picture. What matters is what Mrs. Smith thinks.

This view of shared decision making seems to vest the medical decision-making authority with the patient while relegating physicians to technicians "transmitting medical information and using their technical skills as the patient directs."[20] Thus, while the advocates of "shared decision making" may aspire toward a mutual dialogue between physician and patient, the substantive view informing their ideal reembodies the informative model under a different label.

Other commentators have articulated more mutual models of the physician–patient interaction.[5, 6, 25] Prominent among these efforts is Katz'[31] *The Silent World of the Doctor and Patient.* Relying on a Freudian view in which self-knowledge and self-determination are inherently limited because of unconscious influences, Katz views dialogue as a mechanism for greater self-understanding of one's values and objectives. According to Katz, this view places a duty on physicians and patients to reflect and communicate so that patients can gain a greater self-understanding and self-determination. Katz' insight is also available on grounds other than Freudian psychological theory and is consistent with the interpretive model.[13]

OBJECTIONS TO THE PATERNALISTIC MODEL

It is widely recognized that the paternalistic model is justified during emergencies when the time taken to obtain informed consent might irreversibly harm the patient.[1, 2, 20] Beyond such limited circumstances, however, it is no longer tenable to assume that the physician and patient espouse similar values and views of what constitutes a benefit. Consequently, even physicians rarely advocate the paternalistic model as an ideal for routine physician–patient interactions.[32]

OBJECTIONS TO THE INFORMATIVE MODEL

The informative model seems both descriptively and prescriptively inaccurate. First, this model seems to have no place for essential qualities of the ideal physician–patient relationship. The informative physician cares for the patient in the sense of competently implementing the patient's selected interventions. However, the informative physician lacks a caring approach that requires understanding what the patient values or should value and how his or her illness impinges on these values. Patients seem to expect their physician to have a caring approach; they deem a technically proficient but detached physician as deficient, and properly condemned. Further, the informative physician is proscribed from giving a recommendation for fear of imposing his or her will on the patient and thereby competing for the decision-making control that has been given to the patient.[25] Yet, if one of the essential qualities of the ideal physician is the ability to assimilate medical facts, prior experience of similar situations, and intimate knowledge of the patient's view into a recommendation designed for the patient's specific medical and personal condition,[3–5, 25] then the informative physician cannot be ideal.

Second, in the informative model the ideal physician is a highly trained subspecialist who provides detailed factual information and competently implements the patient's preferred medical intervention. Hence, the informative model perpetuates and accentuates the trend toward specialization and impersonalization within the medical profession.

Most importantly, the informative model's conception of patient autonomy seems philosophically untenable. The informative model presupposes that persons possess known and fixed values, but this is inaccurate. People are often uncertain about what they actually want. Further, unlike animals, people have what philosophers call "second-order desires,"[33–35] that is, the capacity to reflect on their wishes and to revise their own desires and preferences. In fact, freedom of the will and autonomy inhere in having "second order desires" and being able to change our preferences and modify our identity. Self-reflection and the capacity to change what we want often require a "process" of moral deliberation in which we assess the value of what we want. And this is a process that occurs with other people who know us well and can articulate a vision of who we ought to be that we can assent to.[13] Even though changes in health or implementation of alternative interventions can have profound effects on what we desire and how we realize our desires, self-reflection and deliberation play no essential role in the informative physician–patient interaction. The informative model's conception of autonomy is incompatible with a vision of autonomy that incorporates second-order desires.

OBJECTIONS TO THE INTERPRETIVE MODEL

The interpretive model rectifies this deficiency by recognizing that persons have second-order desires and dynamic value structures and placing the elucidation of values in the context of the patient's medical condition at the center of the physician-patient interaction. Nevertheless, there are objections to the interpretive model.

Technical specialization militates against physicians cultivating the skills necessary to the interpretive model. With limited interpretive talents and limited time, physicians may unwittingly impose their own values under the guise of articulating the patient's values. And patients,

overwhelmed by their medical condition and uncertain of their own views, may too easily accept this imposition. Such circumstances may push the interpretive model toward the paternalistic model in actual practice.

Further, autonomy viewed as self-understanding excludes evaluative judgment of the patient's values or attempts to persuade the patient to adopt other values. This constrains the guidance and recommendations the physician can offer. Yet in practice, especially in preventive medicine and risk-reduction interventions, physicians often attempt to persuade patients to adopt particular health-related values. Physicians frequently urge patients with high cholesterol levels who smoke to change their dietary habits, quit smoking, and begin exercise programs before initiating drug therapy. The justification given for these changes is that patients should value their health more than they do. Similarly, physicians are encouraged to persuade their human immunodeficiency virus (HIV)-infected patients who might be engaging in unsafe sexual practices either to abstain or, realistically, to adopt "safer sex" practices. Such appeals are not made to promote the HIV-infected patient's own health, but are grounded on an appeal for the patient to assume responsibility for the good of others. Consequently, by excluding evaluative judgments, the interpretive model seems to characterize inaccurately ideal physician–patient interactions.

OBJECTIONS TO THE DELIBERATIVE MODEL

The fundamental objections to the deliberative model focus on whether it is proper for physicians to judge patients' values and promote particular health-related values. First, physicians do not possess privileged knowledge of the priority of health-related values relative to other values. Indeed, since ours is a pluralistic society in which people espouse incommensurable values, it is likely that a physician's values and view of which values are higher will conflict with those of other physicians and those of his or her patients.

Second, the nature of the moral deliberation between physician and patient, the physician's recommended interventions, and the actual treatments used will depend on the values of the particular physician treating the patient. However, recommendations and care provided to patients should not depend on the physician's judgment of the worthiness of the patient's values or on the physician's particular values. As one bioethicist put it:[36]

> The hand is broken; the physician can repair the hand; therefore the physician must repair the hand—as well as possible—without regard to personal values that might lead the physician to think ill of the patient or of the patient's values…. [At] the level of clinical practice, medicine should be value-free in the sense that the personal values of the physician should not distort the making of medical decisions.

Third, it may be argued that the deliberative model misconstrues the purpose of the physician–patient interaction. Patients see their physicians to receive health care, not to engage in moral deliberation or to revise their values. Finally, like the interpretive model, the deliberative model may easily metamorphose into unintended paternalism, the very practice that generated the public debate over the proper physician–patient interaction.

THE PREFERRED MODEL AND THE PRACTICAL IMPLICATIONS

Clearly, under different clinical circumstances different models may be appropriate. Indeed, at different times all four models may justifiably guide physicians and patients. Nevertheless, it is important to specify one model as the shared, paradigmatic reference; exceptions to use other models would not be automatically condemned, but would require justification based on the circumstances of a particular situation. Thus, it is widely agreed that in an emergency where delays in treatment to obtain informed consent might irreversibly harm the patient, the paternalistic

model correctly guides physician–patient interactions. Conversely, for patients who have clear but conflicting values, the interpretive model is probably justified. For instance, a 65-year-old woman who has been treated for acute leukemia may have clearly decided against reinduction chemotherapy if she relapses. Several months before the anticipated birth of her first grandchild, the patient relapses. The patient becomes torn about whether to endure the risks of reinduction chemotherapy in order to live to see her first grandchild or whether to refuse therapy, resigning herself to not seeing her grandchild. In such cases, the physician may justifiably adopt the interpretive approach. In other circumstances, where there is only a one-time physician–patient interaction without an ongoing relationship in which the patient's values can be elucidated and compared with ideals, such as in a walk-in center, the informative model may be justified.

Descriptively and prescriptively, we claim that the ideal physician–patient relationship is the deliberative model. We will adduce six points to justify this claim. First, the deliberative model more nearly embodies our ideal of autonomy. It is an oversimplification and distortion of the Western tradition to view respecting autonomy as simply permitting a person to select, unrestricted by coercion, ignorance, physical interference, and the like, his or her preferred course of action from a comprehensive list of available options.[34, 35] Freedom and control over medical decisions alone do not constitute patient autonomy. Autonomy requires that individuals critically assess their own values and preferences; determine whether they are desirable; affirm, upon reflection, these values as ones that should justify their actions; and then be free to initiate action to realize the values. The process of deliberation integral to the deliberative model is essential for realizing patient autonomy understood in this way.

Second, our society's image of an ideal physician is not limited to one who knows and communicates to the patient relevant factual information and competently implements medical interventions. The ideal physician—often embodied in literature, art, and popular culture—is a caring physician who integrates the information and relevant values to make a recommendation and, through discussion, attempts to persuade the patient to accept this recommendation as the intervention that best promotes his or her overall well-being. Thus, we expect the best physicians to engage their patients in evaluative discussions of health issues and related values. The physician's discussion does not invoke values that are unrelated or tangentially related to the patient's illness and potential therapies. Importantly, these efforts are not restricted to situations in which patients might make "irrational and harmful" choices[29] but extend to all health care decisions.

Third, the deliberative model is not a disguised form of paternalism. Previously there may have been category mistakes in which instances of the deliberative model have been erroneously identified as physician paternalism. And no doubt, in practice, the deliberative physician may occasionally lapse into paternalism. However, like the ideal teacher, the deliberative physician attempts to *persuade* the patient of the worthiness of certain values, not to *impose* those values paternalistically; the physician's aim is not to subject the patient to his or her will, but to persuade the patient of a course of action as desirable. In the *Laws*, Plato[37] characterizes this fundamental distinction between persuasion and imposition for medical practice that distinguishes the deliberative from the paternalistic model:

> A physician to slaves never gives his patient any account of his illness ... the physician offers some orders gleaned from experience with an air of infallible knowledge, in the brusque fashion of a dictator.... The free physician, who usually cares for free men, treats their diseases first by thoroughly discussing with the patient and his friends his ailment. This way he learns something from the sufferer and simultaneously instructs him. Then the physician does not give his medications until he has persuaded the patient; the physician aims at complete restoration of health by persuading the patient to comply with his therapy.

Fourth, physician values are relevant to patients and do inform their choice of a physician. When a pregnant woman chooses an obstetrician who does not routinely perform a battery of prenatal tests or, alternatively, one who strongly favors them; when a patient seeks an aggressive cardiologist who favors procedural interventions or one who concentrates therapy on dietary changes, stress reduction, and life-style modifications, they are, consciously or not, selecting a physician based on the values that guide his or her medical decisions. And, when disagreements between physicians and patients arise, there are discussions over which values are more important and should be realized in medical care. Occasionally, when such disagreements undermine the physician–patient relationship and a caring attitude, a patient's care is transferred to another physician. Indeed, in the informative model the grounds for transferring care to a new physician is either the physician's ignorance or incompetence. But patients seem to switch physicians because they do not "like" a particular physician or that physician's attitude or approach.

Fifth, we seem to believe that physicians should not only help fit therapies to the patients' elucidated values, but should also promote health-related values. As noted, we expect physicians to promote certain values, such as "safer sex" for patients with HIV or abstaining from or limiting alcohol use. Similarly, patients are willing to adjust their values and actions to be more compatible with health-promoting values.[38] This is in the nature of seeking a caring medical recommendation.

Finally, it may well be that many physicians currently lack the training and capacity to articulate the values underlying their recommendations and persuade patients that these values are worthy. But, in part, this deficiency is a consequence of the tendencies toward specialization and the avoidance of discussions of values by physicians that are perpetuated and justified by the dominant informative model. Therefore, if the deliberative model seems most appropriate, then we need to implement changes in medical care and education to encourage a more caring approach. We must stress understanding rather than mere provisions of factual information in keeping with the legal standards of informed consent and medical malpractice; we must educate physicians not just to spend more time in physician–patient communication but to elucidate and articulate the values underlying their medical care decisions, including routine ones; we must shift the publicly assumed conception of patient autonomy that shapes both the physician's and the patient's expectations from patient control to moral development. Most important, we must recognize that developing a deliberative physician–patient relationship requires a considerable amount of time. We must develop a health care financing system that properly reimburses—rather than penalizes—physicians for taking the time to discuss values with their patients.

CONCLUSION

Over the last few decades, the discourse regarding the physician–patient relationship has focused on two extremes: autonomy and paternalism. Many have attacked physicians as paternalistic, urging the empowerment of patients to control their own care. This view, the informative model, has become dominant in bioethics and legal standards. This model embodies a defective conception of patient autonomy, and it reduces the physician's role to that of a technologist. The essence of doctoring is a fabric of knowledge, understanding, teaching, and action, in which the caring physician integrates the patient's medical condition and health-related values, makes a recommendation on the appropriate course of action, and tries to persuade the patient of the worthiness of this approach and the values it realizes. The physician with a caring attitude is the ideal embodied in the deliberative model, the ideal that should inform laws and policies that regulate the physician–patient interaction.

Finally, it may be worth noting that the four models outlined herein are not limited to the medical realm; they may inform the public conception of other professional interactions as well. We suggest that the ideal relationships between lawyer and client,[14] religious mentor and laity, and educator and student are well described by the deliberative model, at least in some of their essential aspects.

Acknowledgments

We would like to thank Robert Mayer, MD, Craig Henderson, MD, Lynn Peterson, MD, and John Stoeckle, MD, as well as Dennis Thompson, PhD, Arthur Applbaum, PhD, and Dan Brock, PhD, for their critical reviews of the manuscript. We would also like to thank the "ethics and the professions" seminar participants, especially Robert Rosen, JD, Francis Kamm, PhD, David Wilkins, JD, and Oliver Avens, who enlightened us in discussions.

Notes

1. Veatch RM. *A Theory of Medical Ethics*. New York, NY: Basic Books Inc Publishers; 1981.
2. Macklin R. *Mortal Choices*. New York, NY: Pantheon Books Inc; 1987.
3. Ingelfinger FJ. Arrogance. *N Engl J Med*. 1980; 304:1507.
4. Marzuk PM. The right kind of paternalism. *N Engl J Med*. 1985; 313:1474–1476.
5. Siegler M. The progression of medicine: from physician paternalism to patient autonomy to bureaucratic parsimony. *Arch Intern Med*. 1985; 145:713–715.
6. Szasz TS, Hollender MH. The basic models of the doctor-patient relationship. *Arch Intern Med*. 1956; 97:585–592.
7. Weber M; Parsons T, ed. *The Theory of Social and Economic Organization*. New York, NY: The Free Press; 1947.
8. Ballantine HT. Annual discourse—the crisis in ethics, anno domini 1979. *N Engl J Med*. 1979; 301: 634–638.
9. Burke G. Ethics and medical decision-making. *Prim Care*. 1980; 7:615–624.
10. Veatch RM. Models for ethical medicine in a revolutionary age. *Hastings Cent Rep*. 1975; 2:3–5.
11. Stone AA. *Mental Health and Law: A System in Transition*. New York, NY: Jason Aronson Inc; 1976.

12. MacIntyre A. *After Virtue*. South Bend, Ind: University of Notre Dame Press; 1981.

13. Sandel MJ. *Liberalism and the Limits of Justice*. New York, NY: Cambridge University Press; 1982.

14. Fried C. The lawyer as friend: the moral foundations of the lawyer client relationship. *Yale Law J.* 1976; 85:1060–1089.

15. Jones JH. *Bad Blood. New* York, NY: Free Press; 1981.

16. *Final Report of the Tuskegee Syphilis Study Ad Hoc Advisory Panel*. Washington, DC: Public Health Service; 1973.

17. Brandt AM. Racism and research: the case of the Tuskegee Syphilis Study. *Hastings Cent Rep.* 1978; 8:21–29.

18. Krugman S, Giles JP. Viral hepatitis: new light on an old disease. *JAMA.* 1970; 212:1019–1029.

19. Ingelfinger FJ. Ethics of experiments on children. *N Engl J Med.* 1973; 288:791–792.

20. President's Commission for the Study of Ethical Problems in Medicine and Biomedical and Behavioral Research. *Making Health Care Decisions*. Washington, DC: US Government Printing Office; 1982.

21. *Statement on a Patient's Bill of Rights*. Chicago, Ill: American Hospital Association; November 17, 1972.

22. Uniform Rights of the Terminally Ill Act. In: *Handbook of Living Will Laws*. New York, NY: Society for the Right to Die; 1987:135–147.

23. *Bouvia v Superior Court*, 225 Cal Rptr 297 (1986).

24. *Natanson v Kline*, 350 P2d 1093 (Kan 1960).

25. Appelbaum PS, Lidz CW, Meisel A. *Informed Consent: Legal Theory and Clinical Practice*. New York, NY: Oxford University Press Inc; 1987:chap 3.

26. Faden RR, Beauchamp TL. A *History and Theory of Informed Consent*. New York, NY: Oxford University Press Inc; 1986.

27. *Canterbury v Spence,* 464 F2d 772 (DC Cir 1972).

28. Brock D. The ideal of shared decision-making between physicians and patients. *Kennedy Institute J Ethics.* 1991; 1:28–47.

29. Brock DW, Wartman SA. When competent patients make irrational choices. *N Engl J Med.* 1990; 322:1595–1599.

30. Eddy DM. Anatomy of a decision. *JAMA.* 1990; 263: 441–443.

31. Katz J. *The Silent World of Doctor and Patient*. New York, NY: Free Press; 1984.

32. Tannock IF, Boyer M. When is a cancer treatment worthwhile? *N Engl J Med.* 1990; 322:989–990.

33. Frankfurt H. Freedom of the will and the concept of a person. *J Philosophy.* 1971; 68:5–20.

34. Taylor C. *Human Agency and Language*. New York, NY: Cambridge University Press; 1985:15–44.

35. Dworkin G. *The Theory and Practice of Autonomy*. New York, NY: Cambridge University Press; 1988:chap 1.

36. Gorovitz S. *Doctors' Dilemmas: Moral Conflict and Medical Care*. New York, NY: Oxford University Press Inc; 1982:chap 6.

37. Plato; Hamilton E, Cairns H, eds; Emanuel EJ, trans. *Plato: The Collected Dialogues*. Princeton, NJ: Princeton University Press; 1961:720 c-e.

38. Walsh DC, Hingson RW, Merrigan DM, et al. The impact of a physician's warning on recovery after alcoholism treatment. *JAMA.* 1992; 267:663–667.

Moral Relationships Between Nurse and Client: The Influence of Metaphors

Janet L. Storch

Metaphors have been commonly used to characterize the nature of the health professional–client relationship, with particular attention to the moral dimensions of that relationship. Metaphors often highlight significant aspects of a relationship, providing us with concrete ways of thinking about the nature of the relationship. However, any metaphor must be used with caution, recognizing that it has the capacity to enlighten, to mislead, and to constrain our thinking. Given the power that metaphors can exert on our practice, critical reflection on how they can shape the moral dimensions of the client–professional relationship is essential.

In this essay, an overview of the types of nurse–client relationships described in the literature through the use of metaphors is provided. The ways in which various metaphors can assist us with or detract us from a clear understanding of our moral agency and our moral duties to our clients/patients are then examined by considering metaphors that are limiting, misguided, or helpful in clarifying the nature of that moral relationship. Finally, a synopsis of key aspects of this special relationship concludes the essay. In an era when health care delivery is beset by a variety of sociopolitical ideologies, it is timely for nursing to embrace metaphors that articulate the values inherent in its practice.

METAPHORS AND MODELS TO DEFINE RELATIONSHIPS

Before embarking on the discussion, a brief commentary on the use of metaphors is in order. A metaphor is defined as a figure of speech in which one thing is compared to another thing by being spoken of as if it were the other. Although metaphors are commonly used in poetry and in lyrics, as well as in ordinary conversation to embellish discourse, they can be most useful in helping us to see some aspects of life, such as interpersonal relationships, in a way that enhances our understanding. Thus, we are directed to see and to think about that relationship in a particular way. That is, metaphors lead us to emphasize certain aspects of the relationship and minimize others. At the same time, metaphors offer alternative views or ways of seeing a relationship. In this way, metaphors can have a powerful influence on our language, on how we think, and on how we come to understand that aspect of life. In many respects, this influence is positive and enlightening. At the same time, this emphasis can lead to a distortion in thinking because it can overemphasize one view at the expense of other equally valid views that become excluded from consideration. That exclusion itself is significant because it allows us to "not see" the whole picture (Morgan, 1997).

Veatch (1972) and Callaban (1988) are two ethicists who have employed metaphors to facilitate understanding of health professional–patient relationships. Several models and metaphors have been identified in health care and health ethics literature. They are captured in the table on the following page (Table 5.1). Some of these metaphors focus on the comparison of physicians to engineers, to priests, or to contractors (see Veatch, 1972). These metaphors portray medicine as among the first of professions. A more recent discussion, by Emanuel and Emanuel (1992), is based on various approaches in one's relationships with clients rather than on strictly metaphorical comparisons. Consideration of these approaches seems to have been directed towards moving the medical profession forward to keep pace with the changed expectations of the public to be served.

In the discourse about nurse–client relationships that uses metaphorical thinking, there is clearly some "borrowing" of approaches from the literature describing other health professional–patient relationships through model and metaphor. There are also significant contrasts in the types of models and metaphors utilized to understand the nature of the relationship between physicians and patients when compared with those used to characterize nurse–client relationships. In general, nurse–client models and metaphors are more concrete and, therefore, more explicit in their characterization of nursing (e.g., mother, servant). This concreteness can create particular problems for the nursing profession. The nursing profession can be characterized so clearly that images are difficult for the public, other professions, and nurses themselves to shed with ease. It may even be difficult to recognize the distortions the metaphors convey.

METAPHORS AND NURSE–CLIENT RELATIONSHIPS

It seems unlikely that any other vocation or profession has experienced the diversity of imagery and metaphor that nursing has encountered in the Western world over the past century. Initially

Table 5.1

MODELS AND METAPHORS IDENTIFIED IN THE LITERATURE

Physician–Patient Relationships and Health Professional–Patient Relationships

VEATCH 1972	MAY 1975	BAYLES 1981
1. Engineering (Employer)	1. Contract	1. Agency
2. Priestly	2. Covenant	2. Contract
3. Collegial		3. Friendship
4. Contractual		4. Paternalistic
		5. Fiduciary

CALLAHAN 1988	EMANUEL & EMANUEL 1992
1. Contract	1. Paternalistic
2. Covenant	2. Informative
3. Advocate	3. Interpretive
4. Fiduciary	4. Deliberative

Nurse-Client Relationships

SMITH 1950	BROCK 1580
1. Nurse as surrogate mother	1. Nurse as parent surrogate
2. Nurse as technician	2. Nurse as physician surrogate
3. Nurse as contracted clinician	3. Nurse as healer
	4. Nurse as patient advocate or protector
	5. Nurse as educator
	6. Nurse as contracted clinician

WINSLOW 1984	
I. Military metaphor	
2. Legal metaphor (Advocacy)	

FOWLER 1984	MITCHELL 1990
1. Mercantile	1. Domestic (servant)
2. Indentured servant	2. Family (mother surrogate)
3. Engineering	3. Medical (physician extender)
4. Priestly	4. Business (employee)
5. Collegial	5. Advocacy (patient advocate)
6. Contractual	6. Contractual (contracted clinician)
7. Friendship (Aristotelian)	7. Friendship (friend)
8. Covenantal	

the depiction of nursing was through pictures (painted or sketched), often with metaphors as captions (e.g., Angels of Mercy). More recently, the use of written metaphors to describe and analyze nurses and nurse–client relationships has been common. One can only surmise that the penchant for "picturing" the nurse historically is related to a fascination with the female figure. Physicians have also experienced imagery of their roles and relationships with patients, but the images and metaphors of physicians have not been so varied, so gender related, nor so extensive. As noted earlier, the concrete nature of nursing metaphors, such as those depicted in Table 5.1, is also significant. Many of the conclusions about nursing embedded in the minds of readers or viewers have been based upon these metaphors and have been difficult for nursing to overcome. These metaphors are rooted in long-standing historical images.

Historical Images of Professional Nursing

In 1996, the International Council of Nurses, the International Red Cross, and the Red Crescent Museum in Geneva developed an exhibition to capture in images, text, and testimonials the first 30 years (1900-1930) of "… nursing's rise as an intellectual, socially responsible endeavor" (*Profession: Nurse* 1995, p. 11). This exhibition included a wide range of posters, postcards, drawings, paintings, and photographs that depicted nurses and conveyed a sense of the nurse's role and relationship to patients and to society.

The pictures and other material provided images of nurse as mother, sister, friend, lover, guardian angel, or army sergeant. In the accompanying publication, produced by the International Red Cross and Red Crescent Museum, the authors note that these images of nursing (these metaphors of nursing) were widely used during the First World War for purposes of raising funds for the war effort, raising morale, and stimulating patriotic zeal. "A mother figure to all the wounded, the needy and children, a nurse—with or without the red cross or crescent on her uniform—was often perceived as a savior in the glow of fervent patriotism…. Nurses were viewed as moral figures above all suspicion and were therefore used for propaganda purposes …" (*Profession: Nurse*, 1995, p. 26).

Following World War I, as the image of the universal mother and guardian angel gave way to Post War realities, nurses began to be depicted as fighters or soldiers who fought the residual ills of the War and epidemics, and worked in communities with social welfare officers to fight social ills.

The World Wars, and wars of the previous century, had a profound influence on the devel-

opment of nursing. Florence Nightingale's work in founding nursing as a profession was given impetus by the Crimean War. And the influence of military models of health care delivery and hospital organization directed the manner in which nursing unfolded as an independent entity. Only in the latter three decades of the twentieth century has the influence of some of these metaphors begun to fade from view. In fact, some of these historical images or metaphors of nursing continue to have a profound effect on the public's view of nurses, fellow health professionals' understanding of nurse–client relationships, and the views of nurses themselves. Some of these views or perceptions have served to limit the significance of professional nursing.

Limiting Metaphors: Nurse As Parent, Nurse As Servant, Nurse As Friend

Assuming the majority of people hold positive perceptions of parents, and of mothers in particular, the metaphor of *nurse as parent surrogate* or *nurse as mother surrogate* to describe the nurse–client relationship allows us to see some fundamental foundations of that relationship. It is a relationship based upon trust, integrity, promise-keeping, dedication, and nurturance. Taking that metaphor of mother or parent further, one can understand the nurse–client relationship to involve some degree of protection of the client in care, an attempt to help clients gain or regain independence, and a commitment to never abandon a client in need. Inasmuch as this metaphor serves to enlarge understanding about these moral features of the relationship, it is well used.

However, in highlighting some similar characteristics, there can be a tendency to overgeneralize. All features of the nurse–client relationship come to be seen as "parenting" or "mothering" relationships. The ways in which this might distort the nature of the relationship are many. Nursing comes to be seen as largely women's work and as a selfless endeavour. Like mothering, nursing then comes to be viewed as something that anyone can do. In making these assumptions, it becomes easy to discount nursing knowledge, skill, and expertise. The "tender loving care" provided by nurses may appear to be just like mother's care and concern, with little more knowledge required than what arises from trying to be caring and helpful to another.

Mitchell (1990) has labeled the mother/parent metaphor a *family metaphor*. She identifies a primary concern within the metaphor of surrogate mother to be found in "… the arrangement of health care services and relationships according to family roles, with the physician as father, nurse as mother, and patients as dependents …" (page 5). In this scenario the nurse is expected to work (likely harder than anyone else) to maintain harmony in the home, i.e., the hospital. Further, the nurse as helpmate is not accorded power for decision making. This has significant implications for the nurse's ability to exercise his or her moral agency.

The *friendship metaphor* has positive parallels to the family metaphor, including expectations that clients can depend upon nurses and that nurses would value truth-telling and fidelity. It is misleading, however, in that the nurse–client relationship cannot be a relationship of equals, like friendship. Clients are often in a vulnerable state during their health care encounter and there is, by reason of that vulnerability and by reason of the different type and level of knowledge about the client's condition, an asymmetry of power in the healing relationship.

Finally, the *nurse as servant metaphor* adds one level of clarity to the nurse–client relationship, but at the price of potentially serious misconceptions about the relationship. From a positive view, the servant metaphor emphasizes service to others, and in this way captures the moral ideal of service critical to professional roles. In this case, nurses as professionals use their knowledge and skills in service to others The misleading aspects of the metaphor include the implication that nurses will do anything that needs to be done at work, including domestic work (Mitchell, 1990). This has led to the serious exploitation of nurses in the past and to a significant extent in the present. Nurses' responses to such exploitation have been to establish unions for some protection from the arbitrariness of employers. Through unions they have set limits on the work they are required to

do and the times in which they will do it. Nevertheless, in our current era of health care cost constraint, nurses are all too often expected to fill in the gaps when resources are cut.

A serious distortion of the metaphor of nurse as servant is the characterization of the nurse as an *indentured servant* who just "follows orders" (Fowler, 1984). This understanding of the nurse's role and relationship within the health care team led to obedience, in which the nurse cedes his or her moral agency to institutional directives, with the result that both nurse and client suffer. From this indentured servant metaphor, the long history of nurse as handmaiden to the physician has also been prominent. This places the client in a secondary position relative to the nurse–physician, then nurse–client relationship. Indeed, the Nightingale pledge that many nurses took at either capping ceremonies or graduations in times past included the phrase "… with loyalty will I endeavor to aide the physician in his work and devote myself to the welfare of the patient" (Storch, 1982, p. 202). In this sense, devotion to the patient was considered to be realized through loyally aiding the physician (Fowler, 1984). It was not until the middle of the twentieth century that those two commitments (to physician and to patient) were disentangled. By the early 1970s the International Council of Nurses Code of Ethics stated with unmistaken clarity that "The nurse's primary responsibility is to those people who require nursing care" (Storch, 1982, p. 201). Yet, amongst physicians, health administrators and the public, there are still many who wonder why nurses are not "doing nursing" anymore (e.g., Stein, 1990). Whether their puzzlement is written or stated, the source of concern often can be traced to the query about why nurses are not there to "aid" physicians any longer or to follow orders without question(s).

Misguided Metaphors

Use of the *metaphor of technician* or *nurse as engineer* to describe the nurse–patient relationship emphasizes the task aspect of nursing roles. The strength of this metaphor rests in its emphasis on technical competence. Competence is a highly valued dimension of the nurse-patient relationship since "… caring without knowledge remains simply a matter of good intentions …" (Falk Raphael, 1996). Unless the nurse meets the level of technical competence to carry out her tasks, "… the whole relationship begins with a lie" (Pellegrino, 1979, p. 48).

However, emphasizing the technical and task aspects of nursing captures only a fraction of nursing knowledge and skill, and the metaphor of technician limits understanding about the work that nurses do. As "re-engineering" of care-giver roles has become fashionable (Schweikhart and Smith-Daniels, 1996), this distortion of role has led to the devaluing of wholistic nursing practice and, alarmingly, to simplistic solutions to nursing replacement. Since many can see only the "tasks" nurses do, the rest of nursing work remains invisible. For example, in the giving of a medication, what is observed is a pill moving from the nurse's hand to the client's mouth. What is unobserved is the nurse's assessment of the client's condition while that simple act is in progress—respirations, pallor, comfort, degree of mobility, ease of swallowing, skin turgor, evidence of edema, etc.—the mental note taken of a plan of care on-course or one in need of modification (based on expert knowledge of the condition, the drug, and environmental stressors). Verbal and nonverbal communication occur in that simple but highly complex interaction. Opportunities arise to engage in client teaching, support, guidance, and reassurance. Perhaps, most important, is the sense of presence the expert nurse brings to the encounter—a way of being with the client that reflects the depth of care and concern, laced with competence to deliver, for that one individual. Thus, the concrete task observed is not the real work of nursing: the real work of nursing requires knowledge and skill that is all but invisible to the observer. The type of care expert nurses provide must begin with considerable investment in the relationship, involves the use of self, and involves attention to the uniqueness of that client.

These same misguided task-oriented conclusions are operative in the *physician extender* and

physician surrogate metaphors. While there are aspects of medical tasks and medical work that nurses are able to perform, even in performing those tasks nursing work is different. Taking on specific tasks of medicine does not equate to being either a physician extender or a physician surrogate, or a physician for that matter. Nursing roles and relationships are different, with different goals and different processes of care. For example, both physicians and nurses will monitor arterial blood gas results. The physician monitors those results to diagnose cardio-pulmonary dysfunction; the nurse monitors the same results to plan activity, rest, and comfort.

Nursing knowledge increasingly involves many ways of knowing, beyond empirical knowledge and technical skill. It includes knowledge gained through empirics, but also knowledge drawn from ethics, personal knowledge, aesthetics, and sociopolitical knowing (Carper, 1978; White, 1995). Different knowledge and skill lead to different ways of approaching care, and to a different form of nurse–client relationship, including greater attention to "ways of being" in relationship with the clients (Silva, Sorrell and Sorell, 1995).

Helpful Metaphors: Nurse As in a Covenantal Relationship, As Healer, As Advocate

Among the many metaphors applied to nurse–client relationships are several that stand out as characterizing more clearly than others the ideals of what these relationships should be. Use of the metaphor of a *covenantal relationship* emphasizes that nurse and client are "… bound to one another in many ways, not the least of which is morally" (Fowler, 1984, p. 338). As members of a community, and within that community a health care system, nurses are expected to be faithful and to keep their promise of profession, i.e., to use their knowledge and skills to minimize harm and to benefit others.

A convenantal model calls attention to the reciprocal indebtedness of the public and the profession, suggesting that professional power is a gift from the public to the profession given in exchange for its expertise and orientation to the service of others (Bernal, 1992, p. 22).

In emphasizing concepts of relatedness and reciprocity, the covenantal model underscores nursing practice priorities of the 1990s.

The image of *nurse as healer* is a long standing metaphor utilized since the early 1900s to emphasize the healing powers of the nursing presence. Whether a nurse is fully present with a client through the painful journey of being a critically ill patient in ICU or CCU, through an outpatient experience of chemotherapy, or through a long period of rehabilitation at home recovering from a stroke, the professional nurse's ongoing presence can facilitate the individual to move towards restoration and healing. In this way the nurse has a different but complementary role to that of physician.

The *nurse as client advocate* was introduced in the early 1970s and was based on a clearer understanding of nurses' direct accountability (legal and ethical) to clients. Considerable attention in nursing literature (see for example, Donahue, 1978; Abrams, 1978; Curtin, 1979; Gadow, 1980; Kohnke, 1982; Fowler, 1989; Bernal, 1995) has been directed towards identifying the role of advocacy and types of advocacy (e.g., intervening, protecting, informing, supporting, speaking for, coordinating, empowering, etc.) as well as problems for nurses in fulfilling a role as client advocate.

In 1984, Winslow analyzed the shift from a nursing practice based on a military model (characterized by hierarchy and obedience) to one based on a legal model that focused on advocacy for the client in health care. He identified several issues surrounding the nurse as patient or client advocate, including lack of clarity of the concept, the need to revise nursing practice acts to allow for this type of nursing role, the question as to whether clients and their families were prepared to accept advocacy as a nursing role, the potentially adversarial nature of advocacy, and the potential conflicting interests and loyalties inherent in advocacy. Advocacy has served as a powerful metaphor for nursing, although often with only superficial understanding of its real power.

As long as advocacy is confined to legal metaphor it is limiting. However, when it is viewed as "… not simply one more alternative to be added to the list of past and present concepts of nursing … but as embracing all of them …" (Curtin, 1979, p. 2), its real meaning is understood. Benner (1994) characterized client advocacy as involving openness and engagement in moral and clinical reasoning. Drawing upon the work of Gadow (1980), who conceptualized "existential advocacy," Benner contrasts the "narrow legal sense of advocacy" (page 49) with a deeper and more meaningful form of advocacy. She describes this type of advocate as one who "stands alongside, who interprets, and understands …" (page 49)—language congruent with a covenantal relationship. She suggests that this enriched metaphor of client advocacy is manifest in the following way: managing and coordinating services to a client so that all services are directed toward an agreed upon intent to ensure client and family well-being, "… standing in for someone to give them voice … getting appropriate medical intervention for [clients] … and presencing and acknowledging loss and grief" with one who is dying (page 51).

These metaphors of nurse in a covenantal relationship, nurse as healer, and nurse as advocate, approach more closely than the previous metaphors the morally significant aspects of the nurse–client relationship. Their emphasis is on the moral commitment of the nurse to be a comforting presence to clients through difficult health situations; to be in relationship with clients; and to intervene, inform, support, and facilitate their empowerment. This emphasis provides insight into the "special" nature of the nurse–client relationship.

What Metaphors Enable Us to See and Learn

Metaphors used to describe the nurse–client relationship can be instructive and they can be limiting. Their limitations include their potential to further devalue nursing knowledge and skill, to perpetuate stereotypical notions of nurse–client and physician–client relationships, to mislead by suggesting equal partnership in that relationship, to perpetuate the task-oriented view of nursing, and to conflate nurse and physician roles. The strength of metaphors applied to nursing rests in the ability to understand more readily the historical shifts in nursing roles and nurse–client relationships and to appreciate both constancy and change in nurse–client relationships over time. Further, metaphors help to articulate the values in nursing practice in an era when roles are under threat from an economic imperative.

The constant themes of the nurse–client relationship accessed through metaphor are relationships based on the moral foundations of trust, integrity, respect, truth-telling, and promise-keeping. These themes are fundamental to nursing. The covenantal metaphor emphasis on reciprocity and connectedness makes more visible the foundation of the relationship. Metaphors have also served a useful purpose in drawing distinctions between medicine and nursing over time. When used with care, metaphors enable us to see and learn much about the nature of nursing and the nature of the nurse–patient relationship. Most importantly, the moral foundations of that relationship can become more visible and less difficult to articulate and defend.

References

The author wishes to thank Dr. Gwen Hartrick, Dr. Patricia Rodney, and Dr. Rita Schreiber for their critical review of this essay and for their helpful suggestions.

Abrams, Natalie (1978). "A contrary view of the nurse as patient advocate," *Nursing Forum* 17(3): 258–267.

Bayles, Michael D. (1981). *Professional Ethics*. Belmont: CA. Wadsworth Publishing Co.

Baylis, Francoise, Downie, Jocelyn, Freedman, Benjamin, Hoffmaster, Barry, and Sherwin, Susan, eds. (1996). *Health Care Ethics in Canada*. Toronto: Harcourt Brace and Company.

Benner, Patricia (1994). "Caring as ways of knowing and not knowing." In *The Crisis of Care* (pp. 42–62). Edited by Susan Phillips and Patricia Benner. Washington D.C.: Georgetown University Press.

Bernal, Ellen W. (1992), "The nurse as patient advocate." *Hastings Center Report* 22(4): 18–23.

Brock, Dan W. (1980). "The nurse-patient relation: Some rights and duties." In *Nursing: Images and Ideals* (pp. 102–124). Edited by Stuart F. Spicker and Sally Gadow. New York: Springer Publishing Co.

Callahan, Joan, ed. (1988). *Ethical Issues in Professional Life*. New York: Oxford University Press.

Carper, Barbara (1978). "Fundamental patterns of knowing in nursing." *Advances in Nursing Science* 1(1): 13–23.

Curtin, Leah (1979). "Nurse as advocate: A philosophical foundation for nursing." *Advances in Nursing Science* 1(3): 1–10.

Donahue, M. Patricia (1978). "The nurse: A patient advocate?" *Nursing Forum* 17(2): 143–151.

Emanuel, Ezekiel J. and Emanuel, Linda L. (1995). "Four models of the physician-patient relationship." In *Health Care Ethics in Canada* (pp. 163–179). Edited by Francoise Baylis et al. Toronto: Harcourt Brace and Company.

Fowler, Marsha (1984). Ethics and Nursing, 1893–1984: The Ideal of Service, the Reality of History. Doctoral Dissertation, University of Southern California.

_____ (1989). "Social advocacy." *Heart and Lung* 18(1): 97–99.

Gadow, Sally (1980). "Existential advocacy: Philosophical foundations of nursing." In *Nursing: Images and Ideals* (pp. 79–101). Edited by Stuart F. Smith and Sally Gadow. New York: Springer Publishing Company.

Kohnke, Mary (1982). *Advocacy: Risk or Reality*. Toronto: C.V. Mosby.

May, William F. (1975). "Code and covenant or philanthropy and contract." *Hastings Center Report* 5(6): 29–38.

Mitchell, Christine (1990). "The nurse-patient relationship: A source of some moral duties." In Humanities and the Health Professions, Occasional Papers of the Connecticut Humanities Council, No. 8, 3–16.

Morgan, Gareth (1997). *Images of Organizations*. Thousand Oaks: Sage Publications.

Profession: Nurse, Images 1900–1930 (1995). Geneva: Musée International de la Red Cross et du Red Crescent.

RNABC (1997). *The Role of the Nurse in Advocacy.* Vancouver: Registered Nurses Association of British Columbia.

Schweikhart, Sharon Bergman, and Smith-Daniels, Vicki (1996). "Reengineering the work of caregivers: Roles redefinition, team structures, and organizational redesign." *Hospital and Health Administration* 41(1): 19–35.

Silva, Mary, Sorrell, Jeanne, and Sorrell, Christine (1995). "From Carper's ways of knowing to ways of being: An ontological shift in nursing." *Advances in Nursing Science* 18(1): 1–13.

Smith, Sheri (1980). "Three models of the nurse-patient relationship." In *Nursing: Images and Ideals* (pp. 176–188). Edited by Stuart F.

Spicker and Sally Gadow. New York: Springer Publishing Company.

Stein, Leonard, Watts, D.T., and Howell, T. (1990). "The doctor-nurse game revisited." *New England Journal of Medicine* 60(5): 812–816.

Storch, Janet L. (1982). *Patients' Rights: Ethical and Legal Issues in Health Care and in Nursing.* Toronto: McGraw Hill.

Veatch, Robert M. (1972). "Models for ethical medicine in a revolutionary age." *Hastings Center Report* 2(3): 5–7.

White, Jill (1995). "Patterns of knowing: Review, critique and update." *Advances in Nursing Science* 17(4): 78–86.

Winslow, Gerald R. (1984). "From loyalty to advocacy: A new metaphor for nursing." *Hastings Center Report* 14(3): 32–40.

Understanding Trust

Carolyn McLeod

Current health care practitioners are in a different situation than their predecessors when it comes to patient trust. One Canadian physician is quoted as saying, "The profession had more respect [in the past]. Your opinion doesn't count as much with patients any more" (*The Globe and Mail*, F4, 23/11/2002). Physicians and other practitioners cannot take the trust of patients in their opinions for granted.[1] Yet trust provides the moral foundation for any healthy patient–practitioner relationship.[2] The problem is serious. Now how do we solve it? Well, part of the solution (and only part of it[3]) is to teach practitioners how to build and maintain patient trust. This step in turn requires a clear understanding of what trust is; otherwise, advice on how to promote it would surely be empty. My intention here is to provide such understanding, along with a rough guide on how practitioners could use it to foster trust in their relationships with patients.

A THEORY OF TRUST[4]

What is it that we trust in other people? What about them makes us willing to trust? A general answer, for which there is some consensus in ethics, is their competence to do what we trust them to do and their motivation for doing it; surely, we would not trust people unless we thought they had the necessary competence and desire to do what we want them to do. However, controversy exists around the question of how we want people we trust to be motivated to act. Following Annette Baier,[5] many ethicists assume that the relevant motivation is goodwill: we want those whom we trust to be motivated by goodwill towards us. But not all philosophers agree, and some fail to give a clear answer to that question.[6] It is important not to be ambiguous in answering it because part of what makes trust unique from other attitudes, such as mere reliance, *is* the kind of motivation we expect from people we trust. I propose that what we expect is not goodwill, but moral integrity. This virtue involves consistently doing what "one takes oneself to have the most moral reason to do."[7] Moreover, we would want them to generally share our understanding of what counts as a good moral reason.

Thus, our attitude about how we want people we trust to be motivated to act targets both their moral integrity and what they stand for. But there is more still: sometimes that attitude also concerns their perception of their relationship with us. Sometimes, for us to be optimistic that other people will be motivated to honour our trust, we have to expect that they perceive their relationship with us similarly to the way that we perceive it.

THE COMPETENCE OF THE ONE TRUSTED

The idea that trust involves optimism about the competence of the other is not controversial; but let me discuss it nonetheless, specifically as it relates to patient trust. For such trust to occur, optimism about the competence of the practitioner is essential. Consider a sample relationship in this domain.

> For years, Todd has had the same family physician, Dr. Young. He has always depended on Dr. Young to provide him with good medical advice and to perform medical procedures competently. He has kept her as his family physician for so long partly because Dr. Young gives him a lot of information about potential harms and benefits of different procedures or treatments. It is important to Todd that he be informed as much as possible about his health care so that he can be sure he truly wants what he gets.

Todd clearly relies on the competence of Dr. Young. He is optimistic that she is competent to perform medical procedures and to give Todd sound advice as well as detailed information about his health care options. If such optimism were to fade away, so would Todd's trust.

Trusters such as Todd are often unaware of what people they trust have to do to display their competence, and the former are vulnerable as a result. Todd trusts Dr. Young to give him competent advice, even though Todd probably could not tell good medical advice from bad. Bioethicists emphasize the need for patients to trust their practitioners because of the knowledge gap that normally exists between them.[8] Patients are vulnerable in medical encounters in part because of that gap.[9]

Patients trust not only the technical competence of health care professionals, but also their moral competence. One dimension of moral competence is knowing what is morally required in different situations. And another is acting on what is required: that is, being morally virtuous. The latter overlaps with moral integrity as a feature of trust, which I discuss below. The former—moral understanding—is relevant to trust in the competence of health care practitioners in the following ways. Minimally, patients expect practitioners to understand the moral importance of honouring a commitment to provide them with health care. However, many expect greater moral understanding than that. For example, Todd is representative of a growing segment of Western society that trusts physicians to understand the need to respect patient autonomy (along with related issues such as the responsibility to disclose information to patients). It is not enough that health care practitioners have the necessary technical skills and scientific knowledge to be competent practitioners. Even patients who assume that physicians should be paternalistic trust physicians to understand the moral importance of acting in their best interests.

Thus, patients trust health care practitioners to have some moral understanding, or competence, which is part of their more general optimism about the competence of their practitioners to do what they trust them to do.

THE MOTIVATION OF THE ONE TRUSTED

We want people we trust to have not only the ability to do what we trust them to do, but also the motivation to do it. People can be motivated to do things in many different ways. What is the relevant motivation in trust relations? Baier argues that it can neither be something sleazy (e.g., pure selfishness) nor something that implies total indifference to others' welfare. For example, I might think that a surgeon will perform surgery on me competently not because I believe he has any concern for me or because he has moral integrity, but because I know that he does not want to get sued. The language of trust would be out of place in describing my attitude toward him. I do not trust the surgeon; I merely rely on him. Reliance is an attitude toward another's competence where, as long as that person is motivated to do what he is competent to do, it is irrelevant to us what kind of motivation he has for acting. With trust, this issue is not at all irrelevant.

What we trust in others is not simply kindly feeling towards us, however. We can trust others even without being optimistic that they feel kindly toward us; e.g., we may trust them without expecting them to have specific concern for us. For example, it is conceivable that a patient could trust a nurse to be motivated by a commitment to provide her with good health care without assuming that the nurse has kindly feelings for her. Particularly in trust relations between patients and specialists, such as surgeons, kindly feelings need not be a feature of the relationship.

Even if someone does have kindly feelings toward us, knowing that may not be a good reason to trust that person. Suppose that not only is Todd optimistic that Dr. Young respects his autonomy, Dr. Young is committed to doing so (where that requires that she disclose information to Todd about his health status and his health care options). If Dr. Young were to develop reliable and kindly feelings toward Todd and be motivated because of those feelings to be dishonest with him about his health status, she would be betraying Todd's trust. She would be failing to inform him of any potentially serious health problems not because she thinks it is her moral duty to prevent Todd from experiencing distress (Dr. Young is committed to promoting patient autonomy), but because she has a strong desire not to cause Todd any distress. In that case, Dr. Young would be acting on kindly feelings without doing what Todd trusts her to do. Todd's trust in her therefore could not be grounded in kindly feelings.

Trust is usually incompatible with serious forms of deception unless deception is necessary to shield the trusting person from severe harm. If Todd became clinically depressed and suicidal, it might be compatible with his trust in Dr. Young for Dr. Young to withhold information from him about a serious illness, at least temporarily. But even when it is not necessary to deceive others to protect their welfare, kindly feelings can encourage deception if those feelings are strong enough. What we want, ultimately, from people we trust are not kindly feelings, but *a commitment to doing what is right in the circumstances*. In the scenario above, the right thing for Dr. Young to do, both from her perspective and from Todd's, is to disclose information to Todd in a way that is respectful of his autonomy.

One might think it is a bit overblown to say that what we want from people we trust is for them to "do the right thing." It may be that we just want them to make considered judgments in determining how to best serve our interests, as opposed to having their kindly feelings motivate them in ways that might subvert our interests. We might still trust their goodwill but only if it is informed by their judgment. The idea that goodwill of this sort is a component of trust is compelling; nonetheless, it fails to capture one aspect of trust relations. Consider a situation where someone we trust uses her considered judgment to determine our interests and she acts accordingly, but she ignores her responsibilities to others in the process. For example, what if Dr. Young were good at respecting Todd's autonomy, but she also gave preferential treatment to Todd, even over patients who were suffering more than him and who had arrived at Dr. Young's office first? Many people in Todd's place would be appalled, or at least concerned, and insist that was not what they had trusted the physician to do. Presumably, then, I have misconstrued Todd's interests by implying that Dr. Young could satisfy them simply by respecting Todd's autonomy. Assuming that Todd is a decent guy, his interest could not be to have others suffer for his own sake. But even if he were not at all decent, it would not be in his interests to see his physician treating her patients unfairly; Todd may be disturbed by such treatment if only because it suggests to him that one day Dr. Young might treat *him* unfairly! Either way, what Todd trusts Dr. Young to do *is* the right thing. He trusts her to be motivated by judgments that are not merely considered but are also moral.

In summary, we want those we trust to be motivated by moral integrity. We want them to have an enduring commitment to act in a morally respectful way toward us and we want their actions to accord with that commitment. Having integrity means that your actions are integrated with what you stand for, while having moral integrity means that they are integrated with what you stand for morally speaking. When Dr. Young fails to disclose important information to Todd about his health status, she compromises her own moral integrity, and in doing so, betrays Todd's trust.

What the Trusted One Stands for

Because people can stand for very different things, it cannot only be moral integrity that we expect from people we trust. We care about what they stand for, not just about whether they will act on what they stand for. Todd does not trust Dr. Young simply to act on whatever values Dr. Young accepts as the right values. He expects her to endorse specifically the value of respect for patient autonomy. A further feature of trust, therefore, is an expectation that what the one trusted stands for, morally speaking, is similar enough to what we stand for (as far as we know what that is) that we can count on her to do what we trust her to do.

To trust others, we usually require some sense of what they stand for so that we can know whether they are likely to act in the way that we would expect them to. And what that way is depends on what we perceive to be morally acceptable ways to act. For example, what Todd

expects from health care practitioners he trusts is respect for patient autonomy because he believes that is important in health care.

But perhaps it is unrealistic to claim that before patients can trust practitioners, they have to have some idea of what they stand for. Patients often deal with practitioners whom they have never met. How could they assume anything about where their moral commitments lie? But surely they could presume that practitioners will respect the values of their own profession, which, among other things, include benefiting patients and respecting their autonomy. Such a presumption is rebuttable, of course—not *all* health care practitioners embrace those values; however, it is not unreasonable because of how practitioners are taught to behave.

One could add that trust tends to grow or diminish as our knowledge of what others stand for increases. Further, the amount of evidence we need about how similar their values are to our own likely depends on what is at stake for us by trusting them. For example, there is more at stake in trusting a physician to treat us for cancer than in trusting one to give us a flu shot. Presumably, we would want to know more about the values of the physician in the first case than we would in the second before trusting that physician.

The Trusted One's Perception of Our Relationship

A final feature of trust is that we expect people we trust to interpret the nature of our relationship similarly to the way we do. If they conceive of our relationship differently, they may not welcome our trust (just as practitioners may not welcome patients trusting them in certain ways). Adding this feature takes care of cases of unwelcome trust, and it concerns our attitude specifically toward *whether*, as opposed to *how*, people we trust will be motivated to act.

When people do not welcome our trust, they do not object to our optimism about their competence, their moral integrity, or about the fact that we admire what they stand for. Rather, they object to our expectation that they do something for us.[10] For example, practitioners who do not welcome the trust of patients do not wish to do what these patients trust them to do (e.g., make house calls or perform unnecessary procedures).

While some moral commitments demand that we respect the interests of everyone (e.g., our duty not to commit murder), others require only that we behave in a certain way toward people with whom we are in a special kind of relationship. Although I may have a duty to be honest on some level with everyone, I am not morally required, I do not think, to be as honest about my feelings with everyone as I am with people with whom I am intimate. Similarly, I am not morally obligated to be as concerned for the welfare of others as I ought to be for my own family members and close friends. Often what we trust in others, including parents, lovers, and professional people, is that they do something for us that they would not do for just anyone. In other words, we trust them to act on relationship-specific commitments.

Unwelcome trust is a potential problem only in relationships where one expects the other to have what I call *special concern*. When we trust others to have specific concern that they are committed to having toward everyone, unwelcome trust should not be an issue. If we trust them to have special concern—that is, to do only what they are committed to doing in certain kinds of relationships—our trust may be unwanted. It would be unwanted specifically if we expected the trusted person to interpret our relationship differently than the way she does. For example, if a patient trusts a health practitioner to be emotionally attentive in the way that a lover would, but the practitioner does not think of (and does not want to think of) his relationship with the patient as an intimate relationship, the patient's trust would be unwanted. Yet by having such trust in her practitioner, the patient must expect him to think of their relationship as more like an intimate relationship than a patient-practitioner one. Without that expectation, she could not be optimistic that he would be emotionally supportive in the way that he would with a lover.

SUMMARY AND NOTES ON FOSTERING PATIENT TRUST

With that last expectation, we come to a rather complex understanding of trust. It involves optimism about the trusted person's competence and moral integrity, together with two expectations, which concern what that person stands for and her perception of our relationship. This analysis might seem so complex as to be implausible given how pervasive trust is and how easily some of us seem to be able to trust other people. However, it is important to realize that a trusting attitude, and each feature of it, need not be conscious for trust to exist. Because trust *is* so pervasive—we trust people in a myriad of ways every single day—there must be "such a thing as unconscious trust" (Baier 1995, 99).

We are most conscious of what the key elements of trust are when trust is missing; we realize what is important to us in trust relations when we contemplate why we *dis*trust someone. On my account, such reflection should lead to one or more of the following conclusions: that we are pessimistic rather than optimistic about the other's competence or moral integrity;[11] and that we suspect that person does not have certain values in common with us or does not share our perception of our relationship. These seem to be clear avenues toward distrust, and they originate in the theory I have outlined here.

So how can health care practitioners use this theory to try to promote patient trust? The answer is straightforward: they need to make room for each element of trust in their relationships with patients. First, they need to allow for optimism about their own competence and moral integrity by continually displaying each with patients. Of course, they must maintain their competence as health practitioners and also be able to convey to patients that they are competent. The relevant competence includes a kind of moral competence, which practitioners should have to begin with or learn through some training in bioethics. They need to know, for example, how to respect the autonomy of their patients, which is one of the core moral values of all health professions.

Displaying moral integrity with patients requires that practitioners honour their commitments to patients. And since moral integrity involves a general promise to do what is *right*, the commitments they honour cannot be substantially different for patients in similar circumstances. Rightness entails treating like cases alike. Further, if practitioners fail for whatever reason to meet a specific commitment to a patient, they must take some responsibility for the harm or disappointment they have caused.[12] People with integrity take their commitments seriously, which means that they try to remedy situations in which those commitments have been violated.

Second, practitioners must try to encourage the two expectations involved with trust. They could probably promote the expectation of shared values by clearly stating what they value about patient care. For example, they could assure patients that they are committed to promoting their welfare and to respecting their autonomy. And if procedures exist which they would refuse to perform because their conscience prohibits them, they could make those procedures known to patients, thereby setting the boundaries of their trust relationship. At the same time, however, they need to assure patients that they would refer them to practitioners who would consent to the relevant procedures, which is a requirement of most medical associations including the CMA. Exceptions, of course, are cases where the relevant procedures (e.g., prenatal diagnosis for the purposes of sex selection) violate fundamental norms of our society.

To promote the expectation about the nature of their relationship with patients, practitioners could assure patients that they perceive that relationship to be professional. Patients can more easily trust practitioners to honour the sorts of commitments one can reasonably expect them to fulfill (depending on their specific profession) if the practitioners ensure that their relationships with patients remain on a professional level.

Note that caution is necessary in establishing trust when practitioners know or suspect that a patient is in an abusive relationship or has a history of physical or sexual abuse. Survivors of abuse often have problems with trusting, or distrusting, because they have trusted another whom they should have been able to trust, but who betrayed them severely.[13] Rather than perpetuate damage to their trust skills, practitioners should not expect trust from those patients until they give the patients ample evidence that they themselves are trustworthy.[14] Here is an example of what that might mean in practice: in performing a physical examination or procedure, the practitioner could ask the patient frequently if she is all right, rather than simply expect that she will be all right and will not fear being violated again.

Particularly in cases where the ability of patients to trust others has been damaged, the call for practitioners to try to promote patient trust may seem unreasonable. And it may in fact be unreasonable in some cases. But surely that is not always true. And hopefully understanding trust and the different components of it makes it clear what practitioners could do to encourage trust from patients, which is of fundamental importance because of the moral value of trust.

Notes

1. For detailed discussion of the decline in patient trust, see Edmund Pellegrino's "Trust and Distrust in Professional Ethics," *Ethics, Trust, and the Professions*, eds. Pellegrino, Robert Veatch, and John Langan (Washington: Georgetown University Press, 1991), and Onora O'Neill's *Autonomy and Trust in Bioethics* (Cambridge UK: Cambridge University Press, 2002).

2. Without trust, other morally relevant aspects of these relationships (e.g., beneficence and respect for autonomy) would not exist. See Caroline Whitbeck, "Trust," *The Encyclopedia of Bioethics* (2nd ed. New York: MacMillan, 1995).

3. I do not pretend that the burden of a solution should lie entirely with health care practitioners. Other measures, such as using the media to inform the public of the benefit that many practitioners provide

to patients on a daily basis, are also necessary. See O'Neill's *Autonomy and Trust in Bioethics* on using the media to communicate actual information to the public about the work of practitioners.

4. This theory was first published in "Our Attitude Towards the Motivation of Those We Trust," *Southern Journal of Philosophy* 38(3), 2000: 465–479. It reappears in my book, *Self-Trust and Reproductive Autonomy* (Cambridge, Mass: MIT Press, 2002). I wish to thank both *The Southern Journal* and the MIT Press for their permission to reprint parts of these works. The theory I present here is a shortened version of the original.

5. See Baier, "Trust and Anti-Trust," *Ethics* 96 (1986): 231–260.

6. Disagreement comes from Richard Holton, in "Deciding to Trust, Coming to Believe," *Australasian Journal of Philosophy* 72 (March): 63–76. Ambiguity about the relevant motivation with trust exists in Trudy Govier's *Dilemmas of Trust* (Montreal: McGill-Queen's University Press, 1998). She writes that when we trust someone, "we believe in his or her basic integrity; we are willing to rely on him or her," (91) and that when we trust ourselves, we have a firm belief in our "own good character and good sense" (95), or at least a "positive sense of our own motivation" (99). So do we want the trusted one to act with integrity, with good sense, with any kind of positive motivation, or with any motivation compatible with relying on someone?

7. Cheshire Calhoun, "Standing for Something," *The Journal of Philosophy* 92(5): 249.

8. Edmund Pellegrino, "Trust and Distrust in Professional Ethics"; Richard Zaner, "The Phenomenon of Trust and the Patient-Physician Relationship," in *Ethics, Trust, and the Professions*; and Caroline Whitbeck, "Trust."

9. Another important reason is their illness.

10. See Karen Jones, "Trust as an Affective Attitude," *Ethics* 107:4–25.

11. Jones (ibid.) argues that distrust is an attitude of pessimism rather than optimism about the motivation or competence of others.

12. I discuss in detail this backward-looking element of integrity in the longer versions of this paper. See also Margaret Urban Walker's "Picking Up Pieces: Lives, Stories, and Integrity" (*Moral Understandings: A Feminist Study in Ethics*. New York: Routledge, 1998).

13. See Judith Herman, *Trauma and Recovery* (New York: Basic Books, 1992), especially pp. 51, 52.

14. Diane Lepine, "Ending the Cycle of Violence: Overcoming Guilt in Incest Survivors," *Healing Voices: Feminist Approaches to Therapy with Women*, eds. Toni Ann Laidlaw, Cheryl Malmo, and Associates (San Francisco: Jossey-Bass, 1990).

A Relational Approach to Autonomy in Health Care

Susan Sherwin

Respect for patient autonomy (or self-direction) is broadly understood as recognition that patients have the authority to make decisions about their own health care. The principle that insists on this recognition is pervasive in the bioethics literature: it is a central value within virtually all the leading approaches to health care ethics, feminist and other. It is not surprising, then, that discussions of autonomy constantly emerged within our own conversations in the Network; readers will recognize that autonomy is woven throughout the book in our various approaches to the issues we take up. It is, however, an ideal that we felt deeply ambivalent about, and, therefore, we judged it to be in need of a specifically feminist analysis.

In this chapter, I propose a feminist analysis of autonomy, making vivid both our attraction to and distrust of the dominant interpretation of this concept. I begin by reviewing some of the appeal of the autonomy ideal in order to make clear why it has achieved such prominence within bioethics and feminist health care discussions. I then identify some difficulties I find with the usual interpretations of the concept, focusing especially on difficulties that arise from a specifically feminist perspective. In response to these problems, I propose an alternative conception of autonomy that I label "relational" though the terms *socially situated* or *contextualized* would describe it equally well. To avoid confusion, I explicitly distinguish my use of the term *relational* from that of some other feminist authors, such as Carol Gilligan (1982), who reserve it to refer only to the narrower set of interpersonal relations. I apply the term to the full range of influential human relations, personal and public. Oppression permeates both personal and public relationships; hence, I prefer to politicize the understanding of the term *relational* as a way of emphasizing the political dimensions of the multiple relationships that structure an individual's selfhood, rather than to reserve the term to protect a sphere of purely private relationships that may appear to be free of political influence.[1] I explain why I think the relational alternative is more successful than the familiar individualistic interpretation at addressing the concerns identified. Finally, I briefly indicate some of the implications of adopting a relational interpretation of autonomy with respect to some of the issues discussed elsewhere in this book, and I identify some of the changes that this notion of relational autonomy suggests for the delivery of health services.

THE VIRTUES OF A PRINCIPLE OF RESPECT FOR PATIENT AUTONOMY

It is not hard to explain the prominence of the principle of respect for patient autonomy within the field of health care ethics in North America: respect for personal autonomy is a dominant value in North American culture and it plays a central role in most of our social institutions. Yet, protection of autonomy is often at particular risk in health care settings because illness, by its very nature, tends to make patients dependent on the care and good will of others; in so doing, it reduces patients' power to exercise autonomy and it also makes them vulnerable to manipulation and even to outright coercion by those who provide them with needed health services. Many patients who are either ill or at risk of becoming ill are easily frightened into overriding their own preferences and following expert advice rather

than risking abandonment by their caregivers by rejecting that advice. Even when their health is not immediately threatened, patients may find themselves compelled to comply with the demands of health care providers in order to obtain access to needed services from health professionals who are, frequently, the only ones licensed to provide those services (e.g., abortion, assistance in childbirth, legitimate excuses from work, physiotherapy).[2]

Without a strong principle of respect for patient autonomy, patients are vulnerable to abuse or exploitation, when their weak and dependent position makes them easy targets to serve the interests (e.g., financial, academic, or social influence) of others. Strong moral traditions of service within medicine and other health professions have provided patients with some measure of protection against such direct harms, though abuses nonetheless occur.[3] Most common is the tendency of health care providers to assume that by virtue of their technical expertise they are better able to judge what is in the patient's best interest than is the patient. For example, physicians may make assumptions about the advantages of using fetal heart monitors when women are in labor without considering the ways in which such instruments restrict laboring-women's movement and the quality of the birthing experience from their perspective. By privileging their own types of knowledge over that of their patients (including both experiential knowledge and understanding of their own value scheme), health care providers typically ignore patients' expressed or implicit values and engage in paternalism[4] (or the overriding of patient preferences for the presumed benefit of the patient) when prescribing treatment.

Until very recently, conscientious physicians were actually trained to act paternalistically toward their patients, to treat patients according to the physician's own judgment about what would be best for their patients, with little regard for each patient's own perspectives or preferences. The problem with this arrangement, however, is that health care may involve such intimate and central aspects of a patient's life—

including, for example, matters such as health, illness, reproduction, death, dying, bodily integrity, nutrition, lifestyle, self-image, disability, sexuality, and psychological well-being—that it is difficult for anyone other than the patient to make choices that will be compatible with that patient's personal value system. Indeed, making such choices is often an act of self-discovery or self-definition and as such it requires the active involvement of the patient. Whenever possible, then, these types of choices should be made by the person whose life is central to the treatment considered. The principle of respect for patient autonomy is aimed at clarifying and protecting patients' ultimate right to make up their own minds about the specific health services they receive (so long as they are competent to do so). It also helps to ensure that patients have full access to relevant information about their health status so that they can make informed choices about related aspects of their lives. For example, information about a terminal condition may affect a person's decisions to reproduce, take a leave of absence from work, seek a reconciliation from estranged friends or relatives, or revise a will.

Although theorists disagree about the precise definition of *autonomy*,[5] there are some common features to its use within bioethics. In practice, the principle of respect for patient autonomy is usually interpreted as acknowledging and protecting competent patients' authority to accept or refuse whatever specific treatments the health care providers they consult find it appropriate to offer them (an event known as informed choice). Since everyone can imagine being in the position of patient, and most can recognize the dangers of fully surrendering this authority to near strangers, it is not surprising that the principle of respect for patient autonomy is widely endorsed by nearly all who consider it. Despite different theoretical explanations, the overwhelming majority of bioethicists insist on this principle as a fundamental moral precept for health care. Support is especially strong in North America, where it fits comfortably within a general cultural milieu in which attention to the individual

and protection of individual rights are granted (at least rhetorical) dominance in nearly all areas of social and political policy.[6] Both Canadian and U.S. courts have underlined the importance of protection of individual rights as a central tenet of patient–provider interactions, making it a matter of legal as well as moral concern.

Further, the principle requiring respect for patient autonomy helps to resolve problems that arise when health care providers are responsible for the care of patients who have quite different experiences, values, and world views from their own; under such circumstances, it is especially unlikely that care givers can accurately anticipate the particular needs and interests of their patients. This problem becomes acute when there are significant differences in power between patients and the health care professionals who care for them. In most cases, the relevant interactions are between patients and physicians, where, typically, patients have less social power than their physicians: doctors are well educated and they tend to be (relatively) healthy and affluent, while the patients they care for are often poor, and lacking in education and social authority. In fact, according to most of the standard dichotomies supporting dominance in our culture—gender, class, race, ability status— odds are that if there is a difference between the status of the physician and the patient, the physician is likely to fall on the dominant side of that distinction and the patient on the subordinate side. The tendency of illness to undermine patients' autonomy is especially threatening when the patients in question face other powerful barriers to the exercise of their autonomy, as do members of groups subject to systemic discrimination on the basis of gender, race, class, disability, age, sexual preference, or any other such feature. A principle insisting on protection of patient autonomy can be an important corrective to such overwhelming power imbalances.

Moreover, physician privilege and power is not the only threat to patient autonomy. Increasingly, the treatment options available to both patients and physicians are circumscribed by the policies of governments and other third-party payers. In the current economic climate, those who fund health care services are insisting on ever more stringent restrictions on access to specific treatment options; physicians find themselves asked to perform gate-keeping functions to keep costs under control. In such circumstances, where patient care may be decided by general guidelines that tend to be insensitive to the particular circumstances of specific patients, and where the financial interests of the institution being billed for the patient's care may take priority over the patient's needs or preferences, the principle of respect for patient autonomy becomes more complicated to interpret even as it takes on added importance.

The principle of respect for patient autonomy can also be seen as an attractive ideal for feminists because of its promise to protect the rights and interests of even the most socially disadvantaged patients. Feminist medical historians, anthropologists, and sociologists have documented many ways in which health care providers have repeatedly neglected and misperceived the needs and wishes of the women they treat.[7] The ideal of respect for patient autonomy seems a promising way to correct much that is objectionable in the abuses that feminist researchers have documented in the delivery of health services to women and minorities. Most feminists believe that the forces of systematic domination and oppression work together to limit the autonomy of women and members of other oppressed groups; many of their political efforts can be seen as aimed at disrupting those forces and promoting greater degrees of autonomy (often represented as personal "choice") for individuals who fall victim to oppression. For example, many feminists appeal at least implicitly to the moral norm of autonomy in seeking to increase the scope of personal control for women in all areas of their reproductive lives (especially with respect to birth control, abortion, and childbirth, often discussed under a general rubric of "reproductive freedom" or "reproductive choice").

In a world where most cultures are plagued by sexism, which is usually compounded by other deeply entrenched oppressive patterns, fundamental respect for the humanity, dignity, and autonomy of members of disadvantaged groups, though extremely fragile, seems very important and in need of strong ethical imperatives. Feminists strive to be sensitive to the ways in which gender, race, class, age, disability, sexual orientation, and marital status can undermine a patient's authority and credibility in health care contexts and most are aware of the long history of powerful medical control over women's lives. They have good reason, then, to oppose medical domination through paternalism. Promotion of patient autonomy appears to be a promising alternative.[8] Understood in its traditional sense as the alternative to heteronomy (governance by others), autonomy (self-governance) seems to be an essential feature of any feminist strategy for improving health services for women and achieving a nonoppressive society.

PROBLEMS WITH THE AUTONOMY IDEAL

Nonetheless, despite this broad consensus about the value of a principle of respect for patient autonomy in health care, there are many problems with the principle as it is usually interpreted and applied in health care ethics. As many health critics have observed, we need to question how much control individual patients really have over the determination of their treatment within the stressful world of health care services. Even a casual encounter with most modern hospitals reveals that wide agreement about the moral importance of respect for patient autonomy does not always translate into a set of practices that actually respect and foster patient autonomy in any meaningful sense. Ensuring that patients meet some measure of informed choice—or, more commonly, informed consent[9]—before receiving or declining treatment has become accepted as the most promising mechanism for insuring patient autonomy in health care settings, but, in practice, the effectiveness of the actual procedures used to obtain informed consent usually falls short of fully protecting patient autonomy. This gap is easy to understand:

attention to patient autonomy can be a time-consuming business and the demands of identifying patient values and preferences are often sacrificed in the face of heavy patient loads and staff shortages. In addition, health care providers are often constrained from promoting and responding to patients' autonomy in health care because of pressures they experience to contain health care costs and to avoid making themselves liable to lawsuits. Moreover, most health care providers are generally not well trained in the communication skills necessary to ensure that patients have the requisite understanding to provide genuine informed consent. This problem is compounded within our increasingly diverse urban communities where differences in language and culture between health care providers and the patients they serve may create enormous practical barriers to informed choice.

There are yet deeper problems with the ideal of autonomy invoked in most bioethical discussions. The paradigm offered for informed consent is built on a model of articulate, intelligent patients who are accustomed to making decisions about the course of their lives and who possess the resources necessary to allow them a range of options to choose among. Decisions are constructed as a product of objective calculation on the basis of near perfect information. Clearly, not all patients meet these ideal conditions (perhaps none does), yet there are no satisfactory guidelines available about how to proceed when dealing with patients who do not fit the paradigm.

Feminist analysis reveals several problems inherent in the very construction of the concept of autonomy that is at the heart of most bioethics discussions.[10] One problem is that autonomy provisions are sometimes interpreted as functioning independently of and outweighing all other moral values. More specifically, autonomy is often understood to exist in conflict with the demands of justice because the requirements of the latter may have to be imposed on unwilling citizens. Autonomy is frequently interpreted to mean freedom from interference; this analysis can be invoked (as it frequently is) to oppose taxation as coercive and, hence, a violation of personal autonomy. But coercive measures like taxation are essential if a society wants to reduce inequity and provide the disadvantaged with access to the means (e.g., basic necessities, social respect, education, and health care) that are necessary for meaningful exercise of their autonomy. In contrast to traditional accounts of autonomy that accept and indeed presume some sort of tension between autonomy and justice, feminism encourages us to see the connections between these two central moral ideals.

In fact, autonomy language is often used to hide the workings of privilege and to mask the barriers of oppression. For example, within North America it seems that people who were raised in an atmosphere of privilege and respect come rather easily to think of themselves as independent and self-governing; it feels natural to them to conceive of themselves as autonomous. Having been taught that they need only to apply themselves in order to take advantage of the opportunities available to them, most learn to think of their successes as self-created and deserved. Such thinking encourages them to be oblivious to the barriers that oppression and disadvantage create, and it allows them to see the failures of others as evidence of the latters' unwillingness to exercise their own presumed autonomy responsibly. This individualistic approach to autonomy makes it very easy for people of privilege to remain ignorant of the social arrangements that support their own sense of independence, such as the institutions that provide them with an exceptionally good education and a relatively high degree of personal safety. Encouraged to focus on their own sense of individual accomplishment, they are inclined to blame less well-situated people for their lack of comparable success rather than to appreciate the costs of oppression. This familiar sort of thinking tends to interfere with people's ability to see the importance of supportive social conditions for fostering autonomous action. By focusing instead on the injustice that is associated with oppression, feminism helps us to recognize that autonomy is best achieved where the social conditions that support it are in place.

Hence, it provides us with an alternative perspective for understanding a socially grounded notion of autonomy.

Further, the standard conception of autonomy, especially as it is invoked in bioethics, tends to place the focus of concern quite narrowly on particular decisions of individuals; that is, it is common to speak of specific health care decisions as autonomous, or, at least, of the patient as autonomous with respect to the decision at hand. Such analyses discourage attention to the context in which decisions are actually made. Patient decisions are considered to be autonomous if the patient is (1) deemed to be sufficiently competent (rational) to make the decision at issue, (2) makes a (reasonable) choice from a set of available options, (3) has adequate information and understanding about the available choices, and (4) is free from explicit coercion toward (or away from) one of those options. It is assumed that these criteria can be evaluated in any particular case, simply by looking at the state of the patient and her deliberations in isolation from the social conditions that structure her options. Yet, each of these conditions is more problematic than is generally recognized.

The competency criterion threatens to exclude people who are oppressed from the scope of autonomy provisions altogether. This is because competency is often equated with being rational,[11] yet the rationality of women and members of other oppressed groups is frequently denied. In fact, as Genevieve Lloyd (1984) has shown, the very concept of rationality has been constructed in opposition to the traits that are stereotypically assigned to women (e.g., by requiring that agents demonstrate objectivity and emotional distance),[12] with the result that women are often seen as simply incapable of rationality.[13] Similar problems arise with respect to stereotypical assumptions about members of racial minorities, indigenous peoples, persons with disabilities, welfare recipients, people from developing countries, those who are nonliterate, and so on. Minimally, then, health care providers must become sensitive to the ways in which oppressive stereotypes can undermine their ability to recognize some sorts of patients as being rational or competent.

Consider, also, the second condition, which has to do with making a (reasonable) choice from the set of available options. Here, the difficulty is that the set of available options is constructed in ways that may already seriously limit the patient's autonomy by prematurely excluding options the patient might have preferred. There is a whole series of complex decisions that together shape the set of options that health care providers are able to offer their patients: these can involve such factors as the forces that structure research programs, the types of results that journals are willing to publish, curriculum priorities in medical and other professional schools, and funding policies within the health care system.[14] While all patients will face limited choices by virtue of these sorts of institutional policy decisions, the consequences are especially significant for members of oppressed groups because they tend to be underrepresented on the bodies that make these earlier decisions, and therefore their interests are less likely to be reflected in each of the background decisions that are made. In general, the sorts of institutional decisions in question tend to reflect the biases of discriminatory values and practices.[15] Hence, the outcomes of these multiple earlier decisions can have a significant impact on an oppressed patient's ultimate autonomy by disproportionately and unfairly restricting the choices available to her. Nevertheless, such background conditions are seldom visible within discussions of patient autonomy in bioethics.

The third condition is also problematic in that the information made available to patients is, inevitably, the information that has been deemed worthy of study and that is considered relevant by the health care providers involved. Again, research, publication, and education policies largely determine what sorts of data are collected and, significantly, what questions are neglected; systemic bias unquestionably influences these policies. Further, the very large gap in life experience between physicians, who are, by virtue of their professional status, relatively privileged members of society, and some of their seriously disadvantaged patients makes the likelihood of the former anticipating the specific information needs of the latter questionable. While an open consent process will help reduce this gap by providing patients with the opportunity to raise questions, patients often feel too intimidated to ask or even formulate questions, especially when they feel socially and intellectually inferior to their physicians and when the physicians project an image of being busy with more important demands. Often, one needs some information in order to know what further questions to ask, and large gaps in perspective between patients and their health care providers may result in a breakdown in communication because of false assumptions by either participant.

The fourth condition, the one that demands freedom from coercion in exercising choice, is extremely difficult to evaluate when the individual in question is oppressed. The task becomes even trickier if the choice is in a sphere that is tied to her oppression. The condition of being oppressed can be so fundamentally restrictive that it is distorting to describe as autonomous some specific choices made under such conditions. For example, many women believe they have no real choice but to seek expensive, risky cosmetic surgery because they accurately perceive that their opportunities for success in work or love depend on their more closely approximating some externally defined standard of beauty. Similar sorts of questions arise with respect to some women's choice of dangerous, unproven experiments in new reproductive technologies because continued childlessness can be expected to have devastating consequences for their lives. In other cases, women sometimes choose to have abortions because they fear that giving birth will involve them in unwanted and lifelong relationships with abusive partners. Some women have little access to contraceptives and find themselves choosing sterilization as the most effective way of resisting immediate demands of their partners even if they might want more children in the future. Or, some women seek out prenatal diagnosis and selective abortion of cherished fetuses because they realize that they cannot afford to raise a child born with a serious disability, though they would value such a child themselves. Many middle-class Western women choose hormone replacement therapy at menopause because they recognize that their social and economic lives may be threatened if they appear to be aging too quickly. When a woman's sense of herself and her range of opportunities have been oppressively constructed in ways that (seem to) leave her little choice but to pursue all available options in the pursuit of beauty or childbearing or when she is raised in a culture that ties her own sense of herself to external norms of physical appearance or fulfillment associated with childbearing or, conversely, when having a(nother) child will impose unjust and intolerable costs on her, it does not seem sufficient to restrict our analysis to the degree of autonomy associated with her immediate decision about a particular treatment offered. We need a way of acknowledging how oppressive circumstances can interfere with autonomy, but this is not easily captured in traditional accounts.

Finally, there are good reasons to be wary of the ways in which the appearance of choice is used to mask the normalizing powers of medicine and other health-related institutions. As Michel Foucault (1979, 1980) suggests, in modern societies the illusion of choice can be part of the mechanism for controlling behavior. Indeed, it is possible that bioethical efforts to guarantee the exercise of individual informed choice may actually make the exercise of medical authority even more powerful and effective than it would be under more traditionally paternalistic models. In practice, the ideal of informed choice amounts to assuring patients of the opportunity to consent to one of a limited list of relatively similar, medically encouraged procedures. Thus, informed consent procedures aimed simply at protecting autonomy in the narrow sense of specific choice among preselected options may ultimately serve to secure the compliance of docile patients who operate under the illusion of autonomy by virtue of being invited to consent to procedures they are socially encouraged to choose. Unless we find a way of identifying a deeper sense of autonomy than that associated with the expression of individual preference in selecting among a limited set of similar options, we run the risk of struggling to protect not patient autonomy but the very mechanisms that insure compliant medical consumers, preoccupied with the task of selecting among a narrow range of treatments.

FOCUS ON THE INDIVIDUAL

A striking feature of most bioethical discussions about patient autonomy is their exclusive focus on individual patients; this pattern mirrors medicine's consistent tendency to approach illness as primarily a problem of particular patients.[16] Similar problems are associated with each discipline. Within the medical tradition, suffering is located and addressed in the individuals who experience it rather than in the social arrangements that may be responsible for causing the problem. Instead of exploring the cultural context that tolerates and even supports practices such as war, pollution, sexual violence, and systemic unemployment—practices that contribute to much of the illness that occupies modern medicine—physicians generally respond to the symptoms troubling particular patients in isolation from the context that produces these conditions. Apart from population-based epidemiological studies (which, typically, restrict their focus to a narrow range of patterns of illness and often exclude or distort important social dimensions), medicine is primarily oriented toward dealing with individuals who have become ill (or pregnant, [in]fertile, or menopausal). This orientation directs the vast majority of research money and expertise toward the things that can be done to change the individual, but it often ignores key elements at the source of the problems.

For example, physicians tend to respond to infertility either by trivializing the problem and telling women to go home and "relax," or by prescribing hormonal and surgical treatment of particular women, rather than by demanding that research and public health efforts be aimed at preventing pelvic inflammatory disease, which causes many cases of infertility, or by encouraging wide public debate (or private reflections) on the powerful social pressures to reproduce that are directed at women. In similar fashion, the mainstream scientific and medical communities respond to the growth of breast cancer rates by promoting individual responsibility for self-examination and by searching for the gene(s) that makes some women particularly susceptible to the disease; when it is found in a patient, the principal medical therapy available is to perform "prophylactic" double mastectomies. Few physicians demand examination of the potential contributory role played by the use of pesticides or chlorine, or the practice of feeding artificial hormones to agricultural animals. Or they deal with dramatically increased skin cancer rates by promoting the personal use of sunscreens while resigning themselves to the continued depletion of the ozone layer. In another area, health care professionals generally deal with the devastating effects of domestic violence by patching up its victims, providing them with medications to relieve depression and advice to move out of their homes, and devising pathological names for victims who stay in violent relationships ("battered woman syndrome" and "self-defeating personality disorder"), but few actively challenge the sexism that accepts male violence as a "natural" response to frustration and fears of abandonment.[17]

Some qualifications are in order. Clearly, these are crude and imprecise generalizations. They describe a general orientation of current health practices, but they certainly do not capture the work of all those involved in medical research and practice. Fortunately, there are practitioners and researchers engaged in the very sorts of investigation I call for, but they are exceptional, not typical. Moreover, I do not want to imply that medicine should simply abandon its concern with treating disease in individuals. I understand that prevention strategies will not eliminate all illness and I believe that personalized health care must continue to be made available to those who become ill. Further, I want to be clear that my critique does not imply that physicians or other direct care providers are necessarily the ones who ought to be assuming the task of identifying the social and environmental causes of disease. Health care training, and especially the training of physicians, is directed at developing the requisite skills for the extremely important work of caring for individuals who become ill. The responsibility for investigating the social causes of illness and for changing hazardous conditions is a social one that is probably best met by those who undertake different sorts of training and study. The problem is that medicine, despite the limits of its expertise and focus, is the primary agent of health care activity in our society and physicians are granted significant social authority to be the arbiters of health policy. Hence, when medicine makes the treatment of individuals its primary focus, we must understand that important gaps are created in our society's ability to understand and promote good health.

In parallel fashion, autonomy-focused bioethics concentrates its practitioners' attention on the preferences of particular patients, and it is, thereby, complicit in the individualistic orientation of medicine. It asks health care providers to ensure that individual patients have the information they need to make rational decisions about their health care, yet it does not ask the necessary questions about the circumstances in which such decisions are made. The emphasis most bioethicists place on traditional, individualistic understandings of autonomy reinforces the tendency of health care providers and ethicists to neglect exploration of the deep social causes and conditions that contribute to health and illness. Moreover, it encourages patients to see their own health care decisions in isolation from those of anyone else, thereby increasing their sense of vulnerability and dependence on medical authority.

The narrow individual focus that characterizes the central traditions within both medicine and bioethics obscures our need to consider questions of power, dominance, and privilege in our interpretations and responses to illness and other health-related matters as well as in our interpretations of the ideal of autonomy. These ways of structuring thought and practice make it difficult to see the political dimensions of illness, and, in a parallel way, they obscure the political dimensions of the conventional criteria for autonomous deliberation. As a result, they interfere with our ability to identify and pursue more effective health practices while helping to foster a social environment that ignores and tolerates oppression. In both cases, a broader political perspective is necessary if we are to avoid the problems created by restricting our focus to individuals apart from their location.

Feminism offers just such a broader perspective. In contrast to the standard approaches in bioethics, feminism raises questions about the social basis for decisions about health and health care at all levels. Here, as elsewhere, feminists are inclined to ask whose interests are served and whose are harmed by the traditional ways of structuring thought and practice. By asking these questions, we are able to see how assumptions of individual-based medicine help to preserve the social and political status quo. For example, the current taxonomy in Canada designates certain sorts of conditions (e.g., infertility, cancer, heart disease, anxiety) as appropriate for medical intervention, and it provides grounds for ensuring that such needs are met. At the same time, it views other sorts of conditions (e.g., malnutrition, fear of assault, low self-esteem) as falling beyond the purview of the health care system and, therefore, as ineligible to draw on the considerable resources allocated to the delivery of health services.[18] In this way, individualistic assumptions support a system that provides expert care for many of the health complaints of those with greatest financial privilege while dismissing as outside the scope of health care many of the sources of illness that primarily affect the disadvantaged. A more social vision of health would require us to investigate ways in which nonmedical strategies, such as improving social and material conditions for disadvantaged groups, can affect the health status of different segments of the community.[19]

None of the concerns I have identified argues against maintaining a strong commitment to autonomy in bioethical deliberations. In fact, I have no wish to abandon this ideal (just as I have no desire to abandon patient-centered medical care). I still believe that a principle of respect for patient autonomy is an important element of good patient care. Moreover, I believe that appeal to a principle of respect for autonomy can be an important instrument in challenging oppression and it can actually serve as the basis for many of the feminist criticisms I present with respect to our current health care system.[20]

What these criticisms do suggest, however, is that we must pursue a more careful and politically sensitive interpretation of the range of possible restrictions on autonomy than is found in most of the nonfeminist bioethics literature. We need to be able to look at specific decisions as well as the context that influences and sometimes limits such decisions. Many of the troublesome examples I review above are entirely compatible with traditional conceptions of autonomy, even though the patients in question may be facing unjust barriers to care or may be acting in response to oppressive circumstances; traditional conceptions are inadequate to the extent that they make invisible the oppression that structures such decisions. By focusing only on the moment of medical decision making, traditional views fail to examine how specific decisions are embedded within a complex set of relations and policies that constrain (or, ideally, promote) an individual's ability to exercise autonomy with respect to any particular choice.

To understand this puzzle it is necessary to distinguish between agency and autonomy. To exercise agency, one need only exercise reasonable choice.[21] The women who choose some of the controversial practices discussed (e.g., abortion to avoid contact with an abusive partner, cosmetic surgery to conform to artificial norms of beauty, use of dangerous forms of reproductive technology) are exercising agency; clearly they are making choices, and, often, those choices are rational under the circumstances.[22] They also meet the demands of conventional notions of autonomy that ask only that anyone contemplating such procedures be competent, or capable of choosing (wisely), have available information current practice deems relevant, and be free of direct coercion. But insofar as their behavior accepts and adapts to oppression, describing it as autonomous seems inadequate. Together, the habits of equating agency (the making of a choice) with autonomy (self-governance) and accepting as given the prevailing social arrangements have the effect of helping to perpetuate oppression: when we limit our analysis to the quality of an individual's choice under existing conditions (or when we fail to inquire why some people do not even seek health services), we ignore the significance of oppressive conditions. Minimally, autonomous persons should be able to resist oppression—not just act in compliance with it—and be able to refuse the choices oppression seems to make nearly irresistible. Ideally, they should be able to escape from the structures of oppression altogether and create new options that are not defined by these structures either positively or negatively.

In order to ensure that we recognize and address the restrictions that oppression places on people's health choices, then, we need a wider notion of autonomy that will allow us to distinguish genuinely autonomous behavior from acts of merely rational agency. This conception must provide room to challenge the quality of an agent's specific decision-making ability and the social norms that encourage agents to participate in practices that may be partially constitutive of their oppression.[23] A richer, more politically sensitive standard of autonomy should make visible the impact of oppression on a person's choices as well as on her very ability to exercise autonomy fully. Such a conception has the advantage of allowing us to avoid the trap of focusing on the supposed flaws of the individual who is choosing under oppressive circumstances (e.g., by dismissing her choices as "false consciousness"), for it is able to recognize that such choices can be reasonable for the agent. Instead, it directs our attention to the conditions that shape the agent's choice and it makes those conditions the basis of critical analysis.

The problems that I identify with the conventional interpretation of patient autonomy reveal a need to expand our understanding of the types of forces that interfere with a patient's autonomy. On nonfeminist accounts, these are irrationality, failure to recognize that a choice is called for, lack of necessary information, and coercion (including psychological compulsion). Since each of these conditions must be reinterpreted to allow for the ways in which oppression may be operating, we must add to this list recognition of the costs and effects of oppression and of the particular ways in which oppression is manifested. But we must do more than simply modify our interpretation of the four criteria reviewed above. We also need an understanding of the ways in which a person can be encouraged to develop (or discouraged from developing) the ability to exercise autonomy. For this task, we need to consider the presence or absence of meaningful opportunities to build the skills required to be able to exercise autonomy well (Meyers 1989), including the existence of appropriate material and social conditions. In addition, our account should reflect the fact that many decision makers, especially women, place the interests of others at the center of their deliberations. Such an analysis will allow us to ensure that autonomy standards reflect not only the quality of reasoning displayed by a patient at the moment of medical decision making but also the circumstances that surround this decision making.

A RELATIONAL ALTERNATIVE

A major reason for many of the problems identified with the autonomy ideal is that the term is commonly understood to represent freedom of action for agents who are paradigmatically regarded as independent, self-interested, and self-sufficient. As such, it is part of a larger North American cultural ideal of competitive individualism in which every citizen is to be left "free" to negotiate "his" way through the complex interactions of social, economic, and political life.[24] The feminist literature is filled with criticism of such models of agency and autonomy: for example, many feminists object that this ideal appeals to a model of personhood that is distorting because, in fact, no one is fully independent. As well, they observe that this model is exclusionary because those who are most obviously dependent on others (e.g., because of disability or financial need) seem to be disqualified from consideration in ways that others are not. Many feminists object that the view of individuals as isolated social units is not only false but impoverished: much of who we are and what we value is rooted in our relationships and affinities with others. Also, many feminists take issue with the common assumption that agents are single-mindedly self-interested, when so much of our experience is devoted to building or maintaining personal relationships and communities.[25]

If we are to effectively address these concerns, we need to move away from the familiar Western understanding of autonomy as self-defining, self-interested, and self-protecting, as if the self were simply some special kind of property to be preserved.[26] Under most popular interpretations, the structure of the autonomy–heteronomy framework (governance by self or by others) is predicated on a certain view of persons and society in which the individual is thought to be somehow separate from and to exist independently of the larger society; each person's major concern is to be protected from the demands and encroachment of others. This sort of conception fails to account for the complexity of the relations that exist between persons and their culture. It idealizes decisions that are free from outside influence without acknowledging that all persons are, to a significant degree, socially constructed, that their identities, values, concepts, and perceptions are, in large measure, products of their social environment.

Since notions of the self are at the heart of autonomy discussions, alternative interpretations of autonomy must begin with an alternative conception of the self. Curiously, despite its focus on individuals, standard interpretations of autonomy have tended to think of selves as generic rather than distinctive beings. In the traditional view, individuals tend to be treated as interchangeable in that no attention is paid to the details of personal experience. Hence, there is no space within standard conceptions to accommodate important differences among agents, especially the effects that oppression (or social privilege) has on a person's ability to exercise autonomy. In order to capture these kinds of social concerns, some feminists have proposed turning to a relational conception of personhood that recognizes the importance of social forces in shaping each person's identity, development, and aspirations.[27] Following this suggestion, I now explore a relational interpretation of autonomy that is built around a relational conception of the self that is explicitly feminist in its conception.

Under relational theory, selfhood is seen as an ongoing process, rather than as something static or fixed. Relational selves are inherently social beings that are significantly shaped and modified within a web of interconnected (and sometimes conflicting) relationships. Individuals engage in the activities that are constitutive of identity and autonomy (e.g., defining, questioning, revising, and pursuing projects) within a configuration of relationships, both interpersonal and political. By including attention to political relationships of power and powerlessness, this interpretation of relational theory provides room to recognize how the forces of oppression can interfere with an individual's ability to exercise autonomy by undermining her sense of herself as an autonomous agent and by depriving her of opportunities to exercise autonomy. Thus, it is able to provide us with insight into why it is that oppressed people often seem less autonomous than others even when offered a comparable range of choices. Under a relational view, autonomy is best understood to be a capacity or skill that is developed (and constrained) by social circumstances. It is exercised within relationships and social structures that jointly help to shape the individual while also affecting others' responses to her efforts at autonomy.[28]

Diana Meyers (1989) has developed one such theory of personal autonomy. She argues that autonomy involves a particular competency that requires the development of specific skills. As such, it can be either enhanced or diminished by the sort of socialization the agent experiences. Meyers shows how the specific gender socialization most (Western) women undergo trains them in social docility and rewards them for defining their interests in terms of others, thereby robbing them of the opportunity to develop the essential capacity of self-direction. Such training relegates most women to a category she labels "minimally autonomous" (as distinct from her more desirable categories of medially autonomous and fully autonomous). Relational theory allows us to appreciate how each relationship a person participates in plays a role in fostering or inhibiting that individual's capacity for autonomous action by encouraging or restricting her opportunities to understand herself as an autonomous agent and to practice exercising the requisite skills. Such a conception makes clear the importance of discovering the ways in which oppression often reduces a person's ability to develop and exercise the skills that are necessary for achieving a reasonable degree of autonomy.

For instance, relational theory allows us to see the damaging effects on autonomy of internalized oppression. Feminists have long understood that one of the most insidious features of oppression is its tendency to become internalized in the minds of its victims. This is because internalized oppression diminishes the capacity of its victims to develop self-respect, and, as several feminists have argued, reduced (or compromised) self-respect undermines autonomy by undermining the individual's sense of herself as capable of making independent judgments (Meyers 1989; Dillon 1992; Benson 1991, 1994). Moreover, as Susan Babbitt (1993, 1996) has argued, these oppression-induced barriers to autonomy cannot necessarily be rectified simply by providing those affected with more information or by removing explicit coercive forces (as the traditional view assumes). When the messages of reduced self-worth are internalized, agents tend to lose the ability even to know their own objective interests. According to Babbitt, in such cases transformative experiences can be far more important to autonomy than access to alternative information. Feminist theory suggests, then, that women and members of other oppressed groups can be helped to increase their autonomy skills by being offered more opportunities to exercise those skills and a supportive climate for practicing them (Meyers 1989), by being provided with the opportunity to develop stronger senses of self-esteem (Benson 1994; Dillon 1992; Meyers 1989), by having the opportunity for transformative experiences that make visible the forces of oppression (Babbitt 1993, 1996), and by having experiences of making choices that are not influenced by the wishes of those who dominate them (Babbitt 1993, 1996).

Autonomy requires more than the effective exercise of personal resources and skills, however; generally, it also demands that appropriate structural conditions be met. Relational theory reminds us that material restrictions, including very restricted economic resources, on-going fear of assault, and lack of educational opportunity (i.e., the sorts of circumstances that are often part of the condition of being oppressed), constitute real limitations on the options available to the agent. Moreover, it helps us to see how socially constructed stereotypes can reduce both society's and the agent's sense of that person's ability to act autonomously. Relational theory allows us to recognize how such diminished expectations readily become translated into diminished capacities.

The relational interpretation I favor is feminist in that it takes into account the impact of social and political structures, especially sexism and other forms of oppression, on the lives and opportunities of individuals. It acknowledges that the presence or absence of a degree of autonomy is not just a matter of being offered a choice. It also requires that the person have had

the opportunity to develop the skills necessary for making the type of choice in question, the experience of being respected in her decisions, and encouragement to reflect on her own values. The society, not just the agent, is subject to critical scrutiny under the rubric of relational autonomy.

It is important, however, to avoid an account that denies any scope for autonomy on the part of those who are oppressed. Such a conclusion would be dangerous, since the widespread perception of limited autonomy can easily become a self-fulfilling prophecy. Moreover, such a conclusion would be false. Many members of oppressed groups do manage to develop autonomy skills and, thus, are able to act autonomously in a wide variety of situations, though the particular demands of acting autonomously under oppression are easily overlooked (Benson 1991). Some feminists, such as bell hooks (1990) and Sarah Hoagland (1992), have observed that the marginality associated with being oppressed can sometimes provide people with better opportunities than are available to more well-situated citizens for questioning social norms and devising their own patterns of resistance to social convention. Because those who are especially marginalized (e.g., those who are multiply oppressed or who are "deviant" with respect to important social norms) may have no significant social privilege to lose, they are, sometimes, freer than others to demand changes in the status quo. They may be far more likely to engage in resistance to the norms of oppression than are those who derive some personal benefits from oppressive structures (e.g., middle-class, able-bodied, married women).

Still, we must not make the mistake of romanticizing the opportunities available to the oppressed. An adequate conception of autonomy should afford individuals more than the opportunity to resist oppression; it should also ensure that they have opportunities to actively shape their world. A relational conception of autonomy seems better suited than the traditional models to handle the complexities of such paradoxes because it encourages us to attend to the complex ways in which the detailed circumstances of an individual's social and political circumstances can affect her ability to act in different kinds of contexts.

When relational autonomy reveals the disadvantage associated with oppression in terms of autonomy, the response should not be that others are thereby licensed to make decisions for those who are oppressed; this response would only increase their powerlessness. Rather, it demands attention to ways in which oppressed people can be helped to develop the requisite autonomy skills. The best way of course to help oppressed people to develop autonomy skills is to remove the conditions of their oppression. Short of that, long-term social projects can help to provide educational opportunities to counter the psychological burdens of oppression. In the short term, it may be necessary to spend more time than usual in supporting patients in the deliberative process of decision making and providing them with access to relevant political as well as medical information when they contemplate controversial procedures (e.g., information about the social dimensions of hormone replacement therapy).

Relational autonomy is not only about changing the individual, however. It also demands attention to ways in which the range of choices before those who belong to oppressed groups can be modified to include more nonoppressive options, that is, options that will not further entrench their existing oppression (as often happens, for example, when women choose cosmetic surgery or the use of many reproductive technologies). Whereas in traditional autonomy theory only the mode and quality of specific decisions are evaluated, feminist relational autonomy regards the range and nature of available and acceptable options as being at least as important as the quality of specific decision making. Only when we understand the ways in which oppression can infect the background or baseline conditions under which choices are to be made will we be able to modify those conditions and work toward the possibility of greater autonomy by promoting nonoppressive alternatives.

As in health matters, it is important in relational discussions not to lose sight of the need to continue to maintain some focus on the individual. Relational autonomy redefines autonomy as the social project it is, but it does not deny that autonomy ultimately resides in individuals. Our attention to social and political contexts helps deepen and enrich the narrow and impoverished view of autonomy available under individualistic conceptions, but it does not support wholesale neglect of the needs and interests of individuals in favor of broader social and political interests. Rather, it can be seen as democratizing access to autonomy by helping to identify and remove the effects of barriers to autonomy that are created by oppression. A relational approach can help to move autonomy from the largely exclusive preserve of the socially privileged and see that it is combined with a commitment to social justice in order to ensure that oppression is not allowed to continue simply because its victims have been deprived of the resources necessary to exercise the autonomy required to challenge it.

Acknowledgments

This chapter has evolved over the course of the Network interactions and has benefited enormously from Network discussions. I am grateful to all Network members for careful readings of many earlier drafts and stimulating comments. In addition to input from Network members, I have also benefited from the generous attention paid by Keith Burgess-Jackson, Sue Campbell, Richmond Campbell, Carmel Forde, Jody Graham, Carl Matheson, Barbara Secker, and Eldon Soifer.

Notes

1. Some Network members prefer the terms, "contextual" or "situated" as a way of avoiding all confusion with those feminists who reserve the term "relational" to refer exclusively to interpersonal relations. I feel that this usage perpetuates the misleading sense that interpersonal relations are themselves "apolitical." I have, therefore, chosen to insist on a thoroughly political reading of the term "relational" that applies to both interpersonal and more public sorts of relations.
2. While questions of patient autonomy arise in interactions with all health care providers, North American health care delivery is largely structured

around provision of medical services; moreover, physicians control most of the decision making that determines provision of health care services. Hence, much of the subsequent discussion focuses explicitly on patient autonomy in relation to physician authority, even though many of the concerns raised also extend to other (nonmedical) types of health care practice.

3. The most vivid examples appear in the distressing history of medical research with human subjects. See, for example, Katz 1972.

4. I deliberately retain the gendered term in this particular instance since it accurately reflects the connection to the traditional gendered role of patriarchal father who presumes authority to make decisions on behalf of all other family members. Traditional stereotypes of mothering and gender-neutral parenting do not retain this hierarchical flavor.

5. For a review of most of the common interpretations, see Dworkin 1988.

6. Interest in respect for patient autonomy is hardly unique to North America, however. See note 20.

7. See, for example, Corea 1985; Ehrenreich and English 1979; Fisher 1986; Perales amd Young 1988; and White 1990. This is not a straightforward history of constant abuse or one-sided power, however; as Wendy Mitchinson documents in Chapter 6, the relationship between women and their doctors has long been complex and ambiguous.

8. At the very least, we need a more complex analysis of the options for decision making than is provided by the familiar dichotomous structure of patient autonomy versus medical paternalism. See Mahowald 1993 for development of the idea of maternalism as an alternative that is aimed at capturing both these aspects of medical responsibility; see also Sherwin 1992 for a brief proposal of "amicalism."

9. *Informed choice* suggests a wider scope for patient autonomy than *informed consent* in that it includes the possibility of patients' initiating treatment suggestions, where *informed consent* implies that the role of the patient is merely to consent to the treatment proposed by the physician; further, *informed choice* makes more explicit that patients ought also to be free to refuse recommended treatments as well as to accept them.

10. Many of these concerns are not exclusive to feminists; several have also been raised by other sorts of critics. I call them feminist because I came to these concerns through a feminist analysis that attends to the role in society of systems of domi-

nance and oppression, especially those connected with gender.

11. This reduction may be a result of a tendency to collapse the ideal of personal autonomy central to bioethics discussions with the concept of moral autonomy developed by Immanuel Kant.

12. It is often taken as a truism in our culture that emotional involvement constitutes irrationality, that emotions are direct threats to rationality. It is hard to see, however, how decisions about important life decisions are improved if they are made without any emotional attachment to the outcomes.

13. Susan Babbitt (1996) argues that the traditional conception of rationality is defined in terms of propositional understanding in ways that obscure the experiences and needs of oppressed people.

14. For example, research priorities have led to the situation where birth control pills are available only for women and this increases the pressure on women seeking temporary protection against pregnancy to take the pill even when it endangers their health.

15. See Chapter 10.

16. I focus primarily on medicine since it is the dominant health profession and is responsible for organization of most health services in developed countries. Most health professions involve a similar bias toward treatment of individuals, though some (e.g., social work) pride themselves on attending to social structures as well as individual need, and most health professions, including medicine, include subspecialties concerned with matters of public health.

17. See Chapter 9.

18. Because health care is a provincial responsibility, there are differences in the precise services offered from province to province and from one administration to the next within provinces. The examples here are broad generalizations.

19. Such considerations do play a role in health care planning at a governmental level where the focus shifts from medical interventions to the idea of *health determinants*, but here, too, there is excessive attention paid to what the individual can and should be doing ("healthism") and insufficient concern about promoting egalitarian social conditions. See Chapters 3 and 4.

20. When I read an early version of this section of the paper to the Second World Congress of the International Association of Bioethics in Buenos Aires, Argentina, in November 1994, I was struck by how passionately committed local feminists were to retaining a version of the respect for

autonomy principle. They felt that most women in their country had very little authority over decisions about their health care, and so they were struggling to reverse a strongly paternalistic bias on the part of physicians by appeal to the principle of respect for autonomy. While they acknowledged that this principle was not as well-entrenched in their society as it is in North America, they considered it very important to their own feminist health agenda. They see respect for patient autonomy as having profoundly liberatory potential in their own society; this perspective provides clear reason not to dismiss this principle lightly, flawed though it may be.

21. The language of agency and autonomy is quite varied within feminist (and other) discourse. For example, the term *agency* is used throughout the collection *Provoking Agents: Gender and Agency in Theory and Practice* (Gardiner 1995) in ways that sometimes appear to overlap with my usage of *relational autonomy*. Susan Babbitt (1996), on the other hand, seems to use the two terms in ways analogous to the use here.

22. The notion of agency is itself highly contested within current feminist theory. Postmodern accounts seem to deny the possibility of subjectivity in any familiar sense; since agency is traditionally assigned to a single subject, once the subject is eliminated, the possibility of agency seems to disappear as well. I do not address this complex theoretical issue here but continue to rely on common sense understandings of both subjectivity and agency. Readers interested in understanding the feminist debates around agency may consult Gardiner 1995.

23. In addition, we need the conceptual space to be able to acknowledge that restrictive definitions of health sometimes preempt autonomy analysis by limiting the opportunity of some people even to enter the relatively well-funded health care system for assistance with problems (e.g., poverty) that affect their health.

24. The agent imagined in such cases is always stereotypically masculine.

25. Feminist discussion of these and other critiques can be found in Gilligan 1982; Baier 1985; Code 1991; and Held 1993.

26. See Nedelsky 1989 for discussion of this view and its limitations.

27. For example, Baier 1985; Code 1991; and Held 1993.

28. An alternative feminist conception of a relational view of autonomy is provided by Anne Donchin (1998). I see her account as complementary to, not competitive with, this one.

References

Babbitt, Susan. 1993. "Feminism and Objective Interests." In *Feminist Epistemologies*, eds. Linda Alcoff and Elizabeth Potter. New York: Routledge.

———. 1996. *Impossible Dreams: Rationality, Integrity, and Moral Imagination*. Boulder, Colo.: Westview Press.

Baier, Annette. 1985b. "What Do Women Want in a Moral Theory?" *Nous* 19(1): 53–63.

Benson, Paul. 1991. "Autonomy and Oppressive Socialization." *Social Theory and Practice* 17(3): 385–408.

———. 1994. "Free Agency and Self-Worth." *Journal of Philosophy* 91(12): 650–68.

Code, Lorraine. 1991. *What Can She Know? Feminist Theory and the Construction of Knowledge*. Ithaca, N.Y.: Cornell University Press.

Corea, Gena. 1985. *The Hidden Malpractice: How American Medicine Mistreats Women*. New York: Harper Colophon Books.

Dillon, Robin. 1992. "Toward a Feminist Conception of Self-Respect." *Hypatia* 7(1): 52–69.

Donchin, Anne. 1998. "Understanding Autonomy Relationally: Toward a Reconfiguration of Bioethical Principles." *Journal of Medicine and Philosophy* 23.

Dworkin, Gerald. 1988. *The Theory and Practice of Autonomy*. Cambridge: Cambridge University Press.

Ehrenreich, Barbara, and Deirdre English. 1972. *Witches, Midwives, and Nurses: A History of Women Healers*. Glass Mountain Pamphlet, no. 1, Old Westbury, N.Y.: The Feminist Press.

Fisher, Sue. 1986. *In the Patient's Best Interests: Women and the Politics of Medical Decisions*. New Brunswick, N.J.: Rutgers University Press.

Foucault, Michel. 1979. *Discipline and Punish*. New York: Vintage.

———. 1980. *Power/Knowledge*. Ed. Colin Gordon. Brighton, Eng.: Harvester

Gardiner, Judith Kegan. 1995. *Provoking Agents: Gender and Agency in Theory and Practice*. Chicago: University of Illinois Press.

Gilligan, Carol. 1982. *In a Different Voice: Psychological Theory and Women's Moral*

Development. Cambridge, Mass.: Harvard University Press.

Held, Virginia. 1993. *Feminist Morality: Transforming Culture, Society, and Politics.* Chicago: University of Chicago Press.

Hoagland, Sarah Lucia. 1992. "Lesbian Ethics and Female Agency." In *Explorations in Feminist Ethics: Theory and Practice,* ed. Susan Browning Cole and Susan Coultrap-McQuin. Bloomington: Indiana University Press.

hooks, bell. 1990. *Yearning: Race, Gender, and Cultural Politics.* Toronto: Between the Lines.

Katz, Jay, ed. 1972. *Experimentation with Human Beings: The Authority of the Investigator, Subject, Professions, and State in the Human Experimentation Process.* New York: Russell Sage Foundation.

Lloyd, Genevieve. 1984. *The Man of Reason: "Male" and "Female" in Western Philosophy.* Minneapolis: University of Minnesota Press.

Mahowald, Mary Briody. 1993. *Women and Children in Health Care: An Unequal Majority.* New York: Oxford University Press.

Meyers, Diana T. 1989. *Self, Society, and Personal Choice.* New York: Columbia University Press.

Nedelsky, Jennifer. 1989. "Reconceiving Autonomy." *Yale Journal of Law and Feminism* 1(1): 7–36.

Perales, Cesar A., and Lauren S. Young, eds. 1988. *Too Little, Too Late: Dealing with the Health Needs of Women in Poverty.* New York: Harrington Park Press.

Sherwin, Susan. 1992. *No Longer Patient: Feminist Ethics and Health Care.* Philadelphia: Temple University Press.

White, Evelyn C., ed. 1990. *The Black Women's Health Book: Speaking for Ourselves.* Seattle, Wash.: Seal Press.

Chapter 6   CONSENT TO TREATMENT

Informed Consent: Framing the Questions

Paul S. Appelbaum, Charles W. Lidz, and Alan Meisel

What is informed consent? The answer may seem self-evident only to those who have yet to explore the many meanings of the term. Informed consent refers to legal rules that prescribe behaviors for physicians in their interactions with patients and provide for penalties, under given circumstances, if physicians deviate from those expectations; to an ethical doctrine, rooted in our society's cherished value of autonomy, that insures to patients their right of self-determination when medical decisions need to be made; and to an interpersonal process whereby physicians (and often other health-care professionals) interact with patients to select an appropriate course of medical care.

Informed consent is each of these things, yet none of them alone. As a theory based on ethical principles, given effect by legal rulings, and implemented by clinicians, it has been haunted by its complex lineage. When legal principles and ethical values conflict, which should take precedence? When clinical interests appear to be served by neither legal nor ethical concerns, which interests should be compromised and to what degree? The vast literature on informed consent, found in journals and books of medicine, law, philosophy, and public policy, has been stimulated by the need to create a workable doctrine that can accommodate values that to many observers are in an irremediable state of conflict....

1.1 THE CLINICAL SETTING

John Williamson (all names have been altered in this history of an actual case) is a 23-year-old man who was seen in an outpatient surgical clinic of a major health center and diagnosed as suffering from an acute flare-up of chronic pancreatitis. Mr. Williamson's chief complaint was the intense abdominal pain that accompanies pancreatitis. Dr. Johnson, the chief surgical resident, had seen him a number of times before for similar problems. Dr. Johnson and Dr. Ricah, the senior resident, examined him and asked whether the narcotic pain relievers they had previously prescribed were doing him any good.

Patient: No.... I am just getting used to them. Maybe a couple of belts (i.e., drinks) would help me out.

Chief Resident: No, I can guarantee that that will not help.... I've looked at your tests but I still want to look at your X-rays. What I think is that you will do better if we take out part of your pancreas; as long as you understand that this is a serious operation in that, while you probably won't die from it, there is a small chance that you might, although not much. But there are serious side effects from it, like you will probably have some diabetes and have trouble digesting your food. Then I think that we should go ahead and have you talk with your wife about coming in and make plans for you to come in.

Senior Resident: I think that you ought to understand that this is not going to be a cure-all. This is not going to do away with all of your problems. You are still going to have a lot of problems from that pancreas of yours.

Patient: I know that.

A researcher studying informed consent, who made daily rounds with the surgical team, witnessed the above conversation and later that morning interviewed Mr. Williamson.

Researcher: Can you tell me what your problem is?

Patient: It is the pancreas.

Researcher: Have any idea why?

Patient: No, I don't know. The doctor knows really what I'll have to do…. I've been having this problem about two years now. It's getting unbearable. Before, I could live with it, but now I'll take a chance on anything….

Researcher: Can you tell me what they are going to do in this operation?

Patient: They are going to take my pancreas out.

Researcher: The whole pancreas?

Patient: Um-hm…. It is going bad anyway. I'd rather have it out of me than if it really might ruin me on the inside….

Researcher: Think it will make the pain better?

Patient: Well, at least we won't take any chances.

Mr. Williamson was brought into the hospital one week later, after he complained that he was unable to wait the scheduled month before the operation because of the pain. Dr. Johnson described the case on rounds as being one in which he had treated the patient with painkillers for an extensive period of time. He described Mr. Williamson as an ex-alcoholic whose pancreatic deterioration was the result of alcoholism. Dr. Johnson said that he would not make a final decision about going through with the operation until he saw whether or not the X-rays showed that the lesion was limited to an operable area of the pancreas. In his view, the main advantage of the operation was that it would allow Mr. Williamson to be withdrawn from the pain medication. He also said he hoped the patient was telling the truth when he said he had quit drinking, or he would just have the same problem again.

The next day Dr. Johnson revealed to the surgical team on rounds that he planned to do a distal pancreatectomy. "That should benefit him if he has really quit drinking…. He has said that he wants it out. The results are not good with distal pancreatectomies but it is probably worth a try…. He knows we are doing it to get him off medication." The next morning Dr. Ricah told Mr. Williamson that the X-ray had come back and that they planned to do the operation the next week.

While waiting in the hospital for the tests to be completed and for the scheduled surgery, Mr. Williamson generally was told a little bit about what was happening each day. Four days before the scheduled operation, Dr. Johnson told him, "I'd say that there is a 50 percent chance that there will be no pain after the operation and an 80 to 90 percent chance that it will help you. The object is to relieve some of your pain, and as far as that is concerned the only other thing that we're concerned with is that you've got to be sure you don't drink, because that's not helping at all. So we are going ahead Wednesday, O.K.?" Mr. Williamson agreed.

The next day Mr. Williamson asked about his sugar test. The surgeon responded, "Your sugar seems to be normal. I think if we only have to take out half or two-thirds of the pancreas that you should not become diabetic. You may have to watch your diet a little bit, but that is all." In another interview that afternoon it became clear that Mr. Williamson now understood that only part of the pancreas would be removed, but his description seemed to imply that it was being removed to prevent the spread of an infection.

Two days before the operation, during rounds, the following discussion occurred:

Patient: How long will the operation take?

Senior Resident: Four or five hours. It's a pretty long one. I want you to know that we may have to take out your spleen as well as your pancreas.

Patient: What is that?

Senior Resident: Oh, it's an organ that takes care of things like the breakdown of old blood cells and a few things like that. It seems to have something to do with fighting infections, so for people who have it taken out, we usually make a special effort to vaccinate them again. We will try to save it, but the blood vessels that feed it run right along the back of the pancreas and it is much better to take it out than to get all of the bleeding that is sometimes required to save the blood vessels…. Another problem we could have is adhesions.

Patient: What's that?

Senior Resident: Well, because you have had this many operations, things get sticky in there, and we may have trouble with things getting stuck together.

Patient: What about the diabetes thing?

Senior Resident: The chances are that you will not have to take any medicine but you may have to watch your diet a bit.

Although Dr. Johnson was convinced that this operation was a good idea, his senior resident was not, and they argued about it more than once. Dr. Ricah felt the patient was expecting too much from the treatment and it was not going to provide him with the relief he expected. Dr. Johnson contended, "There are risks, but I've explained them to him and I'll explain them to him again tomorrow. I think we can help this kid."

The afternoon before the operation Dr. Johnson did the informed consent disclosure required of him by hospital rules.

Chief Resident: We've talked about everything, I think. We're going to take out that area of the pancreas that is abnormal, and we will probably also have to take out your spleen as well. The problems of the operation are the possibility of bleeding during the operation. Sometimes there is a possibility of infection from the operation. We will cover you with antibiotics, of course, both before and after the operation. When you come out of the operation you'll have a drain in your nose and in your stomach for a few days. It isn't an easy operation but I am fairly confident that we can help you.

Later that evening one of the evening shift nurses went into Mr. Williamson's room to get a consent form signed.

Nurse: John, I have to get your consent, but you did talk to Dr. Johnson about it today, didn't you?

Patient: (nods)

Nurse: First let me tell you what will happen tomorrow. As soon as we're through here, I am going to start an IV on you and then you're going to get a PhisoHex shower; you know that, don't you?

Patient: (nods)

Nurse: (Describes morning shower, blood pressure monitoring, Valium administration, and starting general anesthesia. Reports that the operation will take four or five hours and tells the patient that he will then come back up to the ward and describes some of the postoperative care. About 10 minutes of description.) Well, all I have left is for you to sign this [consent form]. Read it over first. If you have any questions, just ask. (She leaves the room briefly while he reads a general consent form for surgical procedures containing information specific to his situation.)

Patient: Sign here right? (signing)

Nurse: Do you have any questions?

Patient: Not really. (after a moment) I do have one question. Does my spleen have anything to do with my having children?

Nurse: (surprised) No, no, nothing to do with that.

Mr. Williamson had his operation the next morning.

Mr. Williamson's case is in some ways typical of and in some ways quite different from most doctor–patient interactions. The ambiguities in communication and the unspoken motives of all participants is, current research suggests, common to the medical setting. On the other hand, despite important omissions and Mr. Williamson's less-than-perfect understanding of the reasons for and possible consequences of the procedure he was to undergo, quite a bit of information was passed to Mr. Williamson by his physicians. Existing empirical research, as we shall see, indicates that this is not universally the case.

For our purposes, any conclusions we might draw from interaction between these physicians and their somewhat bewildered patient are of much less importance than the questions raised.

1. The discussions Drs. Johnson and Ricah had with their patient, culminating in his encounter with the nurse who brought him a consent form for his signature, are a part of the preoperative routine (some might say ritual) in most medical centers. Asked why they were doing what they did, most of the participants would probably have replied, "I am trying to live up to my responsibilities under the law of informed consent." What is the law of informed consent and how did it evolve into its current form?

2. Had Dr. Johnson been asked whether he would have behaved differently in the absence of a legal requirement for him to discuss certain issues with his patient, he might well have hesitated before responding. "I'm not sure," he might have replied, "because I've just taken for granted that this is something that we have to do. But now that I think about it, I'd feel uncomfortable operating on someone without telling him something about the operation. It's his body, after all. And besides, he'll be more cooperative if he knows what's going on." This response suggests that the conveyance of information from doctor to patient has roots that go deeper than the legal rules that usually dominate most discussions of consent. Basic notions of right and wrong and good and bad seem to be involved. What are the ethical underpinnings of consent in the doctor–patient relationship?

3. Although Drs. Johnson and Ricah may have felt both legal and ethical imperatives to provide Mr. Williamson with certain information concerning his medical care, they were clearly selective. Mr. Williamson was told some of the major risks of surgery, for example, but never that his physicians viewed the operation largely as a maneuver to wean him from the use of painkillers or that they had substantial doubts that the procedure would measurably reduce his pain. There was no discussion at all of possible alternatives to the distal pancreatectomy Dr. Johnson decided to perform. What infor-

mation does the law require physicians to disclose to their patients when it defines what constitutes an informed consent?

4. Mr. Williamson, who had barely completed high school, had obvious difficulty understanding some of the information his physicians communicated to him. In part, this problem may have resulted from the lack of detail he was offered. The discussion of diabetes as a possible consequence of the surgery, for example, was conducted without any effort to explain to Mr. Williamson just what it might mean to cope with a surgically induced diabetic state. But some of Mr. Williamson's confusion stemmed from his own intellectual limitations. Was he able to understand enough of what he was told to make a meaningful decision about surgery? How can one determine who is able to make their own decisions—in legal terms, who is competent to decide for themselves—and who is not? When someone is found not to be competent, what alternative decision-making mechanisms are available?

5. Lurking in the back of the minds of the physicians in this case was the knowledge that some doctors are subjected to suit by their patients on the grounds that informed consent was not obtained. On what basis can such suits be brought and according to what rules are they handled by the legal system?

6. The procedure Dr. Johnson performed on Mr. Williamson is an accepted part of the surgical repertoire, not an innovation that Dr. Johnson decided to test. Furthermore, Dr. Johnson's sole motivation for performing the surgery was to help Mr. Williamson, rather than in a formal way to gather data that might be of assistance to other patients in the future. What if the opposite had been the case? That is, what if Dr. Johnson had been introducing a new surgical procedure and intended to use information about Mr. Williamson's operation as part of a larger body of data to assess the new procedure's utility? Would the ethical or legal rules governing consent change?

Should consent be obtained differently in such circumstances?

The questions stated so far address primarily the theoretical aspects of informed consent from an ethical and legal perspective. Mr. Williamson's case also raises a number of practical questions concerning informed consent in the clinical setting.

7. As we have seen, questions exist about how effective the efforts to communicate with this patient really were, and how much he was able to comprehend, regardless of the communication methods used. What do we know about various methods of disclosure? How much do patients understand as a result? How competent are most patients? Finally, how are decisions about medical care really made?

8. Careful review of the transcripts of Mr. Williamson's discussions with his caregivers suggests some puzzling and troubling issues. For example, Mr. Williamson was given a good deal of information about his treatment over a period of several days. However, he appears to have committed himself to proceed with the surgery well before all the information about it was made available, even before its full extent and major complications were made known to him. (He was unaware that a splenectomy would be part of the procedure until quite late in the process.) What suggestions can we make to Drs. Johnson and Ricah as to how they might better have dealt with Mr. Williamson to ensure a more informed decision?

9. One of the more curious aspects of the interactions was the late appearance on the scene of a nurse bearing a consent form for Mr. Williamson to sign. What purpose do these consent forms have, and are there ways of using them that integrate them more meaningfully into the rest of the informing process?

10. Mr. Williamson consented to have the procedure performed even though he evidently had some serious concerns about the possible results. He signed the consent form, after all, while still entertaining the

possibility that the removal of his spleen might have an adverse impact on his ability to father children. What if he had refused to undergo the procedure? Do we have any understanding of why patients refuse treatment, what role the provision of information to them plays in their refusal, and how refusals might best be responded to?

11. A great deal of ink has been spilled in efforts to determine how Mr. Williamson and his doctors should interact before his consent to surgery is considered legitimate. How would critics of the present process have altered the discussions? Are legal approaches the best way to go about modifying the behavior of both sides?...

A Moral Theory of Informed Consent

Benjamin Freedman

Most medical codes of ethics, and most physicians, agree that the physician ought to obtain the "free and informed consent" of his subject or patient before attempting any serious medical procedure, experimental or therapeutic in nature. They agree, moreover, that a proxy consent ought to be obtained on behalf of the incompetent subject. And informed consent is seen as not merely a legal requirement, and not merely a formality: it is a substantial requirement of morality.

Acceptance of this doctrine, however, requires the solution of a number of problems. How much information need be imparted? At what age is a person mature enough to consent on his own behalf? Can prisoners give a "free and informed consent" to be experimented upon? Lurking behind these and similar questions there are more fundamental difficulties. What are the functions of consent for the competent and the incompetent? What is the sense in which the patient/subject must be "free," "informed," and "competent?" It is by way of an approach to these latter questions that I shall attempt to respond to the more specific questions.[1]

I. CONSENT AND THE COMPETENT

The negative aspects of the doctrine of informed consent have ordinarily been the focus of attention; difficulties in obtaining the informed consent

of the subject/patient render the ethics of experimentation and therapeutic measures questionable. Our common view of informed consent is that, when at all relevant, it represents a minimum condition which ethics imposes upon the physician. It is seen as a necessary condition for medical manipulation, but hardly as a sufficient condition.

The reasons why this is so—why it is not sufficient that an experimenter, for instance, have received informed consent from his subject before proceeding—are quite obvious. The scarcity of medical resources (which includes a scarcity of qualified physician-investigators) forbids us from wasting time upon poorly-designed experiments, or upon experiments which merely replicate well-established conclusions. There seems to be, as well, a limit to the dangers which we (ordinarily) allow subjects to face. We do not, as a matter of policy, think it wise to allow would-be suicides to accomplish their end with the aid of a scientific investigator. Many other reasons could be given for the proposition that a person does not have a right to be experimented upon, even when he has given valid consent to the procedure.

The Right to Consent

But there does seem to exist a positive right of informed consent, which exists in both therapeutic and experimental settings. A person who has the capacity to give valid consent, and who has in fact consented to the procedure in question, has a right to have that fact recognized by us. We all have a duty to recognize a valid consent when confronted with it.

From whence derives this right? It arises from the right which each of us possesses to be treated as a person, and in the duty which all of us have, to have respect for persons, to treat a person as such, and not as an object. For this entails that our capacities for personhood ought to be recognized by all—these capacities including the capacity for rational decision, and for action consequent upon rational decision. Perhaps the worst which we may do to a man is to deny him his humanity, for example, by classifying him as mentally incompetent when he is, in fact, sane. It is a terrible thing to be hated or persecuted; it is far worse to be ignored, to be notified that you "don't count."

If an individual is capable of and has given valid consent, I would argue that he has a right, as against the world but more particularly as against his physician, to have it recognized that valid consent has been given. (The same applies, of course, with still greater force, with regard to *refusals* to consent to medical procedures.) The limited force of this claim must be emphasized: it does not entail a right to be treated, or to be experimented upon. It is a most innocuous right, one which most of us would have little hesitation about granting.

It is, therefore, curious that the literature on informed consent has failed to recognize this right—has, in fact, tacitly denied this right, at least as regards experimentation. In writings on informed consent it seems to have been assumed that if, under certain conditions, it is *doubtful* that valid consent to an experiment has been granted, it is best to "play it safe" ethically. In cases of doubt, we prefer not to take chances: in this case, we will not take a chance upon violating the canons of ethics by experimenting without being certain that the subject has validly consented to the experiment. Since we do not at present know whether a prisoner can give a valid consent, let us not take chances: we call for a

moratorium on prison experimentation. Since we do not know at what age a person has the capacity to give a valid consent, we avoid the problem by setting the age of majority at a point where it is beyond doubt that maturity has been attained. If we must err, we shall ensure that we err in being overly ethical.

The establishment of the innocuous right to have valid consent recognized as such eliminates this expedient. Other writers have conceptualized the conflict as one between a right and, at best, a mere liberty. From the patient's point of view, he has a right to have his health protected by the physician, and a mere liberty to be experimented upon. From the physician-investigator's point of view, he has a duty to protect the subject's health, and a mere liberty to experiment upon the subject (contingent, of course, upon obtaining the subject's consent). A recognition of the claims of personhood and autonomy, however, reveals this to be a conflict between rights and duties. The physician-investigator has a duty to recognize consent when validly offered. When the consent is of doubtful validity, therefore, the physician experiences a conflict between two duties. He will not be ethically well-protected by choosing not to experiment, for there exists the possibility—which, as cases are multiplied, becomes a probability—that he is violating a duty in so choosing. Problems in informed consent present us with a dilemma. It is no longer the case that the burden of proof devolves upon the would-be experimenter. The would-be abstainer-from-experiments may have to prove his case as well.

These considerations give us a new point of departure in investigating problems of informed consent. They show us that there is no "fail-safe" procedure which we can fall back upon in cases of doubt. Rather, what is required is an exhaustive examination of each case and issue, to see whether or not a valid consent has in fact been obtained….

The Requirement of Information

The most common locution for the requirement which I am discussing is "informed consent"—

we require "informed consent" to protect a doctor from legal liability resultant from his therapeutic endeavors, or to ensure the "ethicacy" of an experiment. But I believe "informed consent" to be a serious misnomer for what we do, in fact, want medical practice to conform to.

No lengthy rehearsal of the absurdities consequent upon taking the term "informed consent" at face value is necessary. The claim has been made, and repeated with approval, that "fully informed consent" is a goal which we can never achieve, but toward which we must strive. In order to ensure that fully informed consent has been given, it has seriously been suggested that only medical students or graduate students in the life sciences ought to be accepted as subjects for experimentation. *Reductio ad absurdum* examples of "fully informed consent" have been elaborated, in forms which list all the minutiae of the proposed medical procedure, together with all of its conceivable sequelae. With such a view of "informed consent" and its requirements, it is not surprising to find doctors who claim that since they cannot fully inform patients, they will tell them nothing, but instead will personally assume the responsibility for assuring the subject's safety.

In truth, a *reductio ad absurdum* of this view of "informed consent" need not be constructed; it serves as its own *reductio ad absurdum.* For there is no end to "fully informing" patients. When the doctor wishes to insert a catheter, must he commend to the subject's attention a textbook of anatomy? Although this, of course, would not suffice: he must ensure that the patient understand the text as well. Must he tell the patient the story of Dr. X, that bogey of first-year medical students, who, in a state of inebriation, inserted ("by mistake") his pen-refill instead of the catheter? With, of course, the assurance that *this* physician never gets drunk ("Well, rarely, anyway.") Must the patient be informed of the chemical formula of the catheter? Its melting point?

The basic mistake which is committed by those who harp upon the difficulties in obtaining informed consent (and by critics of the doctrine) is in believing that we can talk about information in the abstract, without reference to any human purpose. It is very likely impossible to talk about "information" in this way; but impossible or not, when we do in fact talk about, or request, information, we do not mean "information in the abstract." If I ask someone to "tell me about those clouds" he will, ordinarily, know what I mean; and he will answer me, in the spirit in which he was asked, by virtue of his professional expertise as an artist, meteorologist, astronomer, soothsayer, or what-have-you. The meteorologist will not object that he cannot tell you the optical refraction index of the clouds, and therefore that he cannot "fully answer" your question. He knows that you are asking him with a given end in mind, and that much information about the cloud is irrelevant *relative to that purpose.*

That this "abstract information" requirement is not in question in obtaining valid consent is hardly an original point, but it is worth repeating. One of the leading court opinions on human experimentation puts it like this: "... the patient's interest in information does not extend to a lengthy polysyllabic discourse on all possible complications. A mini-course in medical science is not required...."[2]

The proper question to ask, then, is not "What information must be given?" That would be premature: we must first know for what purpose information is needed. *Why* must the patient be informed? Put that way, the answer is immediately forthcoming. The patient must be informed so that he will know what he is getting into, what he may expect from the procedure, what his likely alternatives are—in short, what the procedure (and forbearance from it) will mean, so that a responsible decision on the matter may be made. This is the legal stance, as well as, I think, a "common sensical" stance; as Alexander Capron writes, the information component in valid consent derives in law from the recognition that information is "necessary to make meaningful the power to decide."[3] The proper test of whether a given piece of information needs to be given is, then, whether the physician, knowing what he does about the patient/subject, feels that that patient/subject would want to know this before making up his mind. Outré, improbable consequences would not ordinarily, therefore, be relevant information. Exceptionally, they will be: for example, when there is a small risk of impotence consequent upon the procedure which the physician proposes to perform upon a man with a great stake in his sexual prowess. This is only sensible.

Our main conclusion, then is that valid consent entails only the imparting of that information which the patient/subject requires in order to make a responsible decision. This entails, I think, the possibility of a valid yet ignorant consent.

Consider, first, the therapeutic context. It is, I believe, not unusual for a patient to give his doctor *carte blanche* to perform any medical procedure which the physician deems proper in order to effect a cure. He is telling the doctor to act as his agent in choosing which procedure to follow. This decision is neither unwise nor (in any serious sense) an abdication of responsibility and an unwarranted burden upon the physician. We each of us choose to delegate our power of choice in this way in dealing with our auto mechanic or stockbroker.

It may be harder to accept an ignorant consent as valid in the purely experimental context. I think, however, that much of this difficulty is due to our paucity of imagination, our failure to imagine circumstances in which a person might choose to proceed in this way. We might approach such a case, for example, by imagining a Quaker who chooses to serve society by acting as a research subject, but who has a morbid fear of knives and pointed instruments. The Quaker might say to the physician-investigator that he wants to serve science but is afraid that his phobia would overcome his better judgment. He might consequently request that any experiment which would involve use of scalpels, hypodermic needles, and such, be performed without informing him: while, say, he is asleep or unconscious. He might further ask the doctor not to proceed should the experiment involve considerable risk. In such a case, or one similar, we would find an instance of a valid yet ignorant consent to experimentation.

The ostensible differences between the therapeutic and experimental contexts may be resolved into two components: in the therapeutic context it is supposed that the physician knows what the sequelae to treatment will be, which information, by definition, is not available in the experimental situation; and in the therapeutic context the doctor may be said to be seeking his patient's good, in contrast to the experimental context where some other good is being sought. On the basis of these differences it may be claimed that a valid yet ignorant consent is enough permission for therapy, but not for experimentation.

Closer examination, however, reveals that these differences do not necessarily obtain. First, because I believe it would be granted that a valid yet ignorant consent can be given in the "therapeutic-experimental" situation, where a new drug or procedure is being attempted to aid the patient (in the absence of any traditional available therapy). In the therapeutic-experimental situation, as in the purely experimental situation, the sequelae are not known (although of course in both cases some definite result is expected or anticipated). If a valid yet ignorant consent is acceptable in the one, therefore, it must be acceptable in the other.

Secondly, because it is patently not the case that we can expect there to be no good accruing to the subject of an experiment by reason of his participation. There are, commonly, financial and other "tangible" benefits forthcoming (laboratory training, and so on). And it must … be said that the pleasures of altruism are not negligible. The proposed differences between experimentation and therapy do not stand up, and so we must say that if a valid yet ignorant consent is acceptable in the one it must be acceptable in the other. It must be remembered that this statement only concerns itself with one part of the consent doctrine, which is, itself, only one of the requirements which the ethical experiment must satisfy….

Our conclusion, then, is that the informing of the patient/subject is not a fundamental requirement of valid consent. It is, rather, derivative from the requirement that the consent be the expression of a responsible choice. The two requirements which I do see as fundamental in this doctrine are that the choice be responsible and that it be voluntary.

The Requirement of Responsibility

What is meant by saying that the choice must be "responsible?" Does this entail that the physician may at any time override a patient's judgment on the basis that, in the physician's view, the patient has not chosen responsibly? Surely not; to adopt such a criterion would defeat the purpose embodied in the doctrine of consent. It would mean that a person's exercise of autonomy is always subject to review.

Still, some such requirement would appear to be necessary. A small child can certainly make choices.[4] Small children can also be intelligent enough to understand the necessary information. Yet surely we would not want to say that a small child can give valid consent to a serious medical procedure.[5] The reason for this is that the child cannot choose *responsibly*.

We are faced with a dilemma. On the one hand, it appears that we must require that the choice be responsible. To require only that the choice be free would yield counter-intuitive results. On the other hand, if we do require that the choice made be a responsible one, we seem to presuppose some body which shall judge the reasonableness of choices; this represents a paternalism which is antithetical to the doctrine of consent. An elderly patient chooses to forgo further life-saving measures. How are we to judge whether or not this choice is a responsible one?

The path between the horns of this dilemma involves saying that the "responsibility" which we require is to be predicated not on the nature of the particular choice, but on the nature of the patient/subject. What we need to know is whether *he* is a responsible man ("in general," so to speak), not whether the choice which has been made is responsible. In this way, we avoid the danger of upholding as "responsible" only those choices which we ourselves feel are good choices. We can and do admit into the community of responsible persons individuals who make choices with which we do not agree.

In this sense, responsibility is a dispositional characteristic. To say that someone is a responsible individual means that he makes choices, typically, on the basis of reasons, arguments, or beliefs—and that he remains open to the claims of reason, so that further rational argument might lead him to change his mind. It is to say that a person is capable of making and carrying through a life-plan—that he is prepared to act on the basis of his choices. It is to say that a person is capable of living with his life-plan; he can live with the consequences of his choices, he *takes responsibility* for his choices.[6] Of course, none of these are absolutes: all responsible people are at times pigheaded, at times short-sighted, at times flighty. That is to say, all responsible men at times act irresponsibly. Should the lack of responsibility persist, of course, to an extreme degree, we may say that the person has left the community of responsible folk.

Voluntarism and Reward

The other requirement of valid consent is that it be given voluntarily. The choice which the consent expresses must be freely made.

We all know some conditions which, if satisfied, make us say that a consent has been given involuntarily. The case which immediately springs to mind occurs when an individual succumbs under a threat: we call this duress or coercion. But the threat need not be overt; and perhaps there need not be a threat at all to render consent involuntary.

Hence, the major problem currently engendered by the requirement of voluntariness. It is typified by the prisoner who "volunteers" for an experiment in the hope or expectation of a reward: significantly higher wages, an opportunity for job training, better health care while involved in the experiment, a favorable report to his parole board. Is the consent which the prisoner offers a voluntary consent? The problem may be stated more generally thus: At what point does reward render consent involuntary?

The problem of reward is particularly difficult, since it involves questions of degree. Is a prisoner's consent involuntary if the reward for his participation in the experiment is a three-month reduction of sentence? Is it relevant here that the prisoner is serving a twenty-year sentence, rather than a one-to-five-year sentence? Does a possible increase in wages from twenty-five cents per hour to one dollar per hour constitute duress? Should we consider the percentage increase, or the increase in absolute value, or the increase in actual value which the seventy-five-cent disparity represents in the prison environment?

To some, of course, questions like these have little meaning. They have little meaning to those who are indifferent to the demands of justice and autonomy which the consent doctrine represents, to those who are willing to buy guinea pigs, rather than to reward human beings. And they have little meaning for those who are convinced that prisoners are inherently unfree, and who thus would call for a total cessation of prison experimentation. Each of these positions denies, in an *a priori* fashion, freedom to prisoners; each must be rejected. A recognition of the fact that decisions about consent may be over- as well as under-protective forces us to deal with this sort of question, complex though it may be.

As is so often the case, posing the question in a different way may facilitate response. We have been considering the question of how much reward nullifies the validity of consent, how much reward renders the subject unfree. But is it in fact the case that *reward* is the disruptive factor here?

This problem may be clarified by the following examples. Imagine an upper-middle-class individual, who can provide for his family all of their needs and most of the amenities of civilized life. Let us say that this person is offered one hundred dollars to cross the street— if you like, make it one thousand or ten thousand dollars? He chooses to cross the street. Is his choice *involuntary*? Despite the substantial reward, I think most of us would agree that the consent was freely offered (and would that we should have such problems!).

Consider a person who deeply wants to be an astronaut. He is told that as part of the program he must participate in experiments to determine resistance to high-G conditions. Is his consent to this invalid, involuntary? I think not. We would say, this is part of his job; he should have expected it; and if he can't stand the heat, he should get out of the kitchen. In this vein, consider Evel Knievel, a financially prosperous man, who is offered millions of dollars to perform daredevil stunts. His choice may be bizarre, even crazy: but has his reward rendered it unfree?

Finally, consider a man who is informed by his doctor that he will most likely die unless he has open-heart surgery. His "reward" for consenting is his life; the penalty for not consenting is death. Does this mean this man cannot give the doctor valid consent—morally valid consent— to proceed?

There are two distinctions which, I think, go a long way towards dispelling these problems. First, I think it must be granted that natural contingencies ("acts of God," things which come to pass naturally, those contingencies which we cannot hold anyone responsible for) do not render a person unfree, nor do they render unfree the choices which a person makes in light of those contingencies.[7]

That natural contingencies do not render a man unfree is a point which is apt to be forgotten in the present context. I am not—in the morally relevant sense—lacking in freedom because I cannot, unaided, fly through the air, or live on grass. Nor am I unfree because my heart is about to give out. Nor am I unfree when, recognizing that my heart may give out, I choose to undergo surgery. I may, of course, be so crazed by knowing that I am near death's door that I am in a state of general impotence, and hence must have the choice made for me; but general incompetence is not in question here. The distinction between choices forced by man, and choices forced by nature, is, then, of importance.

The second distinction is between those pressures which are, and those which are not, in Daube's words, "consonant with the dignity and responsibility of free life."[8] I would explain this as follows: there are certain basic freedoms and rights which we possess which *entitle* us (morally) to certain things (or states of affairs).

We would all, no doubt, draw up different lists of these rights and freedoms; but included in them would be safety of person, freedom of conscience and religion, a right to a certain level of education, and, for some of us, a right to some level of health care. When the "reward" is such as only to give us the necessary conditions of these rights and freedoms—when all that the reward does is to bring us up to a level of living to which we are entitled, and of which we have been deprived by man—then the "reward," I think, constitutes duress. A reward which accrues to one who has achieved this level, or who can easily achieve it (other than by taking the reward option), and which hence serves only to grant us "luxury" items, does not constitute duress, and hence does not render choice unfree, no matter how great this reward may be.

The rewards above the moral subsistence level are true rewards. In contrast, we may say (with some touch of metaphor) that the "rewards" which only bring us up to the level to which we were in any event entitled are properly viewed as functioning as *threats:* "Do this, or stay where you are:"—when you should not have been "where you are" in the first place.

The astronaut, Evel Knievel, and the upper-middle-class street-crosser are being granted "luxury" items, and hence are capable of giving free consent. But consider a man who will not be admitted to the hospital for treatment unless he agrees to be a subject in an experiment (unrelated to his treatment). Those who feel, as I do, that we are, here and now, morally entitled to medical treatment would agree, I trust, that this illegitimate option coerces the man into agreeing. Or consider a man who has religious scruples against donating blood, who takes his daughter to a hospital for treatment. He is told that the doctors will not treat her unless the family donates a certain amount of blood. His freedom has been nullified; his "consent" to donating blood is morally invalid. Similarly, the college student whose grade is contingent upon his participation in the instructor's psychological experiments is not validly consenting to serve. He is entitled to have his grade based upon his classroom work.

It yet remains to apply this distinction to our original problem, prison experimentation. The application will not be attempted here, for we would first need to be clear in our minds what rights and freedoms a prisoner is entitled to. I would not hesitate to say, though, that when a situation is created whereby a prisoner can only receive decent health care by participating in an experiment, he is being coerced into that experiment. I would have little hesitation in claiming that if subjecting himself to experimentation is the only way in which a prisoner could learn a trade which maybe used "outside," then that prisoner is being coerced, his consent is not free. When we take into account the condition of our society, these would seem to be reasonable entitlements for the prisoner. Other rewards—for example, higher pay—may or may not constitute rewards above the moral subsistence level; if they are, then consent in light of these rewards could be freely offered. Perhaps too much has been said already; judgments like these must be made in an individualized fashion, one which is sensitive to the realities of prison life.

II. CONSENT AND THE INCOMPETENT

In this section will be discussed, first, the question of how the age of majority and minority with reference to valid consent ought to be set; and secondly, the problems associated with the concept of proxy consent.

The Age of Consent

It has been argued that the requirements for obtaining valid consent are that the patient/subject must have consented freely and that he must be a responsible individual. The requirement of voluntariness does not raise any novel problems when applied to minors. Rather, what we usually have in mind when restricting the power of the minor to consent is that he is not, in the sense required, a responsible individual.

I have claimed that to be a responsible individual one must be capable of rationally adopting, following through, and accepting the consequences of a life-plan. The age, therefore, at which society indicates a presumption that individuals can satisfy these conditions can be said to be the age at which society ought to grant the right to give valid consent to serious medical procedures. The examples which spring to mind are the age of conscription and the age of marriageability. At these ages society has indicated that one is capable of acting, in a complex society, as an individual.

This is not an argument like that which says "If you are old enough to fight, then you are old enough to vote." The requirements necessary for being a soldier may be wholly unrelated to the requirements necessary before the franchise may be properly exercised. In contrast, the responsibility which we assume to be possessed by those capable of soldiering and contracting marriage is the same responsibility which is required to make consent valid: the ability to work through and with a life-plan....

But the setting of an age of consent indicates only a presumption and nothing more. The fact that someone has passed the age of consent is not conclusive proof that he is responsible (in the sense required); the fact that someone is below the age of consent is not conclusive proof of irresponsibility. The presumption may be defeated in either direction.

It is clear, for example, that an adult is not, *ipso facto,* responsible. The adult may be insane.

It is equally clear that a minor need not be irresponsible. People mature at different rates. If evidence of responsibility may be supplied on behalf of one below the age of consent, the presumption of irresponsibility should be defeated. The sort of evidence which would be necessary is that which indicates that the person can work through a life-plan. It may be said that this notion is being approached by the law in the special provisions sometimes made for the "emancipated minor." Marriage or economic self-sufficiency are among the common requirements for being considered an emancipated minor. One of the special prerogatives of the emancipated minor is that he may consent on his own behalf to medical care. I would argue that this should be extended to cover participation in experimentation as well.

Proxy Consent

Proxy consent is consent given on behalf of an individual who is himself incapable of granting consent. The major category of those who require proxy consent are minors, but proxy consent may need to be obtained for the insane or the unconscious as well. My comments will nevertheless be restricted to the case of minors, leaving the other cases to be dealt with by implication. In minors, proxy consent is ordinarily granted by the child's parent or guardian; exceptionally, it may be given by another close relative or by an individual appointed by the court for the specific purpose of granting consent to some procedure.

I have argued that the function of informed consent is to respect the autonomy and dignity of the individual. This cannot be the function of proxy consent. The minor patient/subject cannot fully express autonomy and dignity through choices. It may be said that the function of proxy consent is to protect the right of the parents to raise their child as they see fit, to do with the child as they like. But the child is not the property of the parents; parents do not have an absolute right of disposal over the child. In law we recognize constraints upon the parental power, and common morality affirms the justice in this. What then is the function of proxy consent?

I think it would be best to turn this question on its head. By virtue of what right which the child possesses do we require the granting of proxy consent before a medical procedure may be initiated? What *could* be the source of such an obligation? We ordinarily recognize that there is only one fundamental right possessed by minors, a right to be protected and aided in development. "... A child, unlike an adult, has a right 'not to liberty but to custody.' "[9] All other rights which a child possesses, all other duties which we have towards children, are derivative from this single right, and are void when inconsistent with it. Broadly speaking, in consequence of this right, we must do what we may to promote the welfare of the child; we must abstain from doing what will injure the child, physically or otherwise; and, as far as this right goes, we are at liberty to deal with the child in ways which neither help nor hurt.

That proxy consent is ordinarily to be obtained from the parent or guardian of the child is understandable. We feel that the parent has the best interests of the child at heart, and knows how best to seek the child's welfare. It also follows from this right, however, that, when the parent does not have the best interests of the child in mind, the power of proxy consent should be transferred to another. It is on such a basis that society feels justified in removing a child from his parent's custody, and in appointing another to act *in parens patriae*. If this system is to be effective, society must, by and large, act on the basis of shared common views about what the welfare of the child consists of. We cannot allow anything which a parent considers to be a benefit to the child—being boiled in oil to save his eternal soul—to count as action in the child's best interests. This does not preclude a certain amount of leeway in a liberal society as to permitted views of welfare: if most feel that it is better, when the money is available, to send the child to a private school, we yet will not fault an affluent parent who decides to send his child to a public school.

The consequences of these propositions for cases when proxy consent is being sought for the purpose of giving therapy to a child accord well with the way the law handles this subject. The problem situation which arises concerns parents who, because of religious scruples, refuse to consent to needed medical treatment for their child. Jehovah's Witnesses, for example, who believe that blood transfusions are forbidden by the law of God, will not consent on behalf of their child to blood transfusions. Society feels that the benefit of the child is to be found in allowing the procedure. Because of this, the hospital will often turn to a judge, who appoints someone to act *in parens patriae* for the purpose of consenting to the specific procedure....

Proxy consent to experimentation on children is a more complicated matter. In law, there are two kinds of intervention in the person of another which are actionable in the absence of consent: those interventions where harm does, and where harm does not, result. The latter are termed "wrongful" or "harmful touchings" (though no harm has occurred). In other words, the mere *doing* of something to a person without his consent is, in itself, an actionable wrong.

We may say that, corresponding to this division, there are two sorts of experiments: those which do, and those which do not, injure the subject appreciably. Beecher has noted, for example, that "Many thousands of psychomotor tests and sociological studies have been carried out in children during the child's development and have revealed much information of value.... Sound nutritional studies without risk have been carried out. So have certain blood studies."[10] It must be added that many studies of value cannot, due to metabolic and other differences, be carried out in adults with results which will be valid for children.

It is clear, on the basis of the principle of benefit, that proxy consent to dangerous or harmful experiments on children cannot be valid. What about those experiments which carry no appreciable risk—the "wrongful touchings" sort? In an adult, it would seem, the right to autonomy, the right "to be let alone," is sufficient basis for the action of wrongful touching. But the child does not have a right to autonomy, except insofar as some measure of autonomy is necessary to promote the child's development and well-being.

Harmless experiments on children, therefore, which satisfy the other canons of medical ethics—good design, well-trained experimenters, and so forth—could be performed. Parents would not be derelict in their duty should they consent, on behalf of their child, to experiments of this sort. Participation in these experiments [does] not infringe the child's right to welfare, unless they would result in a *harmful* (and not just any) restriction of autonomy.

As I see it, the fundamental problem with those who would forbid *all* experimentation upon children[11] is that they confuse consent in adults with proxy consent for children. These two are fundamentally different requirements. Children are not small adults; our relations with children must not be made to approach as nearly as possible to our relations with adults. There are things which you ought to grant to children which need not be granted to adults: if a child is thirsty you provide him with drink. And there are things which may licitly be done to children which could not be done with adults: if my parents annoy me I may not send them to their room. A child is (morally) a different sort of thing than is an adult; we must adjust our relations with them according to their claims upon us.

CONCLUSION

This paper represents an attempt to formulate what I call a "moral theory" of the requirement of consent to serious medical procedures. The method used involves an interplay between cases and principles, such that each influences the other. Well-established moral intuitions about cases suggested some principles and called for the rejection of others. These principles in turn, once established, enabled the clarification of a proper approach to other, borderline cases.

Under the influence of situation ethics, much of the work on medical ethics has stressed the respects in which cases differ. This has resulted in the development of an *ad hoc* literature on cases which pose difficulty for the doctrine of informed consent. As the cases accumulated the doctrine began to seem more and more amorphous.

In contrast, this paper has sought to unify the doctrine of consent. Principles which are developed through considering the problems raised by prison experimentation in turn suggested solutions to other situations; rather than stressing the differences between the experimental and the therapeutic contexts, their similarities were emphasized. There is, I think, a need for such efforts at unification, as there is a need for a literature which is committed to the unique aspects of different cases.

Acknowledgments

The research for this paper was begun during an internship at the Institute of Society, Ethics and the Life Sciences in the month of June, 1973. I gratefully acknowledge the help of Drs. Daniel Callahan, Marc Lappé, Peter Steinfels, and Robert Veatch, of the Institute, who helped make my internship profitable and enjoyable. My wife Barbara read the manuscript and suggested a number of needed changes.

Notes

1. For examples of a similar method applied to different problems, see Thomas I. Emerson, *Toward A General Theory of the First Amendent* (New York: Vintage Books, 1967).

2. *Cobbs* v. *Grant,* 502 P. 2d 1, 11.

3. Alexander M. Caron, "Legal Rights and Moral Rights," in Hilton, *et al.,* eds., *Ethical Issues in Human Genetics* (Plenum Press, 1978), 228.

4. The counter-suggestion may be made that children cannot *really* make choices. This would, I think, put too great a weight upon the requirement of voluntarism. We would be recruiting the concepts of choice and volition to do a job which they have not been designed for.

5. I am speaking of course in the moral, not the legal, context. It may be that in an emergency a child may, in the absence of his parents, give legally valid consent.

6. This gives us the link between "responsible" in the dispositional sense explained here, and "responsible" in the blame-sense of the word ("I'll hold you responsible for that.").

7. The *caveat* must be added: natural contingencies do not have, as their *sole* result, the rendering of a person unfree, in the sense which vitiates consent: a man's brain tumor can make the man an idiot, schizophrenia can make a man insane, but these do not so much affect a person's volition as they do disturb his entire psychic structure.

8. David Daube, quoted in Henry K. Beecher, *Research and the Individual: Human Studies* (Boston: Little, Brown, 1970), p. 146.

9. *In re Gault.* 387 U.S. 1 (1967).

10. Beecher, p. 67.

11. See, for example, Paul Ramsey, "Consent as a Canon of Loyalty With Special Reference to Children in Medical Investigations," in *The Patient as Person* (New Haven: Yale University Press, 1970).

Being a Burden on Others

Nancy S. Jecker

Individuals facing death are sometimes reluctant to exhaust the income and assets they have accumulated over a lifetime in order to pay for end-of-life care. They also may fear and wish to avoid becoming dependent and reliant on family members for assistance with activities of daily living. In principle, the ethical standard of respecting patients' autonomous choices should support honoring a decision to forgo treatment, irrespective of the reasons for the decision. Nonetheless, our tendency is to discredit decisions to forgo treatment that are made on the basis of the financial or emotional burden treatment places on family members. In this article I ask the following questions: How ought we to think about the various burdens medical treatment imposes on other people? Should patients themselves consider such burdens when making life and death health-care decisions? When they do, should health-care providers and others abide by patients' decisions? I will argue that reasons of justice can support patients' choices to incorporate such considerations into their personal health-care decisions. I will show that respect for patients' well-being and moral integrity can require others to honor patients' preferences made on this basis. Although my defense of these positions is general in spirit and applies to a wide range of health-care decisions, I pay particular attention to the competent patient's refusal of life-extending medical treatment.

THE ARGUMENT FROM JUSTICE

At both macro and micro levels, justice is routinely accepted as a legitimate basis for allowing people to forgo lifesaving medical treatment. Thus, most accept the claim that, under conditions of scarcity, society is permitted to allow people to die in order to use its health-care resources in other ways. For example, if there is not enough of a lifesaving resource to provide it to all in need, we may then choose to withhold it from one patient to provide it to another who is more likely to benefit. Even when there is no natural scarcity of health-care resources, the dollars to pay for health care are themselves scarce. Thus, we regard society as justified in choosing to allocate its limited wealth to various goods, including not only lifesaving treatments but also other kinds of health care and other social goods. These decisions are made not only at a societal level, but also within organizations. For instance, insurance companies formulate policies governing how much money will be devoted to lifesaving treatments—such as coronary by-pass surgery—versus other forms of treatment—such as preventive screening for various forms of cancer. Likewise, hospitals make trade-offs between patients by developing policies about how many Medicaid patients to admit. These decisions have life or death consequences, even though the losers in such decisions are often "faceless victims" (such as the Medicaid patient who is turned away from a hospital and whose medical conditions subsequently worsens). Finally, smaller groups and individuals also participate in distributive decisions with potential life and death ramifications. For instance, an individual or family may subscribe to an insurance plan that does not cover life-prolonging treatments, such as organ transplantation for certain categories of patients, but provides excellent long-term care benefits.

A common feature these choices share is that they require weighing *competing* values against one another. At stake is not simply how to contain costs, but whether to invest limited resources in one way or another. In each of the above examples, distributive choices entail determining which individuals exert a stronger claim, or which of several priorities should be ranked higher. If the job of justice is to weigh competing claims for scarce goods, then justice naturally directs attention to the *opportunity costs* of using health-care treatments. The opportunities forgone by accepting a certain treatment may include not giving resources to other persons, not investing in other forms of health care, or not investing in other social goods. In short, justice situates isolated acts of treating patients in a broader social context, and fastens the individual to a larger network of persons. In this regard, justice exposes the fallacy of viewing ethical dilemmas in medicine apart from the background choices that structure available options.[1]

In the case of life-extending or lifesaving medical care, justice can give ethical warrant to patients' decisions to forgo treatment and be allowed to die. Patients may decline lifesaving care on grounds of justice, when others have overriding claims to lifesaving resources. Justice also may furnish a basis for forgoing lifesaving medical treatment, where accepting such treatment would also entail accepting finite palliative and caregiving resources to which others have a stronger claim. To explore more fully the role of justice in decisions to decline life-extending treatment, consider the following example.

> Joe is a seventy-one-year-old gentleman who has been diagnosed with oat cell carcinoma of the lung. The tumor is fairly widespread. The physicians treating Joe recommend a combination of radiation and chemotherapy. They point out that this usually increases survival by many months and also provides some palliative care. The patient refuses the recommended course of treatment because he is concerned about the costs that would be borne by his family members, including the cost of his wife staying with him near the hospital. At home, Joe would be cared for on a full-time basis by his daughter, who is a nurse. She has agreed to move in with him and take an indefinite leave of absence from her current job.

In considering his options, Joe reflects along the following lines. First, he observes that the family financial and human resources that would be required to pursue additional months of life are scarce. Second, he judges that there are other priorities that have a stronger pull on these resources. For example, his daughter has a young child of her own to care for, and she badly needs to make more time for personal projects that impart meaning and significance to her life. Joe's wife would be financially better able to fend for herself when Joe is gone if the money being spent on medical care were available for her to use. This money was intended to provide financial security in old age, not to be depleted in a short period of time to pay for medical care. Although Joe imagines that, in an ideal world, his resources would be more abundant and his options more robust, the actual choice he faces is how to distribute limited family resources fairly between all.[2]

One consideration at work in Joe's line of reasoning is an ethical ideal that I shall call *just caring*. Just caring requires that persons who care direct their limited resources toward persons or priorities whose claim to be cared for is strongest. When persons who care are blind to justice, they may be tempted to lavish attention on a single object and thereby neglect others who need care more, or as much. In the example described above, the daughter who extends an offer to care for her father responds to her parent's needs in a loving way, but arguably omits considerations of fairness to herself and others to whom she is already devoted. Just caring would require her to restrain her immediate impulse to help her father in order that she might consider the needs of herself and others whom she is called upon to support. Generally speaking, "caring, like loving, needs criteria for it to be helpful caring, just caring, truthful caring, not destructive caring."[3] Thus, it is misleading to think only about caring or loving without concern for justice. Although family members may be disposed to operate "under the canon of mercy, not as an officer of justice,"[4] they should cultivate the ability to step back and consider how to care justly and wisely.[5] Also at work in Joe's reflections is an ethical idea of justice in the family. In situations where life-extending medical treatment is made available by drawing from family wealth or services, the family functions as a commons.[6] A tragedy of the commons occurs when members seek to take more common goods than they are entitled to, or when they refuse to make appropriate sacrifices and contributions. A commons flourishes only when each party is willing to acknowledge resources as shared commodities and respect others' stake in preserving them. To prevent a tragedy from occurring, Joe rightly considers the effect that his individual health-care decisions have for the commons upon which his wife depends. Viewing health-care choices in this light attenuates an exclusive focus on self and prevents persons from becoming morally deaf and dissociated from others. It introduces a role for justice by supporting family members who wish to give up goods in order to secure a fair share for others.

These points make evident that choosing to pursue life-extending medical treatment can place heavy demands on a family's financial and caregiving resources. Family burden is often overlooked in justice debates, but it will increasingly emerge as salient because the demand for family caregiving is expected to grow as the population ages.

OBJECTIONS

One objection that these remarks elicit is that dying patients who place other people's monetary or caregiving needs before their own are simply mistaken in their moral assessment. According to this objection, the dying patient's needs always enjoy pride of place, because life itself is of inestimable value. Thus, when others compete for financial resources or caregiving attention, their needs should be overridden when they are for less weighty purposes. The problem that such reasoning encounters is that it runs deeply counter to our implicit choices and values in many other areas. For example, we implicitly accept that life holds finite value whenever we endanger our lives in ordinary activities, such as crossing the street at a busy intersection, flying in airplanes, and driving automobiles. Likewise, when making health-care decisions, we frequently place the goal of extending life alongside the good of improving life's quality. For example, we prefer medications from which death has resulted, such as oral contraceptives, over safer medications that are less convenient. As noted previously, individuals sometimes opt for health insurance plans that offer limited coverage for certain forms of lifesaving treatment but provide other kinds of benefits. It is simply not true, then, that we can dismiss as misguided a patient's wish to forgo lifesaving treatment in order to avoid becoming a burden to others. Instead, it is consistent with our larger body of beliefs and choices to regard the value of life-sustaining treatment as limited and to allow patients to weigh the emotional and financial costs to others against the cost of giving up additional months of life.

A second objection calls into question the claim that a commons represents a true depiction of family relations. One irritant in this image may be that those who think in accordance with it will be inclined to trammel benevolence and goodwill by introducing a vocabulary of rights and duties into family life. In response, it can be said that love and benevolence need not function as adversaries to rights and duties. Instead, it is possible for these goods to coexist harmoniously: rights and justice improve caring by distinguishing what is wise and helpful caring.

A related concern that the image of a family commons may prompt is that justice is intrusive and out of place in loving relationships; justice entails calculating what people are due and making explicit trade-offs, whereas genuine love must be spontaneous and unconditional. To address this concern, it is important to illuminate the assumptions upon which it is based. First, caring requires separation from justice only if it is imagined that caring is exempt from justice's claims. But the relationships people forge do not make a moral island.[7] Figuring out what one ought, morally, to do is never solely a matter of getting clear about what caring calls for. Instead, caring relationships are circumscribed and undergirded by ethical considerations outside themselves. Second, the idea that the introduction of justice into personal relationships inevitably spoils caring, because it is cold and unfeeling, is based upon the erroneous assumption that justice is a virtue only between strangers. But justice can also be construed as applying to relationships of goodwill between persons who face competing loyalties.[8] On the latter reading, loving relationships occur in the context of multiple commitments, and justice aims to balance fairly the multiple loyalties people have.[9] If my reasoning is sound, then it is possible to view justice as a family virtue and to picture family resources as a commons in which each member holds a stake. This framework gives moral support to taking burdens on other family members into account when making health-care decisions.

THE ARGUMENT FROM HAPPINESS AND INTEGRITY

Thus far, I have argued that justice supports patients' choices to take burdens on others into account when making health-care decisions. I now provide reasons why health-care providers and others should honor patients' choices that are made on this basis. My argument will be that permitting patients to act in accordance with their own moral convictions is a prerequisite to patients' happiness and moral integrity.

Aristotle apparently held that performing noble and good deeds is "a thing desirable for its own sake,"[10] and that those who regularly perform such deeds experience a sense of happiness and well-being. One reason that happiness may be an outgrowth of virtuous activity is that persons who practice virtue develop integrity and self-respect. Integrity describes those who abide by moral standards and dispositions that are their own, and who hold strong and deeply felt convictions.[11] Self-respect refers to having a sure sense of one's own worth.[12] Forgoing health-care resources in order to benefit others is an act of integrity when it indicates that one is living up to one's own sense of justice under conditions where this ideal is tested. By contrast, consuming health-care resources generates shame and guilt and undermines integrity when these actions betray one's moral convictions and dispositions.

These remarks suggest a reason why patients should be permitted to regard the burdens their decisions impose on others as important. Permitting such considerations may be a necessary part of honoring patients' moral autonomy and ability to be self-respecting moral agents. When individuals do what they believe is right, this strengthens their sense of moral self-worth and dignity. By contrast, when persons are compelled to disappoint themselves, this lowers their self-estimation. When patients' moral decisions are overridden, they rightfully perceive this as an insult because it conveys that they are not fully capable moral agents. To the extent that the capacity to reflect on choices and form moral opinions is bound up with individuals' sense of their own identity, those who are made to transgress their own moral beliefs will have a less sure sense of who they are and what they hope to be in the world.

CONCLUSION

I have argued that there is little ethical basis for the unease health providers sometimes feel when patients decline treatment to avoid imposing burdens on others. This leaves us, still, with the lurking question: What is it about taking such burdens into account that troubles so many? I have suggested already that taking burdens to others into account plays havoc with the belief that life is of inestimable value and that we, therefore, must do everything possible to keep patients alive. If there is a price that patients themselves are not willing to pay for additional weeks or months of life, this undermines the belief that life possesses infinite value. Particular lives hold finite, even measurable, value to those who live them. Identifying burdens to others as an ethically valid basis for withdrawing treatment also may prompt unease, because it appears to make a mockery of the cherished idea that human beings are essentially free and unencumbered beings. Patients who consider the burdens they impose on others reveal themselves to be deeply embedded in relationships and social structures to which they owe duties and from which they are entitled to benefits. In point of fact, this perspective hardly makes a mockery of individual autonomy. To the contrary, the idea of autonomy allied with moral responsibility more truly captures original Kantian and Enlightenment views about the function of autonomy in moral life. Kant himself held that individuals become autonomous and self-determined, not by setting themselves free of social and ethical moorings, but by being guided by reason and imposing moral rules and principles upon themselves.[13] On this understanding, a patient who evades her ethical and social responsibilities in reaching treatment decisions is not genuinely autonomous. She is not mastered by her rational and moral self, but succumbs instead to fear of death or weakness of moral will. If this is correct, then the tensions that ethical duties to family members and others introduce into health-care decisions should help to move debates about patient autonomy to a higher ground.

Although I have sketched a partial answer to the question of how we should think about the consideration of burdening others when making health-care decisions, there is a darker side that I have not addressed. Namely, how should we as a society respond to patients who insist that everything possible be done and who simply refuse to take burdens to others into account? How should society answer patients who believe that they are

owed the best and most expensive care that medicine can offer, regardless of the burdens this imposes?

This darker side of considering the costs of medical treatment has received some attention in recent debates about rationing medicine and reforming the health-care system. Yet most attention has focused on macro policy choices, rather than face-to-face encounters among patients, family members, and health professionals. Ultimately, when explicit rationing policies are in place, the darker side of rationing debates will rear its ugly head. A first step to facing squarely the challenges that lie ahead is to accept and support those who humbly and courageously choose to forgo medical treatment on behalf of valued others.

Notes

1. A. C. Baier, "Alternative Offerings to Asclepius." *Medical Humanities Review* 6, no. 1 (1992): 9–19.

2. Adapted from B. A. Brody and H. T. Engelhardt, eds., *Bioethics: Readings and Cases* (Englewood Cliffs, NJ: Prentice-Hall, 1987), 341, case D.

3. M. A. Farley, "Love, Justice and Discernment: An Interview with Margaret A. Farley," *Second Opinion* 17, no. 2 (1991): 80–91.

4. M. Battin, "Choosing the Time to Die: The Ethics and Economics of Suicide in Old Age," in *Ethical Dimensions of Geriatric Care*, ed. S. F. Spicker, S. R. Ingman, and I. R. Lawson, (Dordrecht, The Netherlands: D. Reidel, 1987), 161–90.

5. C. Gilligan. "Remapping the Moral Domain," in *Reconstructing Individualism,* ed. T. C. Heller, M. Sosna, and D. E. Wellerby (Stanford, CA: Stanford University Press. 1986), 237–52; N. P. Lyons, "Two Perspectives: On Self, Relationships, and Morality," *Harvard Educational Review* 53 (1983): 125–45.

6. G. Hardin, "Living on a Lifeboat," in *Moral Issues,* ed. J. Narveson (New York: Oxford University Press, 1983), 167–78; N. S. Jecker, "The Role of Intimate Others in Medical Decisions," *Gerontologist* 30 (1990): 65–71.

7. N. S. Jecker, "Impartiality and Special Relationships," in *Kindred Matters: Rethinking the Philosophy of the Family*, ed. K. Kipnis, D. Meyers, and C. Murphy (Ithaca, NY: Cornell University Press, at press).

8. J. Kilner, "Who Shall Live?: An African Answer," *Hastings Center Report* 14 (June 1984): 18–22; G. Sher, "Other Voices, Other Rooms," in *Women and Moral theory*, ed. E. F. Kittay and D. T. Meyers (Totowa, NJ: Rowman and Littlefield, 1987), 178–89.

9. N. S. Jecker and A. O. Berg, "Allocating Medical Resources in Rural America: Alternative Perceptions of Justice," *Social Science and Medicine* 34 (1992): 467–74.

10. Aristotle, *Nicomachean Ethics,* in *The Basic Works of Aristotle*, ed. R. McKeon (New York: Random House, 1941), 935–1126, at 1102.

11. B. Williams, "Utilitarianism and Moral Self-Indulgence," in B. Williams, *Moral Luck* (Cambridge, England: Cambridge University Press, 1981), 40–53.

12. T. E. Hill, *Autonomy and Self-Respect* (Cambridge, England: Cambridge University Press, 1991).

13. I. Kant, *Groundwork of the Metaphysics of Morals*, trans. H. J. Paton (New York: Harper and Row, 1956). For further discussion of this point, see M. J. Meyer, "Patients' Duties," *Journal of Medicine and Philosophy* 17 (1992): 541–56; E. H. Morreim, *Balancing Act* (Dordrecht, The Netherlands: Kluwer, 1991), chap. 7.

Involving Children in Medical Decisions

Christine Harrison, Nuala P. Kenny, Mona Sidarous, and Mary Rowell

Eleven-year-old Samantha is a bright, loving child who was treated for osteosarcoma in her left arm. The arm had to be amputated, and Samantha was given a course of chemotherapy. She has been cancer-free for 18 months and is doing well in school. She is self-conscious about her prosthesis and sad because she had to give away her cat, Snowy, to decrease her risk of infection. Recent tests indicate that the cancer has recurred and metastasized to her lungs. Her family is devastated by this news but do not want to give up hope. However, even with aggressive treatment Samantha's chances for recovery are less than 20%.

Samantha adamantly refuses further treatment. On earlier occasions she had acquiesced to treatment only to struggle violently when it was administered. She distrusts her health care providers and is angry with them and her parents. She protests, "You already made me give up Snowy and my arm. What more do you want?" Her parents insist that treatment must continue. At the request of her physician, a psychologist and psychiatrist conduct a capacity assessment. They agree that Samantha is probably incapable of making treatment decisions; her understanding of death is immature and her

anxiety level very high. Nursing staff are reluctant to impose treatment; in the past Samantha's struggling and the need to restrain her upset them a great deal.

WHY IS IT IMPORTANT TO INCLUDE CHILDREN IN MEDICAL DECISION-MAKING?

Ethics

Traditionally, parents and physicians have made all medical decisions on behalf of children. However, just as the concept of informed consent has developed over the last 30 years with respect to competent adult patients, so new ways of thinking about the role of children in medical decision-making have evolved.

Ethical principles that provide guidance in the care of adults are insufficient in the context of caring for children.[1–3] Issues related to the voluntariness of consent, the disclosure of information, capacity assessment, treatment decisions and bereavement are more complex, as is the physician's relationship with the patient and the patient's family.[3, 4] Adult models presume that the patient is autonomous and has a stable sense of self, established values and mature cognitive skills; these characteristics are undeveloped or underdeveloped in children.

Although it is important to understand and respect the developing autonomy of a child, and although the duty of beneficence provides a starting point for determining what is in the child's best interest, a family-centred ethic is the best model for understanding the interdependent relationships that bear upon the child's situation.[5] A family-centred approach considers the effects of a decision on all family members, their responsibilities toward one another and the burdens and benefits of a decision for each member, while acknowledging the special vulnerability of the child patient.

A family-centred approach presents special challenges for the health care team, particularly when there is disagreement between parent and child. Such a situation raises profound questions about the nature of the physician–patient relationship in pediatric practice. Integrity in this relationship is fundamental to the achievement of the goal of medicine,[6] which has been defined as "right and good healing action taken in the interest of a particular patient."[7] In the care of adults, the physician's primary relationship is with the particular capable patient. The patient's family may be involved in decision-making, but it is usually the patient who defines the bounds of such involvement.

The care of children, on the other hand, has been described in terms of a "triadic" relationship in which the child, his or her parents and the physician all have a necessary involvement (Dr. Abbyann Lynch, Director, Ethics in Health Care Associates, Toronto: personal communication, 1992). When there is disagreement between parent and child, the physician may experience some moral discomfort in having to deal separately with the child and parent.

The assumption that parents best understand what is in the interest of their child is usually sound. However, situations can arise in which the parents' distress prevents them from attending carefully to the child's concerns and wishes. Simply complying with the parents' wishes in such cases is inadequate. It is more

helpful and respectful of the child to affirm the parents' responsibility for the care of their child while allowing the child to exercise choice in a measure appropriate to his or her level of development and experience of illness and treatment. This approach does not discount the parents' concerns and wishes, but recognizes the child as the particular patient to whom the physician has a primary duty of care. This approach seeks to harmonize the values of everyone involved in making the decision.[6]

Law

The legal right to refuse medical treatment is related to, but not identical with, the right to consent to treatment. The patient's right to refuse even life-saving medical treatment is recognized in Canadian law[8, 9] and is premised on the patient's right to exercise control over his or her own body. Providing treatment despite a patient's valid refusal can constitute battery and, in some circumstances, negligence.

To be legally valid the refusal of medical treatment must be given by a person deemed capable of making health care choices, that is, capable of understanding the nature and consequences of the recommended treatment, alternative treatments and nontreatment. In common law the notion of the "mature minor" recognizes that some children are capable of making their own health care choices despite their age.[10] In common law and under the statutory law of some provinces patients are presumed capable regardless of age unless shown otherwise; in other provinces an age at which patients are presumed capable is specified.[11] When a child's capacity is in doubt an assessment is required.

In the case of children who are incapable of making their own health care decisions, parents or legal guardians generally have the legal authority to act as surrogate decision-makers. The surrogate decision-maker is obliged to make treatment decisions in the best interest of the child. Health care providers who believe that a surrogate's decisions are not in the child's best interest can appeal to provincial child welfare authorities. The courts have the authority to assume a *parens patriae* role in treatment decisions if the child is deemed to be in need of protection. This issue has arisen most commonly with respect to Jehovah's Witnesses who refuse blood transfusions for their children on religious grounds, and courts have authorized treatment in recognition of the state's interest in protecting the health and well-being of children.[12] Every province has child welfare legislation that sets out the general parameters of the "best interest" standard. Courts are reluctant to authorize the withholding or withdrawal of medical treatment, especially in the face of parental support for such treatment.

A special point to consider involves the use of patient restraints. The wrongful or excessive use of restraints could prompt an action of false imprisonment or battery. Restraint can involve the use of force, mechanical means or chemicals. The use of restraint compromises the dignity and liberty of the patient, including the child patient. Restraints should never be used solely to facilitate care but, rather, only when the patient is likely to cause serious bodily harm to himself or herself or to another. If restraint is required, the health care provider should use the least restrictive means possible, and the need for the restraint (as well as its effect on the patient) should be assessed on an ongoing basis.

Policy

The Canadian Paediatric Society has no policy regarding the role of the child patient in medical decision-making. The American Academy of Pediatrics statement on this question articulates the joint responsibility of physicians and parents to make decisions for very young patients in their best interest and states that "[p]arents and physicians should not exclude children and adolescents from decision-making without persuasive reasons."[13]

Empirical studies

As they grow, children develop decision-making skills, the ability to reason using complex concepts, an understanding of death[14] and the ability to imagine a future for themselves.[15] Children with a chronic or terminal illness may have experiences that endow them with insight and maturity beyond their years. Families often encourage children to participate in decision-making. Allowing even young children to make decisions about simple matters facilitates the development of skills that they will need to make more complex decisions later on.[16–18]

Because tools developed to assess the capacity of adults have not been tested with children, health care professionals working with children should be sensitive to the particular capacity of each child. Children are constantly developing their physical, intellectual, emotional and personal maturity. Although developmental milestones give us a general sense of capacities, 2 children of the same age will not necessarily have the same ability to make choices. Even when they are deemed capable of making health care choices, children need support for their decisions from family members and the health care team.

HOW SHOULD I DETERMINE THE APPROPRIATE ROLE OF A CHILD IN MEDICAL DECISION-MAKING?

Most children fall into one of three groups with respect to their appropriate involvement in decision-making.[19, 20]

Infants and Young Children

Preschool children have no significant decision-making capacity and cannot provide their own consent. As surrogate decision-makers, parents should authorize (or refuse authorization) on their child's behalf, basing their decisions on what they believe to be in the child's best interest.

Primary-School Children

Children of primary-school age may participate in medical decisions but do not have full decision-making capacity. They may indicate their assent or dissent without fully understanding its implications. Nonetheless they should be provided with information appropriate to their level of comprehension. Although the child's parents should authorize or refuse to authorize treatment, the child's assent should be sought and any strong and sustained dissent should be taken seriously.[21]

Adolescents

Many adolescents have the decision-making capacity of an adult.[22, 23] This capacity will need to be determined for each patient in light of his or her

- ability to understand and communicate relevant information,
- ability to think and choose with some degree of independence,
- ability to assess the potential for benefit, risks or harms as well as to consider consequences and multiple options, and
- achievement of a fairly stable set of values.[24]

Many children and adolescents, particularly those who have been seriously ill, will need assistance in developing an understanding of the issues and in demonstrating their decision-making capacity. Age-appropriate discussions, perhaps with the assistance of teachers, chaplains, play therapists, nurses, psychologists or others skilled in communicating with children, are helpful. The child's participation may be facilitated by the use of art activities, stories, poems, role-playing and other techniques.[25, 26]

Physicians should ensure that good decisions are made on behalf of their child patients. Although the interests of other family members are important and will influence decision-making, the child's interests are most important and are unlikely to be expressed or defended by the child himself or herself. Anxious, stressed or grieving family members may need assistance in focusing on what is best for the child. This may be especially difficult when a cure is no longer possible; in such cases a decision to stop treatment may seem like a decision to cause the child's death.

Whether or not the child participates, the following considerations should bear upon a treatment decision concerning that child:

- The potential benefits to the child
- The potential harmful consequences to the child, including physical suffering, psychological or spiritual distress and death
- The moral, spiritual. and cultural values of the child's family

THE CASE

For Samantha, resuming aggressive treatment will have a serious negative effect on her quality of life. The chances of remission are small, yet a decision to discontinue treatment will likely result in her death. Because death is an irreversible harm, and decisions with serious consequences require a high level of competence in decision-making,[27] the capacity required would be very high. It has been determined that Samantha does not have this capacity.

Nevertheless, Samantha is included in discussions about her treatment options, and her reasons for refusing treatment are explored.[28] Members of the team work hard to re-establish trust. They and Samantha's parents come to agree that refusing treatment is not necessarily unreasonable; a decision by an adult patient in similar circumstances to discontinue treatment would certainly be honoured. Discussions address Samantha's and her parents' hopes and fears, their understanding of the possibility of cure, the meaning for them of the statistics provided by the physicians, Samantha's role in decision-making and her access to information. They are assisted by nurses, a child psychologist, a psychiatrist, a member of the clergy, a bioethicist, a social worker and a palliative care specialist.

Discussions focus on reaching a common understanding about the goals of treatment for Samantha. Her physician helps her to express her feelings and concerns about the likely effects of continued treatment. Consideration is given to the effects on her physical well-being, quality of life, self-esteem and dignity of imposing treatment against her wishes. Spiritual and psychological support for Samantha and her family is acknowledged to be an essential component of the treatment plan. Opportunities are provided for Samantha and her family to speak to others who have had similar experiences, and staff are given the opportunity to voice their concerns.

Ultimately, a decision is reached to discontinue chemotherapy and the goal of treatment shifts from "cure" to "care." Samantha's caregivers assure her and her family that they are not "giving up" but are directing their efforts toward Samantha's physical comfort and her spiritual and psychological needs. Samantha returns home, supported by a community palliative care program, and is allowed to have a new kitten. She dies peacefully.

Notes

1. Ruddick W. Parents and life prospects. In: O'Neill O, Ruddick W, editors. *Having children: philosophical and legal reflections on parenthood.* New York: Oxford University Press; 1979:124.

2. Nelson JL. Taking families seriously. *Hastings Cent Rep* 1992; 22:6.

3. Hardwig J. What about the family? *Hastings Cent Rep* 1990; 20(2):5–10.

4. Leikin S. A proposal concerning decisions to forgo life-sustaining treatment for young people. *J Pediatr* 1989; 115:17–22.

5. Mahowald M. *Women and children in health care.* New York: Oxford University Press; 1993:187, 189.

6. Hellmann J. In pursuit of harmonized values: patient/parent–pediatrician relationships. In: Lynch A, editor. *The "good" pediatrician: an ethics curriculum for use in Canadian pediatrics residency programs.* Toronto: Pediatric Ethics Network; 1996.

7. Pellegrino ED. Toward a reconstruction of medical morality: the primary of the act of profession and the fact of illness. *J Med Philos* 1979; 4:47.

8. *Malette v. Shulman* [1990], 67 DLR (4th) (Ont CA).

9. Art. 11 CCQ.

10. Rozovsky LE, Rozovsky FA. *The Canadian law of consent to treatment.* Toronto: Butterworths; 1992:53–7.

11. Etchells E, Sharpe G, Elliott C, Singer PA. Bioethics for clinicians 3: Capacity. *Can Med Assoc J* 1996; 155:657–61.

12. R.B. v. Children's Aid Society of Metropolitan Toronto, [1995] 1 SCR 315 (SCC).

13. American Academy of Pediatrics. Informed consent, parental permission and assent in pediatric practice. *Pediatrics* 1995; 95:314–7.

14. Matthews GR. Children's conceptions of illness and death. In: Kopelman LM, Moskop JC, editors. *Children and health care: moral and social issues.* Dordrecht (Holland): Kluwer Academic Publishers; 1989:133–46.

15. Koocher GP, DeMaso. Children's competence to consent to medical procedures. *Pediatrician* 1990; 17:68–73.

16. King NMP, Cross AW. Children as decision makers: guidelines for pediatricians. *J Pediatr* 1989; 115:10–6.

17. Lewis MA, Lewis CE. Consequences of empowering children to care for themselves. *Pediatrician* 1990; 17:63–7.

18. Yoos HL. Children's illness concepts: old and new paradigms. *Pediatr Nurs* 1994; 20:134–45.

19. Broome ME, Stieglitz KA. The consent process and children. *Res Nurs Health* 1992; 15:147–52.

20. Erlen JA. The child's choice: an essential component in treatment decisions. *Child Health Care* 1987; 15:156–60.

21. Baylis F. The moral weight of a child's dissent. *Ethics Med Pract* 1993; 3(1):2–3.

22. Weithorn LA, Campbell SB. The competency of children and adolescents to make informed treatment decisions. *Child Dev* 1982; 53:1589–98.

23. Lewis CC. How adolescents approach decisions: changes over grades seven to twelve and policy implications. *Child Dev* 1981; 52:538–44.

24. Brock DW. Children's competence for health care decisionmaking. In: Kopelman LM, Moskop JC, editors. *Children and health care: moral and social issues.* Dordrecht (Holland): Kluwer Academic Publishers; 1989:181–212.

25. Adams PL, Fras I. *Beginning child psychiatry.* New York Bruner/Mazel; 1988.

26. Kestenbaum CJ, Williams D, editors. *Handbook of clinical assessment of children and adolescents.* New York University Press; 1988.

27. Drane JF. The many faces of competency. *Hastings Cent Rep* 1985; 15(2):17–21.

28. Freyer DR. Children with cancer: special considerations in the discontinuation of life-sustaining treatment. *Med Pediatr Oncol* 1992; 20:136–42.

Health Care Decisionmaking by Children: Is It in Their Best Interest?

Lainie Friedman Ross

Some bioethicists have argued for a role for the family in the patient's health care decision-making, even when that patient is a competent adult.[1] Such a move challenges most of American bioethics, which holds patient autonomy as the primary ethical principle in health care decisionmaking. Ironically, there is an opposite movement in pediatrics, where ethicists and policymakers are seeking to exclude parents from many of their children's health care decisions.[2]

In pediatrics, the doctor-patient relationship traditionally has included three parties: the physician, the child, and his or her parents. Parents were not merely surrogate decision-makers on the grounds of child incompetence, but rather, parents were believed to have both a right and a responsibility to partake in their child's medical decisions.[3] In this paper I will examine the evolving position regarding the role of the child in the decisionmaking process as advocated by the American Academy of Pediatrics (AAP). I will offer both moral and pragmatic arguments why I believe this position is misguided.

RECOMMENDATIONS OF THE AMERICAN ACADEMY OF PEDIATRICS

In 1995, the AAP published its recommendations for the role of children in health care decision-making. The AAP recommended that the child's voice be given greater weight as the child matured. The AAP categorized children as (1) those who lack decisionmaking capacity; (2) those with a developing capacity; and (3) those who have deci-sionmaking capacity for health care decisions.

For children who lack decisionmaking capacity, the AAP recommended that their parents should make decisions unless their decisions are abusive or neglectful. When children have developing decisionmaking capacity, the physician should seek parental permission and the child's assent. In many cases, the child's dissent should be binding, or at minimum, the physician should seek third-party mediation for parent–child disagreement. Although the child who dissents to life-saving care can be over-ruled, attempts should be made to persuade the child to assent for "coercion in diagnosis or treatment is a last resort" (p. 316). When children have decisionmaking capacity, the AAP concluded that the children should give informed consent for themselves and their parents should be viewed as consultants.

A major problem with the AAP recommen-dations is that it assumes decisionmaking capacity can be defined and measured, although the AAP offers no guidance as to what this defi-nition is or how to test for it. Instead, the AAP recommends individual assessment of decision-making capacity in each case. However, since there are no criteria on which to base maturity or decisionmaking capacity, the decision of whether to respect a child's decision is dependent upon the judgment of the particular pediatrician—a judgment he or she has no training to make.

My main concern with the AAP recommen-dations, however, is what should be done when parents and children disagree on health care deci-sions: according to the AAP, if there is parental-child disagreement and the child is judged to have decisionmaking authority, the child's decision should be binding. If the child has developing capacity, various mechanisms to resolve the conflict should be attempted. They propose:

> short term counseling or psychiatric consultation for patient and/or family, "case management" or similar multidisciplinary conference(s), and/or consultation with individuals trained in clinical ethics or a hospital based ethics committee. In rare cases of refractory disagreement, formal legal adjudication may be necessary. (p. 316)

I will ignore the difficulties in determining whether a minor has decisionmaking capacity and assume that some minors are competent to make at least some health care decisions. If autonomy is based solely on competency, then competent children should have decisionmaking autonomy in the health care setting. It is my view, however, that even if children are competent, there is a morally significant difference between competent minors and adults. Competency is a necessary but not a sufficient condition on which to base respect for a minor's health care decisionmaking autonomy.

COMPETENCY OF CHILDREN

The psychological literature divides the process of giving informed consent into three components: the patient's consent is informed (made knowingly), is competent (made intelligently), and is voluntary.[5] Although a survey of the literature reveals scant empirical data, existing data suggest that most health care decisions made by adults and children do not fulfill these three components.[6] The data also suggest that adults and older children do not significantly differ in their consent skills.[7] If competency is the only criterion on which respect for autonomy in health care is based, then this difference in treatment cannot be justified.

No test has been developed that uniformly distinguishes all competent individuals from incompetent individuals. Given that competency is context-specific, it is doubtful whether such a

test could be developed. And even if a nonculturally biased, objective test could be devised, individual testing of every potential patient would exact a high price in terms of efficiency, privacy, and respect for autonomy. Instead, adults have traditionally been presumed competent and children have been presumed incompetent. That is, respect for autonomy in health care uses both a threshold concept of competency and an age-standard.

To some extent the age-standard is arbitrary as there are individuals above the line (older than the legal age of emancipation) who are incompetent and individuals below the line (younger than the legal age of emancipation) who are competent. But the statutes are not capricious: in general, individuals above the line are more likely to be competent than individuals below it.

AUTONOMY OF CHILDREN

One reason to limit the child's present-day autonomy is based on the argument that parents and other authorities need to promote the child's life-time autonomy. Given the value that is placed on self-determination, it makes sense to grant adults autonomy provided that they have some threshold level of competency. Respect is shown by respecting their present project pursuits. But respect for a threshold of competency in children places the emphasis on present day autonomy rather than on a child's life-time autonomy. Children need a protected period in which to develop "enabling virtues"—habits, including the habit of self-control, which advance their life-time autonomy and opportunities. Although many adults would also benefit from developing their potentials and improving their skills and self-control, at some point (and it is reasonable to use the age of emancipation as the proper cut-off), the advantages of self-determination outweigh the benefits of further guidance and its potential to improve lifetime autonomy.

A second reason to limit the child's present-day autonomy is the fact that the child's decisions are based on limited world experience and so her decisions are not part of a well-conceived life plan. Again, many adults have limited world experience, but children have a greater potential for improving their knowledge base and for improving their skills of critical reflection and self-control. As Willard Gaylin explains:

> Surely, part of what goes into our abridgement of the child's autonomy is the recognition that although he may be [competent the limitations of his experience have] distorted his capacity for sound judgement.[9]

By protecting the child from his own impetuosity, his parents help him obtain the background knowledge of the world and the capacities that will allow him to make decisions that better promote his life plans. His parents' attempt to help him flourish may not be achieved, but that does not invalidate their attempt.

A third reason childhood competency should not necessarily entail respect for a child's autonomy is the significant role that intimate families play in our lives. Elsewhere, I have argued that when the family is intimate, parents should have wide discretion in pursuing family goals, goals which may compete and conflict with the goals of particular members.[10] In general, parental autonomy promotes the interests and goals of both children and parents. It serves the needs and interests of the child to have autonomous parents who will help him become an autonomous individual capable of devising and implementing his own life plan. It serves the adults' interest in having and raising a family according to their own vision of the good life. These interests do not abruptly cease when the child becomes competent. If anything, now parents have the opportunity to inculcate their beliefs through rational discourse, instead of through example, bribery, or force.

There are also pragmatic reasons to permit parents to override the present-day autonomy of competent children. First, one can argue for a determination of competency that allows unusually mature children to be emancipated. The problem, as I have already mentioned, is that no such test exists. Second, one can acknowledge

that it is best if parents recognize their child's maturity and treat them accordingly, but deny that this justifies granting competent children legal emancipation. Many parents respect their mature child's decisions voluntarily. Laura Purdy remarks: "It is plausible to think that children's maturity is not completely unrelated to parental good sense."[11] Child liberationists may object because a voluntary approach only encourages parents to respect their children's autonomy, but it does not legally enforce it. However, the voluntary approach is more consistent with a policy to limit the state's role in intrafamilial decisions, which is important for the family's ability to flourish.

HEALTH CARE RIGHTS IN CONTEXT

A final argument against respecting the health care decisions of minors is based on placing the notion of health care rights in context. Most individuals who support health care decisionmaking for children view it as an exception and do not seek to emancipate children in other spheres. But why should a child who is competent to make major health care decisions not have the right to make other types of decisions? That is, if a fourteen-year-old is competent to make life-and-death decisions, then why can't this fourteen-year-old buy and smoke cigarettes? Participate in interscholastic football without his parents' consent? Or even drop out of school?

Child liberationists explore what it means to give children equal rights with adults in all spheres. In recent years, this position has become popular in both academic circles,[12] and the White House.[13] Child liberationists argue that children are the last oppressed group in society. They lament that child-protection and not child liberation remains the legal ideal. They support the view that children have equal rights with their adult counterparts. But the rights that enable adults to flourish are not the same as those needed by children. In general, adults need mostly negative rights (the rights of noninterference and self-determination). Children also need negative rights (the right not to be physically, sexually, or emotionally abused), but they also need a wide variety of positive rights (the right to an education, adequate nutrition, and medical care). Child protectionists justify this difference in treatment on the grounds that children are less powerful, more vulnerable, and more needy of protection; child liberationists claim that such treatment further increases their powerlessness and vulnerability.

What would it mean to endorse equal rights for children? It is a radical proposal with wide repercussions.[14] It would mean that children could make binding contracts, and that there would be the dissolution of child labor laws, mandatory education, statutory rape laws, and child neglect statutes. As such, it would give children rights for which they are ill-prepared and deny them the protection they need from predatory adults. It would leave children even more vulnerable than they presently are.

Endorsement of child liberation would make a child's membership in a family voluntary. For example, Howard Cohen argues that children should be allowed to change families, either because the child's parents are abusive, or because a neighbor or wealthy stranger offers him a better deal.[15] Such freedom ignores the important role that continuity and permanence play in the parent–child relationship—a significance the child may not yet appreciate.[16]

My objection to the child liberationist position should in no way suggest that I do not place great value on freedom. My objection is that respect for an individual's autonomy means respecting her good and bad decisions. Child liberation requires that I respect a child's present-day autonomy regardless of its long-term impact on her developing personhood. Imagine, then, that a fourteen-year-old with new-onset diabetes refuses to take insulin because she fears needles (or because her boyfriend's religious beliefs proscribe medical care) even though she understands that she will die without it. Who is willing to abandon her to her autonomy? The laws that give adolescents the right to consent to treatment often do not give them the right to refuse treatment.[17]

Liberationists may object that adults also make bad decisions, and that physicians often challenge adults whom they perceive to be making bad decisions. The difference is that the competent adult's decision ultimately prevails. In contrast, most health care professionals who care for children would be unwilling to respect the fourteen-year-old diabetic child's treatment refusal. More generally, we would be unwilling to respect a competent child's present-day autonomy whenever she makes a bad decision. But if we are unwilling to respect her autonomy on the basis of content, then we are not respecting her autonomy. To respect only those decisions a child makes with which we agree is not to show respect for the child's autonomy, but to make a farce out of what is meant by respect for autonomy.[18]

THE FAMILY AS THE LOCUS OF DECISIONMAKING

One of my major concerns with the AAP's recommendations is their willingness to involve third parties in the decisionmaking process. My concern is that these decisions undermine the family. Physicians provide only for the child's transient medical needs; his parents provide for all of his needs and are responsible for raising the child in such a way that he becomes an autonomous responsible adult. Goldstein and colleagues at Yale University's Child Study Center expressed their concern that health care professionals sometimes forget where their professional responsibilities end, and described the harm that we do when we think we can replace parents.[19] By deciding that the child's decision should be respected over the parents' decision, physicians are replacing the parents' judgment that the decision should be overridden with their judgment that the child's decision should be respected. To do so makes this less an issue of respecting the child's autonomy, and more about deciding who knows what is best for the child. In general, parents are the better judge as they have a more vested interest in their child's well-being and are responsible for the day-to-day decisions of child-rearing. It behooves physicians to be humble as they are neither able nor willing to take over this daily function.

I do not mean to suggest that children, particularly mature children, should be ignored in the decisionmaking process. Diagnostic tests and treatment plans should be explained to children to help them understand what is being done to them and to garner, when possible, their cooperation. Parents should include their children in the decisionmaking process both to get their active support and to help them learn how to make such decisions. However, when there is parental–child disagreement, the child's decision should not be decisive nor should health care providers, as I have argued, seek third party mediation. Rather, as I have already argued, there are both moral and pragmatic reasons why the parents should have final decisionmaking authority. As such, I believe that the AAP's recommendation to empower competent adolescents to consent and refuse treatment on their own is misguided.

Acknowledgments

This paper is adapted from my Ph.D. dissertation, *Health Care Decision Making for Children*, chapter 4, "Respect for the Child's Autonomy." An earlier version of this paper was published as "Arguments against Health Care Autonomy for Minors," *Bioethics Forum* 11, no. 4 (1995): 22-26. A later version of this paper was presented at the Annual Meeting of the Chicago Clinical Ethics Program, "Do Parents Know Best?" February, 1997.

Notes

1. James L. Nelson, "Taking Families Seriously," *Hastings Center Report* 22, no. 4 (1992): 6–12; Nancy S. Jecker, "The Role of Intimate Others in Medical Decision Making," *The Gerontologist* 30 (1990): 65–71; John Hardwig, "What About the Family? *Hastings Center Report* 20, no. 2 (1990): 510.

2. William Bartholome, "Hearing Children's Voices," *Bioethics Forum* 11, no. 4 (1995): 3–6; Council on Scientific Affairs of the American Medical Association, "Council Report: Confidential Health Services for Adolescents," *JAMA* 269 (1993): 1420–24; Garry S. Sigman and Carolyn O'Connor, "Exploration for Physicians of the Mature Minor Doctrine," *Journal of Pediatrics* 119, no. 4 (1991): 520–25.

3. Allen Buchanan and Dan Brock, *Deciding for Others: The Ethics of Surrogate Decision Making* (New York: Cambridge University Press, 1989).

4. American Academy of Pediatrics, Committee on Bioethics, "Informed Consent, Parental Permission, and Assent in Pediatric Practice," *Pediatrics* 95 (1995): 314–17.

5. Thomas Grisso and Linda Vierling, "Minor's Consent to Treatment: A Developmental Perspective," *Professional Psychology* 9, no. 3 (1978): 412–27.

6. Paul S. Appelbaum, Charles W Lidz, and Alan Meisel, *Informed Consent: Legal Theory and Clinical Practice* (New York: Oxford University Press, 1987); Stanley Milgram, *Obedience to Authority: An Experimental View* (New York: Harper and Row, 1974).

7. Grisso and Vierling, "Minors Consent to Treatment."

8. Laura M. Purdy, *In Their Best Interest? The Case Against Equal Rights for Children* (New York: Cornell University Press, 1992).

9. Willard Gaylin, "Competence: No Longer All or None," in *Who Speaks for the Child: The Problems of Proxy Consent,* ed. Willard Gaylin and Ruth Macklin (New York: Plenum Press, 1982), p. 35.

10. Lainie Friedman Ross, *Health Care Decision Making for Children*, unpublished manuscript, 1996.

11. Purdy, *In Their Best Interest?* p. 78.

12. Howard Cohen, *Equal Rights for Children* (Totowa, NJ.: Rowman and Littlefield, 1980); John Harris, "The Political Status of Children," in *Contemporary Political Philosophy,* ed. Keith Graham (Cambridge, Mass.: Cambridge University Press, 1982), pp. 35–55.

13. Hillary Rodham, "Children Under the Law," *Harvard Educational Review* 43 (1973): 487–514; Rodham, "Children's Rights: A Legal Perspective," in *Children's Rights: Contemporary Perspectives,* ed. Patricia A. Vardin and Ilene N. Brody (New York: Teachers College Press, 1979).

14. Richard Farson, "A Child's Bill of Rights," in *Justice: Selected Readings,* ed. Joel Feinberg and Hyman Gross (Belmont, Calif: Dickenson Publishing Co. 1977).

15. Cohen, *Equal Rights,* p. 66.

16. Joseph Goldstein, Anna Freud, and Albert J Solnit, *Before the Best Interests of the Child* (New York: The Free Press, 1979).

17. Jan C. Costello, "If I Can Say Yes, Why Can't I Say No? Adolescents at Risk and the Right to Give or Withhold Consent to Health Care," in *Child, Parent, and State: Law and Policy Reader,* ed.

S. Randall Humm et al. (Philadelphia: Temple University Press, 1994), pp. 490–503.

18. H. Tristram Engelhardt, Jr., "Freedom vs. Best Interest: A Conflict at the Roots of Health Care," in *Dax's Case: Essays in Medical Ethics and*

Human Meaning, ed. Lonnie D. Kliever (Dallas: Southern Methodist University Press, 1989).

19. Joseph Goldstein et al., *In the Best Interest of the Child* (New York: The Free Press, 1986).

Culture, Power and Informed Consent: The Impact of Aboriginal Health Interpreters on Decision-Making

Joseph M. Kaufert and John D. O'Neil

INTRODUCTION

The signing of a consent agreement prior to surgery or invasive diagnostic or treatment procedures is a pivotal event in the negotiation of trust in the doctor-patient relationship. Most analysts have focused on the legal, ethical or procedural aspects of consent. However, there is growing recognition of the importance of considering political and cultural factors which lie outside the immediate context of the medical encounter and beyond the control of either physician or patient. This chapter will examine the processes through which consent is negotiated when the patient is a Native from one of the remote areas of northern Canada. It will explore the application of ethnomedical approaches emphasizing explanatory models and an interactionist framework to understanding the impact of intermediaries in cross-cultural negotiation of consent.

In our research on cross-cultural communication in urban hospitals, it was apparent that negotiations around the signing of a consent form provided the clearest illustration of the unequal knowledge and power of the clinician and the patient. The clinician's approach to obtaining consent was based primarily on a biomedical understanding of a particular disease and associated treatment procedures; the approach of the Native patient to giving consent was based on experiential and cultural knowl-edge of past and present illnesses, interpretations of the social meaning of hospital regulations and health professional behaviour, and general attitudes defining intergroup relations in the wider society....

MEDIATING CLIENT AND PHYSICIAN EXPLANATIONS OF INVASIVE DIAGNOSTIC PROCEDURES: A CASE EXAMPLE

The case documents the communication with an Aboriginal patient who was asked to consent to gastroscopic and colonscopic examinations. The 46-year-old Cree-speaking woman was referred from a northern nursing station for further investigation of anaemia by a gastroenterologist in Winnipeg. A series of encounters were videotaped at each stage of the diagnostic workup. Several encounters involved the signing of formal consent agreements. In each encounter the physician worked with a Cree-speaking medical interpreter to explain diagnostic and treatment options and negotiate patient consent for examinations of the stomach, small and large intestine.

In the initial encounter, the physician attempted to evaluate the patient's understanding of her own problem and to explain his diagnostic model of the probable cause of anaemia. Specifically he attempted to move from discussing the client's understanding of anaemia (conceptualized by the patient in terms of weakness) to a more complex model linking the loss of blood to the presence of lesions caused by anti-inflammatory medication. Following a cursory explanation of the general diagnosis, the physician moved to a series of diagnostic questions about presence of blood in the patient's stool.

Doctor: She's anaemic and pale, which means she must be losing blood.

Interpreter (Cree): This is what he says about you. You are pale, you have no blood. (Cree term for anaemia connotes bloodless state).

Doctor: Has she had any bleeding from the bowel when she's had a bowel movement?

Interpreter (Cree): When you have a bowel movement, do you notice any blood?

Patient (Cree): I'm not sure.

Interpreter (Cree): Is your stool ever black, or very light? What does it look like?

Patient (Cree): Sometimes dark.

At this point the patient told the interpreter that she did not understand how her "weakness" (anaemia) was related to questions about gastrointestinal symptomatology in the physician's reference to dark stools. Without asking for additional explanation from the physician, the interpreter attempted to link the patient's understanding of her anaemia with the concept of blood loss.

Interpreter (Cree): We want to know, he says, why it is that you are lacking blood. That's why he asked you what your stool looks like. Sometimes you lose your blood from there, when your stool is black.

In discussing the probable etiology of the woman's anaemia, the physician introduced a complex explanatory model which explained gastric or intestinal bleeding in terms of the possible side effects of anti-inflammatory medication for rheumatism. The patient again indicated that she did not understand why the questions about her experience with medication for rheumatism were relevant to the current diagnosis of problems with weakness and blood loss. The interpreter provided an unprompted explanation linking the line of questioning about the side effects of anti-inflammatory drugs with the concept of blood loss.

Interpreter (Cree): He says that those pills you are taking for rheumatism, sometimes they cause you to bleed inside, or you will spit up blood. Not everyone has these effects. This is why he wants to know about your medication.

Following gastroscopy, the physician attempted to explain the results of the gastric studies and at the same time to extend the initial consent agreement to permit colonscopic examination of the lower bowel.

Doctor: Everything looked good. There was no ulcer and no nasty disease in the stomach or the esophagus. No bleeding. You're still anaemic so we still want to find out if there's any bleeding from the lower end.

Interpreter (Cree): He says this about you: there's nothing visible in your stomach. Nothing, no sores, lumps, what they call "ulcers." Nothing from where you swallow. Nothing wrong that can be seen.

Patient: (Nods, but makes no verbal response.)

Doctor: We're going to put a small tube in from the colon. It's only this big. To have a look, to see if there's any abnormality. It won't take too long and it will be very quick and you shouldn't be uncomfortable with it at all. Okay?… So we'll go ahead and do that now while we can.

Interpreter (Cree): He wants to see you over here from where your bowel movements come from. Something will be put there, like the first one (the tube you swallowed), but smaller. So you can be examined "down there." Maybe somewhere "down there," it'll be seen that you are losing blood from there. The reason why you are lacking blood. That's what he's looking for. The cause for your blood loss.

During the exchange the patient's willingness to extend the initial consent agreement to cover the investigation of the lower bowel is inferred from a nod and no real alternative was suggested by the physician. The patient was asked to initial the addition to the consent agreement, without formal translation of the English text.

Colonoscopic and radiological examination of the intestine revealed a benign polyp. The physician recommended that the polyp should be cauterized through a second colonoscopy and asked the patient to sign a consent form for the additional procedure. Although risks and benefits were not formally discussed the interpreter elaborated on the basic diagnostic information provided by the physician. The interpreter also introduced a more formal decision point at which the patient was asked to give her formal consent.

Doctor: We X-rayed the bowel.

Interpreter (Cree): And this is what they did this morning—when you were X-rayed. The pictures of the area you have bowel movements.

Patient (Cree): Yes.

Doctor: And that shows a polyp, a small benign tumor. And I have to take that out.

Interpreter (Cree): This picture they took this morning. He saw it already.

There's something growing there. About this size. And it has to be removed, because you might bleed from there.

Patient (Cree): Yes.

Doctor: Now I can take it out without an operation, by putting a tube inside the bowel, and putting a wire around it and burning the polyp off. That stops the bleeding, no need for an operation.

Interpreter (Cree): He says they can put in a tube like before and burn off the growth.

Patient: (Nods but makes no verbal response.)

Doctor: If she wants to make the arrangements for the hospital admission she can come down and sign the consent form.

Interpreter (English): Will there be complications?

Doctor: There are a few complications but I think it would be difficult to explain them all.

Interpreter (Cree): After this procedure has been done you won't be staying here at the hospital. You'll be able to go home on Saturday. It will be done on Friday, then you'll already be able to go home on Saturday. It won't be long. But it's entirely up to you.

In this exchange, the interpreter is providing more than a simple elaboration of the risks, benefits and rationale for the procedure. The physician assumes that his explanation of the reasons for doing the procedure will be sufficient to obtain the patient's consent. In addition the physician closes the exchange by asserting that it would be too difficult to explain all the possible complications. However, in both instances, the interpreter does not provide a literal translation of the physician's side comments, but attempts to assure the patient and justify the procedure through explanations addressing the patient's concern with the length of her stay and desire to return to her home community. The interpreter assures the patient, "You'll be able to go home on Saturday" emphasizing the expectation that the operation will be minor and she won't be separated from family and home for long. The interpreter's statement linking approval of the consent to the patient's early return to her community occurs in Cree and therefore is not accessible to the physician.

As the end of the encounter the physician included the consent agreement with the hospital admission protocol and assumed it would be signed with the other paper work. The interpreter provided a more direct opportunity for the patient to give or withhold consent.

Interpreter (Cree): Do you want to have this procedure done? Will you consent to have this growth removed—burned? Do you consent to have it done?

Patient (Cree): I don't know.

Interpreter: You know, if it's not removed it may bleed. It may cause problems.

Interpreter (English directed at physician): Dr. _____, isn't it true that if it's not removed, it can bleed and she can become anaemic?

Doctor: That's correct, we feel that your anaemia may result from the bleeding of the polyp.

Interpreter (Cree): If it's not removed, you may end up with cancer. You know? And you will not have an operation. It's harder when a person has an operation. You know? And [this procedure] that he's going to do will get it on time. Before it begins to bleed or starts to grow. You're lucky it's caught on time. And it will bother you when you have a bowel movement. This way there's no danger that this growth will bleed.

Patient (Cree): I still don't know.

Interpreter (Cree): Well if you want to come in for the procedure while you are here? It's all up to you to think about.

Again, the interpreter has assumed responsibility for providing a rationale for the procedure and explaining the potential benefits. Her explanations are also clearly based on her own medical knowledge, and her understanding of the patient's explanatory model. The fear of cancer in the Native community is linked to general understandings about the history of infectious disease epidemics that nearly destroyed Aboriginal society in North America. Cancer is increasingly viewed as the new "epidemic." The interpreter is using her knowledge of these fears to negotiate the patient's consent, but she is also using Cree models of negotiation emphasizing individual autonomy. Her final statement emphasizes her client's ultimate personal responsibility. "It's all up to you to think about."

At this point, the patient accompanied the interpreter and physician to the appointment desk and scheduled the colonoscopy for the following day. After a brief summary of the text (which was printed in English) was provided by the interpreter, the patient signed the consent form. The formal act of signing the form was immediately subordinated to a discussion of specific arrangements for the client's discharge from hospital and travel arrangements for returning to the reserve community.

In this case, consent was negotiated by drawing on expressions of trust by the patient about her relationship with the interpreter. The physician initially assumed that little explanation was required for consent, and indicated his unwillingness to negotiate. Information sharing occurred gradually over the course of the encounter. The interpreter assumed the negotiator's role, based on shared cultural understanding of both biomedicine and Native culture. Throughout the sequence of interaction the interpreter worked to elicit and clarify both the client's and clinician's interpretation of the condition and the program of treatment. However, the interpreter's intervention introduced a third party into the clinician–client relationship. She directly influenced the course of the decision by independently introducing new information about illness and treatment options. She also imposed decision points where the patient could actually exercise her option to consent.

The patient's willingness to allow the interpreter to negotiate consent is also evident in her reluctance to ask the physician direct questions. In response to the interpreter's questions about her understanding, she repeats at several junctures, "I don't know." This provides a cue for the interpreter to introduce further information or elaborate relative risks. The final consent is passive, in the sense that the patient signs the forms without further resistance.

POWER AND CONTROL IN CONSENT DECISIONS AMONG NATIVE CANADIANS

The case study demonstrates the role of interpreter-advocates in redressing cultural and structural constraints for Native people in consent negotiations in urban hospitals (Kaufert and Koolage 1984). In some urban hospitals interpreters have expanded their role beyond narrow language translation functions to assume advocacy roles which empower the client through providing information about the structure of the health care system and elaborating these treatment options.

However, in consent negotiations involving both Indian and Inuit patients, the presence of a language interpreter or patient advocate as an intermediary raises a number of ethical and sociopolitical issues. For example, the involvement of interpreter-advocates in the doctor–patient relationship may shift responsibility and initiative for disclosure from the professional to the intermediary. The translator may exercise control through selective interpretation of information provided by the client. The interpreter may also priorize and filter information about treatment options and associated risks or benefits. The interpreters' function of mediating and priorizing information occurs within a linguistic

and cultural "black box." Within this box the interpreter may actively intervene on the patient's behalf, or use his or her cultural knowledge and personal rapport with the patient to reinforce the clinician's definition of appropriate treatment choices. Consideration of this variable by clinicians in obtaining informed consent is important.

In summary, sociocultural analysis of real interaction sequences in the negotiation of consent between the clinician and client differs fundamentally from legal or ethical analysis of the marker decisions. For Native clients, agreements may reflect the emergence of trust relationships achieved through an extended, incremental process of exchange rather than a formal, final contract. Interactionist and ethnomedical approaches more clearly reveal the communication processes and power relations which are part of the process of translating and priorizing information. Our analysis of the role of Native medical interpreters in both case studies clearly indicates that dyadic clinician–client interaction is strongly influenced by intermediaries. Both confirm that translators, cultural brokers, and personal advocates negotiate shared meanings and influence the balance of power in cross-cultural, clinical communication. As well as demarcating formal legal and ethical decision points, cross-cultural consent agreements also function as integrative rituals through which participants reconcile power imbalance and negotiate clinical trust.

Acknowledgements

The authors would like to acknowledge the special contribution of our colleagues and research associates including William Koolage, Margaret Lavallée, Ellen Haroun, Andrew Koster, and Charlene Ball. We wish to thank Jackie Linklater for her assistance in administering the research program and for help in preparing this manuscript. We also wish to thank Drs. Pat Kaufert, Barney Sneiderman, John Walker, Gareth Williams, and Brian Postl for their editorial assistance. Our initial study of hospital-based interpreters was financed by a grant from the Manitoba Health Research Foundation. Subsequent research on interpretation and health communication in Inuit communities was financed by a grant from National Health Research Programs Directorate of Health and Welfare Canada (Project No. 6607-1305-49).

References

Kaufert, J, and W Koolage. 1984. Role Conflict among Culture Brokers: The Experience of Native Canadian Medical Interpreters. *Social Science and Medicine* 18(3): 283–286.

This manuscript contains sections of a previously published manuscript, "Biomedical Rituals and Informed Consent" originally printed in Weisz, G. (ed.) *Social Science Perspectives on Medical Ethics*, University of Pennsylvania Press, 1991.

Reibl v. Hughes, [1980] 2 S.C.R. 880

Summary prepared by Matthew Herder

Mr. Reibl, a Hungarian immigrant 44 years of age, elected to undergo an internal carotid endarterectomy to remove an occlusion in an artery near his brain that was preventing a significant amount of blood flow through the artery. The operation was performed competently by Dr. Hughes, a fully qualified neurosurgeon. However, following the procedure, Reibl suffered a massive stroke, resulting in the paralysis of his entire right side. He also became impotent.

Dr. Hughes had believed that Mr. Reibl's chances of suffering a stroke would be greater if he did not undergo the procedure. However, the risk of stroke, in the absence of surgery, had not been imminent. Prior to the surgery, Dr. Hughes supposedly explained to Mr. Reibl the specific risks associated with this type of surgery, including death or stroke. But Mr. Reibl did not understand these risks. The trial judge found that the precise purpose for the operation was not sufficiently explained, and that Mr. Reibl was left only with the impression that his headaches and hypertension would decrease, thereby improving his job performance. The only risks Mr. Reibl was cognizant of were those inherent in any surgical procedure, such as infection. Had he known of the more serious risks, Mr. Reibl claimed he would not have gone ahead with the operation, especially in light of the fact that he was only one and a half years away from being eligible for pension benefits from his employer.

The issue for the Supreme Court of Canada concerned liability for failure to meet the requisite standard of disclosure for informed consent. Chief Justice Laskin made several important points in the course of the unanimous judgment for the Court.

At trial, the defendant neurosurgeon had been found liable in both battery and negligence. Chief Justice Laskin opted instead to narrow the scope for battery actions. Specifically, only instances where no consent was given, or where there was complete misrepresentation or fraud, such as an entirely different procedure being carried out than the one consented to, were deemed capable of grounding a battery claim. "[F]ailure to disclose the attendant risks" can only go to negligence, not the fact of consent.

The Chief Justice then went on to consider the standard of disclosure. Following *Hopp v. Lepp*, all material risks must be disclosed to the patient. Chief Justice Laskin explained that whether a risk is material depends on whether the risk is looked at from a reasonable person's perspective (objective standard) or the particular patient's perspective (subjective standard). He noted problems with either standard. Adopting a purely objective standard would effectively "hand over to the medical profession the entire question of the scope of the duty of disclosure." Moreover, it is doubtful whether causation could ever be established using this standard: a reasonable person could never refuse consent if the recommended treatment was consistent with medical opinion. The objective standard reinforces the (false) assumption that all patients would necessarily accede to a doctor's advice. On the other hand, a subjective standard lends itself to problems of hindsight bias. Having suffered injury, it is highly unlikely that any patient would admit that he or she would have undergone the treatment, had he or she been differently apprised of the risks involved. That is, causation is too easily met using a subjective test for disclosure. The appropriate standard, therefore, does not entail a purely subjective or objective assessment of what risks are and are not material.

Chief Justice Laskin continued to refer to the standard as an objective one; however, he introduced certain subjective elements into the standard. "Special considerations affecting the particular patient" play a role in determining whether a risk is material. On the facts here, "the anticipation of a full pension would be a special consideration." Such considerations may also be indicated when the patient asks the doctor specific questions. The Chief Justice added one further caveat. Those special considerations must themselves be reasonable:

> Thus, for example, fears which are not related to the material risks which should have been but were not disclosed would

not be causative factors. However, economic considerations could reasonably go to causation where, for example, the loss of an eye as a result of non-disclosure of a material risk brings about the loss of a job for which good eyesight is required.

In this case, it was evident that Dr. Hughes failed to meet the requisite standard of disclosure and, had Mr. Reibl fully appreciated the risks of stroke and paralysis, he would not have elected to undergo the procedure. Thus, the judgment at trial was restored.

Norberg v. Wynrib, [1992] 2 S.C.R. 226

Summary prepared by Leah Hutt

Ms. Norberg became addicted to the painkiller Fiorinal. She obtained the drug from her sister and various doctors. Eventually, she began seeing Dr. Wynrib, a doctor in his seventies. She lied to him about various injuries in order to obtain prescriptions for Fiorinal. Dr. Wynrib eventually confronted Ms. Norberg about her drug addiction. He made it clear that he would continue her prescriptions only in exchange for sexual favours.

Ms. Norberg stopped seeing him and sought her drugs from other doctors. She returned to Dr. Wynrib when the other doctors reduced her supply and she engaged in a sex-for-drugs relationship with him for approximately two years.

At one point, Ms. Norberg asked Dr. Wynrib for help with her addiction. He advised her to "just quit," which was virtually impossible to do without professional help. Dr. Wynrib stopped writing her prescriptions when she became the subject of a criminal investigation for double doctoring, but he continued to give her pills after sexual encounters. Dr. Wynrib did not use physical force and Ms. Norberg admitted that she played on his loneliness.

After she was charged with double doctoring, Ms. Norberg attended a rehabilitation centre on her own initiative and stopped using drugs for non-medical reasons. She pled guilty to the charges and received an absolute discharge.

Ms. Norberg sought damages against Dr. Wynrib on the grounds of sexual assault, negligence, breach of fiduciary duty, and breach of contract. The issue was whether she should be allowed to recover damages.

Justice La Forest, writing for the majority of the Supreme Court of Canada, disposed of the case on the basis of the assault claim. Dr. Wynrib relied on the defence of consent. Justice La Forest held that an understanding of the power relationship between the parties was important for understanding the notion of consent. Consent will be vitiated in several circumstances, including where there is such a disparity in the relative positions of the parties that the weaker party is not in a position to freely choose.

To address a situation where there is an apparent power imbalance, Justice La Forest outlined a two-step process for determining whether there has been legally effective consent to sexual assault: (1) proof of an inequality between the parties; (2) proof of exploitation. The type of relationship at issue and community standards of conduct may assist in the determination.

There was a marked power imbalance between the parties. Ms. Norberg was vulnerable because of her drug addiction. Dr. Wynrib was in a position of power by virtue of his medical knowledge, his awareness of her addiction, and his authority to prescribe drugs.

Exploitation existed because Dr. Wynrib did not use his medical knowledge to help Ms. Norberg overcome her addiction. Rather, he used her addiction to pursue his own personal satisfaction. The sex-for-drugs relationship was markedly divergent from what the community would consider acceptable.

The inequality between the parties and the exploitative nature of the relationship removed the possibility of Ms. Norberg providing meaningful consent to the sexual contact. Accordingly, Dr. Wynrib was liable for assault.

Dr. Wynrib argued that Ms. Norberg could not succeed against him because of the legal principle that an action cannot arise out of an illegal act. Justice La Forest dismissed the argument, stating that Ms. Norberg acted out of desperation for Fiorinal, and so to apply Dr. Wynrib's argument would be to deny her claim on the same basis that she had succeeded. Further, there was no link between the assault and the double doctoring—she would have suffered the same harm if Dr. Wynrib had been her only drug supplier.

After reviewing damage awards of other sexual abuse and rape cases, Justice La Forest awarded Ms. Norberg general damages (which are meant to compensate Ms. Norberg for her suffering) in the amount of $20,000. He awarded an additional $10,000 in punitive damages (which are meant to punish Dr. Wynrib and deter him and others from engaging in similar conduct).

Justice McLachlin (as she then was), writing for two justices of the Court, also found in favour of Ms. Norberg but did so on the basis that Dr. Wynrib breached his fiduciary duty to her. The characteristics of a fiduciary relation-

ship are: (1) the fiduciary has scope for the exercise of some discretion or power; (2) the fiduciary can unilaterally exercise that power or discretion so as to affect the other person's legal or practical interests; (3) the other person is peculiarly vulnerable or at the mercy of the fiduciary. The hallmark of the relationship is that one party promises to exercise power on the other party's behalf in the best interest of the other.

In this case, the classic characteristics of a fiduciary relationship were present. Dr. Wynrib had the power to advise Ms. Norberg, treat her, and prescribe her drugs. Ms. Norberg was vulnerable because of her patient status, especially in light of her addiction. Dr. Wynrib breached his fiduciary duty to Ms. Norberg when he prescribed drugs that were not required medically, when he failed to assist her in obtaining addiction counselling, and when he placed his own interest in obtaining sexual favours from her in conflict with and above her interest in obtaining treatment.

Justice McLachlin rejected Dr. Wynrib's argument that Ms. Norberg could not succeed because of her own illegal act, stating that Ms. Norberg had done nothing wrong in the context of the relationship. She was a sick person suffering from an addiction. Rather than help her, Dr. Wynrib used his power to keep her in an addicted state and to use her for his own sexual purposes. To apply Dr. Wynrib's argument here amounts to "blaming the victim." The responsibility for sexual exploitation rests solely with the physician, regardless of the patient's conduct.

Justice McLachlin would have awarded $20,000 for the prolongation of Ms. Norberg's addiction, $25,000 for sexual exploitation and $25,000 in punitive damages.

Justice Sopinka also found in Ms. Norberg's favour but on the basis of breach of contract. He rejected the assault claim because, although the sexual contact was against her wishes, Ms. Norberg had consented to it. He found that there may be cases where a doctor, by virtue of his/her status, exercises such control over a patient that the patient's submission cannot be genuine, but that was not the case here, where Ms. Norberg admitted she played on Dr. Wynrib's loneliness to continue obtaining prescriptions. Ms. Norberg's addiction did not interfere with her ability to reason, although it inspired her decision, and she willingly engaged in sexual activity.

The focus of Justice Sopinka's decision was on Dr. Wynrib's conduct in light of his professional duty to Ms. Norberg. The doctor–patient relationship is essentially based in contract. Ms. Norberg's consent to the sexual touching did not release Dr. Wynrib from his duty to her and the state not to mistreat her in a medical way by prolonging her period of addiction without proper treatment. The fact that a patient acquiesces to a form of treatment does not absolve the physician of the duty if the treatment is not in accordance with medical standards. Dr. Wynrib breached his duty to treat Ms. Norberg.

Justice Sopinka also dismissed Dr. Wynrib's argument about Ms. Norberg's double-doctoring offence. He stated that emphasis is now placed on preserving the administration of justice from the taint that would result from approving a transaction the court ought not to countenance. In this case, the administration of justice would suffer no disrepute in the public's eyes if the court assisted Ms. Norberg in this case.

Justice Sopinka would have awarded $20,000 in general damages for Dr. Wynrib's failure to treat Ms. Norberg's addiction. The sexual acts were causally connected to the failure to treat and formed part of the damage assessment. No punitive damages would have been awarded because the basis of liability was the failure to treat, not the sexual acts.

Arndt v. Smith, [1997] 2 S.C.R. 539

Summary prepared by Leah Hutt

Ms. Arndt, while pregnant, was exposed to the virus that causes chickenpox. Her physician, Dr. Smith, did not properly advise her of the related risks of this exposure to the fetus. The baby was born congenitally injured by chickenpox. Ms. Arndt asserted that she would have had an abortion in the second trimester had Dr. Smith adequately explained the risks to the fetus, thus avoiding the costs of raising a disabled child. Dr. Smith argued that Ms. Arndt would not have had an abortion, even if she had been advised of all the risks. Accordingly, the loss claimed was not caused by the failure to advise of the risks.

The trial judge weighed Ms. Arndt's assertion against the facts that she wanted a child: she was sceptical of "mainstream" medical intervention; she did not want an ultrasound scan of the developing fetus; second trimester abortions held increased risks; an abortion required the approval of a committee on health grounds; the risk of

serious injury to the fetus was minimal; and medical professionals would not have supported an abortion. He concluded that, on a balance of probabilities, she would not have had an abortion.

The issue on appeal was whether a subjective or objective test, or some combination of the two, applied to a plaintiff when determining whether the failure to advise of a risk caused the loss claimed. Justice Cory, writing for the majority of the Supreme Court of Canada, held that the court should adopt the modified objective test set out in *Reibl v. Hughes*. The test requires the court to consider what a reasonable patient in Ms. Arndt's shoes would have done in the same situation. A "reasonable patient" is taken to possess reasonable beliefs, fears, desires, and expectations. Questions posed by the patient at the time consent is sought will usually be taken to reveal the patient's concerns.

The majority of the SCC felt that the modified objective test struck a fair balance between a purely subjective approach and a purely objective approach. A subjective approach favours the plaintiff, who will invariably state, with the benefit of hindsight, that she never would have consented if the risks had been disclosed. An objective approach, on the other hand, favours the physician by setting the standard of a reasonable person without the reasonable concerns of the plaintiff.

Justice Cory found that a reasonable person in Ms. Arndt's position would not have had an abortion when the exposure to chickenpox posed a very small increased risk to the fetus. Although Ms. Arndt had made a very general inquiry concerning the risks of her exposure, there was nothing to demonstrate that she had a particular concern about it. The factors considered by the trial judge supported the view that the failure to properly disclose the risks did not affect Ms. Arndt's decision to continue the pregnancy. Therefore, the failure to disclose did not cause the financial losses for which Ms. Arndt claimed.

Chapter 7 COMPETENCE

Competence, Marginal and Otherwise: Concepts and Ethics

Benjamin Freedman

I. RIGHTS AND DEGREES OF COMPETENCE

A society that is sensitive to rights is, for that reason, sensitive to persons. On one level, rights function as a meta-possession: a grounding for the possibility of an individual's possessing anything, a claim that the individual counts, that his wants and interests must be allowed for in our handling of him. Thus, rights serve the function of protecting interests of the personality. Under the regime of rights, desires, inclinations, and so on are given protection.

This model rests upon a notion of the personality as a construct pre-dating the "existence" or "conference" of rights. One cannot guard the valuable before one possesses it. Rights, however, do more than this. Legally or morally, they define the limits of the protected personality. When we determine, through rights, the kinds of interests and desires that we shall protect, we also determine to some degree the manner in which persons shall be protected. Those whose desires remain unexpressed cannot have their desires protected under a regime of rights. Those with bizarre or profoundly deviant desires are unprotected in their pursuits: for example, the man with disturbed ideation, who wishes protection from feared disintegration, or spontaneous combustion.

In response to these circumstances, it is common to appeal to a two-fold nature in rights.[1]

With respect to those who are competent, the expression of their rights typically takes the form of heeding their wishes. The competent tell us what content to give to their rights. A competent person's right to seek medical care will express itself in *his* decisions as to whether he will seek care, for what condition, and in what form. For the incompetent—the voiceless—we are forced to look elsewhere than at their desires, in giving an expression to their rights. One approach to this has us making decisions in terms of the incompetent's "best interests," as determined by his biological and psychological being, on the one hand, and, on the other, by a community consensus concerning the good for man.

On most accounts, though, this dichotomy—the competent and the incompetent—is not exhaustive. Between them lies a middle ground. Epistemologically, we may term this third group those of dubious competence. This appelation, however, tells us nothing about *them*. It merely points up the limits of our knowledge, limits which may be attributed more to laziness than to vagueness of the phenomenon. On the borderline between competencey and incompetency we face a choice of temperament in choosing a term by which to describe this group. For reasons of brevity and optimism, I will term them the marginally competent.

Practically speaking, as there are three main forms of incompetence, so are there three main groupings of the marginally competent. The first form of incompetence relates to age, infants and small children being a paradigm case of legal and moral incapacity. Between the extremes of infancy and adulthood, the individual's competence is developing. Although in some legal matters the distinction between an "infant" and an adult is firm, this bright line exists only in the legal codes, and is no reflection of reality. As Wilson writes, having described age-based limitations upon capacity, "There is a growing belief among many social observers, however, that many older children have the physical and psychological capacities to act with some autonomy in many areas in which they are now denied independence, that they have a moral right to such autonomy, and that they should be granted corresponding legal rights."[2] For our purposes, the operative words in Wilson's remarks are the qualifiers: "*some* autonomy," not full; "*many*" areas, not all. Though vague and culturally parochial, the period including and surrounding adolescence may serve as the focus for this grouping of the marginally competent.

The second form of incompetence is that presumably stable deficit in intellect and adaptation which is known as mental retardation. The incompetent group would include those with no verbal skills and a very low ceiling on presumed ability to learn. The marginally competent would be those, institutionalized or not, who possess some understanding and some ability to use language to express their wants and desires. The marginally competent are numerically by far the most significant class of the retarded. One estimate has it that for every 1,000 births in the United States, 26 children will be mildly retarded, expressed in their marginal adjustment to adult life; three will be moderately retarded, that is, will never surpass the intellectual attainments of the average seven-year-old; and one will be severely retarded.[3] Given a latitudinous reading of incompetency, then, although between two and three percent of the population are mentally impaired, less than one-half of a percent are totally incompetent.

The third source of incompetency is, loosely, mental illness, whatever its etiology. Those who are prepared to admit the propriety of the concept of mental illness at all will admit that the vast majority of the mentally ill are not wholly incompetent. Even at the fairly extreme end of pathology, very bizarre behavior might overshadow a core of the personality which is in touch with the world and can respond to it. After noting that the ideal model for a "proxy" or substituted consent to medical treatment is that of a mother on behalf of her infant, one psychiatrist notes:

> If it is a severely crippled, emotionally incompetent adult, it may well be that we can approximate the mother-infant relationship, but most severely ill mental patients are not at all like infants, and while the intellectual insufficiencies may seem as great, the emotional components of the "self" are often vastly different. Mental illness is a fragmented, irrational combination of intact and destroyed faculties.[4]

It seems clear, then, that collectively the marginally competent constitute a very substantial group, deserving of a moral analysis as searching and rigorous as has been provided to their neighbors, the competent and the incompetent. Topically, too, the problems of the moral status of the marginally competent have been increasingly urgent in recent years. Can a mental patient, or a mentally-disturbed prisoner, consent to psychosurgery? Can an institutionalized retarded person consent to sterilization? How should we relate to the adolescent cancer patient? These difficult problems all arise from the twilight status of the marginally competent. It may be that some of the difficulty could be alleviated by the simple recognition that there is a middle classification between the competent and the incompetent. In some discussions, we may have crippled ourselves with our paucity of ethical frameworks. Countless arguments could be mounted over whether a mule is a horse or a donkey, but the path of wisdom might be to simply call it a mule.

The quandaries of the marginally retarded have great theoretical significance, for it is only by testing and deepening our understanding of competence that we can clarify the status of the marginally competent. In what follows, then, my *method* will be the clarification of the concept of competence. My *goal* is to achieve an understanding of this concept detailed enough to deal with the vagaries of the human condition.

Before beginning that task, let us face squarely the question of whether competency is an empirical or a moral term. Does it describe a fact in the world, or how we evaluate that fact? A little reflection reveals that in some ways it must do both: a psychiatrist may give expert testimony, in his capacity as a trained observer, about a person's competence seen as a factual matter, and the judge may or may not give this testimony practical effect in deciding how we *ought* to treat that person. Competence is not pure description, then, nor pure evaluation; but, perhaps, an evaluation that stems from certain described facts coupled with a moral theory that tells us what those facts mean, how we ought to respond to those facts. A middle step between description and action is always needed, i.e., a moral theory that interprets experience and guides action.

This point—that the ascription of competence has practical implications, and so presupposes a *moral* theory—is surprisingly easy to forget. One of the better writers on questions of competence proposed as his test for competency "the ability to understand and knowingly act upon the information provided." He goes on to say that, "Meaningful decisions concerning this or any other standard, however, can be made only through a careful empirical study of operational results."[5] Yet he never tells us what we should be looking for in these subsequent studies. Should it be the extent to which this standard enhanced the autonomy of the subjects? Or the rational pursuit of their best interests? Should we be looking to see if judgments of competency using this standard accord well with the "intuitive" judgments of psychiatrists, or lawyers, or laymen? We cannot know where to look unless we know what we are looking for. A theory of the values embedded in the ascription of competency, and of its significance, needs to be provided. Insofar as this theory will

be one which is intended to guide conscientious action, it will be of necessity an ethical theory.

II. CRITERIA OF COMPETENCE: THE BACKGROUND UNDERSTANDINGS OF COMPETENCE

A number of tests for competence have been proposed. "Test" or "criterion" in this context signifies a verbal formula, put in terms of a question, the answer to which will determine whether the person in question is competent or not. As my purpose is moral exploration, rather than legal exposition, I will discuss on their merits and without differentiation proposals put forth by scholars as well as tests actually employed by courts in adjudication in this area.

There are several levels at which tests for competency can be discussed. The first I would term the "general" level. It answers the question: What is the *background* understanding of competency, against which we may judge proposals designed to apply to specific problems?

One sort of general background understanding of competency has been adopted by some members of the medical profession. It has been reported[6] that to test competency, psychiatrists and other physicians often use a functional test. That is to say, if the patient functions well within society, as evinced by an examination of his work history, personal relationships, and so on, he is to be judged competent. Failing these characteristics, he is judged incompetent.

Among lawyers, one can discern a fair amount of agreement on a different background principle of competency. Roth, Meisel, and Lidz put the legal understanding as follows:[7] "The test of competency varies from one context to another. In general, to be considered competent an individual must be able to comprehend the nature of the particular conduct in question and to understand its quality and its consequences."

A specific application of this principle may be found in the law of contracts. When is an individual competent to contract? When he can understand the effect of the transaction that the contract effectuates.[8] Given this principle, the question of competence can only be addressed relative to the situation in question. Someone may be competent, in the sense of understanding what is going on, to engage a house painter at an agreed-upon sum. That same person might be incompetent to contract for futures on the commodities exchange, because he is unable to understand the contingencies involved in that transaction.

It is important to note that the legal background understanding of competency is generally considered to comprise two elements.[9] The first is a bare *knowledge* of what you are doing: the fact that you *are* making a contract; an example is the fact that you have agreed to the doctor's removal of your appendix. The second element requires that you *appreciate* the consequences of the act, including its typical attendant pitfalls or dangers: the fact that, after certain services have been provided, you will be legally required to pay a certain sum; the fact that you will have a scar, etc.

It is not immediately apparent what significance is to be attached to the term "appreciate." This might simply be another term for knowing, used specifically to apply to dangers. It might, on the other hand, mean that you not merely know of these dangers, but that you also take them into account in making your decision, that you appraise them in a rational way.

What is at stake in choosing between the "functioning" standard (that background understanding of competency imputed to medicine) and the legal background understanding (that one is competent with regard to a particular transaction if he understands information surrounding that situation and appreciates the consequences of his actions)?

The first point of divergence is that whereas the legal standard is rather narrowly focused upon the possession and appreciation of information as a mark of competence, the medical standard looks more broadly at action and behavior, and, in particular, interaction. Very broadly speaking, the law has had a traditional inclination to look at people as though they were ambulatory neocortexes. This is an unfortunate perspective even for those who agree that ration-

ality is definitive of humanity, and that obedience to the law can only result from rationality. For surely rationality can express itself actively, rather than by bare ratiocination. Further, even given a mentalist perspective on rationality and thinking, the medical standard is forthright in emphasizing that we can only judge rationality through observable behavior; and in drawing the implication that all behavior, not just speech, should be considered evidential.

The second issue between them might be said to concern the proper scope of competency judgments. In looking at "functioning," medicine might be saying that competency is all of a piece, and so needs to be understood in a global fashion. The law, on the contrary, insists upon an individualized standard. One may be competent to consent to treatment but not to experimentation; one may be competent to prepare this will but not to agree to that contract. Rights of self-determination can be conferred in some areas and arenas, but not in others.

The medical view must surely be rejected, particularly in light of the fact of marginal competence. One's functioning itself is not, after all, of a piece: a person can be relatively successful in his work yet fail dismally at forming personal relationships—a deeply neurotic executive. The institutionalized retarded individual might be unable to work but form close and meaningful personal attachments. When attached to the broad scope of behavior at which medicine might look, a global view—one is competent in all things, or in none—can place an unbearable weight of history upon an individual, and lead to the "labeling" of people in an unjust way.

One issue at hand between these two background views, then, is that of individualization. Is a person's competency to be determined by sole reference to the matter at hand, as the law would have it, or with reference to an entire pattern of behavior, as medicine would have us think? Simply put, since situations of choice differ, competence cannot be an across-the-board affair; and, since situations of choice are similar, competence cannot be entirely determined in an ad hoc fashion.

In exploring the question of individualization, we will first need to distinguish between two approaches to competency, those of policy and of concept; a distinction of major importance for analysis.

What is meant by the policy level? A standard of competency is to *achieve* certain practical things, chief among these being the preservation of a balance between freedom and protection. The policy view judges criteria of competence by the results they yield. Good results, results with which society is pleased, are determinative of good criteria for competence.

Yet behind the policy view, and to some degree presupposed by it, is the *conceptual* level. For it, the basic desideratum of a standard is that it mark off the competent from the incompetent. It does no good to be informed that some need to be protected, others need to have their choices respected, and that a good rule will strike a balance. We need to know who *belongs* in each of these categories. The conceptual view supplies a theory of competency, a theory about why some people—whom we term the competent—are granted the privilege of making decisions, even silly decisions, while this privilege is denied to another class of people. The theory will enable us to distinguish between warranted and unwarranted paternalism, on the basis of qualities which differ across populations. It tells us who is entitled to autonomy, and who is entitled to protection.

Once we understand the concepts and policies underlying a given situation, we can assess the type and level of competence desirable. Some situations obviously require different competencies. A justified imputation of criminal liability, for example, must enquire into aspects of the person different from those needed to be able to fix civil liability. To that extent, we must individualize the question of competence.

On the other hand, some situations are sufficiently analogous that a single test of competence might serve for all within the set. The analogies must rest upon similarities between the concepts and/or the policies underlying the situations. A simple example of such a set of situations (or "situation-types"), would be non-capital criminal liability. Consistency demands that at some point the similarity between two situations must be so great that they must both use the same test of competence.

Here is another candidate for a situation-type. It could be argued that the age for consent to medical treatment should not be greater than the age at which one may voluntarily join, or be conscripted into, the armed forces.[10] The age which we fix for service represents society's judgment about when a person is sufficiently mature to be uprooted from his family and to act autonomously, the age at which a person can take responsibility for choices that will govern his entire future course of life. On a conceptual level, it seems that these are the same qualities that are involved in deciding whether to undergo medical treatment.

With regard to policy questions, though, there is clearly a difference between medical consent and armed service. On the one hand, the army might demand physical development of a sort that does not enter into competence for consent; and so a it is quite reasonable that a *later* age for army service might be required than is needed for medical consent. On the other hand, policy considerations might constrain us to limit or qualify the age for consent for reasons that stem from the question of financial obligation. An argument for requiring the consent of a parent to a procedure upon a minor who is living at home is that the parent is obligated to pay for the minor's treatment. (This policy consideration might instead be addressed by placing financial liability for the course of treatment upon the minor in the case in which the parent has not consented; in that way we would not have compromised the true question of the minor's competence, as we would do in the event we set a higher age of competence for this conceptually irrelevant circumstance. Policies, unlike concepts, may be achieved in many different ways.)

With regard to the question of individualization, then, neither the legal nor the medical background understandings of competence are fully satisfactory. From the theory of a situation—its policy and conceptual components—emerges a single test of situation-appropriate competence;

yet several situations may be served by the same theory. Let me develop this notion of theory a bit further in discussing the tests for competency proposed for consent to medical treatment.

III. CRITERIA OF COMPETENCE: CONSENT TO MEDICAL TREATMENT

In some situations, it is not clear how the background understandings of competence may be applied; and in others, the background understandings seem unacceptably simple-minded. As a result, variant tests of competency are developed. The situation with which I will deal concerns competence to consent to medical treatment. I take this case partly because of its intrinsic interest and importance, and partly because of its symbolic significance. Consent to treatment seems an ideal testing-ground for theories concerning the scope and nature of human autonomy. Also, the concepts and policies underlying consent have been explored extensively by courts and scholars.

There are five main tests for competence to consent to or to refuse, treatment, delineated clearly by Roth, Meisel, and Lidz[11] but mentioned by others as well.[12] They are as follows:

1. One is competent to consent to treatment if, in consenting, one achieves a *reasonable result* or is seeking a reasonable outcome.

2. One is competent to consent to treatment if one has followed a rational process in making up one's mind, if one can give or has given *rational reasons* for the choice made.

3. One is competent to consent to treatment if one is *able to express consent* to, or refusal of, that treatment, for whatever reasons and despite the seeming unreasonableness of the outcome.

4. One is competent to consent to treatment if one has the *ability to understand* and knowingly act upon the information which the doctor supplies in the course of "obtaining a consent."

5. One is competent to consent to treatment if one *actually understands* and acts upon the information which is provided by the physi-

cian. (This test differs from the previous one in that our judgment is now made on the basis of the assimilation by the patient of the information provided about this specific procedure. By contrast, the "ability to understand" test could examine the patient's ability to understand, not *this* information, but information of an *equivalent complexity*.)

To make matters a bit more concrete, consider this example: Jones is being seen by Dr. Smith, a psychiatrist. Dr. Smith judges that Jones would benefit from taking Thorazine, a major tranquilizer or anti-psychotic agent. Jones presumably refuses; had he agreed to this "treatment of choice," although in theory he might be competent, incompetent, or somewhere in between, nobody is likely to raise the question in any practical forum. Is Jones competent (in which case presumably his refusal will be effectuated), or incompetent (in which case steps may be taken to initiate proceedings culminating in the legally-sanctioned, forcible administration of the drug)?

This question should be a practical one for psychiatrists. It might be objected that the question of competence is properly one for the courts. While this is of course true, nevertheless someone must initiate the inquiry leading to the proceeding, and psychiatrists are well-placed to do this.

Even with the minimal information given above about Jones, two of the above standards could decide the question of his competence. One would be the reasonable outcome test. Presumably, Dr. Smith would feel that Jones had failed this test, that, in refusing, Jones is *per se* irrational. The test need not lead us to *this* result, however, for although Dr. Smith may be a reasonable man himself, his responses are neither exhaustive or definitive of the repertoire of the reasonable man. A third party, lawyer, psychiatrist, or plumber, might feel that the reasonable man would *always* refuse administration of Thorazine, or, in *Jones's circumstances* would refuse Thorazine. Yet another observer might believe that a reasonable man could swing either way in this choice, that the factors pro and con the administration of the drug are fairly evenly balanced. But the interesting thing about all of these positions is that none of them require more knowledge about Jones. If anything further needs to be learned, it is how the reasonable man would respond.

Nor need we know anything further about this case in order to decide the question of Jones's competence under the third test, that of the "ability to make a choice." *Ex hypothesi,* Jones has chosen to refuse the treatment. Any further knowledge concerning itself with Jones's maturity, intellect, emotional state, and so on, is, for this test, superfluous.

In the case of test two, we would need to ask Jones why he has refused the treatment and, if those reasons are judged to be rational, his refusal is competent. Suppose Jones indicates that he fears delayed side-effects of the drug, or feels that he is "getting better" and his condition will clear up without the drug, or believes his psychiatrist to be incompetent. These all sound like rational reasons. In contrast, he might say that taking the drug will motivate those who are electrically controlling his behavior to turn him off. This, presumably, will be judged an irrational reason, and a conclusive indication that his decision was incompetent.

The fourth test is not interested in why Jones has refused, but in whether he can understand the information which we feel should be relevant to consent or refusal. Is Jones so mentally defective, or so out of touch with reality, that we cannot get this *kind* of material through? The fifth test, that of actual understanding, asks the same question, but this time the object of inquiry is whether Jones understands the information provided about the drug. Operationally these tests would proceed as follows: Jones would be informed either about the therapeutic intervention (the reasons for its recommendation, its risks and alternative methods of treatment if any), or else he would be informed of other matters of an equivalent complexity. Smith would query Jones to elicit whether this information has been assimilated; if it has, Jones's refusal or consent would be binding, in the sense that it

would have been conclusively demonstrated that Jones is competent….

V. A "RECOGNIZABLE REASONS" CRITERION OF COMPETENCY

… Consent is valuable in its protection of freedom. Hence, it is process-centered, and must concern itself with what goes into the decision, and not merely with the result. Since it is a result of our rights to freedom, it is person-centered, and depends upon characteristics of the individual himself.

The last of the criteria to be examined, that of rational reasons, comes closest to satisfying these requirements. Under it, an individual is competent if he can supply rational reasons for his decision. This criterion serves well in that it is process-centered, and in its dependence upon characteristics of the person himself. It can be criticized on the grounds that it is an overly-paternalistic criterion, since it distinguishes between acceptable (rational) and unacceptable reasons for action. This criticism loses its force, however, if latitude is given to the notion of rational reasons, if we are willing to accept as rational reasons arguments which we would not find decisive, but agree are relevant.

Perhaps this point would seem more plausible if instead of speaking of "rational reasons," a phrase which is, anyway, abominably redundant, we spoke of "recognizable reasons." Reasons consist of premises that argue towards a practical conclusion. For a reason to be recognizable, then, it must contain both acceptable premises and a conclusion related to those premises. Since we wish to give latitude to an individual's own value system, one which we do not necessarily share, it is not required that the conclusion "follow" from the premises, in that we believe the premises are *strong* enough to justify the conclusion.

There are two ways in which a person might fail to produce recognizable reasons. The first is by founding his argument upon premises known to be false. This was done by Yetter, for example, in her refusal of a breast biopsy because of her belief that the surgery will affect her reproductive ability. The second is by producing reasons which, even if true and weighted heavily, fail to support the conclusion drawn, e.g., by refusing surgery because it's Tuesday. A *non-sequitur* is not an argument.

That which also allows us to grant freedom of action in our society is the warranted belief that, by and large, one person's choices will be recognizable by others. It is only given this condition that we can empathize with a person's behavior, and it is only given this condition that behavior becomes sufficiently predictable to enable us to live together in society.

Freedom within society is a reciprocal affair, which requires of me that I order my affairs in the light of what others may be expected to do. It therefore presumes a degree of commonality and predictability of motivation. From this concept of freedom there follows some version of the "rational reasons" criterion of competence; for freedom is only possible in the light of the characteristics possessed by recognizable reasons.

It needs to be noticed, however, that a considerable potential for abuse lurks in such a criterion. People, however competent, are not always prepared to give reasons for their choices. We should also recall that rationality can be demonstrated in the way in which a person orders his life, not merely in the verbal justifications he gives for his behavior.

In the light of these considerations, perhaps competence should generally be judged in a dispositional way. If a person has been disposed to be competent—if he has ordered his life within our society, made and carried out long-range plans, and so on—then extraordinarily strong evidence would need to be produced in attempting to prove that he had failed to achieve a competent decision. The reverse would be true for one with dispositional incompetence. The relevant comparison would be with decisions other than medical treatment, but involving equivalent seriousness and complexity, which he has faced; which could, depending on the nature of the proposed medical intervention, require

examination of such traditional aspects of adjustment as work-experience, family life, and ability to run an independent household. Perhaps a strong, but defensible, burden of proof should need satisfaction to treat a "dispositional competent's" decision as incompetent, and vice versa.

With regard to information and its relationship to competence, I am suggesting a reversal of the traditional roles. Traditionally, it was thought that the ascertainment of competence was an issue which needed to be decided prior to the transmittal of information. To the contrary, I believe that information is prior to competence, in that a competent decision includes, but extends beyond, the requirement that the person involved be able to allow the informing process to enter into his decision-making in a substantial way. He must be capable of utilizing the information provided in formulating his reasons.

This burden of informing the person is recognized as a heavy one. If understanding cannot be achieved by the ordinary process, then further methods must be sought. The method of informing chosen must be one designed to enlighten the individual in question. Only when it is clear that no manner of informing the patient will serve does the issue of competence become moot. Since competence is primarily concerned with the manner in which the individual uses the information, the prerequisite to competence is information.

Our discussion also inclines us to an intriguing perspective upon the institutionalized marginally competent. Institutionalization has been said to limit an individual's competence by denying him the opportunity to develop his decision-making capacities and by insulating him from the world of responsibility. Institutionalization does something else as well. It limits the *evidence* of competency. It deprives an individual of a history of successful decision-making, which would have given outside observers confidence in his competency. There is not much which the individual could reasonably do to combat this implication, and so we must act on his behalf: first, by sympathetically examining his attempts at decision-making; second, and more fundamentally, by providing opportunities within the institution for the individual to develop and reveal his capacity to take responsibility for his own actions.

There is no use to assuming competence into existence. Making a decision does not mean a mumbled "yes" or "no"; it assumes an underlying process into which relevant facts about the world enter in a recognizable way. If those relevant facts can by no fashion be communicated, if they cannot be ordered into an argument supporting a conclusion, then competence is not present. Yet a very great wrong is perpetrated in not making the attempt to recognize competence when it is present, albeit veiled. The most serious harm we can visit upon a human being is to tell him that his viewpoint, his innermost self, is of no worth. Whatever the outcome, the very attempt to elicit a competent opinion, if conscientiously carried out, can serve to allay this harm. Whatever the outcome, by entering into his world he is reassured that he is indeed a being of significance to others.

Notes

1. See Freedman, *On the Rights of the Voiceless,* 3 J. Med. & Phil. (1978), and works discussed there.
2. J. Wilson, The Rights of Adolescents in the Mental Health Care System II (1978).
3. R. Allen, E. Fernter & H. Welhofen, Mental Impairment And Legal Incompetence I (1968 Citing Report Of The Presidents Panel On Mental Retardation (1962).
4. Gaylin, *The Problem of Psychosurgery* in W. Gaylin, R. Neville & J. Meister eds., Operation on the Mind 13 (1975).
5. Friedman, *Legal Regulation of Behavior Modification in Institutional Settings,* 17 Ariz L. Rev 80, 95 (1975).
6. Neuwirth, Heister & Goldrich, *Capacity, Competence, Consent: Voluntary Sterilization of the Mentally Retarded*, Col Human Rights L. Rev 452 (1975).
7. Roth, Meisel & Lidz, *Tests of Competency to Consent to Treatment.* 134 Am J. Psych 279 (1977).
8. Allen et al. *supra* note 3, Appendix A, Part 1.
9. *Id.*, 264.
10. Freedman, *A Moral Theory of Informed Consent*, 5 Hastings Centre Rep. (1975).
11. Roth et al., *supra* note 7.
12. *See, eg.,* Friedman, *supra* note 5; G. Annas, L. Glantz & B. Kayz, Informed Consent To Human Experimentation: The Subjects Dilemma 153 (1977).

ECT and Special Problems of Informed Consent

Charles M. Culver and Ronald M. Green

Can a severely depressed patient validly consent to a course of ECT? Can this patient validly refuse consent? Although the requirement of informed consent is a firm part of the ethical practice of medicine, two separate problems make these questions appropriate and urgent where ECT is concerned. One problem is that ECT is usually prescribed for patients who are seriously depressed and whose ability to consent might therefore be open to question. A second problem concerns the therapy itself: ECT has been held by some to be an intrusive physical technique with inherently unacceptable risks and hence beyond the range of rational choice. While these two problems challenge the validity of informed consent to ECT from different directions, both throw open to question the current practice of employing ECT on the basis of patient consent.

DEPRESSION AND COMPETENCE TO CONSENT

The first of these two problems is not unique to ECT. It is encountered frequently in the fields of psychiatry and neurology where the brain, the organ that plays a decisive role in the giving of consent, is often involved in the disease process and may, as with ECT, itself be the direct object of treatment. One might therefore suppose that psychiatry and neurology must be inherently paternalistic when serious mental illness is involved, that is, that they must involve minimal reliance on the patient's expressed wishes regarding treatment and primary reliance on the treatment team's (or family's) judgment concerning what is in the patient's best interests.[1]

In fact, clinical practice does not appear to bear out this supposition. Not only is the patient's consent actively sought in such cases by responsible physicians, but a patient's refusal to consent is usually respected. How can we account for this? Part of the answer seems to be that in the view of most psychiatrists serious mental illness does not usually render a patient incapable of making informed decisions about treatment. Patient A is a case in point.

> *Case 1*. Ms. A, a 71-year-old woman, was admitted to our unit with a moderately severe depression. She had had three other depressive episodes over the past 40 years. The third episode, which occurred 6 years earlier, was the most severe. She was initially given antidepressant medication; when this proved ineffective ECT was recommended. Ms. A consented and received a course of eight sessions of ECT, which resulted in a prompt alleviation of her depression and a return to her usual active life.
>
> Ms. A remained symptom-free for 6 years, but then once again, without any clear precipitant, she became depressed, with a significant sleep disturbance, loss of appetite and weight, and occasional thoughts of suicide. She was hospitalized

and given antidepressant medication, which, as before, proved ineffective. She readily agreed to a course of ECT. Despite her depression Ms. A appeared to her psychiatrists to be capable of understanding her situation and making an informed decision about her treatment. She understood that ECT would almost certainly alleviate her depression as it had before, and she clearly preferred ECT to the options of no further treatment or some combination of continued antidepressant medication with psychotherapeutic support. After only four treatments, her mood improved substantially, her appetite and sleep pattern returned to normal and her suicidal thoughts ceased. She was discharged and 6 months later remained in normal mood.

Ms. A seems to us to illustrate a quite unproblematic use of ECT. Most, but not all, depressed patients appear to be as capable of making an informed decision as she was. However, some patients seem to be unable to give or not give consent at all. Occasionally patients withhold consent when their physicians and relatives believe that it would be most reasonable for them to agree. And, although rarely, a severely depressed patient refuses ECT at a time when it appears that he or she will die without it.

The response of psychiatrists to these cases differs widely. In some instances, treatment is initiated independently of the patient's wishes, while in other cases those wishes are respected. The reasons why one course or another is taken are not always clearly articulated, and this lack of clarity is partly due to the inadequacy of terms used to describe patients whose consent is more problematic than Ms. A's was. When psychiatrists and others discuss these cases, terms such as "competence," "rationality," and "capability" are often used. The terms are often used interchangeably, imprecisely, and in a confusing manner. For example, a patient who considers and then refuses what his or her physicians believe to be a very necessary treatment may be labeled "incompetent."

On further inquiry it is often the case that there is no independent measure of the patient's competence; rather, the label has come from the treatment-refusal decision. Those doing the labeling have moved from their disagreement with the patient's decision to a label that characterizes the patient as globally incompetent. This kind of linguistic move is confusing at best. Patients who make what appear to be unwise treatment decisions often carry out most of their other activities quite competently. But there is a further danger in this too-quick and too-global labeling: it may reassure the physician that a particular paternalistic insistence on treatment is justified when it may not be. This is because it is easier for most of us to think we are treating an incompetent patient (despite his or her protestations) than to think we are forcing our own treatment decision on a competent patient who disagrees with it.

Because of these difficulties we want to suggest a particular use of terminology in dealing with these matters, which we hope will be clarifying, and a certain associated moral reasoning. We suggest first of all that "competent" and "incompetent" not be used as global attributes of a person but rather be applied more narrowly with respect to particular abilities, for example, that a person be described as "competent to do X" only when certain criteria are met. We will say then that a patient is *competent to decide* about having a particular treatment (such as ECT) when the following are satisfied: 1) the patient knows that the physician believes the patient is ill and in need of treatment (although the patient may not agree), 2) the patient knows that the physician believes this particular treatment may help the patient's illness, and 3) the patient knows he or she is being called upon to make a decision regarding this treatment.[2]

These are deliberately "minimal" criteria because the intent, for reasons explained below, is to consider a patient competent to make a treatment decision unless he or she is *clearly* incompetent to do so.

We suggest further that "rational" and "irrational" be used as attributes of the decisions made by patients. Thus while some patients will be deemed incompetent to make treatment decisions, the rest will be considered competent to make decisions that may be judged rational or irrational. An irrational decision is one based on an irrational belief (e.g., a patient does not believe he or she has cancer despite overwhelming evidence that he or she has) or on an irrational desire (e.g., a patient prefers to die rather than have a gangrenous foot amputated but can give no reason for this choice).[3] This use of "irrational," which will be illustrated in some of the examples below, is meant to accord with the way the term is usually employed, not only by psychiatrists but by people in general.

Thus we would view Ms. A as having been competent to make a treatment decision and would also view her decision as a rational one. We now wish to apply the above terminology to other more troublesome cases to see whether it helps clarify and make explicit the way we (and others) believe it appropriate to respond in such cases.

THE PATIENT INCOMPETENT TO MAKE A TREATMENT DECISION

Case 2. Ms. B, a 69-year-old woman with a biopsy-proven unresectable retroperitoneal sarcoma, was admitted to our unit in a profound confusional state that was thought to be a result of delirium, a very severe psychotic depression, or a combination of the two. Approximately 1 year earlier she had been admitted to the hospital with a similar mental syndrome. At that time a retroperitoneal mass had been identified and biopsied during laparotomy. Treatment with ECT at that time (1 year before the present admission) resulted in dramatic clearing of her confusional state and melancholia, enabling Ms. B to resume a satisfying life with her family for a period of about 10 months, when the current confusional state developed.

At this point Ms. B was disoriented to place and time and was severely agitated and restless. She was not able to give understandable answers to most direct questions, and in general her speech consisted of incoherent babbling. An extensive search for a metabolic, pharmacologic, or structural cause for her mental syndrome yielded no positive results. Her retroperitoneal sarcoma appeared to have increased somewhat in size, but this could not be directly correlated with her change in mental function. Her sarcoma was in no way felt to be immediately life-threatening. Her physicians felt that ECT was again indicated but that she was not competent to give informed consent to any treatment procedure. The hospital attorney was of the opinion that ECT could be used if the unanimous informed consent of her three adult children was obtained. Her children did consent, and a course of ECT was again administered. A similar gratifying improvement resulted.

Ms. B was not competent to decide about having ECT according to our criteria: there seemed no way to make her aware that there was a treatment decision to be made, let alone communicate to her why her doctors believed treatment was necessary.

We believe that under these circumstances it is usually sufficient to allow next-of-kin to make treatment decisions about the patient's care. They are usually in the best position to know the patient's values and to apply those values to the decision at hand. Any position about treatment the patient has *previously* expressed (while competent) should of course be given great weight and should almost always be determinative.

It is because we believe that patients incompetent to make a treatment decision can usually be treated with only next-of-kin's consent, while far more stringent criteria must be met to treat patients who competently decide against treatment, that our criteria for competence are so minimal. We want to allow next-of-kin to represent a patient's interests only in those cases in which it is abundantly clear that the patient is simply unable to represent his or her own interests.

COMPETENTLY MADE IRRATIONAL DECISIONS

As we have indicated, patients can be competent to make a decision, but their decisions can be viewed by their physicians and others as irrational. They may tenaciously hold patently false beliefs about themselves or their conditions, or they may have desires we usually consider to be irrational. Nevertheless, in most instances patients' wishes are and should be respected even when they seem significantly irrational.

Nonetheless, psychiatry (and, to a lesser extent, neurology) seems to be distinguished by a somewhat lesser reluctance than other branches of medicine to override the wishes of patients who make seriously irrational decisions. This probably reflects the judgment that such patients not infrequently make irrational decisions that seem part of the disease from which they suffer and that they can very frequently be expected to reverse their wishes after treatment. However, competence should be accorded considerable respect in the treatment of even severe mental illness, and psychiatrists should require a compelling reason to overrule the wishes of a patient displaying minimal competence to make treatment decisions. Where ECT is concerned this means that if a patient understands the reasons for his or her physician's recommendation of ECT and also knows that consent is being elicited for treatment, this is prima facie a strong reason for respecting the patient's wishes, even when the treatment team disagrees. Ms. C illustrates this situation.

Case 3. Ms. C, a rather frail 55-year-old married woman, was admitted to our unit with a 6-month history of a moderately severe depression. She was transferred to us from a community hospital where her local psychiatrist had tried two different antidepressant medications but had stopped both because of her marked hypotensive response to even the usual low starting dosages.

When she came to us Ms. C was markedly depressed. She had lost a moderate amount of weight and was sleeping poorly but maintained a fairly adequate intake of food and water. We recommended ECT to her. However, she firmly and consistently refused. She had had a close friend who had received ECT; while her friend's depression had improved at the time, she had killed herself a year later. Ms. C acknowledged that ECT "may not have been responsible" for her friend's suicide but said she was terrified of it.

We therefore devised a drug regimen in which we gave her a very small nighttime dosage (10 mg) of desipramine, a tricyclic antidepressant, which we later increased slowly in small (10 mg) increments. We also gave her small morning and noontime doses of methylphenidate, a stimulant. She suffered from significant orthostasis, but with close nursing care this problem proved manageable. After 2 to 3 weeks her depression began to respond. In an additional 2 weeks she was feeling quite well again, and her hypotension had ceased to be a significant problem.

In this case Ms. C's physicians and her husband all felt that ECT should be tried. The probability of significant and rapid benefit was very high and the risk was very small (see below). The alternative to ECT seemed to be a high probability of continued suffering for a long period of time with only slim hope that further alternative treatment might help. The patient's not choosing ECT for the reason she gave seemed on balance irrational to us. However, the harm she risked by not choosing ECT did not seem extreme enough to justify our considering any more coercive efforts.[4] We viewed her as having competently made a decision that was irrational but that should be respected.

In actual fact, we encounter very few patients who refuse ECT. Why should this be so? Probably the most important reason is that we generally suggest ECT only when antidepressant medications have been given an adequate (3–5 week)

trial and have failed. Thus ECT-eligible patients have typically been suffering from depression for some time and want to relieve their pain. If we suggested ECT much earlier—for example, as an alternative to trying medications—we would probably encounter more refusals.

Does the fact that someone is suffering a great deal make suspect their consent to a procedure that holds out a very high probability of relief? We believe it explains *why* they usually consent but it does not invalidate that consent; if one were to make that claim, one would have to disallow the majority of patient consents in medicine. Gall bladders and appendices are removed at times of pain, and probably fewer patients refuse these procedures than refuse ECT. Our patients who consent to ECT seem to make that decision for reasons analogous to those used by patients generally: they dislike very much the suffering associated with being depressed, and while they may have some misgivings about undergoing ECT they would prefer undergoing the treatment to the alternative of continued depression. Assuming that ECT is an acceptable treatment (see below), there seems no other rational basis on which it *could* be chosen, either by the patient or by someone representing his or her interests.[5]

However, there are rare cases involving competent patients in which coercive paternalistic intervention occurs and seems justifiable. These are essentially all cases in which ECT appears to be necessary to save the patient's life. Ms. D is an example.

Case 4. Ms. D, a 69-year-old married woman, was admitted to our unit with a depressive illness of 6 months' duration. Approximately 1 year before admission she was discovered on a routine examination elsewhere to have an elevated lactic dehydrogenase. A liver-spleen scan was done and showed her spleen to be enlarged. No further studies were carried out.

Approximately 6 months before her hospitalization Ms. D's husband suffered a heart attack and was subsequently confined to a nursing home. She stated in retrospect that her "world went to pieces" at that time. She gradually became depressed and experienced characteristic changes in appetite, weight, and sleep. She refused to seek medical attention. Eventually her husband called his lawyer, who summoned the police to her home, where they found her in a state of neglect and brought her to the emergency room at her local hospital. She was admitted and noted to be depressed, but was alert, oriented, and cooperative. Positive physical findings included anemia, leukopenia, hypoproteinemia, and a further increase in spleen size. She was seen by a consulting psychiatrist, who thought she was significantly depressed and recommended treatment with tricyclic antidepressant medication. She agreed to take the medicine, but did not improve. The patient's internist recommended a bone marrow examination and other laboratory studies. Ms. D refused for reasons that she would not clearly discuss, saying only that she "didn't want to bother." She was transferred to our medical center for a further attempt at evaluation and possible treatment.

Our evaluation confirmed the above impressions. She was seen by a neurologist and by a hematologist, who recommended a CT scan, an EEG, a lumbar puncture, and a bone marrow examination. The patient's clinical condition continued to deteriorate, and she began refusing most food and fluids. She refused to allow most of the recommended diagnostic tests to be performed. Repeated efforts by us and by her family to obtain her consent for these studies were unsuccessful and were now met by her saying that "I deserve to die."

We felt she was indeed at risk of death through malnutrition and electrolyte disturbance resulting from inadequate fluids and nutrition. Her husband

and son were informed of the seriousness of the situation. Her son obtained an attorney, went to court, and on the basis of the clinical details we provided, obtained temporary legal guardianship of his mother. He then authorized us to proceed with the diagnostic procedures deemed necessary. These were done despite her objections. The hematology consultant concluded that the most likely hematologic diagnosis was myelofibrosis. Her long-term prognosis from this disorder was thought to be questionable, but her prognosis for the next several years was quite good.

Her son authorized us to proceed with ECT for her now severe melancholia. She was treated initially without her consent and over her stated objections.

After the second treatment she gave verbal consent to further treatments; after the fourth treatment she became brighter in mood, began eating well, and was much more verbal. After a total of 10 treatments Ms. D reported that she felt quite well. She exhibited a mild post-ECT delirium, which subsequently cleared. She was able to express appropriate feelings of sadness about her husband's illness. She told us that she was very grateful we had treated her. At her last follow-up visit, several months after discharge, she was doing quite well.

We viewed Ms. D as entirely competent to make a treatment decision according to our criteria: she knew that her doctors believed she had a very serious depressive illness and that they further believed that ECT was necessary to save her life. She clearly knew that she was being asked to consent to ECT. However, she refused consent, giving no reason other than her belief that she deserved to die. This choice of non-treatment seemed seriously irrational to us and almost certainly a reflection of her profound depressive illness. Thus we believed that paternalistically forcing treatment on her was justified—that one can universally advocate such an intervention when the harm or evil one is probably fore-stalling is so great, the evil one is perpetrating is probably so much less, and the patient's refusal is significantly irrational (2).

Because we viewed Ms. D as competent to decide, we made every effort to obtain her consent to treatment. When this was not forthcoming it was only after much discussion among members of the treatment team and the patient's family that (legal) measures were instituted to allow coercive treatment. Thus her wishes (not to have treatment) were taken very seriously and forced us into a searching examination of our own reasoning. Of course, physicians should engage in a similarly thoughtful weighing of risks and benefits whenever any treatment is recommended to and discussed with a patient. However, if the patient does not consent, we believe open discussion with other staff and family members is called for (except in genuine emergency situations) before paternalistic intervention is ever justified. This requirement is stringent but seems desirable whenever a patient competently makes a decision with which his or her own doctors disagree, and it shows why the consent process is so important when ECT (or any other treatment) is involved.

IS ECT AN INHERENTLY IRRATIONAL TREATMENT?

A quite different challenge to the validity of consent to ECT is posed by those critics who contend that by its very nature this treatment is not rationally choice-worthy. This appears to be the view, for example, of Friedberg, who has characterized ECT as the deliberate infliction of brain damage, which results in serious mental impairment in the form of memory loss and disorientation (6, 7). He considers ECT so un-choice-worthy as therapy that he challenges the moral integrity of physicians who offer it.

Friedberg's rather one-sided and simplistic view of ECT is not shared by the majority of psychiatrists who deal with depressed patients, and it is not borne out by objective studies on the effi-cacy or side effects of this treatment. The pre-ponderance of evidence suggests that ECT usu-ally effects a dramatic amelioration of depression and that it does so in the overwhelming majority of cases with little or no long-term impairment of memory or other injurious sequelae (8–10). In fact, many psychiatrists feel that ECT is so safe, rapid, and efficacious that to refuse to suggest it to seriously depressed patients (who run a signif-icantly high risk of death because of their illness) is itself irresponsible.

Nonetheless, it seems clear that we do not yet know with sufficient precision the frequency of the significant persistent memory loss that does apparently rarely follow ECT, and we do not know anything about patient characteristics (e.g., age, sex, type of lateralization of brain functions) that may increase its likelihood. Many more studies of the kind reported by Squire (11) are needed.

However, it must be emphasized that the issue of the rationality of consenting to ECT does not depend on obtaining any more factual information than we now have. For example, suppose that Friedberg's very negative portrayal of ECT were exactly correct; it would still not follow that it would be irrational for a patient to choose it or immoral for a physician to offer it. This is because it is not usually considered irra-tional to take major steps (including even killing oneself) to escape persistent and unbearable pain, and severe depressive illness frequently involves psychic pain of this sort. Thus a patient who chose to undergo some mild brain damage, which would result in mild persistent memory deficits, in order to escape from severe psychic pain that could not be relieved in any other way would not be making an inherently irrational decision.

However, no critic who has examined the evidence (even the same evidence cited by Friedberg; see Frankel's report [9]) believes that Friedberg's very negative appraisal of ECT is correct. The overwhelming majority of patients incur no residual memory loss at all. Thus the best description of the choice confronting the patient is the following:

1. Continued depression on the one hand (or whatever condition it is hoped ECT might alleviate) with, usually, a continuation of prior attempts at therapy, or
2. ECT on the other hand, which is characterized by certain probable benefits (excellent chance of alleviation of depression; usually lesser chance of alleviation of other conditions) and certain risks (very good to excellent chance of no residual effects; lesser chance [perhaps 10%–50% but not yet known] of minor memory problems that may persist 6–12 months; rare chance [perhaps less than 1% but not exactly known] of moderate to marked memory problems that may persist for longer than a year and in extremely rare cases be chronic and disabling). The risk of memory impairment should be adjusted upward in the case of bilateral ECT and downward with right unilateral ECT.

We believe it is this information which should be given to the patient in the early stage of the informed consent procedure. We hope the day will soon arrive when we can be more precise in communicating the magnitude of the risks involved, but we believe the above summarizes the research literature coupled with our own experience. We have found little difficulty in informing patients of these risks and benefits. We do not believe that our current lack of precise knowledge makes the patient's decision inordinately difficult; many treatments for which we ask consent in medicine contain a much greater zone of uncertainty about outcome than does ECT.

CONCLUSIONS

ECT appears to be an eminently rational treatment for patients to choose in many clinical situations. The vast majority of very depressed (and other) patients do consent to having ECT when it is recommended, and there seems no basis on which to question the validity of their consent.

However, there are a few patients from whom consent is not forthcoming. A few of these are patients who are incompetent to make a treatment decision at all and their next-of-kin must usually be relied upon.

Finally, some patients do refuse ECT. In some cases their refusal seems rational, e.g., when it objectively seems possible but not probable that ECT will help their condition and/or (very rarely) when ECT itself holds a high risk of morbidity. Usually, given the type of clinical situations in which ECT is recommended, a patient's refusal seems irrational to the treatment team. However, except in extreme cases involving a probable risk of death in the near future without ECT, physicians treating depressed patients will not err morally by respecting their patients' informed decisions about treatment.

Notes

1. For a general discussion of paternalistic medical interventions and when they are and are not justified, see Gert and Culver's work (1, 2).
2. These criteria are similar to the criteria employed in most jurisdictions to ascertain that a person has competently made a will: the individual must know he or she *is* making a will, know what his or her assets are, and know who his or her natural heirs are. See Roth and associates' discussion (3) for a useful elaboration of various meanings that have been attached to "competence."
3. The following would be regarded as irrational desires: the desire to die, to suffer pain (physical or mental), to be disabled, or to be deprived of freedom, opportunity, or pleasure. It is not always irrational to desire these things, but it is irrational to desire them without some adequate *reason*. It is sometimes difficult to decide on the adequacy of a person's reason for acting on what would otherwise be an irrational desire. For a fuller account of rationality, see Gert's discussion (4, pp. 27–37).
4. For a full elaboration of the features of a case that determine when paternalistic intervention is justifiable, see Gert and Culver's work (2).
5. Using the analysis and terminology proposed by Gert and Duggan (5), we would say that while the decision to consent to medical procedures is often made in the presence of coercive incentives (e.g., suffering and risk of death), it is nonetheless voluntary, i.e., the patient has the ability to will to have or not to have the treatment depending on whether such coercive incentives are or are not present.

References

1. Gert B, Culver CM: Paternalistic behavior. *Philosophy and Public Affairs* 6:45–57, 1976.
2. Gert B, Culver CM: The justification of paternalism. *Ethics* 89:199–210, 1979.
3. Roth LH, Meisel A, Lidz CW: Tests of competency to consent to treatment. *Am J Psychiatry* 134:279–284, 1977.
4. Gert B: *The Moral Rules*. New York, Harper & Row, 1975.
5. Gert B, Duggan TJ: Free will as the ability to will. *Nous* 13: 197–217, 1979.
6. Friedberg J: Electroshock therapy: let's stop blasting the brain. *Psychology Today* 9(8):13–23, 1975.
7. Friedberg J: Shock treatment, brain damage, and memory loss: a neurological perspective. *Am J Psychiatry* 134:1010–1014, 1977.
8. Fink M: Myths of "shock therapy." *Am J Psychiatry* 134:991–996, 1977.
9. Frankel FH: Current perspectives on ECT: a discussion. *Am J Psychiatry* 134:1014–1019, 1977.
10. Greenblatt M: Efficacy of ECT in affective and schizophrenic illness. *Am J Psychiatry* 134:1001–1005, 1977.
11. Squire LR: ECT and memory loss. *Am J Psychiatry* 134:997–1001, 1977.

Mental Competence and Value: The Problem of Normativity in the Assessment of Decision-Making Capacity

Louis C. Charland

THE DUAL NATURE OF COMPETENCE

The right of an individual to make his or her own medical treatment decisions goes to the heart of what it means to be an autonomous individual. However, there exist circumstances where that right needs to be curtailed. This can occur when an individual is deemed mentally incompetent to make his or her own decisions. Children below a certain age are usually considered incompetent, as are individuals subject to medical or psychiatric conditions that compromise decision-making capacity. Judgments regarding mental competence are often based on special operationalised standards developed to assess it. This article is about the nature of those standards, why they must incorporate elements of value and rationality, and how to reconcile this normative dimension of competence with the requirement that assessments of competence be sufficiently objective. The problem is not only theoretical, but also practical. For in the end, when competence is assessed, either individual freedom is protected or it is violated. You cannot get much more practical about the ethics of autonomy than that.

It is reasonable to require that standards designed to assess competence be objective. Similar tests should yield similar judgments in like cases. The standards employed should be sufficiently objective to be replicable in a manner that yields consistent results across like cases. Anything less would be unjust to those whose competence is at issue. The problem is that objectivity of this sort is both difficult to formulate theoretically and difficult to realise practically. Aside from the fact that existing laws relating to competence vary across jurisdictions, which implies that general criteria must be flexible, there is the deeper problem of how to formulate objective standards for something that is inherently normative. Not surprisingly, standards for competence tend to be extremely open-ended. They tend also to vacillate between specifying what competence is and prescribing what it should be. This is not surprising, since competence is neither pure description nor pure evaluation. It is rather a mixture of both. As one commentator explains: "a psychiatrist may give expert testimony, in his capacity as a trained observer, about a person's competence seen as a factual matter, and the judge may or may not give this testimony practical effect in deciding how we ought to treat that person."[1] Thus in the former case the issue is whether the individual is competent, while in the latter it is whether the individual *should* be considered competent. The dual nature of the concept of competence raises special problems for the requirement that assessments of competence be objective.

One approach to the problem of objectivity is essentially to try to define it away. The strategy is to limit assessment to so-called cognitive capacities and mechanisms alone; for example, the ability to store and retrieve information, to process information, and to appropriately identify what count as the relevant pieces of information. Very basically, the capacities involved are memory, reasoning, and understanding. Many accounts of competence also mention the notion of appreciation. Appreciation consists in an individual's ability to apply his or her current understanding of a given medical condition and its treatment options to him- or herself. It is one thing to understand what schizophrenia is, but quite another to recognise that this information applies to you.

Most existing tests for competence are designed to assess abilities such as those mentioned above. The fact that these abilities are characterised as cognitive is usually deemed essential to the objectivity of the proposed operationalised standards for assessing them. Defining competence in exclusively cognitive terms thus provides a strategy for addressing the

problem of objectivity. So defined, competence has little or nothing to do with value. That makes it easier to view it as an objective commodity. Whether or not such a vision is ethically desirable, it is in any case empirically inadequate. The reason is that decision-making capacity is inextricably normative. There is no such thing as mental competence without value, and normative considerations associated with value cannot be eliminated from the assessment of decision-making capacity. Moreover, the manner in which values figure in competence is not gratuitous. Simply having values is not enough. A certain kind of rationality is also required.

There are a few important precedents that address the relationship between mental competence and value.[2] They are largely the work of philosophers, and two have had an impact far beyond the confines of what is normally considered the province of philosophy. One is referred to in a major legal case.[3] The other is now a matter of United States government policy.[4] Sadly, both initiatives have gone largely unnoticed in academic philosophical circles. It is time to introduce these developments in the philosophy of mental competence to a wider audience.

Unfortunately, the philosophical literature on competence is riddled with problems. Its diverse strands form a tangled web of mutually incompatible terms and distinctions combined in arguments that regularly miss their targets. Introducing two distinctions will help to make some exegetical sense of this terrain. The first distinction is between putative decisions and actual decisions. A putative decision is one that is currently being entertained but has not yet been made. An actual decision is one that is no longer being entertained but has been made. The second distinction is between internal as opposed to external rationality. External rationality has to do with the outcome of actual decisions. Internal rationality has to do with the coherence of putative decisions within a set of values and beliefs.

The assessment of decision-making capacity is normative because value and rationality are involved. Specifically, mental competence is normative because it involves assessing the internal rationality of a putative decision against a background set of values and beliefs. Therefore, the idea that competence can be entirely objective is misguided, and the attempt to downplay or ignore the role of value in competence is wrongheaded. So is the strategy of restricting competence and its standards to what is purely cognitive and mechanistic. None of this means giving up on objectivity entirely. As is common in this area, objectivity is provided by insisting on rigorous operationalised measures for all standards and tests. Together with third-party consensus and agreement, this is about as much as can be reasonably expected in this domain.

RECOGNISABLE REASONS

In a landmark publication, the philosopher Benjamin Freedman states that competence requires alluding to "an individual's own value system."[5] Making value a component of competence invites the question of whether rationality might also play a role in competence. Freedman explicitly links value and rationality. He alludes to both in his discussion of recognisable reasons, his proposed criterion for competency.

Along with many others, Freedman believes that understanding and appreciation are necessary for competence. However, according to him they are not sufficient. In this respect he departs from established tradition. According to Freedman, in order to be deemed competent, an individual must not only understand and appreciate the nature and consequences of the decision at hand, the individual must also be able to provide recognisable reasons for it.[6] Freedman initially flirts with the idea of calling those reasons "rational," but eventually opts for the less redundant formulation that they be termed "recognisable." He does so partly in order to accommodate the fact that an assessor can recognise the legitimacy of a subject's reasons for a decision without having to share or agree with those beliefs.

Recognisable reasons take the form of arguments. Thus for a reason to be recognisable, "it must contain acceptable premises and a conclusion related to those premises."[7] The obvious objection to this proposal, which Freedman anticipates, is that it risks being overly paternalistic: anybody whose reasons you do not deem recognisable will on those grounds be deemed incompetent by you. To remedy the problem, Freedman qualifies what counts as a recognisable reason. He writes: "Since we wish to give latitude to an individual's own value system, one which we do not necessarily share, it is not required that the conclusion 'follow' from the premises."[8] The point is that reasons do not have to logically *entail* the decision they are reasons for in order to be considered recognisable. It is sufficient that they be capable of providing a strong justification for that decision.

In order to be considered recognisable, reasons must at least be relevant to the decision they are reasons for. But relevant in what light? No doubt, reasons are considered relevant to a decision partly according to the values and standards of those assessing competence. However, more importantly, the reasons must also be relevant in light of the individual's own value system. Conflict between the two standards is of course possible. What is unclear is how to resolve it, and in whose favor. On this point Freedman is almost entirely silent. All we are told is that an individual's reasons can be deemed recognisable by others who do not necessarily share that person's values. This, it seems reasonable, is what it means to give "latitude" to an individual's own value system. The proposal is admittedly vague. But it is at least capable of satisfying an important kind of legal consideration. For example, blood transfusions are contrary to the religious value system held by adherents of the Jehovah's Witness faith. Nevertheless, in some jurisdictions the courts have recognised the right of Jehovah's Witnesses to make such choices, even if they result in death.[9] The religious reasons for such refusals were deemed sufficiently strong to count as recognisable reasons even though the presiding judge was not a Jehovah's Witness and probably did not share or agree with that value system.

There are two other features of Freedman's account that are worth noting here. First, he claims that it is process-centered. By this he means that it is concerned with what "goes into the decision, not merely with the result."[10] Second, he claims it involves a reversal of the traditional roles ascribed to information and competence. He writes:

> Traditionally, it was thought that the ascertainment of competence was an issue which needed to be decided prior to the transmittal of information. To the contrary, I believe that information is prior to competence, in that competence includes, but extends beyond, that the person involved be able to allow the informing process to enter into his decision-making in a substantial way. He must be capable of utilizing the information provided in formulating his reasons ... [C]ompetence is primarily concerned with the manner in which the person uses the information.[11]

Both of these points are worth pondering. Consider first the claim that competence is process-centered.[12] The idea is that the actual consequences of a decision should not be a factor in assessing competence. It is not necessary for the decision to have been made and for its consequences to have been assessed in order to determine whether or not the individual is competent to make that decision. Dealing with the putative decision, one that remains to be made but has not yet been made, is sufficient. Here it is important to keep in mind that an assessment of competence is required in order to determine whether a person is even capable of making a decision. Competence needs to be assessed before a decision is made. Obviously, then, the actual decision a person actually makes cannot be what is assessed for competence.

Competence then has to do with our capacity to make decisions and that is independent of the consequences of the actual decisions we make. Now in evaluating the consequences of a decision we may wish to inquire into its rationality. But the term is ambiguous. On the one hand,

there is a sense in which the rationality of a decision can be assessed before it is made. On the other hand, there is a sense in which the rationality of a decision can be assessed only after it has been made. In assessing the rationality of an actual decision, we often want to look at its consequences. Call this "the external sense of 'rationality'." Rationality in that sense requires appealing to what goes on outside the mind, so to speak. It requires looking beyond the internal mental processes involved in reasoning to the actual external consequences of decisions once they have been made.

According to Freedman, it is possible to assess the rationality of a putative decision without looking at its actual consequences or results. Yet he also wants to maintain that rationality somehow is a component of competence and he does refer to rationality in his account of recognisable reasons. Call this "the internal sense of 'rationality'." Internal rationality has to do with whether the putative decision an individual is entertaining coheres with his or her system of values in a manner that satisfies the recognisable reasons criterion. Note that while this conception of competence refers to the content of the putative decision involved, the assessment of competence is restricted to the internal processes that underlie decision-making and does not require reference to the external consequences of that decision. As indicated in the passage quoted above, the recognisable reasons model requires alluding to the content of decisions. Competence then cannot be assessed without alluding to content in that sense. The requirement is sensible, since it would appear to be impossible to assess the reasons for a decision without knowing what that decision is about. There are, however, some who seem committed to denying this, as we shall see in the following section.

To sum up, Freedman's recognisable reasons account of competence is as interesting as it is cryptic. Nevertheless his strategy is clear. First, assessing competence requires inquiring into an individual's ability to make a putative decision by getting him or her to provide reasons for that decision. Those reasons are specified in the form of an argument with premises and conclusion. Second, assessing the internal rationality of a putative decision requires that we interpret that decision and the reasons for it against the background of the individual's own values and not simply our own. Third, competence is a matter of process. Fourth, competence does not require alluding to the consequences of the actual decision that is made, nor does it require an evaluation of its external rationality. All that is required for competence is internal rationality.

AN ENDURING SET OF VALUES

In a classic discussion on the topic of competence, Alan Buchanan and Dan Brock say quite a bit more about the place of value in mental competence than does Freedman. While Freedman talks of a system of values, Buchanan and Brock refer instead to "a *set of values* or *conception of what is good.*"[13] Elsewhere they speak of "relatively stable values or a conception of the good life."[14] At times they also speak of an individual's "underlying and enduring values."[15] One virtue of their account is that it is far more explicit than Freedman's about how value fits into competence. To see this, we need first to review their overall account of competence.

According to Buchanan and Brock, competence is a threshold concept. Either you are competent or you are not. Like virtually everyone else working in the area, they also maintain that competence is decision-relative. Thus "a person may be competent to make a particular decision at a particular time, under certain circumstances, but incompetent to make another decision or even the same decision, under different conditions."[16] Buchanan and Brock's theory of competence has three components: (1) understanding and communication; (2) reasoning and deliberation; (3) a set of values or conception of the good. Understanding is said to consist in part of basic conceptual, linguistic and cognitive abilities. It requires "the capacities to receive, process, and make available for use the information relevant to particular decisions."[17] As the

following passage states, it also involves the notion of appreciation.

> Understanding is not merely a formal or abstract process, but also requires the ability to appreciate the nature and meaning of potential alternatives—what it would be like and "feel" like to be in possible future states and to undergo various experiences—and to integrate this appreciation into one's decision making."[18]

The capacity for appreciation is one reason why competence requires value. For otherwise how could an individual evaluate the nature and personal meaning of the alternatives he or she faces? You cannot rank and weigh alternatives unless you have a set of values. Here then is one reason why a set of values is required for competence.

For much the same reasons, values are also required for reasoning and deliberation. These capacities "require the capacity to draw inferences about the consequences of making a certain choice and to compare alternative outcomes based on how they further one's good or promote one's ends."[19] Of course, those two subcomponents also rely on understanding and the information it provides. Buchanan and Brock say they require "applying the decision-maker's values."[20] This is because in order to deliberate and reason about alternatives we need some way to rank and attach weights to those alternatives. Without values, that task is impossible. Therefore, on the whole, competence requires a set of values or a conception of the good. This is necessary "in order to be able to evaluate particular outcomes as benefits or harms, goods or evils, and to assign different relative weight or importance to them."[21]

Buchanan and Brock are careful to qualify the sense in which competence requires values. They note:

> [S]ufficient internal consistency and stability over time in the values relative to a particular decision are needed to yield

and enable pursuit of a decision outcome; for example, a depressed patient subject to frequent mood changes may repeatedly consent to electroconvulsive treatment, but then change his or her mind before treatment is carried out.[22]

The point is that "sufficient value stability is needed to permit, at the very least, a decision that can be stated and adhered to over the course of its discussion, initiation, and implementation."[23] This is not meant to deny the fact that personal values change and evolve over time, or that people undergo radical changes in some of their most cherished desires and preferences. Neither does it rule out the fact that individuals may be ambivalent about which values they hold. No doubt, there will always be difficult cases and that is something this account needs to deal with. Changes in values in radical end-of-life circumstances are likely to be one problem area. Mental disorders of certain kinds are another. Nevertheless, the fact remains that in many less complex circumstances the requirement that an individual's values be minimally consistent and relatively stable is reasonable. So "competence does not require a fully consistent set of goals, much less a detailed 'lifeplan' to cover all contingencies."[24] All that is required are that the values in question be relatively stable and minimally consistent.

Like Freedman, Buchanan and Brock want to give latitude to an individual's own values when assessing competence. They also grant that conflicts can arise between an individual's stated values and the values of those appointed to assess their competence. For example, people can sometimes entertain decisions that appear contrary to their own self-interests and which, if enacted, would compromise their well-being. In such cases, it is important to weigh the need to protect an individual's well-being against his or her right to self-determination. Among the difficulties is the risk of setting too high a standard for competence and ruling persons incompetent who ought not to be declared so. There is also the risk of setting too low a standard of compe-

tence and thereby failing to protect individual well-being. In the end, the challenge is to avoid succumbing to either of these two errors.[25] This sort of balancing act is impossible without some appeal to value. On the one hand, there are the values of the individual whose competence is being assessed. And, on the other hand, there are the values of those assessing competence.

It should be evident by now that there are important parallels between Buchanan and Brock, and Freedman on the place of value in competence. The parallels in the case of rationality are not as clear and there the exegetical situation is more complicated. Buchanan and Brock argue that so-called outcome accounts of competence need to be rejected. They characterise those as ones that "look solely to the content or outcome of the decision—for example, the standard that the choice be a reasonable one, or be what other reasonable or rational persons would chose."[26] On the face of it, this would appear to be tantamount to a rejection of Freedman's model, since it appeals both to the content of decisions and to what counts as recognisable reasons for those decisions. The problem is that Buchanan and Brock appear to have conflated the notions of content and outcome. They also appear to have conflated external and internal rationality. Yet, like Freedman, they also claim to be committed to an account of competence given in terms of process. To sort things out, we look first at the alleged disagreement over content.

PROBLEMS WITH CONTENT

We have seen that according to Freedman assessing competence requires alluding to the content of the putative decision involved. This is because competence is a matter of how an individual uses information and this is impossible to determine without adverting to what the decision is about. Like Freedman, Buchanan and Brock want to embrace a process account of competence. However, because of the stand they take on the issue of content, their account appears to be incompatible with Freedman's. Thus, in stating the overall aim of their project they say their intention is "to focus primarily on the process of reasoning, not on the content of the decision itself."[27] I believe that Buchanan and Brock are mistaken in thinking they need to reject the notion of content entirely: their account requires a notion of content for just the same reasons as Freedman's. If this is right, then there is more consensus in the literature on competence than even its proponents seem to have realised. However, in order to set the record straight we will have to introduce two additional players, Charles Culver and Bernard Gert.

Recall the fact that Freedman rejects the idea that the actual results of decisions should play a role in determining competence. A version of that condition is the view that someone is competent to consent to something if in consenting he or she achieves a reasonable outcome.[28] On their side, Culver and Gert also reject the idea that the results or outcomes of decisions should be determining factors in competence. As we saw, so do Buchanan and Brock. So everyone seems to be in agreement. Unfortunately, in rejecting the outcome of a decision as an operative factor in competence, Culver and Gert also introduce complications that confuse the overall picture of how decisional content works its way into a process account of competence.

Culver and Gert propose the concept of a kind of decision, which they sharply distinguish from an actual decision.[29] According to them, competence has to do with the former and not the latter. They propose the following definition of competence:

> [A] patient is competent to decide whether to consent or refuse treatment if she adequately understands and appreciates the information given to her during a properly conducted consent process. This definition of competence does not include within it any reference to whether the patient *decided* to consent to or refuse, nor does it indicate whether the patient's consent or refusal seems, on either subjective or objective grounds, to

be wise or foolish, rational or irrational, impulsive or deliberate.[30]

In other words, competence is "determined by the ability of the patient to understand and appreciate all of the relevant information, but independent of the actual decision the patient makes."[31] It is a matter of an individual's "ability to carry out certain mental tasks."[32]

It is now possible to say why Buchanan and Brock do not need to abandon the notion of content in espousing a process account of competence and why, like Freedman, they need a notion of content to ground their account of competence. The reason for the trouble is that they fail to distinguish a putative decision from an actual one. A putative decision is one you are entertaining and deliberating about but have not yet made. An actual decision is one you have made. A putative decision cannot have an *actual* outcome or result, only an actual decision can. However, a putative decision can have an *expected* outcome or result.[33] But in order for this to be the case, the putative decision must have a content in this sense: a semantic interpretation that specifies what the decision is about. The content of a decision in this semantic sense is distinct from its outcome. Therefore, Buchanan and Brock are mistaken to conflate the two. They are also mistaken that a process account of competence can do without alluding to the semantic content of decisions. It follows that in so far as competence is meant to be process-centered and requires content, there are no incompatibilities between the account provided by Buchanan and Brock and the account provided by Freedman.

Where does this leave Culver and Gert? They agree that only an actual decision can have an outcome or result. They also agree with the others that the actual results or outcomes of decisions should not play a role in competence. On the matter of content, however, the situation is more problematic. In fact, they never mention content. Their focus is the notion of a kind of decision as opposed to a particular individual decision.[34] They depart from tradition in selecting a different unit of analysis for the theory of competence. Unfortunately, their alternative does not appear to be satisfactory.

KINDS OF DECISIONS

Culver and Gert provide the following characterisation of what it means to speak of a kind of decision:

> [T]wo decisions are of the same kind with regard to competence when a person who understands and appreciates the pertinent information relevant to deciding in one way—for example, consenting to a treatment—also understands and appreciates the pertinent information relevant to deciding in the other—refusing the very same treatment … [I]f we accept that a patient is competent to make a kind of decision—for example, he is competent to consent to a treatment in specific circumstances—then we must accept that he is competent to refuse the very same treatment in these same circumstances.[35]

No argument is given in favor of this characterisation. The authors simply assert that it is common to many standard accounts. Maybe so, but which ones? It is certainly inconsistent with at least the accounts of Buchanan and Brock, and Freedman. For according to them, competence is decision-relative in quite a strict sense. Recall that "a person may be competent to make a particular decision at a particular time, under certain circumstances, but incompetent to make another decision or even the same decision, under different conditions."[36] Decision relativity is incompatible with Culver and Gert's notion of a kind of decision. Since decision relativity is apparently here to stay, it is the notion of a kind of decision that will have to be abandoned.

First, note that what is involved in decision relativity is a particular instance of a decision, not a general kind of decision. Second, simply to assert that consent and refusal are the same kind of decision seems to beg the question whether they should be treated as such. In fact, Buchanan

and Brock explicitly distinguish the two. They argue that "consent to a low-risk life-saving procedure by an otherwise healthy individual should require only a minimal level of competence, but refusal of that same procedure by such an individual should require the highest level of competence."[37] What varies here is not simply the level of competence required, with the kind decision remaining unchanged. Indeed, the reason the level of competence must vary is that the two decisions and their associated conditions are not the same. They are in fact two different particular decisions, not one general kind of decision. Thus, to declare a *priori* that the conditions for treatment and refusal decisions are the same is to beg the issue at hand. Considered individually, such decisions commonly have different conditions associated with them. Therefore, to focus on kinds of decisions as opposed to individual particular decisions as Culver and Gert suggest is not only incompatible with the spirit of a decision-relative account of competence, it also begs the issue at hand. Consent and refusal are not the same kind of decision. The reason is that they have different expected consequences and associated risks and benefits. This is sufficient to count them as different decisions.

A related problem with the notion of a kind of decision proposed by Culver and Gert is that it is semantically empty. As we have seen, when you deliberate or reason about an individual particular decision there needs to be something you are deliberating about, a specified semantic content. However, Culver and Gert never mention content. In their discussion they are concerned with the case where an individual is being asked to consent to or to refuse treatment. But if the unit of analysis being assessed is a kind of decision, then what is being assessed is this general kind of decision to consent to or to refuse that kind of treatment, not a particular decision to choose or refuse a particular treatment. Decisions of the latter sort are concrete enough. But ones of the former sort appear strangely empty. They do not have a specific semantic content. How then can competence be assessed? The answer is, it cannot. If Culver and Gert are right, then the basic unit of analysis in a competency assessment really turns out to be a sort of abstract place-holder without any specified semantic content. What after all is the semantic content of a kind of decision? What is such a decision about? Suppose a treatment X is involved. Then what is at issue in competency assessment on Culver and Gert's account is this: deciding to consent-to-or-refuse X. But the true object of a competency determination is more fine-grained and concrete than this. It is a particular decision to do a particular thing at a given time. I see no alternative but to conclude that the notion of a kind of decision proposed by Culver and Gert is inadequate as a unit of analysis for the purposes of assessing competence.[38]

A ROLE FOR RATIONALITY

By now it should be clear that there is no incompatibility between endorsing a process account of competence and espousing a notion of decisional content. It should also be clear that a process account of competence requires an appeal to value. In this section, we look more closely at how a process account of competence can incorporate rationality.

To start, it is worth pointing out that Culver and Gert explicitly argue that the assessment of competence should not rest on the rationality of an individual's decision. This is obviously incompatible with the thesis that internal rationality is a condition of competence. The problem is easily resolved. Very simply, Culver and Gert conflate internal and external rationality. They consider all rationality to be external, a feature of actual decisions. Because they do not distinguish actual from putative decisions, it is impossible for them to countenance the possibility that rationality might be a component of competence in the internal sense suggested by Buchanan and Brock, and Freedman. They are right that rationality in the external sense should not be considered a condition of competence, but they are wrong that rationality in the internal sense is not important.

Freedman explicitly endorses an internal account of rationality to complement his process account of competence. So do Buchanan and Brock, once the confusion between decisional content and outcomes is resolved. In the following passage they appear to endorse a version of the recognisable reasons model:

> A crude but perhaps helpful way of characterising the proper aim of the evaluator of the competence of a seemingly harmful or bad patient choice is to think of him or her addressing the patient in this fashion: 'Help me try to understand and make sense of your choice. Help me to see whether your choice is reasonable, not in the sense that it is what I or most people would choose, but that it is reasonable for you in light of your underlying and enduring aims and values.' This is the proper focus of a process account of competence.[39]

So according to Buchanan and Brock, competence involves appealing to the reasonableness of the putative choice in question. Like Freedman, they believe that this determination is internal to the reasoning process. It is now time to try to look more closely at internal rationality and its role in the recognisable reasons account of competence. A putative decision is rational in the internal sense if: (a) it coheres with an individual's enduring aims and values; (b) it is justified in light of those values and their associated beliefs; and (c) the proposed justification is deemed appropriate by the third party responsible for assessing competence. Again, the reasons offered do not have to entail the proposed decision. It is sufficient that they be recognised as an appropriate justification for selecting that option by the assessors. The reasons do not even have to be true, nor do the assessors have to believe they are true. All that is required is that the individual in question believes them to be true.

Consider again the example of the Jehovah's Witnesses and blood transfusions. A Jehovah's Witness's putative decision to refuse a life-saving transfusion may appear unreasonable when assessed against the general public's values and beliefs regarding the preservation of life. But the system of values that define the Jehovah's Witness faith constitutes a strong justification for that decision, one that is recognisable to a suitably disposed third party, and one that coheres with the overall set of values and beliefs associated with that faith. If, as some legal precedents suggest we must, we opt to give latitude to a Jehovah's Witness's value system in assessing his or her competence to make treatment decisions, then it is possible to count those decisions as competent even though they may ensue in death. The Jehovah's Witness's reasons for refusing transfusions are recognisable even to those who might not share them. They are rational in light of, and internal to, the Jehovah's Witness faith. That does not mean that assessments of competence must necessarily collapse into subjectivity. It is not too hard to imagine satisfactory objective means of determining whether a Jehovah's Witness's decision to refuse a transfusion is made in conformity with his or her religious principles and with a basically sound mind. The Jehovah's Witness who refuses a transfusion on the grounds that he or she is Jesus Christ is just as incompetent to make that decision as a severely schizophrenic patient who says the same thing.

ASKING "WHY?"

It is time to leave the realm of philosophical theory and to turn to more practical matters. Having articulated the case for including considerations of value in the assessment of mental competence, we are left with the challenge of how to devise operationalised measures which do that. The traditional approach to competence requires understanding and appreciation. However, if the arguments provided here are correct, then this is not enough. In order to judge competence we need to know more than simply the fact that a patient understands and appreciates the nature of a putative decision. Those conditions only capture a person's abilities to comprehend what the relevant facts of a situation are. If value is going to count as a component of competence we also need to know why a person proposes to choose as they do. This is because it

is primarily values that define goals and aspirations and, thereby, direct conduct.

In determining whether an individual understands and appreciates the nature of a certain decisional task we normally ask questions such as: "Do you understand what this decision is about?" "Do you appreciate what will happen if you choose this rather than that?"[40] Such "What?" questions deal with facts. Answers to them are assessed by determining whether the person involved can demonstrate that he or she has those facts right. Let us grant that all of this is more or less amenable to objective scrutiny. "Why?" questions are a different matter. They are also notoriously absent from competency assessment tools, probably because of their association with questions of value and rationality. "Why?" questions delve into a person's reasons for wanting to choose as he or she does, and that often involves inquiring into that person's values. Assessing the answers to "Why?" questions is likely to be more complicated than assessing the answers to "What?" questions. At the very least, the criteria are going to be different.

The recognisable reasons criterion requires that we ask "Why?" To see the point of that condition imagine the following situation. Patient X understands what is involved in the putative decision to do Y. Patient X also appreciates what it means to opt in favor of the putative decision to do Y. Therefore, so far as understanding and appreciation are concerned, patient X is competent. But now imagine that when asked why she wants to opt to do Y, patient X says "I am inclined to choose Y because I am Jesus Christ!" Is patient X competent? Not likely. Is she incompetent? Perhaps. But there are at least grounds for overriding the usual presumption of competence and inquiring into this individual's competence. The point is that without asking this last question one would probably never come to that inquiry. For it is perfectly conceivable that someone might satisfy the understanding and appreciation conditions and yet at the same time choose to do Y for irrational reasons. It is worth noting that the rare instances when "Why?" questions are employed in assessments of competence; it is not specifically to inquire into the grounds for competence. It is rather to screen out impediments to competence such as pathological extremes of affect, psychosis and the like. However, "Why?" questions do much more. They not only help isolate factors outside competence that may impede or compromise it, they also capture factors that are constitutive of competence, namely, reasons. Thus, "Why?" questions are the clinical key to reasons.

To sum up, considerations of value could probably be incorporated into assessments of competence employing specially tailored "Why?" questions. Such reason-seeking probes should be accompanied by carefully defined operationalised criteria for evaluating what counts as the coherence of a putative decision with an individual's overall set of values, and what counts as a recognisable reason. This is obviously more a strategy than a solution. But it is a start.

CONCLUSION

The aim of this discussion has been to try and clarify the place of value and rationality in the theory and assessment of mental competence. With a few interpretive adjustments, it is possible to make a convincing case for the thesis that there is a lot more consensus in the literature on this topic than might at first appear to be the case. In particular, there is agreement that assessments of competence cannot be carried out independently of certain considerations of value and rationality. This poses problems for the requirement that assessments of competence be objective. Buchanan and Brock say that competence is not something that can be determined scientifically.[41] They are right about this, but that does not mean giving up entirely on objectivity, as they also seem to suggest.

Third party agreement is probably the best and only way to address the requirements of objectivity involved in the assessment of decision-making capacity. This might seem unsatisfactory to those versed in the philosophical intricacies of the problem of objectivity. However, keep in mind that in addition to being objective to some degree, operationalised criteria for assessing competence must also be sufficiently general and flexible to apply across different jurisdictions (such as different states or provinces in the case of some federations). Precision of a certain sort is therefore not desirable. It is also unrealistic. After all, the purpose of philosophical inquiry here is to facilitate problem-solving in a practical domain, not to paralyse it by setting impossible goals and standards. The onus is on those who desire more objectivity in that domain to specify how it might be attained in a manner that meets the practical exigencies of the task.

Notes

1. Freedman, B (1981), Competence, Marginal and Otherwise, *International Journal of Law and Psychiatry* 4, 53–72: p. 55.
2. For an account of the evaluative contribution of emotion to competence see Charland, LC (1999). Appreciation and Emotion: Theoretical Reflections on the MacArthur Treatment Competence Study, *Kennedy Institute Journal of Ethics* 8(4), 359–377; and Charland, LC (1998), Is Mr. Spock Mentally Competent: Competence to Consent and Emotion, *Philosophy, Psychiatry, Psychology* 5(1), 67–95.
3. Freedman's recognisable reasons criterion is referred to in *US v Charters,* F 2d, No. 86-5568, United States Court of Appeals Fourth Circuit, Sept. 18, 1988 *per* Murnaghan Circuit Judge.
4. Both Buchanan and Brock were consulting members of the President's Commission for the Study of Ethical Problems in Biomedical and Behavioral Research and co-authors of its report, *The President's Commission for the Study of Ethical Problems in Medicine and Biomedical and Behavioral Research.* (1982) Making Health Care Decisions, Vol 1 Washington: US Government Printing Office). In that document "a set of enduring values" is listed as a condition of competence.
5. Freedman, *op cit*, p. 61.
6. For an intriguing view of competence that incorporates elements of responsibility in addition to value and rationality see: Elliott, C (1991), Competence as Accountability, *Journal of Clinical Ethics* 2(3), 167–171. Elliott argues that competence should be construed as accountability.
7. Freedman, *op cit*, p. 61.
8. *Ibid*, p. 61.

9. In Canadian law there is the case of *Mallete v Shulman* (1990) 72 OR (2d) 417 (CA).

10. Freedman, *op cit*, p. 61.

11. *Ibid*, p. 62.

12. A similar point is made in: Buchanan, AE, and Brock, DW (1989), *Deciding for Others: The Ethics of Surrogate Decision Making*. Cambridge, Cambridge University Press. The details differ somewhat from Freedman's account.

13. Buchanan and Brock, *op cit*, p. 25.

14. *Ibid*, p. 84.

15. *Ibid*, p. 32.

16. *Ibid*, p. 18.

17. *Ibid*, p. 24.

18. *Ibid*, p. 24.

19. *Ibid*, p. 25.

20. *Ibid*, p. 25.

21. *Ibid*, p. 25

22. *Ibid*, p. 25.

23. *Ibid*, p. 25.

24. *Ibid*, p. 25.

25. *Ibid*, pp. 40–1.

26. *Ibid*, p. 49.

27. *Ibid*, p. 84.

28. Freedman, *op cit*, p. 59; see also: Roth, LH, Meisel, A, Litz, W (1977), Test of Competency to Consent, *American Journal of Psychiatry* 134, 279–284.

29. Culver and Gert (1990), The Inadequacy of Competence. *Millbank Quarterly*, pp. 620, 629, respectively.

30. *Ibid*, p. 621; emphasis added.

31. *Ibid*, p. 634; emphasis added.

32. *Ibid*, p. 621.

33. See, for example, Buchanan and Brock, *op cit*, p. 85.

34. Culver and Gert, *op cit*, pp. 619–620; see also Buchanan and Brock, *op cit*, p. 65.

35. Culver and Gert, *op cit*, p. 620.

36. Buchanan and Brock, *op cit*, p. 18.

37. *Ibid*, p. 52.

38. See Cale, Gita S (1999), Risk-Related Standards of Competence, *Bioethics 13(2)*. 131–148, for a recent discussion of the problem of asymmetry in the area of competence.

39. *Ibid*, p. 56.

40. There are a number of interesting "Why?" questions in Paul Appelbaum and Tom Grisso's MacCAT-T assessment tool. The manual and assessment tool are contained in an appendix to T, Grisso and Appelbaum, PA (1998), *The Assessment of Decision-Making Capacity: A Guide for Physicians and Other Health Professionals*. Oxford: Oxford University Press.

41. Buchanan and Brock, p. 47.

Nothing Matters: Depression and Competence in Clinical Research

Carl Elliott

Madness need not be regarded as an illness. Why shouldn't it be seen as a sudden—more or less sudden—change of character?
— Ludwig Wittgenstein

I hope I am the one.
— Patient with major depression, on being told that ECT carries a 1 in 3000 chance of death.

I

People sometimes do inexplicable things when they are clinically depressed. They make self-destructive choices, alienate their friends, damage their marriages, lose their motivation and creativity at work. A recurring theme in memoirs of depression, typically written during periods of clarity, is the writer's sense of regret and often astonishment at the things she did and said when she was clinically depressed.[1] In *Darkness Visible*, William Styron remembers with some embarrassment his refusal to have dinner with the members of a French academy who had just presented him with a major literary prize.

Strangely enough, physicians, researchers and bioethicists have generally paid little attention to depression when it comes to evaluating competence. This is especially true for clinical research.

Depressed patients are often asked to take part in research protocols, and sometimes this research carries risks. A depressed patient might be enrolled in a protocol to evaluate a new antidepressant, for example, or in a protocol that requires a washout period, in which their current medication will be discontinued. Many Institutional Review Boards enthusiastically approve protocols testing new antidepressants against placebo controls, in which a depressed patient may be taken off his medication for six to 12 weeks. I have seen at least one placebo-controlled antidepressant protocol that called for patients with major depression to be taken off their medication for a year. Any of these situations entail risks, primarily the risk that the depressed patient's condition will worsen. The potential harm can be considerable, and at the extreme end of the spectrum includes the risk of suicide.

Competence to consent to research is one of the most widely and thoroughly discussed issues in bioethics, of course.[2–6] But most clinical research protocols involving depressed patients do not even specify that the patients' competence needs to be evaluated before they are enrolled in the protocol. The reason depression is not considered a warning sign of incompetence, or so I suspect, is that depression is not ordinarily thought to be the type of disorder that would interfere with competence. It is only the rare depressed patient who is psychotic, and while depression may often interfere with a person's memory and concentration, very often this interference is not severe enough to raise any warning flags. Most accounts of competence focus on intellectual capacity and abilities to reason and depression is primarily a disorder of mood. According to conventional thinking, depression is primarily about despair, guilt and a loss of motivation, while competence is about the ability to reason, to deliberate, to compare and to evaluate. These latter abilities are ones that depression is thought to leave intact.

I believe this view of competence is misguided. Depression may well impair a patient's competence to consent to research. Perhaps most crucially, it can impair a person's ability to evaluate risks and benefits. To put the matter simply, if a person is depressed, he may be *aware* that a protocol carries risks, but simply not *care* about those risks. This sort of intellectual impairment can be as important a part of competence as the more detached, intellectual understanding that most accounts of competence emphasize. If I am right, then clinical investigators need to take special precautions in allowing researchers to enroll depressed patients in research protocols.

II

Competence is conventionally defined as the ability to perform a task—in this case, to consent to enroll in a research protocol.[7, 8] What counts as competence to consent, then, will then depend on what one counts as the abilities relevant to the task in question. According to a widely accepted account of competence, the 1983 U.S. *President's Commission Report*, the relevant abilities are (1) the ability to reason and deliberate, (2) the ability to understand and communicate information, and (3) the possession of values and goals.[9] As conceptualized within this framework, a potential research subject takes in the relevant information, weighs it according to his goals and values, and then reasons his way to an informed decision.

I believe that accounts of competence like these are incomplete. If competence to consent to research is defined simply as the ability to make a decision to enroll in a research protocol, we are still left with the problem of what *counts* as that ability—whether a person is incompetent by virtue of making a poor decision, or by virtue of making an irrational decision, or by virtue of coming to his decision in an unsystematic, illogical or erratic way. But since even competent people are sometimes stubborn, obtuse or unreasonable, we need an account of competence that explains why we sometimes feel that a person can be competent and make bad, irrational or even unreasonable choices.

What we really want to know when we ask if a patient is competent is whether he is able to make a decision *for which he can be considered accountable*. What we want to know is whether the decisions that a person makes—whether they are good decisions or bad ones, rational or irrational—are decisions for which that person can legitimately be considered responsible. This is why we define certain mental abilities as relevant: we realize that certain conditions or disorders impair a person's mental abilities such that he is not a morally responsible agent. He can make decisions, but we would not feel comfortable calling him to account for that decision. But since we recognize that a person generally has the right to make even unsound decisions, a judgment about competence ensures that whatever decision a person makes, it is truly *his* decision: a decision for which he can finally be held accountable….

Once we conceptualize competence this way, it becomes clear that it is not just intellectual ability that is relevant to competence. A person's emotional state can also affect her decisions in ways that might lead us to say that she cannot be judged fully accountable for them. The criminal law recognizes this, for example, and often grants leniency when a person acts under severe emotional distress. We often make decisions in the heat of anger or under the cold weight of despair that are uncharacteristic, that we would not have made otherwise, that we later regret and for which we feel we should not be considered fully accountable. Likewise, we often recognize that it would be unfair to hold a person to a decision that he or she made in the face of overwhelming fear. In emotional extremes, we value, think and behave differently—sometimes so differently that we might later feel that the decisions we have made are not decisions for which we can be held completely and unproblematically responsible.

While bioethicists as a whole have not paid much attention to depression, the importance of emotion and mood for competence has not been lost on those who are trained in psychiatry.[10–14] For instance, some accounts of competence stipulate that a person must "appreciate" the consequences of her choice, rather than simply understand them factually, the term "appreciate"

implying a fuller, deeper comprehension of how that decision will affect the patient's life.[15, 16] A patient who can flatly recite the effects of treatment may still seem to fail to appreciate fully just how the treatment is going to affect his or her health. Nor can affect be completely divorced conceptually from cognition. Bursztajn and his colleagues have pointed out how a patient's affect can influence competence by altering his or her beliefs.[17] For example, a depressed patient, convinced that his situation will never change, may refuse treatment based on the unrealistic belief that it will not help him.

However, while some patients may have affective disorders that disrupt their cognitive, rational, decision-making abilities, a slightly different sort of depressed patient presents other problems. This is the depressed patient who is capable of understanding all the facts about his illness and the research protocol in which he is enrolling, and who appreciates the risks and the broader implications of the protocol on his life, but who, as a result of his illness, is not *motivated* to take those risks into account in the same way as the rest of us. These patients, for example, might realize that a protocol involves risks, but simply not *care* about the risks. Some patients, as a result of their depression, may even *want* to take risks.[18]

Could depression lead some patients to overestimate the side effects of interventions and underestimate the likelihood of benefit?[17–20] While there are no good empirical studies examining the question of whether depressed patients are more likely than nondepressed patients to consent to risky or uncomfortable research,[21] Lee, Ganzini and their colleagues have studied the effects of depression and its treatment on the preferences of elderly patients for life-sustaining medical therapies.[22, 23] In one study of 43 depressed patients, a subgroup of 11 severely depressed patients were more likely to choose life-sustaining therapies after their depression had been treated than they were while depressed.[24] This suggests that severe depression might affect the way some patients evaluate risks and benefits, but it is not clear whether evaluation of life-sustaining therapy is similar enough to evaluation of research risks to bear much comparison.

Nonetheless, it seems unlikely that severely depressed patients are in the best position to make important decisions about their welfare. The Royal College of Psychiatrists in the United Kingdom is one of the few bodies to recognize this explicitly, offering the example of a patient with depressive delusions who consents to risky research because he thinks he is guilty and deserves to be punished.[25] Given the sense of hopelessness and worthlessness that characterizes some severely depressed patients, it doesn't seem unreasonable to be concerned about their decision-making. The novelist William Styron describes his own agonizing depressive episode as like "the diabolical discomfort of being imprisoned in a fiercely overheated room. And because no breeze stirs this cauldron, because there is no escape from this smothering confinement, it is entirely natural that the victim begins to think ceaselessly of oblivion."[26]

III

It might not seem controversial to say that mood and emotion affect a person's decision-making. For some people it seems clear that a person who is paralyzed by a fear she admits is unfounded, or who is soaring in a grandiose euphoria brought on by bipolar disorder, or who is gripped by depression-induced despair, is not exactly in the ideal position to make medical decisions. But not everyone agrees…. [E]ven among writers who agree that emotion is an important part of decision-making, it is only the rare one who has tried to say *why* this is so.[27] It is not such an easy question to answer. Even if we concede that emotion and mood are part of ordinary decision-making, it is also normal for a person's mood to change from one time to another, and it is not immediately obvious why a depressed mood should invalidate a patient's competence….

Nonetheless, I believe there are at least two good arguments for the conclusion that some *severely* depressed patients are incompetent to

consent to research, each of which is persuasive for a slightly different type of patient. The first might be called the argument from *identity*. When a person is caught in the grip of depression, his values, beliefs, desires and dispositions are dramatically different from when he is healthy.[28] In some cases, they are so different that we might ask whether his decisions are truly his. A decision may not be truly his in the sense that it reflects dispositions and values that are transient and inconsistent with much more deeply ingrained traits of his character. One might say, "I wasn't myself," when looking back on a time of despondency, and a caricature of the identity argument would hold that we should take this declaration literally: I was not myself, so that decision is not mine. Yet underneath that caricature is a grain of truth. If a person is so deeply depressed that his decisions are wildly inconsistent with his character, it seems problematic to abide by his decisions, particularly if the depression is dramatic and reversible.[29]

Here is where the notion of competence as accountability is helpful. If a person were to behave badly while mentally ill—say, in a full-blown manic episode—we would very likely feel it unfair to hold him fully responsible for what he has done.[30] His behavior was uncharacteristic; he would never have acted this way if he had not been manic; his mania was temporary and reversible with lithium. His actions in the manic state were not truly *his*. The same goes for the depressed patient who is asked to consent to research: his mental state is such that his behavior and choices do not seem to be truly his. If something untoward were to happen to him during the research, for instance, we could not in good conscience say that he bears the full responsibility for undergoing that risk….

The identity argument presupposes a person with a stable character and entrenched dispositions who, while depressed, makes decisions so uncharacteristic that we feel bound to question whether those decisions were truly hers. However, sometimes this break between the depressed and predepressed personality is not so dramatic. Some patients are chronically depressed, and others are depressed periodically. It would not be plausible to argue that the decisions of these depressed patients do not reflect their underlying characters—characters which are closely tied to their depression. Yet there comes a point where, if a person appears largely insensitive to her own welfare, we might feel that she is incompetent to consent to research. Why should this be so?

One answer lies in what might be called the argument from *self-interest*. Our ordinary relationships with other people are based on certain assumptions about their thoughts and behavior. One of these assumptions is that other persons have some minimal concern for their own welfare. For example, the assumption that other people ordinarily both have some minimal degree of self-interest and are best positioned to judge their own interests lies at the heart of the institution of informed consent.

However, if we have reason to believe that severely depressed patients do not have this minimal degree of concern, then a fundamental assumption underlying informed consent is undermined. We justify exposing patients to the risks of research by the assumption that the patient is evaluating that risk with some degree of concern for her welfare. A competent evaluation of risks involves taking into account one's own well-being—not necessarily taking it as an overriding or supremely important concern, but at least taking it into account. If a person is so depressed that she fails to take her interests into account in deciding whether to take a risk, then we can hardly feel comfortable saying that she is accountable for taking that risk....

What sort of practical conclusions should we draw from all these observations about depression? First, it seems clear that we need to see more empirical research on the ways in which severe depression might affect psychological factors relevant to competence. For example, it would be important to know the extent to which severe depression affects how much a person cares about his or her own well-being and how it might affect a person's willingness to expose himself or herself to potential harm....

Secondly, these arguments suggest that we may need to alter our conventional ways of assessing competence. As I have argued, many conventional accounts of how competence should be assessed downplay the importance of emotional factors. However, if my arguments are convincing, it may not be enough for psychiatrists or researchers to evaluate competence simply by testing a person's memory and reasoning ability, such as with a Mini Mental Status Exam. Rather, it may be that evaluations should also be concerned with a person's affective and motivational state: whether a person's mood has dramatically changed recently, how concerned a patient appears to be about her own well-being, how carefully she looks at risks and benefits and so on. Of course, we will also need to find sound and uniform ways of assessing these affective and motivational factors.

Finally, on a more practical level, these arguments should lead us to rethink the conduct of clinical trials testing new treatments for major depression. For example, if it is concluded that severe depression does impair competence to consent, clinical research protocols involving subjects with depression will need to require explicitly that the competence of subjects be evaluated before entering the study. This would make studies of severe depression look more like studies testing new anti-psychotic drugs, which generally require that subjects either be competent to consent or that consent be obtained from an appropriate surrogate.

Also, this view of competence should make us rethink studies involving relatively poor risk–benefit ratios.... For example, sometimes severely depressed patients are enrolled in placebo-controlled studies in which their depression is likely to worsen as a result of receiving a placebo. Researchers argue that exposing competent adults to these sorts of risks is justified at least in part by the institution of informed consent, with the corresponding presumption that potential subjects understand the risks of the protocol, consent to them and can be judged accountable for undertaking them.[31] But if severely depressed patients are incompetent, exposing them to the risk of having their illness worsen is much more difficult to justify….

Notes

1. See, for instance, Elizabeth Wurtzl, *Prozac Nation: Young and Depressed in America* (New York: Houghton Mifflin, 1994); John Bentley Mays, *In the Jaws of the Black Dogs: A Memoir of Depression* (New York: Viking, 1995); William Styron, *Darkness Visible: A Memoir of Madness* (New York: Random House, 1990).

2. Paul Appelbaum, Charles Lidz and Alan Meisel, *Informed Consent: Legal Theory and Clinical Practice* (New York: Oxford University Press, 1986).

3. James Drane, "The Many Faces of Competency." *Hastings Center Report* 15:2(1985):17–21.

4. Willard Gaylin, "The Competence of Children: No Longer All or None," *Hastings Center Report* 12:2(1982):33–28.

5. C. Lidz, A. Meisel, E. Zerubavel, M. Carter, R. Sestak and L. Roth, *Informed Consent: A Study of Decisionmaking in Psychiatry* (New York: The Guilford Press, 1984).

6. Albert Jonsen. Mark Siegler and William Winslade, *Clinical Ethics*, 3rd edition (New York: Macmillan, 1992).

7. Ruth Faden and Tom Beauchamp, *A History and Theory of Informed Consent* (New York: Oxford University Press, 1986).

8. Allan Buchanan and Dan Brock, *Deciding for Others: The Ethics of Surrogate Decision Making* (Cambridge: Cambridge University Press, 1989).

9. US President's Commission for the Study of Ethical Problems in Medicine and Biomedical and Behavioral Research, *Making Health Care Decisions: The Ethical and Legal Implications of Informed Consent in the Patient-Practitioner Relationship* (Washington: US Government Printing Office, 1983).

10. C.M. Culver, R.B. Ferrell and R.M. Green, "ECT and the Special Problems of Informed Consent," *American Journal of Psychiatry* 137:5(1980):586–591.

11. T.H. Gutheil and H. Bursztajn, "Clinician's Guidelines for Assessing and Presenting Subtle Forms of Patient Incompetence in Legal Settings," *American Journal of Psychiatry* 143:8(1986):1020–1023.

12. K.W.M. Fulford and K. Howse, "Ethics of Research with Psychiatric Patients: Principles, Problems and the Primary Responsibility of Researchers," *Journal of Medical Ethics* 19(1993):85–91.

13. L. Ganzini, M.A. Lee, R.T Heintz and J.D. Bloom, "Is the Patient Self-Determination Act Appropriate for Elderly Persons Hospitalized for Depression?" *Journal of Clinical Ethics 4* (1993):46–50.

14. Jan Marta, "The PSDA and Geriatric Psychiatry: a Cautionary Tale," *Journal of Clinical Ethics* 4 (1993):80–81.

15. Thomas G. Gutheil and Paul Appelbaum, *Clinical Handbook of Psychiatry and the Law* (New York: McGraw-Hill, 1982).

16. Paul Appelbaum and Loren Roth, "Competency to Consent to Research: A Psychiatric Overview," *Archives of General Psychiatry* 39(1982):951–958.

17. H. Bursztajn, H.P. Harding, T.G. Gutheil and A. Brodsky, "Beyond Cognition: The Role of Disordered Affective States in Impairing Competence to Consent to Treatment." *Bulletin of the American Academy of Psychiatry and the Law* 19:4(1991):383–388.

18. The epigraph at the beginning of this chapter is one example. It is taken from Culver et al., "ECT and the Specials Problems of Informed Consent," pp. 586–591.

19. L. Ganzini, M.A. Lee, R.T. Heintz and J.D. Bloom, "Do-Not-Resuscitate Orders for Depressed Psychiatric Inpatients," *Hospital and Community Psychiatry* 43:9(1992):915–919.

20. M.D. Sullivan and S.J. Youngner, "Depression, Competence and the Right to Refuse Lifesaving Medical Treatment," *American Journal of Psychiatry* 151:7(1994):971–978.

21. Hirschfeld, Winslade and Kraus believe there are such studies, but they fail to mention that the study they cite included only three patients with depression. See R. Hirschfeld, W. Winslade and T. Krause, "Protecting Subjects and Fostering Research: Striking the Proper Balance," *Archives of General Psychiatry* 54:2(1997):121–123. The study they cite (among others) which they apparently believe supports the claim that to consider severely depressed patients incompetent is to violate their autonomy is B. Stanley, M. Stanley, A. Lautin, J. Laine and N. Schwartz, "Preliminary Findings in Psychiatric Patients as Research Participants: A Population at Risk?" *American Journal of Psychiatry* 138(1981):669–671.

22. M.A. Lee and L. Ganzini, "Depression in the Elderly: Effect on Patient Attitudes toward Life-Sustaining Therapy," *Journal of the American Geriatric Society* 40:10(1992):983–988.

23. M.A. Lee and L. Ganzini, "The Effect of Recovery from Depression on Preferences for Life-Sustaining Therapy in Older Patients," *Journal of Gerontology* 49:1(1994):15–21.

24. Ganzini et al., "The Effect of Depression Treatment on Elderly Patients' Preferences for Life-Sustaining Medical Therapy," *American Journal of Psychiatry* 151: pp. 1631–1636.

25. Royal College of Psychiatrists, *Guidelines for Ethics of Research Committees on Psychiatric Research Involving Human Subjects* (London: Royal College of Psychiatrists, 1989).

26. Styron, *Darkness Visible: A Memoir of Madness.*

27. One notable exception is Louis Charland in his innovative paper, "Is Mr. Spock Mentally Competent?: Competence to Consent and Emotion," *Philosophy, Psychiatry and Psychology* 5(March 1998), pp. 68–81.

28. A.E. Buchanan and D.W. Brock, *Deciding for Others.*

29. A. Shamoo and D. Irving, "The PSDA and the Depressed Elderly: 'Intermittent Competency' Revisited," *Journal of Clinical Ethics* 4(1993):74–79.

30. For a fuller discussion of this sort of case, see my own book: Carl Elliot, *The Rules of Insanity: Moral Responsibility and the Mentally Disordered Offender* (Albany, NY: State University of New York Press, 1996).

31. Loren Roth and Paul Appelbaum. "Obtaining Informed Consent for Research with Psychiatric Patients," *Psychiatric Clinics of North America* 6:4(1983):551–565.

Cynthia's Dilemma:
Consenting to Heroin Prescription

Louis C. Charland

INTRODUCTION

Heroin prescription involves the provision of medically prescribed heroin in the treatment of heroin addiction.[1] Research undertaken on that treatment modality raises complex ethical problems. One that has not been sufficiently addressed is whether the subjects considered for that research are able to consent to it. There are really two problems. First, how can an individual who is addicted to heroin voluntarily consent to participate in research where their drug of choice is offered free of charge? Second, even granting that voluntary consent is possible, is a heroin-dependent individual mentally competent to make decisions of this sort? When I put these questions to Cynthia, a recovering heroin addict at a local clinic, her reaction was disbelief and amazement. "That's crazy," she said, "if you're addicted to heroin, then by definition you can't say 'No' to the stuff." Cynthia's response can be expressed in the form of a dilemma that, in her honor, I will call Cynthia's Dilemma.

This paper is about Cynthia's Dilemma and the ethical conundrum it poses for research on heroin prescription. I will argue that the problems raised by the dilemma are serious, but I will also suggest some possible avenues of response. The source of the dilemma lies in the nature of heroin addiction. Heroin addicts suffer from a compulsive need to seek and use heroin. As a result, they have an impaired decisional capacity to make choices about heroin. Ethical and clinical discussions of heroin prescription seem to have missed this point entirely.

Heroin prescription provides an interesting perspective from which to view the role of value in mental competence (Brock and Buchanan 1987). It also shows why competence must involve some sort of accountability (Elliott 1991). There are also interesting parallels between addiction and depression that are relevant. It has been argued that severely depressed patients may not be competent to consent to research because they care too little about risks (Elliott 1997). The problem with heroin addiction is just the opposite. Heroin addicts care too much about benefits. They care too much about heroin. Clinical tests of the competence of depressed subjects to consent to research have recently been carried out (Appelbaum et al. 1999). I will argue that similar tests should be carried out in the case of heroin prescription. The main conclusion of the paper is that we should not presume that heroin addicts are competent to consent to heroin prescription. In fact, we should assume they are incompetent unless proven otherwise.

WHAT IS HEROIN PRESCRIPTION?

Heroin prescription[2] was employed as a treatment modality in the management of opiate dependence in the United States in the early 1900s (Bayer 1976). It has also been available on a limited basis in Britain since the early 1960s (Brewer 1995; Marsden et al. 1998; Metrebian et al. 1998). Indeed, the first controlled clinical trial devoted to heroin prescription appears to have been conducted in Britain (Hartnoll et al. 1980). Since then, due largely to an alarming increase in the rate of HIV transmission among injectable drug users, several Western governments and public-health authorities have urged that heroin prescription be investigated more fully. Thus there is now a call to move beyond the use of heroin prescription as a limited form of innovative therapy to possibly wider and more systematic treatment interventions of that type. This is the reasoning that led to the famous "Swiss Trials." Between 1992 and 1996 the Swiss government undertook a full-scale study of different therapies for treating heroin addiction. A total of 1,146 individuals were originally enrolled in the study, which was spread over 18 sites (Uchtenhagen, Gutzwiller, and Dobler-Mikola 1997). Another large-scale study is currently underway in the Netherlands (Van den Brink, Hendricks, and van Ree 1999). In Australia, extensive preparations for a large-scale trial were finalized only to be aborted by direct political intervention (Wodak 1997). Finally, in Canada calls for research into heroin prescription by public-health authorities have

been getting increasingly strident (Fisher and Rehm 1997; Miller 1998; Matas 2001; College of Physicians and Surgeons of British Columbia 1995). A recent series of articles and letters in the prestigious journal *Science* testify to the important public profile of heroin prescription today (Bammer et al. 1999a; 1999b; Rushe 1999; Caltrider 1999).

Requests for research into heroin prescription have been bolstered by results from the Swiss experiment. One of the Swiss study sites generated particularly impressive outcomes. In the Geneva Trial, participants were randomized to a treatment arm that received injectable heroin and a control group that was eligible for any other available treatment option (Perneger et al. 1998). Subjects in the experimental group injected heroin under supervised conditions up to three times a day for six months. At the end of the trial, participants in the experimental group showed a marked decrease in illicit drug use and criminal behavior compared to those in the control group. There were also important improvements in health status, including a significant reduction in HIV risk behaviors. Retention rates were impressive, with all but one of the participants in the experimental group still enrolled at the end of the trial. The researchers concluded that heroin prescription was both feasible and clinically effective.

It is important to recognize that the participants in the Geneva Trial were in very poor mental and physical health and living in obvious social distress. They were men in their 30s with an average 12 years of chronic heroin addiction. All had a history of repeated treatment failure and had to be active in their addiction at the time of enrollment. In general, all had a high prevalence of mental disorders with health status scores 1-2 SD below population norms. The details are grim indeed. In the experimental group (n = 27), 4 of the subjects were infected with HIV, 1 had developed AIDS, 22 suffered from severe depression, 25 suffered from severe anxiety, and 18 had a history of at least one suicide attempt. Social-status indicators are equally telling, with 21 of the subjects unemployed for 12 months or more and 7 with previous activity in the commercial sex trade. These are the subjects that received heroin. Health and social status figures for the control group (n = 24) are comparable, although slightly lower in a few instances. The primary diagnosis of the Geneva subjects was heroin dependence. But they obviously suffered from other serious psychiatric conditions. In the terminology of research ethics, they would easily qualify as vulnerable. This will be important in what follows.

Methodologically, the Geneva trial did have limitations. Most of these the authors note themselves. The most significant weakness is highlighted by the World Health Organization's (WHO) evaluation of the Swiss experiment (World Health Organization 1999). The WHO report states that improvements in the health and social status of study participants cannot be directly causally attributed to the administration of heroin itself, but may instead have been a result of the overall treatment program. Improved trial designs that attempt to meet this objection have since been developed (Bammer and Douglas 1996; Van den Brink, Hendricks, and van Ree 1999). Another important issue mentioned in the WHO report is the role of local politics and public opinion in jurisdictions where heroin prescription is envisaged. Switzerland has it own particular sociopolitical climate, and it is hard to generalize from the feasibility of heroin prescription there to other jurisdictions. The same is true with the Netherlands and other European countries where research on heroin prescription is currently being considered or already underway.

The impact of social and political factors on the feasibility of heroin prescription should not be underestimated. Pressures of that sort make heroin-prescription research very unlikely in countries like the United States where key elements of public and professional opinion still remain in the grip of the "War on Drugs" (Angell and Kassirer 1994; Kleber 1994). A good indication of this is a recent consensus statement by the National Institutes of Health (NIH) on "Effective Treatment for Opiate Addiction" (NIH Consensus Conference 1998). In stark contrast to the European developments outlined above, the NIH statement makes no reference to heroin as a possible treatment drug. Instead, the focus is on improved training for physicians, removal of unnecessary barriers to methadone maintenance, and insurance coverage for treatment programs. In its concluding statement the Panel recommends that "all persons dependent on opiates should have access to methadone hydrochloride maintenance therapy under legal supervision, and the U.S. Office of National Drug Control Policy and U.S. Department of justice should take the necessary steps to implement this recommendation." Apparently, methadone maintenance may not be readily nor uniformly available in the United States (Ciment 1998). The barriers responsible for this are very likely the same ones responsible for the omission of heroin in the NIH statement.

THE ETHICS OF HEROIN PRESCRIPTION

The absence of any mention of heroin prescription in the NIH Panel consensus statement means that opiate addicts in the U.S. are being denied a treatment modality that is viewed as promising by other Western jurisdictions. This is arguably a violation of justice. There are other important ethical issues raised in the relevant literature. Highlights include the quarrel that pits harm reduction against abstinence (Erikson et al. 1997; Jurgen 1997); the debate over whether addiction should be viewed as a social or a medical problem (ten Have and Spoken 1985); the argument that existing resources are better spent elsewhere (Gaughwin and Ryan 1999); and the worry that there is a risk of promoting the message that heroin addiction is acceptable (Bammer et al. 1999a). These are just a few scattered themes and examples.

Evidently, there is an interesting literature on the ethics of heroin prescription. No resolution of those issues will be attempted here. For present purposes, what deserves mention is what those discussions omit. Nothing is said about whether the subjects targeted for heroin prescription are capable of competent voluntary consent to heroin. Consent is mentioned, but usually only to say it is important to seek it and to stress that subjects must be properly informed (Gaughwin and Ryan 1999; Koran 1973; Ostini et al. 1993; ten Have and Spoken 1985). Everyone appears to assume that competent voluntary consent to heroin use is possible. There is no indication of any serious worry that prescription subjects might suffer from decisional impairments that compromise their capacity to consent. In addition, no mention is made of the fact that individuals like these are particularly vulnerable to exploitation if promised free heroin. There are therefore two serious omissions in discussions of the ethics of heroin prescription. The capacity to give competent voluntary consent is presumed when it should not be, and no allowance is made for the fact that prospective subjects are particularly vulnerable to offers of free and legal heroin.

A good example of how competence to consent and vulnerability have been overlooked in discussions of heroin prescription is the WHO evaluation of the Geneva Trial. The WHO experts note that the project was approved by the Ethics Committee of the Swiss Academy of Medical Sciences. Indeed, the report simply states that "participation in the study was voluntary" (WHO 1999, 4). The perspective of the Geneva researchers is no different. Summarizing their enrollment procedures, they write,

> during this (initial) visit, the psychiatrist confirmed the patient's eligibility, explained program procedures, obtained informed consent, performed the baseline assessment, and allocated the patient to either immediate or delayed admission by using computer generated random numbers placed in sealed envelopes. (Perenger et al. 1998, 13)

Again, everyone seems to be assuming that competent voluntary consent to heroin prescription is possible. In the words of an early defender of heroin prescription, "administering heroin to addicts who volunteer for research and provide informed consent would not violate medical ethics" (Koran 1973, 657). If Cynthia is right, however, the presumption that heroin addicts are capable of competent voluntary consent to heroin is simply wrong. Let us see why.

CYNTHIA'S DILEMMA

The main premise of Cynthia's Dilemma is that either

1. prospective heroin-prescription subjects are heroin dependent; or
2. they are not heroin dependent.

If (1) is true and subjects *are* heroin dependent, then they cannot participate in the trial, since they are incapable of competent voluntary consent. If (2) is true and subjects are *not* heroin dependent, then they cannot participate in the trial, since they do not qualify. Either way, therefore, subjects cannot participate, from which it follows that the trial cannot be conducted. The key to the dilemma is the claim that because they are heroin dependent, prescription subjects are incapable of competent voluntary consent. To understand the force of this point, we need to look more closely at the nature of addiction.

Why should a diagnosis of heroin dependence preclude the ability to give competent voluntary consent to heroin? The answer lies in the *Diagnostic Statistical Manual of Mental Disorders*. There *substance dependence* is described as "a cluster of cognitive, behavioral, and physiological symptoms indicating that the individual continues use of the substance despite negative consequences. There is a pattern of repeated self-administration that usually results in tolerance, withdrawal, and compulsive drug taking behavior" (American Psychiatric Association 1994, 176). Compulsive drug-taking behavior is a clinical defining feature of substance dependence. Drug taking in this context extends to seeking as well as using. The individual is completely obsessed with the substance they are addicted to. Virtually all daily activities and relationships are organized around procuring and securing their drug of choice. In the words of Alan Leshner, these individuals suffer from "an uncontrollable compulsion to seek and use drugs" (Leshner 1999, 3).

The notion of compulsion is critical to understanding addiction. It is well known that chronic heroin addicts like those in the Geneva Trial no longer take their drug simply because they want to experience its euphoric effects. They also have powerful cravings for it and need to take it to prevent withdrawal. In Leshner's words, "continued repetition of voluntary drug taking begins to change into involuntary drug taking, ultimately to the point that the behavior is driven by a compulsive craving for the drug" (3). This is what Cynthia meant when she said that a heroin addict cannot say "No" to heroin. The compulsive drug taking that defines addiction is a direct physiological consequence of dramatic neuroadaptations produced in the reward pathways of the brain (Koob and Le Moal 1997; Nestler and Aghanjanian 1997; Powledge 1999). The powerful reinforcing effect of social and personal factors that accompany drug use only make those compulsions more acute. The fact that in many cases the brain is permanently altered by addictive drugs is worth noting. It means that recovery for some individuals may require years of maintenance on a replacement drug. This is the rationale behind methadone maintenance.

Compulsion is one clinical defining feature of addiction that compromises decision-making capacity (College on Problems of Drug Dependence 1995, 170–71; Gorelick, Pickens, and Bonkovsky 1999, 179; Leshner 1997; 1999). But it is not the only one. Intoxication and withdrawal are two others. When intoxicated the addict is no longer in the throes of active compulsion. They are instead in a state that resembles delirium (National Bioethics Advisory Commission 1998, 6). Withdrawal is also often considered to be tantamount to delirium (National Bioethics Advisory Commission 1998, 6). There are therefore two different kinds of decisional impairment involved in addiction. First, there is compulsion, which compromises the voluntary nature of choice. Second, there are intoxication and withdrawal, which compromise

the ability to comprehend choices. Compulsion results in volitional impairment, while delirium results in cognitive impairment. A helpful way to interpret this difference is to say compulsion results in disordered desires, while delirium results in disordered beliefs (Elliott 1996, 2–3). However, it is important to remember that addiction is a combination of both compulsion and delirium, locked in a tragic alternating cycle. As tolerance sets in and greater amounts of the drug are required to achieve the same effects, the individual's life literally spirals out of control (Koob and Le Moal 1997, 53 fig.1).

So what does a clinical diagnosis of heroin dependence mean? First, it means that decisions that relate directly to heroin use are susceptible to powerful physiological and psychological compulsions that usually nullify any semblance of voluntary choice. This is one reason why heroin addicts cannot be considered accountable for their decision to use heroin. Second, even if voluntary choice was somehow possible, heroin addicts are still not competent to consent to its use. This is because chronic heroin addiction results in radical changes in personal values that make seeking and using heroin the overriding goal of the addict's life. Quite literally, the addict's brain has been hijacked by the drug (Leshner 1997). Addicts are no longer themselves and in that sense can no longer be considered accountable for their decision to use heroin.

The decisional impairments that result from chronic heroin addiction are therefore complex. They also fluctuate (National Bioethics Advisory Commission 1998, 7). Compulsion is absolutely central to the decisional impairments in addiction. But addiction is not simply a compulsive disorder. As mentioned above, it also results in fundamental changes in personal values. These usually last as long as the person remains actively addicted. There are interesting implications here for the theory of competence. Someone whose life revolves around compulsively seeking and using a drug despite negative consequences can hardly be considered mentally capable of rationally weighing the risks and benefits of using it. Yet the ability to rationally weigh risks and benefits is generally considered to be an important condition of competence. We have seen that addiction lends credence to the view that competence requires some sort of accountability (Elliott 1991). It is time to focus on the argument that addiction compromises competence because it alters a person's values (Brock and Buchanan 1987).

VALUE AND ACCOUNTABILITY

If the Geneva Trial research protocol were submitted to a North American ethics review board today, the issue of competency would almost certainly be raised as a potential problem. Certainly, existing clinical ethical guidelines suggest that it should (National Bioethics Advisory Commission 1998; College on Problems of Drug Dependence 1995). They specifically warn that special care should be taken when administering substances prone to being abused to persons with past or present problems with substance disorders.

The ethics of research involving the administration of alcohol is important to consider in examining heroin prescription. Numerous concerns have been raised about research that involves giving alcohol to subjects who suffer from alcohol abuse or dependence (Koocher 1991; Model, Glazer, and Mountz 1993; National Advisory Council on Alcohol Abuse and Alcoholism 1998; Stricker 1991). Surprisingly, although alcohol and heroin are alike in many relevant respects, similar reservations have not been expressed in the case of heroin. Recall how unproblematic the consent of the Geneva subjects was thought to be. The discrepancy is puzzling. If the competency of alcoholics to consent to research with alcohol is suspect, then why not the competency of heroin addicts to consent to heroin-prescription research? In order to answer that question, we need to specify what counts as competence. A good place to start is the MacArthur model developed by Appelbaum and Grisso (Appelbaum and Grisso 1995; Grisso et al. 1995; Grisso and Appelbaum 1995; Appelbaum and

Grisso 1998). It is one of the most sophisticated models available and has the benefit of having been empirically validated. So let us see how our Swiss subjects would have fared if their eligibility to consent had been assessed using the MacArthur model.

According to the MacArthur model competence is comprised of four distinct components:

1. the ability to understand a choice;
2. the ability to appreciate a choice;
3. the ability to rationally manipulate information; and
4. the ability to communicate a choice.

Since the Geneva subjects were clearly able to communicate a choice, that condition will be ignored in what follows. There are several important features that the MacArthur model shares with other leading accounts in the field. First, there is the fact that mental competence is held to be decision specific. Dan Brock and Alan Buchanan put the point this way: "a person may be said to be competent to make a particular decision at a particular time, under certain circumstances, but incompetent to make another decision, or even the same decision, under different conditions" (Brock and Buchanan 1987, 18). Second, competence is stipulated to be a threshold concept. Either you are competent or you are not.

Now consider consenting to heroin prescription with the MacArthur model in mind. Understanding in this case revolves around whether or not an individual can be said to comprehend the relevant facts involved in a particular decision. Appreciation builds on what is comprehended in understanding and extends to the acknowledgment that those facts pertain to oneself. Thus it is one thing to understand what heroin dependence is, but quite another to recognize and acknowledge that those facts apply to oneself. In alcohol dependence this distinction is especially pertinent, since alcoholics typically deny they are "alcoholic" even though they may understand perfectly well what alcoholism is. Heroin addicts, on the other hand, generally seem to appreciate the fact that they are addicted, even though they may deny the negative consequences of their addiction. So far, it is not unreasonable to grant that the subjects in the Geneva trial may have satisfied the understanding and appreciation conditions of the MacArthur model. If there is a problem with competence, then it must lie elsewhere. The only possibility left is the ability to manipulate information rationally. This involves

a. reasoning logically from premises to conclusion; and
b. evaluating the risks and benefits of prospective decisions.

This last task requires the capacity to assign preferences to anticipated decisional outcomes as well as the capacity to weigh and balance their respective merits. That requires values.

The role of value in mental competence is controversial. On the positive side there are those who argue it is an essential ingredient of competence. For example, Brock and Buchanan have argued that "a competent decision-maker … requires a *set of values* or *conception of the good* that is at least minimally consistent, stable, and affirmed as his or her own" (Brock and Buchanan 1987, 25; emphasis in original). According to them, values are required "in order to be able to evaluate particular outcomes as benefits or harms, goods or evils, and to assign different relative weight to them" (25). Reasoning and deliberation, they say, require "applying the decision-makers' values" (25). Values are also mentioned in the President's Commission discussion of mental competence (President's Commission for the Study of Ethical Problems in Medicine and Biomedical and Behavioral Research 1982, 47). Nevertheless, despite these important precedents, not everyone is equally impressed with the status of value in competence. In their recent book, Appelbaum and Grisso acknowledge that values play a role in competence. They note that in evaluating risks and benefits "one needs to weigh the desirability of various potential consequences, based on one's own subjective values" (1998, 55). However, other than that they have little to say about the matter. The case of heroin prescription

calls for a more refined examination of how exactly values interface with mental competence.

Brock and Buchanan argue that a stable core of enduring values is required for competence. However, they are careful to allow for lapses in consistency and stability. They limit themselves to a requirement of "minimal" stability and consistency. At the very least, a person must have a limited set of enduring values that count as their own. The reason is that a choice that does not—at least minimally—reflect a person's real likes and dislikes cannot be said to be *their* choice. A helpful way to interpret this claim is to say that competence requires some sort of accountability (Elliott 1991). According to Elliott, the essence of accountability is whether "the decision truly belongs to the patient" (169). His point is that "what we really want to know when we ask if a person is competent is whether that person is able to make decisions for which he can legitimately be judged accountable" (169). Now how can a person with no minimally stable real values of their own be held accountable for their decision? It is hard to see how a decision made in such circumstances could reflect a person's real wants and dislikes. There is an important sense in which a choice made in such circumstances does not really belong to the person who makes it. It is not truly theirs. Therefore, they cannot be held accountable for it. Heroin prescription thus provides an interesting illustration of Elliott's thesis that competence requires accountability.[3] Let us now consider how it helps illustrate Brock and Buchanan's claim that an enduring set of values is required for competence.

Consider again our hypothetical competency assessment. Did the Geneva subjects have the requisite core of enduring values to count as competent? And are the values they have really their own? Empirical research on addiction suggests that in both cases the answer is "No" (Koob and Bloom 1988; Leshner 1999). Remember that the brain of a heroin addict has almost literally been hijacked by the drug. The set of values that governs their daily decisions and behavior is no longer really theirs. Everything they decide and do eventually reduces to seeking and using their drug of choice. So if chronic heroin addicts can be said to have enduring values at all, most of them are ultimately controlled and defined by their clinical condition. The drug doesn't always have the first say, but it usually has the last word. It follows that chronic heroin users cannot reasonably be said to have a set of enduring values that is really theirs on which to base decisions about their heroin use. To that extent, they are unable to manipulate information rationally in the sense required, particularly when decisions about their own heroin use are involved. Hence, they cannot be said to be mentally competent when decisions about their drug of choice are at stake.

CARING TOO MUCH

A helpful way to illustrate the decisional biasing that occurs in addiction is to compare it to a related phenomenon in depression. Recall the argument that severely depressed individuals may not be competent to consent to research because they care too little about risks (Elliott 1997). Because of their condition, severely depressed subjects cannot rationally weigh the risks and benefits associated with their decision to consent. The reason is that their sense of value is warped and biased by depression, so *risks are underweighted*. Their decision is not truly theirs, and so they cannot be held accountable for it. Therefore they are not competent to consent. The heroin addict's situation is just the opposite. Because of their condition, addicted subjects cannot rationally weigh the risks and benefits associated with their decision to consent. But their sense of value is warped and biased by addiction, so *benefits are overweighted*. Their decision is not truly theirs, and so they cannot be held accountable for it. It follows that they are not competent to consent.

Therefore, like the severely depressed subject, the addicted individual is apparently not competent to consent to research. In both cases the decision in question is not truly their own. The depressed subject is disposed to care too little, while the addicted subject is disposed to

care too much. Among other things, both suffer from a marked deficiency in the evaluative capacities that govern emotion (Charland 1998a; 1998b). Their choices do not adequately reflect their real enduring values, because the brain mechanisms and systems that govern evaluation have been disrupted and reoriented. This is a good example of how considerations associated with emotion can be important in assessing competence. Indeed, the relevance of emotion to mental competence is starting to receive increased attention (Appelbaum 1998; Elliott 1999). There are also intimate links between emotion and addiction that deserve further study (Elster 1999).[4]

We have seen that there are good reasons for believing that an enduring set of values is a prerequisite of competence. The values of severely depressed individuals and addicted persons are seriously compromised, which suggests their competence is as well. But in the kind of unipolar depression we are discussing, the reorientation in values that occurs is a relatively entrenched and uniform feature. The resulting impairment in decisional capacity is equally entrenched and uniform. The situation with heroin addiction is markedly different. The impairment in decisional capacity is indeed entrenched, and in that respect depression and addiction are analogous. However, in the case of addiction the reorientation in values is not uniform. In the words of the National Bioethics Advisory Commission, substance dependence is a disorder that is characterized by "fluctuating capacity" (National Bioethics Advisory Commission 1998, 7). Thus addiction and chronic unipolar depression are not analogous. The difference arises from the daily dynamics of craving and withdrawal that are characteristic of addiction. This phenomenon is especially prevalent with addiction to a drug like heroin because of its relatively short half-life. Heroin addicts such as the Geneva subjects sometimes have to inject heroin up to two or three times a day.

The philosopher Jon Elster has written eloquently about some of the decision-theoretic options available to model the dramatic shifts in goals and values that characterize addiction (Elster 1999). His discussions of "preference reversal" and "hyperbolic discounting" are particularly helpful in modeling the changes in motivational state that accompany and precipitate relapse. It is because goals and values wax and wane in this way that ambivalence is such a pervasive feature of addiction. Indeed, according to Elster, ambivalence is the hallmark of addiction (10, 74). The addict desperately wants to quit but usually fails. They say they really value and desire a life without drugs but usually end up behaving in a manner that shows they really value and desire the opposite. Life is a relentless seesaw where long-term goals and values repeatedly collapse under the whiplash of craving and compulsion.

A MOMENT OF CLARITY?

The decisional impairments in heroin addiction fluctuate cyclically even though they also exhibit some uniformity. Insofar as they fluctuate, is it possible there may be a point on the continuum of drug use when an addict is competent to consent to heroin? Is there perhaps a moment of clarity between craving and intoxication? It would be rash to dismiss this possibility a priori. Some, indeed, have argued there are such moments. Let us see how plausible the suggestion is.

One set of guidelines on substance-abuse research acknowledges most of the problems with consent described above but claims that there are nonetheless moments when addicts might be competent to voluntarily consent to consume a substance of abuse. The claim is made that "while addicts do exhibit 'loss of control' over their drug use, the 'loss of control' in addiction is not complete" (College on Problems of Drug Dependence 1995, 171). The argument is the following:

> Research has shown ... that when offered a choice between using drugs to experience their pharmacological effects or avoiding drugs to obtain other commodities important to the individual, addicts

often elect not to use drugs…. In other words, using drugs excessively is not entirely outside the realm of the addict's own control but is in part determined by other conditions. Also, addicts make many responsible decisions during their daily lives that involve avoiding drug use. (171)

Only one study is referred to in defense of this point (Higgins et al. 1993). Unfortunately, its relevance is questionable. It deals with cocaine abuse, and of course our topic is heroin dependence. The problem is that cocaine is generally not thought to produce the same sort of dependence as heroin.[5] So it is probably inadvisable to automatically extrapolate from the former case to the latter. Moreover, even granting the study is relevant, it still provides a very weak basis for the general conclusion it is meant to support. Competence is too fine grained a matter for generalizations of this sort (Appelbaum and Grisso 1995; 1998; Brock and Buchanan 1987). The safest course of action is to presume that in the absence of any studies showing that heroin addicts are competent to voluntarily consent to heroin, there is no reason to believe that they are. Fortunately, it is true that addicts sometimes do have a moment of clarity—some would say revelation—when they decide to stop using their drug and commit themselves to recovery (James 1929, 201–04, 320–21). But that decision relates to treatment, and our topic is research.

ALTERNATIVE STRATEGIES

I have argued that the research subjects typically sought for heroin prescription cannot satisfy the requirements for informed consent outlined here. By virtue of their clinical condition, they cannot satisfy the third condition for competent choice outlined in the MacArthur Study: the ability to manipulate information rationally. Heroin-dependent individuals do not possess this ability where heroin is concerned. Either they are completely biased in favor of it by compulsion, or they are condemned to seesaw ambivalently, up to several times a day, between intoxication and craving. In the former case, neither their basic values nor their choices are truly theirs. And in the latter, fluctuations in values and preferences make a decision truly made at one time just as truly nullified at another. It is hard to escape the conclusion that heroin-prescription research violates existing North American ethical standards for clinical research. The only safe assumption is that these subjects are incompetent to consent until proven otherwise.

However, an ethical analysis does not simply end with the declaration that a given treatment intervention or research protocol may be unethical. In many cases much work remains to be done. Heroin prescription is a good example. As we saw, there is apparently a strong need to investigate the medical prescription of heroin as a treatment alternative. In closing, it is interesting to speculate on two possible strategies that might circumvent the problem posed by our dilemma. Because guidelines and regulations governing the medical prescription of heroin and other opiates vary across different jurisdictions, the following remarks will be restricted to general ethical and policy features of the proposed strategic alternatives.

One strategy is simply to grant that prospective subjects for heroin trials are incompetent and then investigate options for surrogate decision making. If prospective subjects considered for heroin trials are willing to enroll, then what harm is there in letting them participate? An appropriate, perhaps independent, surrogate authority could be invoked to certify or deny decisions to enroll. Although adequate follow-up data is lacking, the Geneva Trial participants appear to have had a low-risk experience with important positive benefits. If the risk-benefit ratio of future trials minimizes risks and maximizes benefits in this way, it may be ethically appropriate to permit enrollment using some form of surrogate consent. Willing participants would then be asked to assent to heroin prescription, but their assent would be subject to the approval of a surrogate authority appointed to ensure their best interests are not jeopardized.

A second strategy might be to focus on the notion of risk and build on the idea that competence should be assessed using a sliding scale (Brock and Buchanan 1987, 51–65). Very basically, the sliding-scale approach to competence dictates that when risks are low, standards for competence should be low; and when risks are high, standards for competence should be high. There are precedents for this strategy. For example, in a recent discussion on alcohol research, we are told that "the critical ethical issue related to the administration of ethanol to research subjects involves the degree to which the benefits to the subject or society outweigh the risks to the research participants" (Dolinsky and Baber 1997, 1092). We are also told that "almost all of the studies that have evaluated research participants following exposure to ethanol administration have failed to identify adverse effects on subsequent drinking behavior or psychosocial adjustment" (Dolinsky and Baber 1997, 1092). The implication is that the medical administration of ethanol to alcoholics or problem drinkers may be ethically permissible when the risks to participants are suitably low or nonexistent. Can a similar argument be made for heroin prescription?

Suppose the risks associated with heroin prescription are minimal, or at least not superior to those the addict will encounter in their daily life. What does this mean for competence? According to the second strategy, it means that standards for competence can be set low, since risks are low. Could they be set low enough to permit some form of competent consent? The answer, probably, is no. This is because the subjects sought for heroin prescription invariably suffer from serious psychiatric disorders other than addiction. In Dolinsky and Baber's discussion of ethanol administration, we are told that "subjects with serious psychiatric conditions are usually excluded from studies because of the potential confounding effect of the psychiatric disorder or the potential for the psychiatric state to be exacerbated" (1093). It is not unreasonable to suggest that this provision should also be applied to heroin prescription. I leave the reader to ponder the merits of these two strategies.

CONCLUSION

Heroin prescription as undertaken in the Geneva Trial would appear to violate existing North American ethical standards for clinical research. This is because the subjects considered for such trials fail to satisfy the required standards for competent voluntary consent. It follows that the Geneva Trial would probably be unethical according to existing North American standards. I hasten to add that this is not meant to be an indictment of the personal ethics or professional integrity of the Swiss researchers, nor indeed anyone else currently considering or conducting heroin-prescription research. However, it does strongly suggest that the issue of consent to heroin prescription needs to be revisited. Some form of systematic empirical testing of the sort that has been carried out for depression is probably necessary. In the meantime, we should not presume that heroin-prescription subjects who are active in their addiction are capable of competent voluntary consent to heroin-prescription research. Quite the contrary, we should assume they are incompetent to consent unless proven otherwise.

Notes

1. Like many of the authors I will be discussing, I will use the terms *addiction* and *substance dependence* interchangeably. There are, however, occasions when it is helpful to distinguish the two; for example, when distinguishing the kind of dependence that occurs when opioids are prescribed for pain relief and when they are used for pleasure-seeking and euphoric effects (Stimmel 1997, 53–56). Furthermore, I will also use the terms *decision-making capacity* and *mental competence* interchangeably. As noted in the recent report by the National Bioethics Advisory Commission, they are often used to denote the same thing (National Bioethics Advisory Commission 1998, 13 n. 4). Finally, although heroin can be administered in different forms, the focus of this discussion will be the prescription of injectable heroin.

2. Some authors refer to the medical provision of heroin as "heroin prescription" (Bammer et al. 1999). Others refer to "heroin maintenance" (Perneger et al. 1998) or "heroin substitution" (Jurgen 1997). The terms are often used interchangeably but probably should not be. To characterize what is involved in the medical provision of heroin as "substitution" seems slightly disingenuous. Is the point simply that legal heroin is being substituted for illegal heroin? Or perhaps the idea is that one mode of administration (injection) is being substituted for another (smoking)? Referring to heroin "maintenance" seems more plausible, since subjects in these studies are in fact being "maintained" on heroin. These distinctions become important when the medical administration of heroin is examined in light of the debate between harm reduction and abstinence. The term *prescription* has the advantage here. It is neutral between the provision of heroin to maintain an individual on opiates and prevent withdrawal (goal: harm reduction) and the provision of heroin where the purpose is to taper the individual off opiates entirely (goal: abstinence).

3. Elliott appears to identify accountability and responsibility. For example, he writes: "If a person is accountable for his decision, the credit for that decision justifiably rests with him. Any praise, blame, merit, or demerit that the decision carries can reasonably be said to belong to him, because the decision was truly his" (Elliott 1991, 169). Whether accountability should be identified with responsibility in this way is questionable. Distinguishing practical, or factual, responsibility from moral responsibility is probably advisable here. The sense of accountability I have in mind is the former, more practical and factual one. However, the entire matter needs to be revisited in detail. Elliott's contributions to the theory of competence have certainly not received the attention they merit.

4. One important link is the amygdala, a brain structure that is widely believed to be central to emotion (Damasio 1994; LeDoux 1996; Panksepp 1998). The amygdala is also said to be intimately involved in addiction (Leshner and Koob 1999). The connection is plausible, since both addiction and emotion are closely tied to pleasure and reward. It would not be surprising if they shared some of the same brain systems and pathways.

5. For example, compare the discussion of cocaine and heroin addiction in *Management of Alcohol, Tobacco, and Other Drugs: A Physician's Manual* (2000, 171–88 and 221–82).

References

American Psychiatric Association. 1994. *Diagnostic and statistical manual of mental disorders*, 4th ed. Washington: American Psychiatric Association.

Angell, M., and J.P. Kassirer. 1994. Alcohol and other drugs: Toward a more rational and consistent policy. *New England Journal of Medicine* 331(8): 537–39.

Appelbaum, P. S. 1998. Ought we to require emotional capacity as part of decisional competence? *The Kennedy Institute Journal of Ethics* 8(4): 377–89.

Applebaum, P. S., and T. Grisso. 1995. The MacArthur Treatment Competence Study (I): Mental illness and competence to consent to treatment. *Law and Human Behavior* 19: 105–26.

———. 1998. *Assessing competence to consent to treatment: A guide for physicians and other health care professionals.* Oxford, U.K.: Oxford University Press.

Appelbaum, P. S., T. Grisso, E. Frank, S. O'Donnel, and D. J. Kupfer. 1999. Competence of depressed patients to consent to research. *American Journal of Psychiatry* 156(9): 1380–84.

Bammer, G., and R. M. Douglas. 1996. The ACT heroin trial proposal: An overview. *Medical Journal of Australia* 164: 690–92.

Bammer, G., A. Dobler-Mikota, P. M. Flemming, J. Strang, and A. Uchtenagen. 1999a. The heroin prescribing debate: Integrating science and politics. *Science* 284(5418): 1277–79.

———. 1999b. [Response.] *Science* 284(5418): 531.

Bayer, R. 1976. Heroin maintenance: An historical perspective on the exhaustion of liberal narcotics reform. *Journal of Psychedelic Drugs* 8(2): 157–65.

Brewer, C. 1995. Recent developments in maintenance prescribing and monitoring in the United Kingdom. *Bulletin of the New York Academy of Medicine* 72(2): 359–70.

Brock, D., and A. Buchanan. 1987. *Deciding for others: The ethics of surrogate decision-making.* Cambridge, MA: Cambridge University Press.

Caltrider, W. 1999. Prescribing heroin [Letter]. *Science* 285(5418): 533.

Charland, L. C. 1998a. Appreciation and emotion: Theoretical reflections on the MacArthur treatment competence study. *The Kennedy Institute Journal of Ethics* 8(4): 359–76.

———. 1998b. Is Mr. Spock mentally competent? Competence to consent and emotion. With commentaries and replies. *Philosophy, Psychiatry and Psychology* 5(1): 67–86.

Ciment, J. 1998. Clash in U.S. over methadone treatment. *British Medical Journal* 317(7164): 968.

College of Physicians and Surgeons of British Columbia. 1995. *No further harm: Report of the temporary advisory sub-committee on narcotics harm reduction.* College of Physicians and Surgeons of British Columbia Policy Manual.

College on Problems of Drug Dependence. 1995. Special report: Human subjects issues in drug abuse research. *Drug and Alcohol Dependence* 37: 167–75.

Damasio, A. 1994. *Descartes' error: Emotion, reason, and the human brain.* New York: Putnam.

Dolinsky, Z. E., and T. F. Babor. 1997. Ethical, scientific, and clinical issues in ethanol administration research involving alcoholics as human subjects. *Addiction* 92(9): 1087–97.

Elliott, C. 1991. Competence as accountability. *Journal of Clinical Ethics* 2(3): 167–71.

———. 1996. *The rules of insanity: Moral responsibility and the mentally ill offender.* Albany: State University of New York Press.

———. 1997. Caring about risks: Are severely depressed patients competent to consent to research? *Archives of General Psychiatry* 54: 113–16.

———. 1999. *Bioethics, culture, and identity: A philosophical disease.* London: Routledge.

Elster, J. 1999. *Strong feelings: Emotion, addiction, and human behavior.* Cambridge, MA: MIT Press.

Erikson, P. G., D. M. Riley, Y. W. Cheung, and P. A. O'Hare, eds. 1997. *Harm reduction: A new direction for drug policies and programs.* Toronto: University of Toronto Press.

Fisher, B., and J. Rehm. 1997. The case for a heroin substitution trial in Canada. *Canadian Journal of Public Health* 88(6): 367–70.

Gaughwin, M. D., and P. Ryan. 1999. Heroin addiction: The science and ethics of the new treatment pluralism. *Medical Journal of Australia* 170: 129–30.

Gorelick, D. A., R. W. Pickens, and F. O. Bonkovsky. 1999. Clinical research in substance abuse: Human subject issues. In *Ethics in psychiatric research: A resource manual for human subjects protection,* ed. H. A. Pincus, J. A. Lieberman, and S. Ferris, 177–94. Washington: American Psychiatric Association.

Grisso. T., and P. S. Appelbaum. 1995. The MacArthur treatment competence study, 111: Abilities of patients to consent to psychiatric and medical treatment. *Law and Human Behavior* 19: 149–74.

Grisso, T., P. S. Appelbaum, E. Mulvey, and K. Fletcher. 1995. The MacArthur treatment competence study, II: Measures of abilities related to consent to treatment. *Law and Human Behavior* 19: 127–48.

Hartnoll, R., M. C. Mitcheson, A. Battersby, et al. 1980. Evaluation of heroin maintenance in controlled trial. *Archives of General Psychiatry* 37: 877–81.

Higgins, S.T., A. J. Budney, W. K. Bickel, et al. 1993. Achieving abstinence with a behavioral approach. *American Journal of Psychiatry* 150: 763–69.

James, W. 1929. *The varieties of religious experience.* New York: Modern Library.

Jurgen, R. 1997. Heroin substitution in Canada: A necessary public health intervention. *Canadian Journal of Public Health* 88(6): 365–66.

Kleber, H. D. 1994. Our current approach to drug abuse—Progress, problems, and proposals. *New England Journal of Medicine* 330(5): 361–65.

Koob, G. F., and F. C. Bloom 1988. Cellular and molecular mechanisms of drug dependence. *Science* 242: 715–23.

Koob, G. F., and M. Le Moal. 1997. Drug abuse: Hedonic homeostatic dysregulation. *Science* 278(5335): 52–58.

Koob. G. F., P. P. Sanna, and F. E Bloom. 1998. Neuroscience of addiction. *Neuron* 21: 467–76.

Koocher, G. P. 1991. Questionable methods in alcohol research. *Journal of Consulting and Clinical Psychology* 59: 246–48.

Koran, L. H. 1973. Heroin maintenance for heroin addicts: Issues and evidence. *New England Journal of Medicine* 288(13): 654–60.

LeDoux, J. 1996. *The emotional brain.* New York: Simon and Schuster.

Leshner, A. 1997. Addiction is a brain disease, and it matters. *Science* 278(5335): 45–47.

———. 1999. Science-based views of drug addiction and its treatment. *Journal of the American Association* 282(14): 1314–16.

Leshner, A., and G. F. Koob. 1999. Drugs of abuse and the brain. *Proceedings of the Association of American Physicians* 111(2): 99–108.

Management of alcohol, tobacco, and other drugs: A physician's manual. 2000. Toronto: Center for Addiction and Mental Health.

Marsden, J., M. Gossop, Michael, M. Farrell, and J. Strang. 1998. Opioid substitution: Critical issues and future directions. *Journal of Drug Issues* 27(1): 243–64.

Matas, R. 2001. Addicts to get heroin under research project. *The Globe and Mail,* 8 November, A10.

Metrebian, N., W. Shanahan, B. Wells, and G. V. Stimson. 1998. Feasibility of prescribing injectable heroin and methadone to opiate-dependent users: Associated health and harm reductions. *Medical Journal of Australia* 168(12): 596–600.

Miller, J. S. 1998. *Hepatitis and injection drug use in British Columbia: Pay now or pay later?* Provincial Health Officer. Government of British Columbia, Canada.

Modell, J. G., F. B. Glaser, and J. J. M. Mountz. 1993. The ethics and safety of alcohol administration in the experimental setting to individuals who have chronic, severe alcohol problems. *Alcohol and Alcoholism* 28: 189–97.

National Advisory Council on Alcohol Abuse and Alcoholism [Prepared for the National Institute on Alcohol Abuse and Alcoholism]. 1998. *Recommended Council guidelines on ethyl alcohol administration in human experimentation.* Bethesda: U.S. Department of Health and Human Services.

National Bioethics Advisory Commission. 1998. *Research involving persons with mental disorders that may affect decisionmaking capacity,* Vol. 1, *Report and recommendations of the National Bioethics Advisory Commission.* Rockville: National Institutes of Health.

Nestler. E. J., and G. K. Aghanjanian. 1997. Molecular and cellular basis of addiction. *Science* 278(5335): 58–63.

NIH Consensus Conference, National Consensus Development Panel on Effective Medical Treatment for Opiate Addiction. 1998. Effective treatment for opiate addiction. *JAMA* 280(22): 1936–43.

Ostini, R.. G. Bammer, P R. Dance, and R. E. Goodwin. 1993. The ethics of experimental heroin maintenance. *Journal of Medical Ethics* 19: 175–82.

Panksepp, J. 1998. *Affective neuroscience.* Oxford, U.K.: Oxford University Press.

Perneger, T. V., F. Giner, M. del Rio, A. Mino. 1998. Randomized trial of heroin maintenance programme for addicts who fail in conventional drug treatments. *British Medical Journal* 317: 13–18.

Powledge. T. M. 1999. Addiction and the brain. *Bioscience* 49(7): 513–19.

President's Commission for the Study of Ethical Problems in Medicine and Biomedical and Behavioral Research. 1982. *Making health care decisions*, vol. 1. Washington: U.S. Government Printing Office.

Rushe, S. 1999. Prescribing heroin [Letter]. *Science* 285(5418): 532–33.

Stimmel, B. 1997. *Pain and its relief without addiction: Clinical issues in the use of opioids and other analgesics.* New York: Haworth Medical Press.

Stricker, G. A. 1991. Ethical concerns in alcohol research. *Journal of Consulting and Clinical Psychology* 59: 256–57.

ten Have, H. and P. Spoken. 1985. Heroin addiction, ethics, and the philosophy of medicine. *Journal of Medical Ethics* 11: 173–77.

Uchtenhagen, A., F. Gutzwiller, and A. Dobler-Mikola. 1997. *Programme for a medical prescription of narcotics: Final report of the research representatives.* Berne: Swiss Federal Office of Public Health.

Van den Brink, W., V. M. Hendricks, and J. M. van Ree. 1999. Medical co-prescription of heroin to chronic, treatment resistant methadone patients in the Netherlands. *Journal of Drug Issues* 29(3): 587–607.

Wodak. A. D. 1997. Public health and politics: The demise of the ACT heroin trial. *Medical Journal of Australia* 167: 348–49.

World Health Organization. 1999. *Report of the external panel on the evaluation of the Swiss scientific studies of medically prescribed narcotics to drug addicts.* Geneva: World Health Organization.

Who Holds the Leash?

Carl Elliott

Are heroin addicts competent to consent to research studies where they will receive heroin prescriptions? Louis Charland thinks not, and I would be hard-pressed to make that case any more persuasively and elegantly than he has made it himself. Instead, I want to amplify his arguments by putting them in a slightly different way.

When we judge a person's competence to give informed consent, as Charland points out, what we are really doing is making a judgment of accountability. We are asking the question: Can this person be held accountable for his deci-sion? Can the credit or blame for the decision—the moral responsibility, really—be legitimately attributed to this person? We don't hold small children fully accountable for their decisions and actions, nor persons with certain sorts of mental illnesses, nor certain others whose mental capacities have been distorted or impaired by drugs, illness or injury. Nor, in fact, would we typically judge many of these people capable of informed consent. Aristotle thought that a person could be exonerated from moral responsibility from his or her actions for two reasons: ignorance or compulsion; "I didn't know what I was doing" or "I couldn't help doing it." A similar formulation lies behind the institution of informed consent. For informed consent to be valid, it must be given knowingly and freely. Ignorance or compulsion renders it null and void.

Lying in the background of our ordinary judgments of responsibility is a certain picture of the human being. Part of that picture is the assumption that the person is fully conscious, self-governing, possessed of a certain kind of self-regard, and so on. Most people meet these standards, and most are held morally responsible for most of their actions. When something emerges to disrupt that picture, however, we are inclined to start asking questions about responsibility. Something like this lies behind the suspicion motivating Charland's questions about the heroin addict's capacity to consent. If a person is this driven to use heroin, can we honestly say that the decision to use it is hers? She has "decided" to use it, of course, at least in some sense of the word; but we are tempted to put "decide" here in scare quotes, and to describe that decision using the language of mechanism rather than agency: she was compelled to decide as she did, she was driven to do it, the physical craving forced her, she was in the grip of her addiction.

There are really two related but distinct intuitions at work here. One is the sense that an addiction to a drug is different from a mere desire to use it, and that an important difference between addictive and ordinary desires is the strength and intensity of the addictive desire. The stronger a desire, the more likely we are to feel that a person might have little choice but to give in to it, at least under certain circumstances. A second intuition at work is the sense that, at least at some level, a person in the grip of an addiction is "not herself." Whatever her character or mental makeup, whatever combination of values and desires and traits make her who she is, they are disrupted or deranged (perhaps only temporarily) by her addiction. She is no longer in full control of herself. She must go where her addiction leads her, because the addiction holds the leash.

Something about addictions in particular often leads us to conceptualize them as somehow "external" to the person, rather than as a part of a person's "internal" mental life. Addictions (or so we often think) can take on a life of their own, refusing to be controlled by the person herself, leading her to take actions and make decisions wildly contrary to her own best judgments. Once we conceptualize addictions in this way (and often, it seems to me, there is good reason to do that) Charland's question is inevitable. Can a heroin addict really be held accountable for her decision to enroll in a study in which she will be given free heroin? Is she holding the leash, or does the leash hold her? I have been convinced by Charland's argument that the addict cannot be held accountable, and that she cannot competently consent. Others may disagree, but Charland has nicely set the philosophical terms for that disagreement. If heroin addicts can give competent consent, then we need a very different way to conceptualize addiction.

References

Charland, L. C. 2002. Cynthia's dilemma: Consenting to heroin prescription. *American Journal of Bioethics* 2(2):37–47.

Starson v. Swayze 2003 SCC 32, (2003) 225 D.L.R. (4th) 385

Summary prepared by Shelia Wildeman

This judgment concerns the interpretation and application of Ontario's legal test for capacity to make treatment decisions under the *Health Care Consent Act*, S.O. 1996, s. 4(1), particularly as this plays out in the psychiatric context. That test applies to all persons facing proposed medical treatment in Ontario, including persons involuntarily committed to psychiatric hospital. It states:

> 4(1) A person is capable with respect to a treatment … if the person is able to understand the information that is relevant to making a decision about the treatment … and able to appreciate the reasonably foreseeable consequences of a decision or lack of decision.

In *Starson v. Swayze*, the Supreme Court of Canada affirmed the rulings of both courts below to overturn a decision of Ontario's Consent and Capacity Board that Starson was incapable of deciding whether to accept or refuse certain medical treatments proposed by his psychiatrists. Those treatments included neuroleptic medication, mood stabilizers, anti-anxiety medication, and anti-Parkinsonian medication (the last was proposed for relief of certain side effects of the neuroleptics).

Starson, an unusually gifted thinker in the area of theoretical physics, was involuntarily committed to psychiatric hospital in 1999 by disposition of the Ontario Review Board following a criminal court finding that he was not criminally responsible for two counts of uttering death threats. He had a history of psychiatric admissions reaching back to 1985. His most consistent diagnosis was bipolar disorder. Once in hospital, Starson refused the above medications, consenting to psychotherapy only.

Both the six-judge majority and three-judge dissent in this Supreme Court judgment agreed that under Ontario's test for capacity to make treatment decisions, persons are not held to a "best interests" standard and so may make decisions that are contrary to physicians' advice. In addition, both the majority and dissent noted that a patient need not agree with a physician's precise diagnosis to be considered capable. Moreover, the majority emphasized that legal determinations of capacity in the psychiatric context must avoid the "tendency to conflate mental illness with lack of capacity," which "occurs to an even greater extent when involuntary commitment is involved." Patients with mental disorders are presumptively entitled to make their own treatment decisions, absent rebuttal of that presumption on a balance of probabilities.

However, the majority and dissent differed markedly in their portrayal of the facts of this case and on the fundamental question of whether the initial reviewing judge (Justice Molloy of the Ontario Superior Court) was correct in reversing the Board's decision. The judgment of Justice Molloy was twofold: first, the Board's determination of incapacity was unreasonable given the evidence before it; and second, the Board's interpretation of the statutory test was incorrect.

Justice Major, writing for the majority, affirmed both bases on which Justice Molloy's decision rested. Thus on the one hand, the Board's conclusion was unreasonable given the evidence before it. In the first place, the Board had found that Starson was in "almost total" denial of his illness; on this basis it reasoned that he could not relate information to his own disorder or understand the consequences of this decision. In contrast, Justice Major found that while Starson refused to accept any psychiatric diagnosis, there was sufficient evidence (from Starson and in letters from third parties) that he "clearly recognized" that he had "mental problems" and also recognized that his "perception of reality" differed from that of others. Starson thus demonstrated an ability to grasp "the objectively discernible manifestations of the illness" in a form sufficient to meet the test for capacity. Here Justice Major's analysis proceeded from his endorsement of the principle that to be considered capable, "a patient is not required to describe his mental condition as an 'illness', or to otherwise characterize the condition in negative terms."

Second, the Board had found that Starson failed to appreciate the benefits and risks of the treatments in issue. In contrast, Justice Major found that there was no clear evidence either to rebut Starson's claim that previous treatments had not helped him, or to establish that the proposed treatments offered him better prospects. Thus the Board had no basis on which to conclude that the proposed medications offered "likely benefits" that Starson was unable to appreciate. Furthermore, Justice Major found that Starson did appreciate the primary intended effects of these medications, and rejected them. These included the dulling of his perception and slowing or "normalizing" of his thought, to produce in him a condition he deemed "so boring it would be like death." The evidence did not disprove Starson's assertion that the proposed drug treatments would prevent him from engaging with theoretical physics, which was what gave his life meaning. Thus he appreciated the intended benefits, but valued these differently than his doctors did. As to risks of non-treatment, Justice Major focused on the disputed nature of the evidence on the likelihood of deterioration. Moreover, he emphasized that as Starson was not directly asked whether he appreciated the possibility of deterioration, the presumption that he possessed the ability to appreciate that risk was not rebutted.

The majority also upheld Justice Molloy's opinion that the Board had committed a fundamental error of law in its interpretation of the legal test for capacity. Specifically, the Board's reasons reflected an illegitimate adherence to a "best interests" standard. This was evident in its concluding that Starson was "unable" to appreciate certain consequences that had not necessarily been discussed with him (e.g., future dispositions of the Ontario Review Board). Such perceived inability might more properly indicate a failure to inform on his doctors' part. In addition, Justice Major took from the Board's expression of "great sadness" at Starson's situation the "tenor" of a best-interests orientation.

The dissent, written by Chief Justice McLachlin, argued that the Board clearly met the test of reasonableness in its application of the test to the evidence. First, the evidence amply supported the finding that Starson's denial of his illness was "almost total." This was implicit in Starson's failure to see his symptoms as an illness: he was in denial "about mental illness generally" as well as the presence of illness in his case. Such denial amounted to a delusional misapprehension of the facts of his situation, from which the Board reasonably inferred a failure to understand or appreciate the information relevant to the decision. This along with other evidence also established a reasonable basis on which to conclude that Starson was unable to appreciate the potential benefits and risks of treatment. Chief Justice McLachlin focused in part on the doctors' suggestions that despite their attempts, Starson was incapable of engaging with these issues. Further, contrary to the findings of Justice Major, Chief Justice McLachlin found sufficient evidence that the proposed treatment offered Starson a reasonable prospect of improvement, which prospect he failed to appreciate. Finally, the evidence indicated that Starson was unable to appreciate the links between his refusal and such risks as the unlikelihood of return to his previous intellectual functioning, the possibility of further deterioration, and continued incarceration in hospital. As to error of law, Chief Justice McLachlin found no convincing basis on which to conclude that the Board had illegitimately applied a best-interests standard.

PART 3

Ethics in the Realm of Health Care Policies

Placebo-Controlled Trials in Schizophrenia: Are They Ethical? Are They Necessary?

Charles Weijer

1. INTRODUCTION

… Ethicists and scientists appear, at times, to occupy entirely different spheres of discourse. Since the time of the Nuremberg Code, ethicists have preoccupied themselves with questions of informed consent, confidentiality, and, to a lesser degree, risk benefit analysis and justice; medical scientists have busied themselves with the selection of proper controls, sample size calculations, outcome measures and stopping rules for trials. Controversy over the proper use of placebo controls in schizophrenia research has proven to be a source of challenge—and, at times, frustration—because any analysis rooted solely in science or ethics will be lacking. The proper selection of a control arm in medical studies has implications simultaneously for both disciplines. If standards for the conduct of schizophrenia research are to be addressed comprehensively, the demands of both science and ethics must be taken seriously.

2. HISTORICAL BACKGROUND AND THE *DECLARATION OF HELSINKI*

The debate over the proper role for placebo controls in medical research flared in 1994, with the publication of an article entitled "The continuing unethical use of placebo controls" in the *New England Journal of Medicine* (Rothman and Michels, 1994). Reminiscent of Beecher's famous essay critical of unethical research practices (Beecher, 1966), Rothman and Michels cited numerous examples of clinical trials using a placebo control despite the existence of effective treatment. Such studies, they charged, violated one of the basic tenets of human experimentation articulated in the *Declaration of Helsinki*: "In any medical study, every medical patient—including those of a control group, if any—should be assured of the best proven diagnostic and therapeutic Method" (World Medical Association, 1995). "Nevertheless," they concluded, "studies that breach this provision of the *Declaration of Helsinki* are still commonly conducted, with the full knowledge of regulatory agencies and institutional review boards" (Rothman and Michels, 1994).

The placebo controversy spilled over from the United States into other countries. In Canada, for example, Elliott and Weijer (1995) singled out the use of placebos in schizophrenia and depression research for criticism. Effective and rigorously tested treatment for these two diseases has existed for decades. "Why," they asked, "do psychiatric researchers intentionally give mentally ill patients substandard treatment?" (Elliott and Weijer, 1995). The answer, remarkably enough, is that the Therapeutic Products Directorate—Canada's counterpart to the US Food and Drug Administration—requires that "new psychiatric drugs must be tested against placebo, and shown to be better" (Elliott and Weijer, 1995). Like Rothman and Michels, the authors declare the practice unethical, and base this conclusion, in part, on the *Declaration of Helsinki*.

The reaction from some clinical researchers was: "Shoot—or at least amend—the messenger." Lasagna (1995) retorted that placebos are not the problem, the problem is the *Declaration of Helsinki*. The requirement cited above, he pointed out, not only prohibits the use of placebo controls, but prohibits all clinical research when effective treatment exists.

> I see very little room in this statement for clinical research with a putative new therapy. Unless one is dealing with a disease or symptom for which *no* accepted therapy exists, the "best proven … therapeutic method," which must be guaranteed for *all* subjects (control or not), is the most effective available therapy. By definition, an untested medication cannot be the "best therapeutic method," because its potential efficacy can only be speculated on before a convincing controlled trial. (Lasagna, 1995)

Thus, he argued, it is the *Declaration of Helsinki*—and not the practice of research—that must be altered.

Is the *Declaration of Helsinki* completely misguided? Or, is it a poorly worded expression of a central principle in research ethics: the medical care of subjects ought not be disadvantaged by research participation? An examination of other ethical codes and guidelines favors the latter interpretation. The guidelines of the Medical Research Council of Canada (MRC) state that "[p]articular care must be taken, however, in such studies with patients to ensure that the subject's best interest is never sacrificed to that of the randomized study" (Medical Research Council of Canada, 1987). The US Office for Protection from Research Risk (1993) IRB Guidebook cautions researchers that "[a] design involving a placebo control should not be used where there is a standard treatment that has been shown to be superior to placebo by convincing

evidence." Canada's new Tri-Council Policy Statement on Ethical Conduct for Research Involving Humans, set to replace the current MRC guidelines in May 1998, articulates a similar standard: "The use of placebo controls in clinical trials is generally unacceptable when standard therapies or interventions are available for a particular patient population" (Medical Research Council of Canada, Natural Sciences and Engineering Research Council of Canada, and Social Sciences and Humanities Research Council of Canada, 1998). Finally, and perhaps most telling, the long awaited revision of the *Declaration of Helsinki* (1996) adds the following clarification to the text quoted above: "This does not exclude the use of placebo in studies where *no proven diagnostic or therapeutic method exists*" [emphasis added].

3. CLINICAL EQUIPOISE AND THE ETHICS OF RANDOMIZED CONTROLLED TRIALS

At stake in the placebo debate is a fundamental question of the ethics of randomized controlled trials (RCT): when is it ethical to initiate an RCT? Freedman (1987) provides the most authoritative answer to the question with his notion of clinical equipoise. The principle of clinical equipoise requires that at the start of an RCT there must exist honest, professional disagreement in the community of expert practitioners as to the preferred treatment. This disagreement can arise in various ways. In one scenario, there is a standard treatment but preliminary evidence arises that a new drug may be superior to the existing treatment. In another scenario, the clinical community may be split in their preference for two different treatments; each "faction" having evidence to support their endorsement of one treatment over the other. Whatever the source of the uncertainty, the purpose of an RCT is to resolve the dispute and "the trial must be designed in such a way as to make it reasonable to expect that, if it is successfully concluded, clinical equipoise will be disturbed" (Freedman, 1987).

Clinical equipoise is a robust principle, in part, because it is both a moral and epistemological principle. It has implications for not only the initiation of RCTs but also their design, including the question of what control ought to be used. In general, according to clinical equipoise, the placebo control is used properly in evaluating first-generation treatments for a medical condition. Once effective treatment exists, second-generation treatments ought to be tested against best available therapy. In a subsequent article, Freedman (1990) gives more specific guidance and spells out five conditions in which the use of a placebo control is justified:

(1) there is no standard treatment;
(2) standard treatment is no better than placebo;
(3) standard treatment is placebo;
(4) the net therapeutic advantage of standard treatment has been called into question by new evidence; and
(5) effective treatment exists, but is not available due to cost or short supply.

Two additional cases deserve to be mentioned explicitly. First, it is permissible to use a placebo control in a population of patients who have failed to respond to standard treatment, provided that no effective second-line treatment exists. Second, a treatment added on to a standard regimen might be compared to placebo provided that all patients in the trial receive the standard regimen.

How might an Institutional Review Board (IRB; in Canada, a Research Ethics Board) determine whether placebo is justified in a particular schizophrenia study? Clearly, the onus would fall on the investigator to demonstrate that one of the above conditions is satisfied in the circumstances of the study. If the IRB lacks the expertise to judge such claims authoritatively, it ought to consult with expert practitioners not involved in the conduct of the study (and without any other conflict of interest) and the medical literature.

For example, the IRB might consult Kane's review article on the treatment of schizophrenia in the *New England Journal of Medicine* (Kane, 1996). In this authoritative review, the author concludes that antipsychotic drugs have been proven effective for the treatment of schizo-

phrenia and that "[a]lthough antipsychotic drugs have an array of adverse effects, their therapeutic index is high" (Kane, 1996). Risperidone is a first-line treatment for schizophrenia and

> [i]f compliance is established and the drug is ineffective, a different class of antipsychotic drug should be tried. A second failure would be an indication for the use of clozapine.... Clozapine is at present the best treatment for patients with refractory psychosis. (Kane, 1996)

Once the acute episode has resolved, Kane concludes that maintenance treatment is well established and those recovering from a first episode ought to be treated for 2 years and those who have had two or more episodes should be treated for 5 years or more.

Admittedly, the standard of care for schizophrenia, as for other diseases, is a moving target as new treatments are developed at a rapid rate. But if, for the purposes of illustration, the IRB considers the above description an accurate depiction of the standard of care, when might it legitimately consider a placebo-controlled trial in schizophrenia permissible? Three circumstances in which the use of placebo may be acceptable suggest themselves immediately: (1) a trial of an add-on treatment to first-, second- or third-line treatment for schizophrenia, e.g., risperidone+new drug versus risperidone+placebo; (2) a trial in treatment-refractory patients (i.e., those who fail to respond to clozapine), e.g., new drug versus placebo; and (3) a trial examining the efficacy of prolonged maintenance therapy for patients who have been in full remission for 2 years following a first episode of illness or for 5 years following two or more episodes of illness, e.g., "standard" drug versus placebo....

4. CONCLUSION

... Ethicists and clinician-investigators both support the goal of advancing knowledge of the treatment of schizophrenia, but disagree as to the means that may be legitimately employed to achieve it....

The title of this paper posed two questions regarding the use of placebo controls in schizophrenia research: Are they ethical? Are they necessary? The answer to each of these questions is a qualified "No." While the use of placebo controls may be acceptable in carefully defined circumstances, e.g., testing an add-on to a standard regimen or evaluating a drug in a treatment-resistant patient population, in most cases the use of an active control in schizophrenia research is ethically and scientifically preferable.

Acknowledgment

This work is supported by a Medical Research Council of Canada Scholar Award and Operating Grant.

References

Beecher, H.K., 1966. Ethics and clinical research. *New Engl. J. Med.* 274, 1354–1360.

Elliott, C., Weijer, C., 1995. Cruel and unusual treatment. *Sat. Night* 110 (10), 31–34.

Freedman, B., 1987. Equipoise and the ethics of clinical research. *New Engl. J. Med.* 317, 141–145.

Freedman, B., 1990. Placebo-controlled trials and the logic of clinical purpose. *IRB: Rev. Hum. Subj. Res.* 12 (6), 1–6.

Kane, J.M., 1996. Schizophrenia. *New Engl. J. Med.* 334, 34–41.

Lasagna, L., 1995. The Helsinki Declaration: timeless guide or irrelevant anachronism? *J. Clin. Psychopharmacol.* 15, 96–98.

Medical Research Council of Canada, 1987. *Guidelines on Research Involving Human Subjects.* Minister of Supply and Services, Ottawa.

Medical Research Council of Canada, Natural Sciences and Engineering Research Council of Canada, and Social Sciences and Humanities Research Council of Canada, 1998. *Tri-Council Policy Statement on Ethical Conduct for Research Involving Humans.* Minister of Supply and Services, Ottawa.

Office for Protection from Research Risk, 1993. *Protecting Human Subjects: Institutional Review Board Guidebook.* US Government Printing Office, Washington, DC.

Rothman, K.J., Michels, K.B., 1994. The continuing unethical use of placebo controls. *New Engl. J. Med.* 331, 394–398.

World Medical Association, 1995. Declaration of Helsinki [1964, rev. 1975, 1983, 1989]. In: Reich, W.T. (Ed.), *Encyclopedia of Bioethics*, rev. ed. Simon and Schuster/Macmillan, New York, 2765–2767.

A Critique of Clinical Equipoise: Therapeutic Misconception in the Ethics of Clinical Trials

Franklin G. Miller and Howard Brody

The Hypericum Depression Trial Study Group published in 2002 the results of a randomized trial comparing hypericum (St. John's Wort), sertraline (Zoloft), and placebo in the treatment of major depression.[1] In the study, funded by the National Institutes of Health, 340 subjects from twelve participating centers were randomized to three trial arms for an eight-week period, with careful monitoring to assure that patients who worsened significantly or who became suicidal were removed from the study and received adequate treatment. Neither hypericum nor sertraline was found to be superior to placebo on the primary outcome measures. The authors noted, "From a methodological point of view, this study can be considered an example of the importance of including inactive and active comparators in trials testing the possible antidepressant effects of medications. In fact, without a placebo, hypericum could easily have been considered as effective as sertraline."[2]

What can we conclude about the ethics of this trial? One dominant viewpoint in research ethics would have prohibited the study. On this viewpoint, a randomized trial is ethical only in circumstances of "clinical equipoise"—a genuine uncertainty within the medical community as to whether (in this case) any of the three treatment arms are superior to the other two. No such uncertainty exists. Approximately twenty-five clinically available antidepressants, including sertraline, have been shown to be superior to placebo.[3] Moreover, the majority opinion within psychiatry probably holds that sertraline is definitely superior to hypericum for major depression, even if hypericum has potential for the treatment of mild to moderate depression. But another widespread viewpoint would hold that the trial was ethically sound. Depressed individuals widely use hypericum, a "natural" agent, despite the lack of proven efficacy. Accordingly, a rigorous evaluation offered scientific, clinical, and social value. According to the report of trial results, the study was approved by institutional review boards (IRBs) at twelve sites and subjects provided written informed consent.

But if clinical equipoise is a basic requirement for ethical research, how could all these review boards be blind to the unethical nature of this trial? And how could two such radically divergent viewpoints exist, without research ethics being widely regarded as in a state of crisis?

THERAPEUTIC MISCONCEPTIONS

The prevailing ethical perspective on clinical trials holds that physician-investigators can discharge their "therapeutic obligation" to patients in the context of randomized clinical trials (RCTs) as long as treatments being tested scientifically satisfy clinical equipoise. We contend that this ethical perspective is fundamentally flawed. An ethical framework that provides normative guidance about a practice should accurately characterize the practice. The prevailing

ethical perspective fails this test: All sound ethical thinking about clinical research, and the regulatory framework for review of protocols for clinical investigation, depends on a basic distinction between research and therapy. But the claims in the prevailing ethical perspective on clinical trials conflate research and therapy. These claims are that the ethics of the physician-patient relationship must govern RCTs, that physicians who conduct these trials have a "therapeutic obligation" to patients enrolled in them, and that RCTs must be compatible with some form of equipoise.

Certainly, investigators and ethicists recognize that clinical trials are scientific experiments, which differ from standard medical care. They also recognize that they are subject to regulatory requirements which do not apply to routine medical practice. However, the prevailing ethical framework views clinical trials through a therapeutic lens. The mainstream ethical approach to clinical trials attempts to have it both ways: to view the clinical trial as a scientific experiment, aimed at producing knowledge that can help improve the care of future patients, and as treatment conducted by physicians who retain fidelity to the principles of therapeutic beneficence and therapeutic non-maleficence that govern the ethics of clinical medicine. The doctrine of clinical equipoise has emerged as the bridge between medical care and scientific experimentation, allegedly making it possible to conduct RCTs without sacrificing the therapeutic obligation of physicians to provide treatment according to a scientifically validated standard of care. This constitutes a "therapeutic misconception" concerning the ethics of clinical trials, analogous to the tendency of patient volunteers to confuse treatment in the context of RCTs with routine medical care.[4] As Paul Appelbaum has recently observed, "In fact, this confusion between the ethics of research and of ordinary clinical care appears rampant in the world of clinical trials."[5]

The therapeutic misconception in the ethics of clinical trials is reflected in the language commonly used within the clinical research enterprise.

Clinical trials are often described as "therapeutic research," and investigators are regarded as having a "therapeutic intent." Research participants who are being studied because they have a medical condition under investigation are referred to as "patients," and investigators as "physicians" or "doctors," without qualification.

To demonstrate our contention about the mainstream approach to the ethics of clinical trials, we will offer an intellectual reconstruction of some of the history of research ethics since the 1970s. This history is characterized by incoherence resulting from commitment to two incompatible positions, each approaching research ethics in a fundamentally different way. The therapeutic misconception about the ethics of clinical trials has emerged from the "similarity position," which argues that ultimately, the ethics of clinical trials rest on the same moral considerations that underlie the ethics of therapeutic medicine. The "difference position" argues that the ethics of clinical trials must start with the realization that medical research and medical treatment are two distinct forms of activity, governed by different ethical principles.

The reigning ethical paradigm for clinical trials has coexisted with clinical trials practice that departs from its guidance. Clinical equipoise, the cornerstone of the similarity position, rules out placebo-controlled trials whenever there is a proven effective treatment for the disorder under investigation.[6] However, IRBs have routinely approved such placebo-controlled trials. These two anomalies—unappreciated theoretical incoherence and conflict between the theoretical paradigm and the practice of ethical review of clinical trials—call for critical examination of the similarity position and the doctrine of clinical equipoise.

THE DISTINCTION BETWEEN RESEARCH AND THERAPY

In 1979, Robert Levine summarized "the most important achievements of the National Commission" for the Protection of Human Subjects of Biomedical and Behavioral Research in "correcting the conceptual and semantic errors that had undermined virtually all previous attempts to develop rational public policy on research involving human subjects."[7] Two portions of Levine's summary capture the essential ingredients of the difference position: recognizing the distinction between research and therapy and, accordingly, abandoning the distinction between therapeutic and nontherapeutic research.

Clinical research shares with medical care the fact that both are performed by physicians in clinical settings, and both often use similar diagnostic and treatment interventions. When the commission began its work, physicians commonly regarded clinical research and medical therapy as inextricably connected. One authority quoted by Levine claimed that "Every time a physician administers a drug to a patient, he is in a sense performing an experiment." But the commission recognized the importance of determining the boundaries between routine medical practice and research. For Levine, the commission's conceptual breakthrough came with the realization that the physicians of the day were thinking about clinical research in the wrong way, and that the boundary between research and therapy was clear rather than fuzzy. The commission came to hold that clinical research is fundamentally different from medical practice.[8]

Clinical medicine aims at providing optimal medical care for individual patients. Ethically, it is governed by the principles of therapeutic beneficence and therapeutic nonmaleficence. Therapeutic beneficence directs physicians to practice medicine with primary fidelity to promoting the health of particular patients. According to therapeutic nonmaleficence, the risks of medical care to which a patient is exposed are to be justified by the prospect of compensating medical benefits for that patient. The physician uses scientific knowledge to care for the patient and engages in therapeutic experimentation with the aim only of finding optimal treatment. It is not part of the role of the physician in providing medical care to develop scientific knowledge that can help future patients.

Clinical research, in contrast, is not a therapeutic activity devoted to the personal care of patients. It is designed for answering a scientific question, with the aim of producing "generalizable knowledge." The investigator seeks to learn about disease and its treatment in *groups* of patients, with the ultimate aim of improving medical care. Scientific interest in any particular patient concerns what can be learned that is applicable to other patients. In view of the nature and purpose of clinical research, the principles of beneficence and nonmaleficence applicable to clinical research lack the therapeutic meaning that guides their application to medical care. Clinical research is dedicated primarily to promoting the medical good of future patients by means of scientific knowledge derived from experimentation with current research participants—a frankly utilitarian purpose.

A major reason for distinguishing research from therapy is to underscore that clinical research has an inherent potential for exploiting research participants.[9] Exploitation also may occur in clinical medicine—venal physicians sometimes perform medically unnecessary procedures for the sake of profit, for example. Yet when physicians of integrity practice medicine, physicians' and patients' interests converge. The patient desires to regain or maintain health or to relieve suffering; the physician is dedicated to providing the medical help that the patient needs.

In clinical research, by contrast, the interests of investigators and patient volunteers are likely to diverge, even when the investigator acts with complete integrity. Patient volunteers, especially in clinical trials, typically seek therapeutic benefit, though they also may be motivated by altruism.[10] Investigators are interested primarily in developing scientific knowledge about groups of patients. Regardless of investigators' motivations, patient volunteers are at risk of having their well-being compromised in the course of scientific investigation. Clinical research involves an inherent tension between pursuing rigorous science and protecting research participants from harm.[11]

Historically, the ethical distinction between research and therapy emerged out of concern about exploitive abuses of patients in clinical research. Reflection on this dark history gave rise to a major development in the ethics of clinical research: the requirement for independent, prospective review and approval of research protocols.[12] Prior independent review was considered necessary for clinical research because of the divergence between the interests of the investigator and the research participant. Self-regulation by physician-investigators could not be trusted in the research context to the same extent that self-regulation by physicians was appropriate in the therapeutic context. The basic rationale for prospective, independent research review depends on the distinction between research and therapy.

The point of distinguishing research and therapy is not to make an invidious comparison, implying that clinical trials are more risky or ethically problematic than routine clinical practice. Indeed, there is some evidence that patients receive more favorable medical outcomes in many clinical trials,[13] and clinical medicine is certainly rife with ethical problems. Further, since research is more carefully regulated than medical practice, it is quite likely that fewer ethical violations occur in research. To say that two activities are ethically different is not to say that either is inherently better than the other.

ABANDONING THE DISTINCTION

The distinction between research and therapy is most likely to be obfuscated in the context of clinical trials, which test the safety or efficacy of investigational and standard treatments. Since patients may derive medical benefit from trial participation, especially in phase III RCTs (the final stage of testing, which many investigational drugs never even reach), clinical trials are often characterized as "therapeutic research."

Nonetheless, the process of treatment in RCTs differs radically from routine clinical practice.[14] Consider the contrast between the hypericum-sertraline trial and routine medical care for depression. If a physician treated 340 patients for major depression, she would not decide which drug to administer by flipping a coin. If the physician elected to use sertraline, she would judge each case individually to determine dose, when to change the dose, and whether to prescribe a second antidepressant or recommend other treatment. We would expect to find considerable variation in the treatment administered to those 340 patients after eight weeks or so. From the vantage point of therapy, this is what it means to provide care to patients.

From the vantage point of research, such variation would wreak havoc on experimental design and the validity and generalizability of findings. So when patients are randomized to one or another experimental drug, and are treated according to relatively inflexible protocols, the activity is very different from therapeutic medicine.

In many other ways, too, routine aspects of research deviate from what would be required by the duties of therapeutic beneficence and nonmaleficence. Volunteer patients and physician investigators are often ignorant of assignment to the experimental or control treatment, which may be a placebo. Trials often include interventions such as blood draws, lumbar punctures, radiation imaging, or biopsies that measure trial outcomes but in no way benefit participants. RCTs often contain a drug "washout" phase before randomization to avoid confounding the evaluation of the investigational treatment with the effects of medication that patients were receiving prior to the trial. These various features of research design promote scientific validity; they carry risks to participants without the prospect of compensating therapeutic benefit.

For these reasons, Levine argued that the second major contribution of the commission was to abandon the "illogical" distinction between therapeutic and nontherapeutic research, which previous policymakers thought was essential to the proper regulation of research and the protection of human subjects.[15] Because research and therapy are distinct activities, and the ethics of therapeutic medicine therefore cannot be automatically extended to guide research, it is mistaken to label research as "therapeutic" or "nontherapeutic," as if that made any fundamental ethical difference. Many research trials consist of a complex mix of therapeutic and nontherapeutic elements—the placebo-controlled trial being only one obvious example—such that labeling the trial as a whole as "therapeutic" or "nontherapeutic" is misleading. In addition, the therapeutic-nontherapeutic distinction diverts attention from key ethical issues. Consider a nontherapeutic trial in which one interviews subjects and takes saliva samples, and a therapeutic trial in which one is testing a new cancer drug that has some promise for creating remission, but also has potentially life-threatening toxicity. Is the latter trial less in need of stringent regulatory oversight because it is "therapeutic"? Or does the therapeutic-nontherapeutic distinction distract the observer from those aspects of the trials that assume far greater moral weight, such as the level of risks and the potential vulnerability of subjects?

Once one understands the distinction between research and therapy, one realizes that "therapeutic" research is still research, and that the ethical rules appropriate to it are those appropriate for clinical research generally. Even though the patient may derive benefit from treatment being evaluated, the basic goal of the activity is not personal therapy, but rather the acquisition of generally applicable scientific knowledge. The basic goal and nature of the activity determines the ethical standards that ought to apply.

Writing in 1993, Jay Katz affirmed the vital importance of the distinction between research and therapy and deplored its blurring in practice: "The astronomical increase in clinical research has, in practice, not led to a clear demarcation between therapy and research, bioethical theories notwithstanding. This vital distinction remains blurred when physician-investigators view subjects as patients, and then believe that patients' interests and not science's are being served by participation in randomized clinical trials that are so commonly conducted in today's world."[16] One of the reasons investigators (and bioethicists) have failed to appreciate the distinction between research and therapy is that the similarity position has conceived the ethics of clinical trials within the context of the physician–patient relationship.

CHARLES FRIED AND THE SIMILARITY POSITION

In 1974, Fried published *Medical Experimentation: Personal Integrity and Social Policy,* which launched the similarity position within bioethics.[17] Fried assumed that answers to ethical dilemmas in research would have to be found within the ethics of therapeutic medicine. He defended fidelity to the interests of the individual patient against a model in which "medicine is to be viewed as caring for populations."[18] What made the RCT ethically suspect was that it seemed to him a prime example of population-focused—rather than individualized—and utilitarian medicine.

Fried devoted most of his book to defending patients' "rights in personal care."[19] Returning to medical research, he took issue with trials in which patients were randomized to receive either the experimental intervention or standard care. Fried coined the term "equipoise" to describe the ethically necessary condition for conducting an RCT: physician-investigators must be indifferent to the therapeutic value of the experimental and control treatments evaluated in the trial. The basic idea of equipoise had previously been articulated by Bradford Hill, a pioneer in the development of RCTs.[20] But what Fried objected to primarily in RCTs was not randomization per se, but the fact that no informed consent had been obtained. Fried saw the threat of "care for groups" (instead of "care for individuals") as residing primarily in the idea that it was legitimate to enroll subjects in an RCT without explicit, informed consent because the results of the trial would provide new medical knowledge that would improve the lot of future patients.[21] Because Fried was concerned chiefly about informed consent, an essential ingredient of both medical research and therapeutic medicine, he saw no problem in applying the ethics of medical therapy to medical research.

In the 1970s, the "respect for patient autonomy" movement was gaining steam as a replacement for the old Hippocratic ethic of paternalistic beneficence. Since both Fried and the National Commission seemed on the surface to be championing patient autonomy, it was easy to miss the point that they were proposing two fundamentally different strategies for approaching the ethics of clinical trials. Put another way, so long as the bioethics debate of the moment has to do with whether research ethics requires all competent subjects to give fully informed consent, any fundamental divergence between the similarity and the difference positions is likely to be obscured.

THE EMERGENCE OF CLINICAL EQUIPOISE

During the 1980s, philosophers interested in research ethics recognized a tension between the obligation of physicians to offer optimal care to their patients ("the therapeutic obligation") and the provision of medical treatment in the context of clinical trials. Don Marquis addressed this problem in a 1983 essay, "Leaving Therapy to Chance."[22] The title is significant, suggesting that the RCT is a form of therapy rather than an ethically distinct activity. Marquis began his essay, "Consider this dilemma: according to an argument that is hard to refute, the procedure for conducting randomized clinical trials of anti-cancer drugs is incompatible with the ethics of the physician–patient relationship. If this problem is to be resolved, then either a key procedure for achieving scientific knowledge in medicine must be given up or unethical behavior by physicians must be tolerated."[23] In framing this "RCT dilemma," Marquis assumed that the appropriate ethic for clinical trials was that of the (therapeutic) physician–patient relationship.

Fred Gifford, following the lead of Marquis, examined the RCT dilemma in greater depth: "The central dilemma concerning randomized clinical trials (RCTs) arises out of some simple facts about causal methodology (RCTs are the best way to generate the reliable causal knowledge necessary for optimally informed action) and a *prima facie* plausible principle concerning how physicians should treat their patients (always do what it is most reasonable to believe will be best for the patient)."[24] Neither Marquis nor Gifford found what they regarded as a satisfactory solution, and neither considered the possibility that the difference position could dismiss the "RCT dilemma" as misguided to begin with.

In a landmark 1987 article, Benjamin Freedman offered a solution to the RCT dilemma that gained widespread acceptance within bioethics. He argued that the tension between ethically legitimate scientific experimentation and the therapeutic obligation of physicians could be overcome by the principle of "clinical equipoise."[25] Freedman agreed with Fried and Marquis that ethical clinical trials had to be compatible with therapeutic beneficence and nonmaleficence. But he argued that Fried's formulation of equipoise was too constraining. Freedman called Fried's original concept "theoretical equipoise" (sometimes called "individual equipoise") and contrasted it with his favored concept of "clinical equipoise" (sometimes called "collective equipoise"). In the latter sense of equipoise, any individual investigator or physician might have reasons to believe that one arm of the RCT offers a therapeutic benefit over the other arm, but the medical profession as a whole remains divided. According to Freedman, an RCT is ethical so long as the professional community has not yet reached a consensus, which recognizes that "medicine is social rather than individual in nature."[26] When, and only when, clinical equipoise is satisfied will patients enrolled in a clinical trial be assured that they will not be randomized to treatment known to be inferior. Freedman thus asserted in a later article that clinical equipoise is "grounded in the normative nature of clinical practice, the view that a patient is ethically entitled to expect treatment from his or her physician—an entitlement that cannot be sacrificed to scientific curiosity."[27]

The bioethics community perceived Freedman's concept of clinical equipoise as both a theoretical and a practical advance. Theoretically, it appeared to offer a more intellectually compelling argument than Fried's initial formulation. Practically, it would permit useful RCTs that would otherwise be ethically proscribed to go forward. Since it appeared to solve the RCT dilemma by accommodating the conduct of clinical trials with the therapeutic obligation of physicians to offer optimal medical care, clinical equipoise gained wide currency as a fundamental concept of the ethics of clinical trials.[28] The persuasive way in which Freedman fortified the similarity position diverted attention from the fact that clinical equipoise collapsed the distinction between research and therapy.

The similarity position and clinical equipoise have been popular not only among bioethicists, but also among investigators. We speculate that this ethical perspective helps to address investigators' psychological needs. Physician-investigators, after all, went to medical school, not investigator school. To think of research with patients outside the ethical framework of the physician–patient relationship, as the difference position requires, may be difficult and threatening to them. Clinical equipoise offers a formula that seems to allow them to mix both physician and investigator roles—even if the psychological comfort is purchased at the price of ethical obfuscation.

The anomaly therefore exists that much of today's bioethical thinking accepts clinical equipoise as an outgrowth of the similarity position, while the Federal regulations grew out of the work of the National Commission, which largely endorsed the difference position. One would imagine that sooner or later proponents of clinical equipoise would realize the need to defend this doctrine from the charge that it conflates the ethics of clinical trials with the ethics of medical care. But this is precisely what has not yet happened.

THE CASE OF PLACEBO-CONTROLLED TRIALS

Although the similarity position, bolstered by clinical equipoise, became the reigning paradigm in the ethics of clinical trials, its dominion over practice was limited. This divorce between theory and practice has been particularly pronounced in the case of placebo-controlled trials. Freedman and his colleagues argued that the use of placebo controls is unethical whenever proven effective treatment exists for the medical condition under investigation in a clinical trial because those randomized to placebo would receive treatment known to be inferior.[29]

Despite the clear implications of clinical equipoise for the ethics of placebo-controlled trials, numerous trials, such as the hypericum-sertraline trial, continued to use placebo controls despite proven effective treatment. Placebo controls have typically been used in trials of new treatments for a wide range of chronic conditions—including mood and anxiety disorders, asthma, stable angina, hypertension, and migraine headaches—all of which can be treated with medication of proven efficacy.

There are two explanations for this incoherence between theory and practice. First, the FDA has encouraged the use of placebo controls in trials concerning these and other chronic conditions.[30] Active-controlled trials designed to test the equivalence of the experimental treatment with a standard treatment suffer from serious methodological limitations. Whenever active-controlled trials show no statistically significant difference between the investigational treatment and an active comparator, two conclusions are possible. Either both were effective in the trial sample of patients, or neither was effective. Without the use of a placebo control, such trials lack internal validity. Accordingly, the FDA has insisted that pharmaceutical companies use placebo controls in trials of new treatments for conditions characterized by fluctuating symptoms and high rates of placebo response.[31] Second, the U.S. federal regulations governing human subjects research do not provide any explicit guidance on the use of placebo controls.[32] IRBs have been free to approve such placebo-controlled trials, provided that they meet regulatory requirements for a favorable risk-benefit ratio, including the potential value of knowledge to be gained and informed consent.

For the most part, this lack of fit between theory and practice received little critical attention until the publication in 1994 of an article in the *New England Journal of Medicine* entitled "The Continuing Unethical Use of Placebo Controls."[33]

Kenneth Rothman and Karin Michels castigated the practice of placebo-controlled trials in the face of proven effective treatment and the role of the FDA in encouraging these trials. They cited the Declaration of Helsinki, which relies heavily on the similarity position, as prohibiting this widespread "unethical" practice.

Their article stimulated a lively debate over the ethics of placebo-controlled trials. Freedman and his colleagues attacked "the placebo orthodoxy" in a two-part article that challenged the scientific value of placebo-controlled trials and reiterated that they are unethical when proven effective treatments exist because they contravene clinical equipoise.[34] Other commentators, writing in leading medical journals, defended more or less extensive use of placebo-controlled trials on methodological and ethical grounds.[35] Without directly challenging the doctrine of clinical equipoise, they implied that clinical equipoise provides erroneous ethical guidance for placebo-controlled trials. Accordingly, the debate over placebo-controlled trials jeopardizes the reigning ethical paradigm of the similarity position and clinical equipoise.

CRITIQUE OF THE SIMILARITY POSITION AND CLINICAL EQUIPOISE

Our reconstruction of the recent history of the ethics of clinical trials has traced the emergence and dominance of the similarity position. This history also reveals cracks in the foundation of this ethical paradigm. Simultaneous endorsement of the difference position, reflected in the federal regulatory system and the Belmont Report, and the similarity position, which invokes the doctrine of clinical equipoise, has left the ethics of clinical trials in a state of incoherence. Although this incoherence has not received critical attention, it becomes apparent once the assumptions underlying the similarity position and clinical equipoise are challenged. In addition, the divorce between research ethics theory and clinical trials practice in the case of placebo-controlled trials suggests that a critique of the similarity position and clinical equipoise is overdue.

We contend that clinical equipoise is fundamentally mistaken because "the RCT dilemma," for which it was proposed as a solution, is false. Clinical equipoise and all other forms of equipoise make sense as a normative requirement for clinical trials only on the assumption that investigators have a therapeutic obligation to the research participants. The "therapeutic obligation" of investigators, forming one horn of the RCT dilemma, constitutes a therapeutic misconception about the ethics of clinical trials. The presumption that RCTs must be compatible with the ethics of the physician–patient relationship assumes erroneously that the RCT is a form of therapy, thus inappropriately applying the principles of therapeutic beneficence and nonmaleficence that govern clinical medicine to the fundamentally different practice of clinical research. It is impossible to maintain fidelity to doing what is best medically for patients in the context of RCTs because these are not designed for, and may conflict with, personalized care. Although ethically appealing, the project of bridging the gap between therapy and research via the doctrine of clinical equipoise is doomed to fail.

The insight that the RCT contravenes the ethics of the physician–patient relationship led Samuel Hellman and Debra Hellman to argue that the RCT is unethical and that other methods of evaluating treatments should be employed.[36] This stance, however, would deprive patients and society of the benefits that flow from rigorous scientific evaluation of experimental and standard treatments. The more reasonable conclusion is that RCTs should be governed by ethical norms appropriate to clinical research, which are distinct from therapeutic beneficence and therapeutic nonmaleficence.

Clinical equipoise is neither necessary nor sufficient for ethically justifiable RCTs. The use of placebo controls when proven effective treatment exists violates clinical equipoise; however, when methodologically indicated, their use is no different in principle from any research intervention that poses risks to subjects without the prospect of benefiting them.[37] In many cases, the risks of withholding effective treatment are excessive, and the use of placebo controls would thus be unethical. Nevertheless, it is the unacceptable level of risk, not the violation of investigators' alleged "therapeutic obligation," that makes these trials unethical. In other cases, including the hypericum-sertraline trial, use of placebo controls when proven effective treatment exists is ethically justifiable.

By conflating the ethics of clinical trials with the ethics of therapeutic medicine, proponents of the similarity position may also contribute to the lack of adequate informed consent. If investigators view the ethics of clinical trials through a therapeutic lens, they may explicitly or implicitly foster the therapeutic misconception among research participants—that is, the tendency of participants in trials to confuse clinical trials with medical care. Research participants need to know that the overall activity is aimed not at their own ultimate benefit, but at discovering new knowledge to help future patients. If they think that clinical trial participation is a form of therapy, then they cannot give informed consent. Moreover, unlike the therapeutic context, the patient-subject cannot delegate the decision to the physician-researcher. In the therapeutic setting, a patient can decide to trust the physician to choose the best treatment because the physician has the patient's best interests at heart. The investigator has the interests of future patients at heart, and so cannot decide for the subject whether or not to participate in the research. To be trustworthy, investigators must themselves understand clearly the ways in which clinical research differs from clinical practice and convey this forthrightly to potential research subjects.

It is worth pondering, however, the practical consequences that might ensue if physicians, investigators, patients, and ethicists understood clinical trials without distortion by therapeutic misconceptions. Would recruitment of participants for valuable clinical trials become substantially more difficult, slowing progress in medical care? The fact that clinical trials are no longer seen as a mode of therapy leaves unchanged the real prospect of therapeutic benefits offered to patients from trial participation, including the opportunity to receive promising investigational agents, ancillary medical care, expert diagnostic evaluations, and education about their disorder. Nonetheless, some patients might be less inclined to participate in clinical trials when they appreciate the differences between these scientific experiments and medical care.

To attract enough subjects, researchers might have to pay people for their participation, as researchers in industry-sponsored clinical trials already do with increasing frequency. Payments would add to the cost of conducting clinical trials, but it might help prevent the therapeutic misconception among trial participants.[38] To be paid signifies that the trial participant is not merely a patient seeking therapy. If additional expenditure is necessary to motivate clinical trial participation, then this is a price worth paying for enhanced professional integrity and informed consent.

AN ALTERNATIVE ETHICAL FRAMEWORK

In view of the theoretical and practical problems associated with the similarity position and its logical offspring, clinical equipoise, an alternative framework for the ethics of clinical trials is needed. The most promising recent treatment of research ethics has been developed by Ezekiel Emanuel, David Wendler, and Christine Grady.[39] They propose seven ethical requirements for all clinical research: (1) scientific or social value; (2) scientific validity; (3) fair subject selection; (4) favorable risk-benefit ratio; (5) independent review; (6) informed consent; and (7) respect for enrolled research participants. This framework is built on the difference between research and therapy and on the core value of *protecting research participants from exploitation.*

Yet even this formulation of an ethical framework appropriate to clinical research testifies to the hold of the similarity position. The authors endorse clinical equipoise, claiming it is implied by the requirements of value, validity, and risk-benefit ratio. We contend, by contrast, that the endorsement of clinical equipoise renders incoherent any account that arises from the difference position. The most important next step for research

ethics is to develop this "non-exploitation" framework systematically in a way that avoids any conflation of clinical research with medical care.

Those who agree that physician-investigators who conduct clinical trials are not governed by therapeutic beneficence still might argue that clinical equipoise provides important methodological guidance for justifying clinical trials. Freedman and his colleagues have argued that clinical equipoise is both an ethical and a scientific principle: "That principle can be put into normative or scientific language. As a normative matter, it defines ethical trial design as prohibiting any compromise of a patient's right to medical treatment by enrolling in a study. The same concern is often stated scientifically when we assert that a study must start with an honest null hypothesis, genuine medical uncertainty concerning the relative merits of the various treatment arms included in the trial's design."[40] Nevertheless, whatever is valid methodologically in clinical equipoise—the honest null hypothesis—can be stated more clearly and without confusion with the therapeutic obligation, by appeal to the requirement of scientific value: no research participants should be exposed to the risks of valueless research. Clinical trials must be designed to answer valuable scientific questions. If the answer is already known or the question is trivial, then there is no honest null hypothesis, and a clinical trial should not be conducted. But this is logically independent of whether all the patients enrolled in the trial would receive medical treatment that is believed by the expert medical community to be at least as good as the standard of care.

This alternative framework provides accurate ethical guidance concerning clinical research without presuming that the ethics of therapeutic medicine should govern clinical trials. We illustrate this by applying the seven ethical requirements to the example of the hypericum-sertraline trial.

Scientific or social value and scientific validity.
The study has social value owing to the widespread use of herbal remedies. Since the efficacy

of hypericum in treating depression (especially major depression) was uncertain, there was an honest null hypothesis that hypericum would be no better than placebo. It would have been unreasonable to design the trial as an active-controlled superiority trial, since it is highly unlikely that hypericum could be shown to be more effective than sertraline. An active-controlled equivalence trial would lack "assay sensitivity" because the finding that the reduction in symptoms of depression experienced by those trial participants receiving hypericum was not significantly different for those receiving sertaline would not validly support the inference that hypericum was effective.[41] It would remain possible that neither treatment was effective in the study sample—as was in fact shown. The study, therefore, was properly designed as a three-arm placebo-controlled trial.

Fair subject selection. There is no evidence to suggest that particularly vulnerable patients were recruited inappropriately for this study, which included a sample representative of depressed patients.

Favorable risk–benefit ratio. Risk–benefit assessment of research protocols ultimately comes down to a matter of judgment. With respect to the use of the placebo control—the aspect of the trial that violated clinical equipoise—the risks to participants from an eight-week trial, with careful exclusionary criteria and monitoring, were not excessive and were justifiable by the anticipated value of the knowledge to be gained from the research. Hence, the placebo component of the study had a favorable risk–benefit ratio. Eliminating the placebo would have made the risk-benefit ratio unfavorable by virtue of undermining the scientific validity of the research.

Independent review, informed consent, and respect for enrolled research participants. The report of the study asserted that IRB approval was obtained at all sites and that all subjects gave informed consent. In addition, the described procedures for monitoring subjects for possible risk of harm indicated an acceptable level of respect.

In sum, this study was ethically justifiable despite violating clinical equipoise; moreover, had it been designed in accordance with clinical equipoise, it would have been methodologically deficient and therefore ethically questionable.

Charles Weijer, a leading advocate of clinical equipoise and the similarity position, has recently claimed that "Placebo-controlled trials in the context of serious illnesses such as depression or schizophrenia are ethically egregious precisely because no competent physician would fail to offer therapy to a patient with the condition."[42] Although we agree that depression is a serious illness, the hypericum-sertraline trial demonstrates that there is nothing "ethically egregious" about the use of placebo controls in trials of treatment for depression, as long as the ethical requirements for clinical research are satisfied. Whether or not one agrees that, all things considered, the placebo control was ethical in this trial, the ethical justification of placebo controls has nothing to do with the therapeutic practice of competent physicians. In any case, the alternative ethical framework with its seven requirements provides adequate guidance for clinical trials without appeal to the incoherent doctrine of clinical equipoise and without conflating the ethics of research with the ethics of therapy.

References

1. Hypericum Depression Trial Study Group, "Effect of *Hypericum Perforatum* (St John's Wort) in Major Depressive Disorder: a Randomized Controlled Trial," *JAMA* 287 (2002):1807–1814.
2. Ibid., 1813.
3. S.M. Stahl, *Essential Psychopharmacology of Depression and Bipolar Disorder* (New York: Cambridge University Press, 2000).
4. P.S. Appelbaum, L.H. Roth, C.W. Lidz, P. Benson, and W. Winslade, "False Hopes and Best Data: Consent to Research and the Therapeutic Misconception," *Hastings Center Report* 17, no. 2 (1987):20–24.
5. P.S. Appelbaum, "Clarifying the Ethics of Clinical Research: a Path Toward Avoiding the Therapeutic

Misconception," *American Journal of Bioethics* 2, no. 2 (2002):22.

6. B. Freedman, "Placebo-Controlled Trials and the Logic of Clinical Purpose," *IRB* 12, no. 6 (1990):1–6.

7. R.J. Levine, "Clarifying the Concepts of Research Ethics," *Hastings Center Report* 9, no. 3 (1979):21–26.

8. National Commission for the Protection of Human Subjects of Biomedical and Behavioral Research, *The Belmont Report* (Washington, D.C.: U.S. Government Printing Office, 1979), p. 3.

9. E.J. Emanuel, D.Wendler, and C. Grady, "What Makes Clinical Research Ethical?" *JAMA* 283 (2000):2701–2711.

10. J. Sugarman, N.E. Kass, S.N. Goodman, P. Perentesis, P. Fernandes, and R.R. Faden, "What Patients Say About Medical Research," *IRB* 20, no. 4 (1998):1–7.

11. F.G. Miller, D.L. Rosenstein, and E.G. DeRenzo, "Professional Integrity in Clinical Research," *JAMA* 280 (1998):1449–54.

12. R.R. Faden and T.L. Beauchamp, *A History and Theory of Informed Consent* (New York: Oxford University Press, 1986):200–232.

13. D.A. Braunholtz, S.J.L. Edwards, and R.J. Lilford, "Are Randomized Clinical Trials Good For Us (in the Short term)? Evidence for a 'Trial Effect,'" *Journal of Clinical Epidemiology* 54 (2001):217–224.

14. J.W. Berg, P.S. Appelbaum, C.W. Lidz, and L.S. Parker, *Informed Consent: Legal Theory and Clinical Practice,* 2nd edition (New York: Oxford University Press, 2001):280–283.

15. R.J. Levine, *Ethics and Regulation of Clinical Research,* 2nd ed. (New Haven: Yale University Press, 1986):8–10.

16. J. Katz, "'Ethics and clinical research' revisited: a tribute to Henry K. Beecher," *Hastings Center Report* 23, no. 5 (1993):36.

17. C. Fried, *Medical Experimentation: Personal Integrity and Social Policy* (New York: American Elsevier, 1974).

18. Ibid., 5.

19. Ibid., 94.

20. A.B. Hill, "Medical ethics and controlled trials," *British Medical Journal* 1 (1963):1043–1049.

21. C. Fried, *Medical Experimentation: Personal Integrity and Social Policy* (New York: American Elsevier, 1974): 8.

22. D. Marquis, "Leaving therapy to chance," *Hastings Center Report* 13, no. 4 (1983):40–47.

23. Ibid., 40.

24. F. Gifford, "The Conflict Between Randomized Clinical Trials and the Therapeutic Obligation," *Journal of Medicine and Philosophy* 11 (1986):347–366.

25. B. Freedman, "Equipoise and the Ethics of Clinical Research," *NEJM* 317 (1987):141–145.

26. Ibid., 144.

27. B. Freedman, "Placebo-Controlled Trials and the Logic of Scientific Purpose," *IRB* 12, no. 6 (1990):5.

28. T.L. Beauchamp, and J.F. Childress, *Principles of Biomedical Ethics* 5th edition (New York: Oxford University Press, 2001):323–327.

29. B. Freedman, K.C. Glass, and C. Weijer, "Placebo Orthodoxy in Clinical Research. II: Ethical, Legal and Regulatory Myths," *Journal of Law, Medicine & Ethics* 24 (1996):252–259.

30. R. Temple and S. E. Ellenberg, "Placebo-Controlled Trials and Active-Control Trials in the Evaluation of New Treatments: Part 1: Ethical and Scientific Issues," *Annals of Internal Medicine* 133 (2000):455–63.

31. T.P. Laughren, "The Scientific and Ethical Basis for Placebo-Controlled Trials in Depression and Schizophrenia: an FDA Perspective," *European Psychiatry* 16 (2001):418–423.

32. Department of Health and Human Services. Protection of Human Subjects. Code of Federal Regulations. 45CFR46, 1991.

33. K.J. Rothman and K.B. Michels, "The Continuing Unethical Use of Placebo Controls," *NEJM* 331 (1994):394–8.

34. See B. Freedman, K.C. Glass, and C.Weijer, "Placebo Orthodoxy in Clinical Research. I: Empirical and Methodological Myths," *Journal of Law, Medicine & Ethics* 24 (1996):243–51; and B. Freedman, K.C. Glass, and C.Weijer, "Placebo Orthodoxy in Clinical Research. II: Ethical, Legal and Regulatory Myths," *Journal of Law, Medicine & Ethics* 24 (1996):252–259.

35. R. Temple and S.E. Ellenberg, "Placebo-Controlled Trials and Active-Control Trials in the Evaluation of New Treatments: Part 1: Ethical and Scientific Issues," *Annals of Internal Medicine* 133 (2000):455–63; E.J. Emanuel and F.G. Miller, "The Ethics of Placebo-Controlled Trials-a Middle Ground," *NEJM* 345 (2001):915–919.

36. S. Hellman and D.S. Hellman, "Of Mice But Not Men: Problems of the Randomized Controlled Trial," *NEJM* 324 (1991):1585–1589.

37. F.G. Miller and H. Brody, "What Makes Placebo-Controlled Trials Unethical?" *American Journal of Bioethics* 2, no. 2 (2002):3–9.

38. N. Dickert and C. Grady, "What's the Price of a Research Subject? Approaches to Payment for

Research Participation," *New England Journal of Medicine* 341 (1999):198–203.

39. See E.J. Emanuel, D. Wendler, and C. Grady, "What Makes Clinical Research Ethical?" *JAMA* 283 (2000):2701–2711.

40. B. Freedman, K.C. Glass, and C.Weijer, "Placebo Orthodoxy in Clinical Research. II: Ethical, Legal and Regulatory Myths," *Journal of Law, Medicine & Ethics* 24 (1996):253.

41. R. Temple and S.E. Ellenberg, "Placebo-Controlled Trials and Active-Control Trials in the Evaluation of New Treatments: Part 1: Ethical and Scientific Issues," *Annals of Internal Medicine* 133 (2000):455–63.

42. C. Weijer, "When Argument Fails," *American Journal of Bioethics* 2, no. 2 (2002): 10.

Proxy Consent for Research on the Incompetent Elderly

Barry F. Brown

In the past decade, the ethical issues of research with the elderly have become of increasing interest in gerontology, medicine, law, and bio-medical ethics. In particular, the issue has been raised whether the elderly deserve special protection as a dependent group (Ratzan 1980). One of the most profound difficulties in this area of reflection is that of the justification of proxy consent for research on borderline or definitely incompetent patients.

Some diseases of the elderly, such as Alzheimer's disease, cause senile dementia: devastating for the patient and family and, in future, a considerable burden for society. This condition, in turn, renders a patient incapable of giving informed, voluntary consent to research procedures designed to learn about the natural history of the disease, to control it, and to find a cure. The research must be done on human subjects, since there is not as yet a suitable animal model; indeed some feel that there never can be such a model. A protection of the patient, rooted in concern for his best interests, from procedures to which he cannot give consent gives rise to a paradox: "If we can only perform senile dementia research using demented patients, but should not allow them to participate because they are incompetent, then we are left in a quandary. We cannot ethically conduct senile dementia research using demented patients because they are incompetent; but we cannot technically perform it using competent subjects because they are not demented" (Ratzan 1980: 36). Such a position seems to protect demented patients at the expense of their exposure, as a class, to prolonged misery or death.

If the patient cannot give consent, is the proxy consent of relatives ethically valid? That is, do the relatives have the moral right or capacity to give consent for procedures that may not offer much hope for the patient in that they may not offer a direct benefit to him?

Such procedures have by recent convention been called non-therapeutic. They might offer a possible benefit for other sufferers in the future, but little hope of benefit for *this* patient, here and now.

At present, an impasse has developed regarding such research. It appears that such procedures might be illegal under criminal laws on assault. If the research is strictly non-therapeutic, then no benefit is to be found for the patient-subject. If the requirement of therapeutic experimentation is that a direct, or fairly immediate, improvement in the patient's condition is the sole benefit that could count, then it is difficult to see how this could be discovered. For unlike the case of a curable disease or research on preventive measures for childhood diseases, such as polio, the Alzheimer's patients suffer from a presently terminal illness. Studies of the causation of this condition may hold little or no hope of alleviating the condition in them. There appears to be no present or future benefit directly accruing to them. Others may benefit, but they likely will not. Thus, it seems, there is no benefit in view.

If, in fact, such procedures, even relatively innocuous ones, are illegal, then such research cannot go ahead. If so, such persons will remain "therapeutic orphans" just as surely as infants and children unless proxy consent is valid. If proxy consent is also legally invalid, then the legal challenge to this impasse may be either legislative or judicial. In either case, ethical arguments must be offered as justification for the case that proxy consent is or ought to be legally valid. The following explorations are a contribution to that debate.

Can some kind of benefit for the demented be found in research that offers no immediate hope of improvement? I believe that it can, but the nature of that benefit will be unfamiliar or unacceptable to those who are sure that there are only two mutually exclusive alternatives: a utilitarian conception of the social good pitted against a deontological notion of the individual's rights.

Contemporary biomedical ethics routinely employs three principles in its effort to resolve such dilemmas (Reich 1970; Beauchamp & Childress 1983). These are the principle of beneficence, which demands that we do good and prevent harm; the principle of respect for persons (or the principle of autonomy), from which flows the requirement of informed consent; and the principle of justice, which demands the equitable distribution of the benefits and burdens of research. But the first two obviously conflict with each other in human experimentation: the principle of beneficence, which mandates research to save life and restore health, especially if this is seen as directed to the good of society, is in tension with the principle of respect for persons, which requires us to protect the autonomy of subjects. Moreover, the principle of beneficence requires us not only to benefit persons as patients through research, but also to

avoid harming them as research subjects in the process. So there is an internal tension between moral demands created by the same principle. Finally, demented patients are no longer fully or sufficiently autonomous. Standard objections to paternalism do not apply. Consequently paternalism of the parental sort is not inappropriate, but rather necessary in order to protect the interest of the patient.

Simple application of these principles, therefore, will not provide a solution. Underlying the manner in which they are applied are radically different conceptions of the relationship of the individual good to the societal or common good.

In the present framework of philosophical opinion, there appear to be two major positions. On the one hand, some consequentialist arguments for non-therapeutic research justify non-consensual research procedures on the grounds that individual needs are subordinate to the general good conceived as an aggregate of individual goods. This good, that of the society as a whole, can easily be seen to take precedence over that of individuals. This is especially so if the disease being researched is conceptualized as an "enemy" of society. On the other hand, a deontological position argues that the rights of the individual take precedence over any such abstract general good as the advancement of science, the progress of medicine, or the societal good. In this view, to submit an individual incapable of giving or withholding consent to research procedures not for his own direct benefit is to treat him solely as a means, not as an end in himself. In this debate, one side characterizes the general good proposed by the other as much too broad and inimical to human liberty; the other sees the emphasis on individual rights as excessively individualistic or atomistic.

There are strengths and weaknesses in both approaches. The consequentialist rightly insists on a communal good, but justifies too much; the deontologist rightly protects individual interests, but justifies too little. I contend that if we are to resolve the dilemma concerning the incompetent "therapeutic orphan," it is necessary to go between these poles. In order to do so, I wish to draw upon and develop some recent explorations concerning non-therapeutic research with young children. In at least one important respect, that of incompetence, children and the demented are similar. We ought to treat similar cases similarly. I wish also to argue that research ethics requires: (1) a conception of the *common good* that is at once narrower than that of society as a whole and yet transcends immediate benefit to a single individual; and (2) a conception of the common good that sees it not in opposition to the individual good but including it, so that the good is seen as distributed to individuals.

THE LESSON OF RESEARCH WITH CHILDREN

As to the first, we may learn much from the discussions concerning research with children, particularly as they bear upon the distinction between therapeutic and non-therapeutic experimentation. In the 1970s a spirited debate took place between the noted ethicists Paul Ramsey and Richard McCormick on the morality of experimentation with children (Ramsey 1970, 1976, 1977; McCormick 1974, 1976). Ramsey presented a powerful deontological argument against non-therapeutic experimentation with children. Since infants and young children cannot give consent, an essential requirement of the canon of loyalty between researcher and subject, they cannot be subjected ethically to procedures not intended for their own benefit. To do so, he contended, is to treat children solely as means to an end (medical progress), not as ends in themselves (Ramsey 1970).

McCormick, arguing from a natural law position similar to that developed in the next section, argued that since life and health are fundamental natural goods, even children have an obligation to seek to preserve them. Medical research is a necessary condition of ensuring health, and this is a desirable social goal. Consequently children, as members of society, have a duty in social justice to wish to accept their share of the burdens of participating in research that promise benefit to society and is of minimal or no risk. Thus the par-

ents' proxy consent is a reasonable presumption of the child's wishes if he were able to consent (McCormick 1974).

There are two major puzzles generated by this debate over non-therapeutic research in children. First, Ramsey stressed that the condition to which a child may be at risk need not reside within his skin, but could be an epidemic dread disease. Thus, testing of preventive measures such as polio vaccine on children is justified; indeed it counts for Ramsey as therapeutic. This is interesting for several reasons. First, the therapeutic benefit may be indirect or remote, not necessarily immediate. Second, it embodies the concept of a group or population at risk smaller than society as a whole. Third, it apparently allows for considerable risk. There was a risk of contracting polio from the vaccine. Although the risk might have been slight statistically, the potential damage was grave. By Ramsey's own account, a slight risk of grave damage is a grave risk. Thus, he was prepared to go beyond the limit of minimal or no risk on the grounds that the polio vaccine was *therapeutic,* while McCormick attempted to justify *non-therapeutic* research on children, but confined the risk to minimal or none. It is odd that in the subsequent protracted debate, this difference was not contested.

The second major puzzle arises from McCormick's view that fetuses, infants, and children ought to participate in low- or no-risk non-therapeutic research in order to share in the burden of social and medical progress in order that all may prosper. Note that only *burdens* are to be shared, not benefits. This is because the topic by definition was non-therapeutic experimentation. By putting it this way he seemed to many to be subordinating the interests of such subjects to a very broadly construed societal good. But let us remember that the argument for such research in the first place was that without it, infants and children would be "therapeutic orphans." That is, without pediatric research, there could be fewer and slower advances in pediatric therapy.

Although not of direct benefit, such research is intended for the long-term benefit of children, and is thus indirectly or remotely therapeutic. It is not conducted for "the benefit of society" or for "the advancement of medical science"; it is for children in the future. Otherwise, it could be carried out on adults. Thus, such research should be construed as done not in view of broad social benefit but for the benefit of children as a group or a sub-set of society. Of course, if advances are made in medicine for the sake of children, society benefits as well, but this is incidental and unnecessary. The sole justification is provided by the benefits now and to come for *children*. At the same time, such benefits set one of the limits for such research: it should be confined to children's conditions, and should not be directed at conditions for which the research may be done on competent persons.

THE COMMON GOOD OF A DISEASE COMMUNITY

Some of the hints arising from the foregoing debate can now be developed. It is indeed wrong to experiment on an incompetent person for "the benefit of society" if the research is unrelated to that person's disease and he is made a subject simply because he is accessible and unresistant. But is it necessarily unethical to conduct experiments on an incompetent person which attempt to discover the cause of the condition which causes the incompetence, and which may cure it or prevent it in others, even if he will not himself be cured?

In a "third way" of conceptualizing the relation between the individual and the group, the good in view is neither that of society as a whole nor that of a single individual. It involves the group of persons with a condition, such as Alzheimer's disease. Here I turn to a conception of the common good articulated by John Finnis of Oxford. Finnis defines the common good not as the "greatest good for the greatest number" but as "a set of conditions which enables the members of a community to attain for themselves reasonable objectives, or to realize reasonably for themselves the value(s) for the sake of which they have reason to collaborate with

each other (positively and/or negatively) in a community" (Finnis 1980: 155).

The community may be either the complete community or the political one, or it may be specialized, such as the medical community, the research community, or the community of children with leukemia, and so on. The common good is thus not the sum total of individual interests, but an ensemble of conditions which enable individuals to pursue their objectives or purposes, which enable them to flourish. The purposes are fundamental human goods: life, health, play, esthetic experience, knowledge, and others. Relevant to this discussion are life, health, especially mental integrity, and the consequent capacity for knowledge, all of which are threatened by diseases which cause dementia.

For my purposes, the community should be considered to be, at a minimum, those suffering from Alzheimer's disease. They have, even if they have never explicitly associated with each other, common values and disvalues: their lost health and the remaining health and vitality they possess. It could be said with McCormick that if they could do so, they would reasonably wish the good of preventing the condition in their relatives and friends.

But the community may be rightly construed more broadly than this. It naturally includes families with whom the patients most closely interact and which interact in voluntary agencies devoted to the condition, the physicians who treat them, the nurses, social workers, and occupational therapists who care for them, and the clinical and basic researchers who are working to understand, arrest, cure, and prevent the disease.

The participation of the patient, especially the demented patient, may be somewhat passive. He is a member of the specialized community by accident, not by choice, unless he has indicated his wish to become a research subject while still competent. Efforts to determine what a demented or retarded person would have wished for himself had he been competent have been made in American court decisions involving an incompetent patient's medical care. These "substituted judgment" approaches may have some worth, especially if the patient had expressed and recorded his wishes while still competent.

An individual might execute a document analogous to a human tissue gift—a sort of pre-dementia gift, in which he would officially and legally offer his person to medical research if and when he became demented. This might alleviate the problem of access to some extent, but it has its own difficulties. A pre-dementia volunteer cannot know in advance what types of research procedures will be developed in future, and so cannot give a truly informed consent except to either very specific procedures now known or to virtually anything. Such a pre-commitment may give some support to the decision to allow him to be a subject. But that decision, I contend, is justified by the claim, if valid, that it is for the common good of the dementia-care-research community, of which he is a member and to which, it is presumed, he would commit himself if he were capable of doing so at the time.

It is true, of course, that one might not ever have wished to participate in research procedures. In this case, the individual should be advised to register his or her objection in advance, along the lines that have been suggested for objection to organ donation in those countries that have a system of presumed consent for such donation. This can be achieved by carrying a card on which such an opt-out is recorded, or by placing one's name on a registry which might be maintained by support organizations. I suggest that unless one opt out in this manner, in the early stages of the disease, he or she be considered to have opted-in. That is, there should be a policy of presumed consent. In any event, as experience with organ retrieval has shown, in the final analysis it is the permission of relatives that is decisive in both those cases in which an individual has consented and those in which he or she has not made his or her wishes known.

The other members of the community may not all know each other. They do, however, have common values and, to a considerable degree, common objectives. There can be a high level of deliberate and active interaction, especially if there is close communication between the researchers, family, and volunteers in the voluntary health agencies.

What, then, is the ensemble of conditions which constitute the common good of the Alzheimer's community? Insofar as the purposes of collaboration include the effort to cure or to alleviate the disease, the common good would embrace, in addition to caring health professionals, a policy of promoting research, its ethical review, a sufficient number of committed clinical and scientific researchers, the requisite physical facilities and funding (some or all of which may be within other communities such as hospitals and medical schools), availability of volunteers for research, an atmosphere of mutual trust between research and subject, and finally ongoing research itself. This list is not exhaustive.

If access to the already demented is not allowed, and if this is essential for research on the disease to continue, it may well be impossible to find the answers to key questions about the disease. The common good of the Alzheimer's community would be damaged or insufficiently promoted. Since the goods of life and mental health are fundamental goods, this insufficiency would be profound.

One essential aspect of this common good is distributive justice. Each patient-subject shares not only in the burdens of research in order that all may prosper, but also the benefits. The benefits are not necessarily improved care or cure for the subject, but generally improved conditions for all such patient-subjects: a more aggressive approach to research, improved knowledge of the disease, increased probabilities for a cure, and others. Since the individual participates wholly in that good, he will be deprived of it in its entirety if it is not pursued. The common good is not so much a quantity of benefits as a quality of existence. It can therefore be distributed in its fullness to each member of the community. So, too, each can suffer its diminution.

Richard McCormick (1974) left his description of the common good unnecessarily broad and sweeping. According to some natural law theorists (Maritain 1947) the common good is always a distributed good, not simply the sum of parts. It is construed as flowing back upon the individual members of the community, who are not simply parts of a whole but persons, to whom the common good is distributed in its entirety. Thus, not only can the common good of which McCormick speaks be narrowed to that of children as a group (equivalent to Ramsey's population at risk) but the benefits of such research can be seen as redistributed to the individuals of the group. The benefits are not to be taken in the sense of an immediately available therapy, but in the sense of improved general conditions under which a cure, amelioration, or prevention for all is more likely.

CONCLUSION

Some of these observations can now be applied to the case of the elderly demented. First, the debate showed the inadequacy of the simple distinction between therapeutic and non-therapeutic experimentation, which has been challenged on several grounds in past years. For example, May (1976: 83) includes diagnostic and preventive types of research under therapeutic experimentation, whereas Reich (1978: 327) observes that the terms "therapeutic" and "non-therapeutic" are inadequate because they do not seem to include research on diagnostic and preventive techniques. In the area of the development of experimental preventive measures such as vaccines for epidemic diseases, and in the area of diseases in which research is carried out on terminal patients with little or no expectation of immediate benefit for these patients, the distinction is somewhat blurred. In each case, there is a defined population at risk: one without the disease but at great risk of contracting it, the other with a disease but with little hope of benefiting from the research.

Such types of research seem to constitute an intermediate category: the "indirectly therapeutic," involving the hope of either prevention or alleviation or cure. This category as applied to dementia shows some characteristics of therapeutic experimentation in the accepted sense, since it is carried out on persons who are ill and it is directed to their own illness. But it also shares some properties of non-therapeutic research, since it is not for their immediate treatment and, therefore, benefit. The good to be achieved is more remote, both in time and in application, since it is less sharply located in the individual than is therapy as such.

It must be admitted that there is a difference between the testing of a vaccine for prevention of disease in young, healthy children and research on elderly, seriously ill patients. In the former, the child-subjects will benefit if the vaccine is successful, or at least be protected from harm. In the latter, the subjects will not benefit by way of prevention or cure of their disease, but rather simply by being part of a community in which those goals are being actively pursued. The identification of the demented patient's good with that common good is doubtless less concrete than the identification of the child's good with that of his peers. But it seems to me that underlying both these cases is a notion of the common good required to justify all cases of research that do not promise a hope of direct benefit to a person who is, here and now, ill.

Years ago, Hans Jonas (1969) noted that a physician-researcher might put the following question to a dying patient: "There is nothing more I can do for you. But there is something you can do for me. Speaking no longer as your physician but on behalf of medical science, we could learn a great deal about future cases of this kind if you would permit me to perform certain experiments on you. It is understood that you yourself would not benefit from any knowledge we might gain; but future patients would." Although greatly vulnerable and deserving of maximum protection, such a patient might be ethically approached to be a research subject, because the benefits to future patients are in a way a value to him: "At least that residue of identification is left him that it is his own affliction by which he can contribute to the conquest of that affliction, his own kind of suffering which he helps alleviate in others; and so *in a sense it is his own cause"* (Jonas 1969: 532, emphasis mine).

In this case, the individual apprehends a good greater than his personal good, less than that of society: that of his disease class, which is *his* good. Of course, the identification of which Jonas speaks is psychological; he would likely not agree with the approach herein outlined and might require that such participation be through a conscious, free choice of the patient. Nevertheless, it is a real, objective good which justifies his choice and prevents us from asking him to participate in research unrelated to his disease. Can a relative, a son or daughter perhaps, ethically make that decision for an incompetent, demented Alzheimer's patient? If so, it is because, in a sense, it is the patient's cause, the patient's good as a member of a community which justifies that choice. It is not a matter of enforcing a social duty or minimal social obligation here, but seeking a good that lies in the relationship one has to others with the same disease. That same good, as noted above, limits the participation of the subject to research related precisely to his disease, not to anything else.

What is the implication of this for risk and the limits of risk? As has been seen, some wish to allow for exposure of subjects to greater than minimal risk provided only that it is classified as "therapeutic" (though the subjects are not ill). Others, in spite of the fact that the research is intended for the benefit of a group at risk, classify it as non-therapeutic and limit the acceptable risk to minimal levels. Are these the only alternatives? One advisory group has allowed, in the case of the mentally incompetent, for a "minor increase over minimal risk" in such circumstances (National Commission for the Protection of Human Subjects 1978: 16). This is presumably permitted because the research is "of vital importance for the understanding or amelioration of the type of disorder or condition of the subjects" or "may reasonably be expected to benefit the subjects in future" (17). But what counts as minor increase in risk? Proposed research into Alzheimer's might involve invasive procedures such as brain biopsies, implantation of electrodes, spinal taps, and injections of experimental drugs. Are these of greater risk than that specified by the National Commission simply because they are invasive of the human

brain? Or is there clear statistical risk of serious added damage to the brain? These are matters for empirical study. The invasiveness per se should not rule out a procedure. The major limitations should be whether the procedure is painful, causes anxiety, or adds to the already serious damage to the brain. If research involving procedures of greater risk than "minor increase over minimal" is ever to be justified, it must be so by the intent to avert the proportional evils of death or mental incapacity. If these are insufficient, then I fail to see what grounds might be available upon which to base a case for legislative change.

It is clear, then, that should such research be acceptable, it also demands that stringent protective procedures be established in order to ensure that the demented are not drafted into research unrelated to their disease class. This is because the standard, being broader than that of "direct or fairly immediate benefit," is open to an accordionlike expansion, and therefore to abuse. Such safeguards could include: rigorous assurance that the proxy's consent (in reality, simply a permission) is informed and voluntary, the provision of a consent auditor, and various layers of administrative review and monitoring, from a local institutional review board up to a judicial review with a guardian appointed to represent the patient-subject's rights. These procedures may prove to be onerous. But we are on dangerous ground, and as we try to avoid overprotection, which may come at the expense of improved therapy for all, we must also avoid opening up a huge door to exploitation.

References

Beauchamp, T.L., & Childress, J.F. *(1983).* *Principles of Biomedical Ethics.* 2nd ed. New York: Oxford University Press.

Finnis, J. (1980). *Natural law and natural rights.* Oxford: Clarendon Press.

Jonas, H. (1969). Philosophical reflections on experimenting with human subjects. In T. Beauchamp and L. Walters (Eds.), *Contemporary issues in bioethics.* 2nd ed. Belmont, CA: Wadsworth.

Maritain, J. (1947). *The person and the common good.* New York: Charles Scribner's Sons.

May, W. (1976). Proxy consent to human experimentation. *Linacre Quarterly, 43,* 73–84.

McCormick, R. (1974). Proxy consent in the experimentation situation. *Perspectives in Biology and Medicine, 18,* 2–20.

McCormick, R. (1976). Experimentation in children: sharing in sociality. *Hastings Center Report, 6,* 41–46.

National Commission for the Protection of Human Subjects (1978). *Report and recommendations: Research involving those institutionalized as mentally infirm.* Washington, DC.

Ramsey, P. (1970). *The patient as person.* New Haven: Yale University Press.

Ramsey, P. (1976). The enforcement of morals: Non-Therapeutic research on children. *Hastings Center Report, 4,* 21–30.

Ramsey, P. (1977). Children as research subjects: a reply. *Hastings Center Report, 2,* 40–41.

Ratzan, R. (1980). "Being old makes you different": The ethics of research with elderly subjects. *Hastings Center Report, 5,* 32–42.

Reich, W. (1978). Ethical issues related to research involving elderly subjects. *Gerontologist, 18,* 326–37.

Swinging on the Pendulum: Shifting Views of Justice in Human Subjects Research

Anna Mastroianni and Jeffrey Kahn

Justice has long been one of the central principles in the ethical conduct of research on human subjects. But its application, as reflected in federal policies pertaining to human subjects research, has undergone a remarkable shift over a relatively short span of time. Understanding this shift is important not only for interpreting claims about justice in human subjects research, but also for assessing the status and adequacy of policies for protecting subjects.

In the 1970s, these policies emphasized the protection of human subjects from the risks of harm in research, and justice was seen as part of this protection. Since the early 1990s, however, justice as applied in research ethics has emphasized the need to ensure access to the potential benefits that research has to offer. That such a dramatic shift could occur so quickly is extraordinary, especially in light of the understanding, coalescing over the same period, that subjects have an inadequate understanding of the research in which they are participating and are inadequately protected by existing practices and policies. The tension between these developments offers an important lesson for research protection as the context of human subject research becomes more complex. Our goal here is to attempt to understand how the pendulum has swung from protection to access, where in its arc we are, and where we should be.

JUSTICE IN THE BELMONT ERA: PROTECTION FROM EXPLOITATION

The development of human subject protection policy in the United States was driven by a history of exploitation of subjects, most notably by research on "vulnerable" subject populations that came to light between the mid-1960s and the early 1970s. The landmark examples were the Willowbrook State School hepatitis vaccine research on institutionalized children; the Jewish Chronic Disease Hospital cancer research, involving the injection of cancer cells into elderly nursing home residents; and the so-called Tuskegee Syphilis Study, which bad been under way for decades but was exposed to an appalled nation in 1972.[1] Those examples contributed to a sense that human subjects research in the United States permitted scandalous practices—inadequate attempts to inform subjects about research and obtain their consent, exploitive recruitment strategies, the use of vulnerable subject populations, and a willingness to expose subjects to significant risk without any potential for direct medical benefit. Further, there was a sense that the risks and benefits of research were split apart—the risks were borne by subjects, the benefits accrued to others.

Thus the early history of U.S. research ethics policy focused on the risks rather than the benefits of research, and on preventing subjects from being exposed to unacceptable or exploitive levels of risk, particularly without the prospect of offsetting direct medical benefits. *The Belmont Report*, issued by the National Commission for the Protection of Human Subjects of Biomedical and Behavioral Research in 1978, identified justice as requiring the fair distribution of the burdens and benefits of research in subject selection and recruitment; in practice, however, justice was interpreted as requiring the prevention of any further exploitation of vulnerable groups.[2] The emphasis was realized through the promulgation of research policies that staked much on protection and that singled out particular groups—namely, prisoners, children, and pregnant women and fetuses—for additional protections.

Prisoners were deemed vulnerable because of the nature of their living environment. Adequate informed consent, it was believed, was not possible when subjects lived in a setting that constrained the autonomy on which the concept of informed consent is based. This view actually ran counter to information collected by the National Commission, which found in interviews with prisoners who participated in research that the prisoners wanted to be enrolled in studies and were highly motivated research subjects, for a variety of reasons—the opportu-

nity to earn a few extra dollars, the perks that might come with research participation, access to more frequent and potentially improved health care, and a belief that participating in research offered a way for them to make a contribution to society. Most interesting was the finding that it was not the least powerful and arguably most vulnerable prisoners who participated in research, but the most powerful.[3] Prisoners often viewed research as an opportunity to be seized rather than a hazard to be avoided; they apparently did not worry that anyone was taking advantage of them. Even so, policies were promulgated, and remain in place today, that made it impossible to perform research on prison populations unless the research either offers a prospect of direct medical benefit to the individual subjects themselves, as in clinical trials for HIV infection, or aims at understanding or improving the prison environment, such that it would potentially benefit prison populations generally.

Children were deemed vulnerable because of similar concerns about informed consent and the potential for taking advantage of their reliance on others. Such concerns were vividly illustrated in the infamous Willowbrook case, where hepatitis vaccine research was performed on institutionalized, mentally retarded children whose parents seemed to have little choice but to agree to their children's participation—thereby picking out the most vulnerable from among the potential pool of children. The rules developed to prevent this sort of exploitation limited research in which children could participate to studies involving either minimal risk or direct medical benefit.

Pregnant women and fetuses were deemed especially vulnerable and deserving of protection. Influenced by the abortion debate and memories of thalidomide, policymakers protected pregnant women from research that carried risk of harm to protect them and their fetus. The implementation of this policy was expanded in practice to include not only pregnant women but also women of childbearing capacity, both to prevent unwitting risk to fetuses and to protect the future health of the women. This practice represented the logical conclusion of a regulatory culture and process that emphasized the protection of subjects from risk as paramount.

FROM PROTECTION TO ACCESS

The research regulatory culture that emphasized protection from risk in the 1970s began to shift during the late 1980s and early 1990s. Due to a growing belief that research increasingly offered real benefits, the application of justice in research began to emphasize the fair distribution of the benefits of research instead of its risks. Advocacy groups, particularly those representing the interests of people with AIDS and women's health groups, argued this view to great effect before Congress and elsewhere. The thrust of their position was that fairness demands not only protection from the risks of research, but increasingly demands the opportunity for inclusion in research. The shift was taking place: from justice as protection to justice as access.

The HIV/AIDS advocacy community was at the forefront of making the case for justice as access. As the first clinical trials for AZT were being undertaken, groups like ACT-UP organized rallies protesting the limited enrollments in them. At a time when subjects were sharing their research medication with friends to spread around whatever potential benefit could be had from these drug trials, protestors were marching in large cities across the country carrying placards proclaiming "Clinical trials are health care too!"[4] Such a sentiment, conflating research participation with medical care, represented not just a shift in emphasis but a total reversal of the ethics of research from protection to access.

Through the late 1970s and 1980s, there was a growing sense that cutting edge therapy could be found in research participation, particularly for cancer, where the best therapeutic outcomes were thought to be in research protocols, and where standard treatment modalities were largely viewed as less effective. It was certainly true that the benefits from the major investments in biomedical research were being realized and applied. The problem was that those benefits were limited to the populations represented in the subject populations—largely although not exclusively adult males. Whatever the complex of reasons for excluding women, racial and ethnic minorities, and children from research participation, the policy was largely predicated on protection from harm and exploitation. But as advocates began to point out, such policies had the effect not only of preventing harm and exploitation, but also of preventing benefit—resulting, claimed one commentator, in a climate that protected some groups to death.[5] Exclusion denies access to the benefits of research at two levels—first to the individuals who may themselves receive the direct medical benefit of research participation, and more notably to the groups from which the subjects come.

There are numerous examples of the research system's failure to provide equitable benefits to women. Among the most notable is the United States Physicians Study, a longitudinal study that assessed the effectiveness of low dose aspirin for preventing heart attacks.[6] It yielded strong evidence of success, but it couldn't be applied outside the research population, comprised exclusively of men, because women are not merely smaller versions of men. Similarly, children are not merely smaller versions of adults, and racial and ethnic groups may differ from each other in disease pathology, drug response, and the like.

The realization that policy and practice had emphasized protection and a denial of the real and perceived benefits of research pushed the pendulum of research policy toward recognizing the importance of access to the benefits of biomedical research, by means of policies requiring inclusion in research set against a background of protection. In 1994, less than twenty years after the first federal policies on research protections were promulgated, the NIH issued the first policy requiring *inclusion* of particular groups in research—the Guideline on Inclusion of Women and Minorities in Research.[7] The guideline represents an unprecedented sea change in thinking about the ethics of research on human subjects.

IMPLEMENTING JUSTICE IN POLICY

The implementation of the 1994 NIH guideline flipped the presumption about research participation from exclusion to inclusion. Researchers were and are now required to include representative populations of women and minorities in their protocols unless there are special reasons for excluding them. It would make no sense, for example, to include women in a clinical trial testing a new drug for prostate cancer, nor would it be reasonable to conduct research on conditions in racial or ethnic groups in which those conditions are not found.

Policy on the participation of children in research is following a similar path, driven by similar arguments. In an effort to protect children, children have been excluded from research that carried greater than minimal risk unless the research also had the potential to provide direct medical benefit to the subjects. Thus federal regulations (subpart D of 45 CFR 46) bar the participation of children in phase I drug trials, which are used to assess the safety of new drugs before their approval. But excluding children from such research has meant there is limited information about the safety of drugs in pediatric populations. This information has instead been pieced together after the drugs are approved and marketed for adults: children have received drug doses based only on the most general calculations of their size relative to the adults for whom drugs are approved, and on the clinical experience (read "trial and error") of pediatricians who have begun to try the drugs on children.

Recent directions from both the NIH and the Food and Drug Administration are changing the presumption from exclusion to inclusion, and requiring a special justification to exclude children.[8] The change in approach has not been completely achieved, however. Reversing the presumption about participation has resulted in a policy that reflects the tension between ensuring access to the benefits of research and protecting subjects from research harms. The dictates of subpart D, as currently written, do not easily coexist with a policy of inclusion. It appears that the long-standing commitments to protection will be weakened as part of the trend toward assuring access to the benefits of research.

Changes in the rhetoric of health policy are further evidence of the emphasis on access to the benefits of research, reaching to the highest levels of our government. Richard Klausner, director of the National Cancer Institute, testifying before Congress in 1998 about the need for large increases in the overall NIH budget (which were eventually granted), argued that substantial additional resources were required "to ensure that all people who wish to participate in a clinical trial are able to do so."[9] The comment both presupposes that there is a real benefit to be had by the subjects of clinical research and reflects a remarkable commitment to universal access to research participation, particularly in a country where there is no similar commitment concerning basic health care.

Klausner's commitment has now been realized in policy, at least for those who have health insurance or are eligible for Medicare. In 1999, United Healthcare, one of the largest managed care organizations in the country, became the first third-party payer to agree to pay the costs associated with their subscribers' participation in clinical trials.[10] The decision was hailed as a major step in removing one of the substantial barriers to participation in clinical trials, since the policy of most health insurers has been to deny payment for the costs of clinical trial participation on the grounds that the treatment rendered is experimental. Whether the change in policy is a function of a changed view of the benefits of research participation, a response to the demands of its customers, or a commitment to supporting the research that yields the clinical advances on which health care depends, it certainly delivers a message to patients. If your insurance company thinks research is worth paying for, it must be worth participating in. Not long after the decision was announced, then-President Bill Clinton directed the Health Care Financing Administration to ensure that all Medicare recipients would enjoy similar access to clinical trial participation, leaving it to policy-makers to determine the conditions under which patients would be eligible for such a benefit.[11] This theme even became part of the rhetoric of the presidential campaign when Al Gore incorporated a reference to access to research participation in his standard stump speech on health care issues.[12]

The final piece of evidence that the pendulum has swung fully from protection to access is the waiver of informed consent in research in emergency settings, written into federal regulations in 1996.[13] The waiver is the ultimate endorsement of an emphasis on the benefits of research since it suggests that research participation is so beneficial, to individuals and society, that we must guarantee access even for those unable to consent. With this step we have now backed away from the cornerstone concept of informed consent, dating back to the Nuremberg era, in the protection of research subjects.

A NEW ERA IN THE PROTECTION OF HUMAN SUBJECTS?

What are the implications for research oversight of the swing from protection to access? The protection of the rights and interests of research subjects is rightly the preeminent concern in research oversight, but how do we ensure that protection is adequately balanced against access? There is ample evidence that even in an environment stressing protection there are serious shortcomings in the process of informed consent,[14] and subjects are persistently confused about the distinction between research and clinical care[15] and the benefits they stand to realize by participating in research.[16] Thus an overemphasis on the benefits of research participation can undermine the reality that research inherently carries risk and very often holds no benefits to the subject.

It is a confusing time to be a subject—or to be thinking about becoming one. The media presents stories about the need for more research and research funding alongside reports of serious harms to subjects in research trials. The death of Jesse Gelsinger in a gene transfer study at the University of Pennsylvania resulted in a swirl of reportage, congressional hearings, university investigations, and new restrictions and

reporting policies for gene transfer research.[17] The *Seattle Times* recently reported on alleged conflicts of interest and failures to obtain informed consent in two clinical trials in which some subjects died unexpectedly, both at Seattle's Fred Hutchinson Cancer Research Center.[18] The *Los Angeles Times* ran a story on "seven deadly drugs" that were fast-tracked to approval by the Food and Drug Administration and were subsequently withdrawn from the market after they were discovered to have serious side effects, sometimes leading to death.[19] And it was recently reported that the FDA has asked for an additional $36 million in the next fiscal year to increase its "emphasis on high-risk trials, such as those enrolling vulnerable populations (mentally impaired and pediatric populations, for example) and sponsor-investigators who have a proprietary interest in the product under study."[20] How do we reconcile these divergent messages to subjects, investigators, IRBs, and institutions, and properly balance the requirements of justice in research? If we fail to answer this question adequately we risk a serious erosion of trust in the research enterprise.

LOOKING AHEAD

Accountability for balancing protection and access falls to those at every level in the conduct of research: the physicians who refer their patients to investigators, the investigators themselves, the IRBs that oversee research, and the institutions where research is performed. Policymaking does not occur in a vacuum; regulatory and spending decisions respond to the perceived needs and expressed desires of the public. Without trust from the public, there can be no research, as there will be no research subjects willing to participate and no willingness on the part of the public to support research with tax dollars. Research is a privilege not to be presumed or exploited, but earned through building and maintaining the public trust. This requires a careful balancing of access and protection.

Recent announcements by the Department of Health and Human Service's Office of Human

Research Protections focus on conflicts of interest in research—at base an effort to secure public trust by ensuring that investigators are not motivated to overlook subjects' protection.[21] The Institute of Medicine recently completed a study recommending, among other things, the accreditation of IRBs.[22] But both of these steps seem to be aimed at assuring that paperwork requirements are met, which is at best a weak proxy for assuring adequate protection of subjects. Thus both efforts seem to miss the point—certification and oversight provide a way of inspecting the implementation of policies aimed at protection rather than a way of exercising them. And thus these approaches encourage us to overlook the nagging, recurring, and fundamental shortcomings in research protections that continue to undermine the trust central to any effort to protect the rights and interests of research subjects, including ensuring their access to the benefits of research.[23]

In the current research climate, the pendulum may have swung as far as it can toward an emphasis on benefits. When a pendulum has finished swinging in one direction, it inevitably starts back in the other, and it eventually comes to a rest in the middle. But the direction in which research ethics policy is swinging at any given time will be a function of how well we manage the balance between policies and practices at either of its two ends. Increasing policy attention to conflicts of interest, reporting, and regulatory oversight of the research environment seems to imply that the pendulum has begun its swing back toward an emphasis on protection. But paperwork requirements are not enough, and may distract us from efforts that will modulate the swing. What remains to be seen is how far the pendulum will go, and whether we have the tools to control it.

Notes

1. J. Jones, *Bad Blood* (New York: Free Press, 1993).
2. National Commission for the Protection of Human Subjects of Biomedical and Behavioral Research, *The Belmont Report: Ethical Principles and Guidelines for the Protection of Human Subjects of Research* (Bethesda, Md.: Department of Health, Education, and Welfare, 1978).
3. National Commission for the Protection of Human Subjects of Biomedical and Behavioral Research, *Report and Recommendations: Research Involving Prisoners* (Bethesda, Md.: Department of Health, Education, and Welfare, 1976); V. Cohn, "Prisoner Test Ban Opposed," *Washington Post,* 14 March 1976.
4. R. Shilts, *And the Band Played On: Politics, People, and the AIDS Epidemic* (New York: St. Martin's Press, 1987).
5. R.A. Charo, "Protecting Us to Death: Women, Pregnancy, and Clinical Research Trials," *Saint Louis University Law Journal* 38, no. 1 (1993): 135–87.
6. J.E. Manson et al., "Aspirin in the Primary Prevention of Angina Pectoris in a Randomized Trial of United States Physicians," *American Journal of Medicine* 89 (1990): 772–76.
7. "NIH Guidelines on the Inclusion of Women and Minorities as Subjects in Clinical Research," *Federal Register* 59 (28 March 1994): 14508.
8. "NIH Policy and Guidelines on the Inclusion of Children as Participants in Research Involving Human Subjects," *NIH Guide*, 6 March 1998, <www.nih.gov/grants/guide/1998/98.03.06>.
9. R. Pear, "Medical Research to Get More Money from Government," *New York Times,* 3 January 1998.
10. G. Kolata and K. Eichenwald, "Insurers Come In from the Cold on Cancer," *New York Times,* 19 December 1999.
11. R. Pear, "Clinton to Order Medicare to Pay New Costs," *New York Times*, 7 June 2000.
12. J. Dao, "Gore Urges Doubling of Funds in War against Cancer," *New York Times,* 2 June 2000.
13. "Waiver of Informed Consent Requirements in Certain Emergency Research," *Federal Register* 61 (2 October 1996): 51531; "Protection of Human Subjects; Informed Consent," *Federal Register* 61 (2 October 1996): 51498.
14. Advisory Committee on Human Radiation Experiments, "Research Proposal Review Project," in *The Human Radiation Experiments* (New York: Oxford University Press, 1996), 439–58; C.H. Braddock, "Advancing the Cause of Informed Consent: Moving from Disclosure to Understanding," *American Journal of Medicine* 105 (1988): 354–55; E.D. Kodish et al., "Informed Consent in the Children's Cancer Group: Results of Preliminary Research," *Cancer* 82 (1988): 2467–81.
15. Advisory Committee on Human Radiation Experiments, "Subject Interview Study," in *The*

Human Radiation Experiments (New York: Oxford University Press, 1996): 459–81; N.E. Kass er al., "Trust: The Fragile Foundation of Contemporary Biomedical Research," *Hastings Center Report* 19 (1989): 25–29.

16. PS. Appelbaum, L.H. Roth, and C.W Lidz, "The Therapeutic Misconception: Informed Consent in Psychiatric Research," *International Journal of Law and Psychiatry* 5 (1982): 319–29; C. Daugherty et al., "Perceptions of Cancer Patients and Their Physicians Involved in Phase I Trials," *Journal of Clinical Oncology* 13 (1995): 1062–72.

17. D.S. Greenberg, "Stricter Regulation Proposed for U.S. Gene Therapy Trials," *Lancet* 355 (1977): 2000.

18. D. Wilson and D. Heath, "Uninformed Consent," *The Seattle Times,* 11–15 March 2001.

19. D. Willman, "How a New Policy Led to Seven Deadly Drugs," *Los Angeles Times,* 20 December 2000.

20. *Health News Daily,* 11 April 2001.

21. J. Brainard, "U.S. Agency Seeks Power to Fine Universities That Violate Rules on Human Research Subjects," *Chronicle of Higher Education,* 24 May 2000.

22. S.G. Srolberg, "Experts Call for New Rules on Research," *New York Times,* 18 April 2001.

23. J.P Kahn and A.C. Mastroianni, "Moving From Compliance to Conscience: Why We Can and Should Improve on the Ethics of Clinical Research," *Archives of Internal Medicine* 161 (2001): 925–28.

Going to the Roots of the Stem Cell Controversy

Søren Holm

INTRODUCTION

The ability to produce and culture human embryonic stem cells has raised hopes for a range of new cell based therapies, but has at the same time created intense national and international debate.

The purpose of this paper is to describe the scientific background to the current ethical and legislative debates about the generation and use of human stem cells, and to give an overview of the ethical issues that are central to these debates. Because the paper is intended to be reasonably comprehensive the presentation and analysis of each individual argument must necessarily be rather brief.[1]

THE SCIENTIFIC BACKGROUND TO THE STEM CELL CONTROVERSY

Three partially independent scientific developments underlie the current debates about stem cell research. These are 1) the discovery of methods to derive and culture human embryonic stem cells, 2) the discovery of nuclear replacement techniques, and 3) the discovery of new and previously unsuspected potentialities of stem cells in the adult human body.

A stem cell is a non-differentiated cell that can divide and multiply in its undifferentiated state, but which can also give rise to more specialised differentiated cells. It has been known for a long time that adult human tissues contain stem cells that can replenish cells lost through normal wear and tear or through trauma or disease. This fact has been utilised as a basis for a number of different treatments including bone marrow and skin transplants.

It has been known that cells from the inner cell mass of the early embryo are stem cells (since we know that they must necessarily be able to become every cell in the body during the development from embryo to adult individual), but no method existed by which these embryonic stem cells could be grown in culture in the laboratory in a way that preserved their stem cell character.

In 1998 researchers at the University of Wisconsin published a method for deriving and culturing human embryonic stem cells indefinitely.[2] This development made it possible to create stable human stem cell lines and generate (in principle) unlimited quantities of any particular embryonic stem cell, and thereby the possibility to 1) standardise research into human stem cells, and 2) create reproducible stem cell therapies.

Almost at the same time as the Wisconsin group developed the method for culturing human embryonic stem cells, a group at the Roslin Institute in Scotland developed methods for the cloning of adult mammals using nuclear replacement techniques.[3] The techniques basically worked by removing a cell from an adult animal, and then taking the cell nucleus from the adult cell and placing it in an ovum from which the original nucleus has been removed. This procedure reprogrammes the adult nucleus to an embryonic state and creates a cell that is more than 99% genetically identical with the original adult cell from which the nucleus was taken.[4] It is, however, not the ability to reproduce a fully-grown mammal by nuclear replacement that is of main interest to the stem cell debate. It is the combination of nuclear replacement techniques and embryonic stem cell culture. When these two techniques are combined it becomes possible to produce embryonic stem cells that are almost genetically identical to any given adult human being.

Research into the potentialities of the remaining stem cells in the adult human body has all progressed apace in recent years. Stem cells have been found in a number of tissues in which it was previously "common knowledge" that they did not exist (e.g., neuronal stem cells in the brain),[5] many kinds of adult stem cells[6] have been cultured, and adult stem cells have been shown capable of transdifferentiation into different kinds of cells than the cells of the tissues in which they originated.[7] These discoveries have opened the possibility that adult stem cells may be used in a range of stem cell therapies far beyond what was thought possible.[8]

At present there are thus three research programmes that are pursued in stem cell research: 1) research on adult stem cells, 2) research on embryonic stem cells from embryos produced through IVF techniques, and 3) research on embryonic stem cells produced through nuclear replacement techniques.[9]

All three research programmes are directed at 1) increasing our knowledge about basic cell biology, 2) creating new therapies through stem cell culture and control of cell differentiation, and 3) producing commercially viable stem cell products either by the direct patenting of stem cell lines, or by combining stem cell technology with genetic engineering or other patentable interventions.

As we will see below, much of the discussion on stem cells is concerned with the ethical issues raised by each of these programmes, and with whether or not these ethical issues should influence decisions about regulation and/or funding of the research programmes.

THE EXPECTED BENEFITS FROM STEM CELL RESEARCH

Stem cell research is undoubtedly going to increase our knowledge about basic cell biology considerably, but this is not the benefit of stem cell research that excites most people. The really exciting thing about stem cell research is in the therapeutic potential of stem cells.

If we can develop methods to grow human stem cells in unlimited quantities, and if we can further learn how to control their differentiation, then a whole range of therapeutic possibilities become (theoretically) available.[10] The most immediate therapeutic gains are likely to be in the area of cell therapy. Many diseases are caused by, or accompanied by, loss of specific cell types. The lost cell types could be produced in the laboratory and later implanted to cure or alleviate the disease.

Further into the future it may become possible to grow whole organs from stem cells and use these for transplantation, removing the need for organ donation; and even further into the future we may be able to use stem cells for rejuvenating therapies leading to an increased life-span.

The therapeutic potential of stem cells spans such a wide range of diseases and conditions that it will constitute a major medical breakthrough if only even a small percentage of the most likely uses (e.g., in the area of cell therapy) become a reality. Even if stem cell therapy turned out only to be effective in myocardial infarction it would still alleviate huge amounts of human suffering.

These very large, and very likely benefits of stem cell research indicate the prohibition of certain kinds of stem cell research needs strong justification. The ethical and regulatory debates have therefore concentrated on whether such justification can be found.

THE ETHICAL ISSUES

Stem Cells and Embryos

One of the main ethical issues discussed concerning stem cell research originates in the fact that embryonic stem cells have to be generated from embryos that are destroyed in the process. This means that stem cell research again raises the question of whether there are any ethical limits concerning the destruction of human embryos for research or therapeutic purposes, as well as the more fundamental question of the moral status of the human embryo. If human embryos have any moral status we need a good justification to destroy them, and the greater their moral status the more important or weighty the justification has to be.[11]

The question of the moral status of the embryo was not resolved during the abortion debate nor during the debates about various forms of assisted reproductive technologies. It is unlikely to be resolved during the current debates about stem cells, since no really new arguments seem to be forthcoming.[12]

If one looks at the legislation about abortion and assisted reproductive technologies it is evident that no jurisdiction has legislation which is compatible with the view that human embryos

are just things with no moral status, and that no jurisdiction has legislation compatible with the view that embryos have the same moral status as born human beings. Most legislations implicitly or explicitly adopt some kind of middle position, although it is often unclear to what extent this represents a considered view or whether it is the result of a political compromise.

The important question with regard to regulation or legislation therefore becomes how the use of embryos for stem cell research and therapy can be fitted into a legislative structure that either relies on a view that embryos have some moral value, or is a direct result of political compromise. Giving some moral status to embryos does not automatically rule out embryonic stem cell research, since it can be argued that the likely benefits in terms of reduction of human suffering and death in many cases outweigh the sacrifice of a (small?) number of human embryos.[13]

All of the ethical questions concerning the use of embryos would be by-passed if it became technically possible to produce cells equivalent to embryonic stem cells, without the creation of embryos. This could, for instance, be the case if other methods for re-programming nuclei from adult cells became available.

PPL Therapeutics PLC has claimed to have done this using bovine cells and is working towards doing it with human cells, but very few details have been released because of commercial concerns.[14]

The Spare Embryo

In arguments about the use of embryos for stem cell research the distinction between embryos produced for research and spare embryos left over after IVF and other forms of assisted reproduction has also been invoked. It has been argued that the use of spare embryos is less problematic than the use of embryos produced for research, and that at present the use of specifically produced embryos for stem cell research should not be allowed.[15] No new arguments to support or refute this distinction have, however, been forthcoming in the stem cell debate.[16]

Women and the Need for Ova

If stem cells are to be produced from embryos that are not "spare" after IVF, the ova for this production must come from women.[17] In the initial research phase the number of ova needed will be relatively small, but for stem cell therapy the number may become very large. If, for instance, a specific therapy is based on nuclear replacement from the intended recipient in order to ensure perfect immunological compatibility, at least one ovum will be needed for each patient (and probably more since techniques for nuclear replacement are unlikely to become 100% effective any time soon).

This raises general problems concerning how we can ensure that the ova are obtained without coercion or exploitation of the ova donors, sellers or providers, but also more specific questions about how a new practice of non-reproduction-related ova procurement would influence the status of women in society.

At an even more general level there is a connection to the debate about the rights and wrongs of the commodification of human body parts.[18]

Stem Cells Produced Using Ova from Other Species

One way of solving the problem of shortage of ova, and the potential ethical problems in using women as donors of ova for these purposes, is to use ova from other species (e.g., bovines) in the creation of stem cells by means of nuclear replacement techniques.

It is, as yet, unknown whether the use of ova from other species is technically possible, and if possible whether the stem cells produced would be functionally and immunologically equivalent to stem cells produced using human ova. The technique has been patented by the American firm Advanced Cell Technology, but there is still doubt in the scientific community whether it actually works.[19]

The additional ethical problems created by this different source of ova can, however, be argued to be small as long as the resulting embryos are only used for stem cell production and not for reproductive purposes.[20]

On some lines of argument the ethical problems may actually be less than if human ova are used, since it could be argued that the embryos produced are not really human embryos. If the moral status of human embryos is based in their being human, then the moral status of these "less than human" embryos could be argued to be less important.

Slippery Slopes towards Reproductive Cloning

A classical slippery slope argument has been prominent in the specific debate about whether the creation of stem cells by means of cell nuclear replacement techniques should be allowed. Opponents of this technique have claimed that allowing this would put us on a slippery slope towards reproductive cloning. The slope that is imagined is of a technical nature. If all the technical problems in the first steps of cell nuclear replacement techniques are solved successfully then it becomes both easier and more tempting (because certain risks have been reduced) to try to use nuclear replacement techniques for reproductive cloning.

This is clearly not a problem if reproductive cloning does not raise any serious ethical problems because in that case there is no slope, slippery or not.[21]

If reproductive cloning is ethically problematic the question then becomes how to respond to the existence of the slope. The slope has to be taken seriously by politicians as a policy problem. Whatever the analysis of bioethicists as to the cogency of the belief that reproductive cloning is a serious ethical problem, there is no doubt that this belief is shared by many people and by many politicians.

The political reaction to the perceived slippery slope depends on whether it is seen as a possible threat to the positive development of stem cell research (as it is perceived by the government in the UK and a number of other European countries), or whether it is seen as a possible tool to justify the prohibition of stem cell research by nuclear replacement as part of a more comprehensive ban on all kinds of human cloning (as it is perceived by the government in the US).[22]

If the slope is seen as a possible threat to the acceptance of stem cell research the logical response is to legally prohibit human reproductive cloning, and to try to convince the public that such a prohibition will be effective.[23] Whether legal prohibition can be effective given the possibilities for international reproductive tourism to more permissive jurisdictions is, however, questionable.[24]

The Presentation of Stem Cell Research— Promising Too Much Too Early?

The public presentation of the benefits of stem cell research has often been characterised by the promise of huge and immediate benefits. Like with many other scientific breakthroughs the public has been promised real benefits within 5–10 years, i.e., in this case significant stem cell therapies in routine clinical use.[25] Several years have now elapsed of the 5–10 years and the promised therapies are still not anywhere close to routine clinical use.[26] There are similarities to the initial enthusiastic presentation of gene therapy in the late 1980s and the later problems encountered, and some reason to fear that stem cell therapies will have an equally long trajectory between theoretical possibility and clinical practice. It is likely that many of the current sufferers from some of the conditions for which stem cell therapies have been promised will be long dead before the therapies actually arrive.[27]

It is clearly ethically problematic to raise false expectations in seriously ill people, and even more problematic if this is partly done from self-interest (e.g. to promote one's own research in the media). But the problem may go deeper because the optimistic predictions and the targeting of these predictions on certain groups of diseases also have a function in the political arena where public policy is decided. When gene therapy was initially promoted, and the public and political resistance overcome, gene therapy was promoted as a treatment for the unfortunate people suffering from genetic disorders. Gene therapy was put forward as their only hope of cure and alleviation. Today we do know however, that most gene therapy projects are not directed towards genetic disease, but towards the treatment of common diseases (partly for commercial reasons). The groups that were used as symbolic "battering rams" to gain political and public acceptance of the gene therapy, have not yet benefited significantly from gene therapy, and many of the people having rarer forms of genetic disorders are unlikely ever to benefit.

SCIENTIFIC UNCERTAINTY, ETHICAL UNEASE AND THE FORMULATION OF PUBLIC POLICY

At the current point in time it is not known which (if any) of the three main lines of research described above is going to be most successful in terms of a) generating scientific knowledge about cell biology, and b) generating new stem cell based therapies for common diseases. That each is, at least at the moment, seen as a viable approach with regard to therapy is attested by the fact that many biotech firms have been founded aiming at exploiting each of the approaches.[28]

The question is important because it has been argued that there is no need to permit more ethically contentious ways of generating stem cells, if the same benefits can be realized using less contentious stem cells, either adult stem cells or stem cells from aborted foetuses.[29]

What factors could we use to decide whether one line of research is more promising than another?[30] One possibility is to think about what characteristics a stem cell should have in order to be therapeutically useful and then try to decide which of the research programmes is most likely to be able to lead to the production of such cells, and if more than one can produce the required cells, which one will progress fastest to the goal.[31] We do know (some of) the characteristics that the therapeutically optimal stem cell should display:

1. No immunological rejection
2. Immediate availability
3. Availability in large numbers
4. Controlled differentiation to desired cells

5. Controlled integration into existing tissues and biological niches leading to normal function
6. No other biological risks

From a theoretical point of view embryonic stem cells created by nuclear replacement should be able to fulfil most of these requirements. We know that they can become all types of cells, and we know that they are immunologically perfectly compatible. We are, however, not yet able to control their differentiation into all desired cell types, and there may be situations of acute organ or cell failure where we do not have the necessary time to grow a sufficient number of cells to initiate therapy in time.

Embryonic stem cells derived in other ways have the disadvantage of not being immunologically perfectly compatible, but they do, on the other hand, offer the advantage of being potentially immediately available from a stem cell bank in the necessary quantities. Adult stem cells are immunologically compatible, but it is still uncertain whether we can derive all types of cells from adult stem cells, and they may also not be available in sufficient quantities in acute cases.

No type of stem cell therefore fulfils all the criteria for a therapeutically optimal stem cell. How should we evaluate this evidence in order to decide what research programmes to pursue?

At approximately the same time, the American National Bioethics Advisory Commission and a British government expert group reviewed the evidence and came to two rather different conclusions. The National Bioethics Advisory Commission concluded that:

> Currently, we believe that cadaveric fetal tissue and embryos remaining after infertility treatments provide an adequate supply of research resources for federal research projects involving human embryos. Therefore, embryos created specifically for research purposes are not needed at the current time in order to conduct important research in this area.
> [...]
> We conclude that at this time, because other sources are likely to pro-

vide the cells needed for the preliminary stages of research, federal funding should not be provided to derive ES cells from SCNT. Nevertheless, the medical utility and scientific progress of this line of research should be monitored closely.[32]

Whereas the British Chief Medical Officer's Expert Group concluded that:

> For some people, particularly those suffering from the diseases likely to benefit from the treatments that could be developed, the fact that research to create embryos by cell nuclear replacement is a necessary step to understanding how to reprogramme adult cells to produce compatible tissue provides sufficient ethical justification for allowing the research to proceed.[33]

What was a fact for one group of experts was clearly not a fact for the other. What is at play here is a different evaluation of the available scientific evidence, but possibly also a different approach to the decision of whether a line of research should be deemed "necessary." Is a particular line of research only necessary if it is the only way to get the knowledge we need for stem cell therapies, or is it necessary if scientific progress will otherwise be slowed down and will be much more costly, but will eventually lead to stem cell therapies any way even if this particular line of research is not pursued?[34]

The policy-maker is thus left with a very difficult problem. If we knew that adult stem cell research could deliver therapies for all the conditions where stem cell therapy seems to be a possibility, then there would be a straightforward policy argument for choosing only to support this ethically uncontentious research programme. If the same goal can be obtained in two ways, and if one of them is less contentious than the other it makes good political sense to choose the uncontentious one.[35] If on the other hand there was unequivocal certainty that research using embryonic stem cells was necessary for the development of stem cell therapies for one or more important diseases, a relatively strong consequentialist argument would offer itself based on a moral imperative to reduce human suffering, and this could be combined with appeals to consistency in those jurisdictions that already allow some kinds of embryo research.

Because there is scientific uncertainty each of these two lines of argument is, however, considerably weakened because an opponent can always point to uncertainty about the underlying empirical premises concerning whether embryonic stem cell research is necessary or not.

CONCLUSION

It should by now be evident that many of the most discussed ethical issues in connection with stem cell research are minor variants of issues that have been discussed in reproductive ethics since the beginning of modern bioethics in the late 1960s and early 1970s. Many arguments in the stem cell debate, for instance, merely re-iterate arguments for or against giving moral status to embryos, or arguments concerning the validity of the distinction between "spare" embryos and embryos produced specifically for research. The underlying points of contention in these recycled arguments have not been resolved during the abortion debate, or during the debates about assisted reproductive technologies, and they are unlikely to be resolved now. Each side has arguments that it sees as compelling, but which the other side rejects utterly. It is probably this re-ignition of old debates that has added to the heat of the stem cell debates, because neither side can give ground without fearing a knock on effect on the political accommodations or compromises reached in the abortion and the assisted reproduction areas.

If we take all of these already well known debates into account it seems that there is a rough hierarchy of contentiousness ordering the different ways of producing human stem cells according to how many issues each raise. This would look something like the following (with the most contentious first):

Embryonic stem cells created by nuclear replacement

Embryonic stem cells from embryos created for research

Embryonic stem cells from spare embryos

Adult stem cells

This proposed hierarchy is not very illuminating for ethical analysis, but it may well influence public policy.

There are, however, also a few issues raised by the stem cell debate that are not as well worn. The most interesting of these are the questions surrounding how public policy should be formed in an area where there is 1) agreement about the value of the goal of a particular kind of research (i.e., the creation of effective stem cell therapies), 2) genuine scientific uncertainty about exactly what line of research is most likely to achieve this goal, and 3) disagreement about the ethical evaluation of some of these lines of research but not about others. This question is perhaps more a question of political or legal philosophy than a question of ethics, but it is nevertheless an issue that should be of interest to those bioethicists who want their elegant analyses transformed into public policy.

Notes

1. One major topic has been left out of this paper because of space constraints. That is the question of intellectual and actual property rights in human stem cell lines and the techniques by which they are produced. This is a huge topic on its own, actualising all the issues of ownership of the human body, body parts and human genetic material.

2. J.A. Thomson, J. Itskovitz-Eldor, S.S. Shapiro, M.A. Waknitz, J.J. Swiergiel, V.S. Marshall, J.M. Jones. Embryonic stem cell lines derived from human blastocysts. *Science* 1998; 282: 1145–1147.

3. I. Wilmut, A.E. Schnieke, J. McWhir, A.J. Kind, K.H. Campbell. Viable offspring derived from foetal and adult mammalian cells. *Nature* 1997; 385: 810–813.

4. The mitochondria in this cell come from the ovum, and contain their own genetic material. It is thus

only if both nucleus and ovum come from the same woman that 100% genetic identity is achieved.

5. C.B. Johanson, S. Momma, D.L. Clarke, M. Risling, U. Lendahl, J. Friesen. Identification of a neural stem cell in the adult mammalian central nervous system. *Cell* 1999; 96: 25–34.

6. In this paper "adult stem cell" will be used for any stem cell derived from a human being after birth.

7. D.L. Clarke, C.B. Johansson, J. Wilbertz, B. Veress, E. Nilsson, H. Karlstrom, U. Lendahl, J. Friesen. Generalized potential of adult neural stem cells. *Science* 2000; 288: 1559–1561; P.A. Zuk, M. Zhu, H. Mizono, J. Huang, J.W. Futrell, A.J. Katz, P. Benhaim, H.P. Lorenz, M.H. Hedrick. Multilineage cells from human adipose tissue: implications for cell-based therapies. *Tissue Engineering* 2001; 7: 211–228.

8. Two recent papers cast some doubt on these possibilities for transdifferentiation, but their validity and relevance is contested. N. Terada, T. Hamazaki, M. Oka, M. Hoki, D.M. Mastalerz, Y. Nakano, E.M. Meyer, L. Morel, B.E. Petersen, E.W. Scott. Bone marrow cells adopt the phenotype of other cells by spontaneous cell fusion. *Nature* 2002; 416: 542–545; Q-L. Ling, J. Nichols, E.P. Evans, A.G. Smith. Changing potency by spontaneous fusion. *Nature* 2002; 416: 545–548. N. Dewitt, J. Knight. Biologists question adult stem-cell versatility. *Nature* 2002; 416: 354.

9. The term "research programme" is here used in the sense given to it by Lakatos, i.e., a group of concrete research endeavours kept together by a common core of relativity stable assumptions about the goals of research, the proper research methodologies and the most fruitful research topics. What distinguishes the three stem cell research programmes from each other is primarily different beliefs about what kind of stem cell is going to be the basis for the most progressive (i.e., productive in terms of scientific and commercial results) research. I. Lakatos. 1974. Falsification and the methodology of scientific research programmes. In *Criticism and the Growth of Knowledge*. I. Lakatos and A. Musgrave, eds. Cambridge. Cambridge University Press: 91–196.

10. R.P. Lanza, J.P. Cibelli, M.D. West. Prospects for the use of nuclear transfer in human transplantation. *Nature Biotechnology* 1999; 17: 1171–1174; E. Fuchs, J.A. Segre. Stem Cells: A New Lease of Life. *Cell* 2000; 100: 143–155.

11. R.M. Doerflinger. The ethics of funding embryonic stem cell research: a Catholic viewpoint. *Kennedy Institute of Ethics Journal* 1999; 9: 137–150.

12. L.H. Harris. Ethics and politics of embryo and stem cell research: Reinscribing the abortion debate. *Women's Health Issues* 2000; 10: 146–151; D.C. Wertz. Embryo and stem cell research in the USA: a political history. *TRENDS in Molecular Medicine* 2002; 8: 143–146.

13. G. McGee, A. Caplan. The ethics and politics of small sacrifices in stem cell research. *Kennedy Institute of Ethics Journal* 1999; 9: 151–158.

14. PPL Therapeutics PLC. 2001. *Interim Report 2001*. Edinburgh. PPL Therapeutics PLC.

15. See for instance the report from the American National Bioethics Advisory Commission. National Bioethics Advisory Commission. 1999. *Ethical Issues in Human Stem Cell Research.* Rockville. NBAC. A number of jurisdictions have legislation concerning assisted reproductive technologies that allow research on spare embryos, but prohibit the creation of embryos for research purposes.

16. On the cogency of the distinction see S. Holm. The spare embryo – A red herring in the embryo experimentation debate. *Health Care Analysis* 1993; 1: 63–66.

17. Unless it is possible to use ova obtained from aborted foetuses, dead women, or ovaries removed as part of surgical interventions. The first two of these alternative sources of ova may in themselves raise ethical issues but these are beyond the scope of this paper.

18. L.S. Cahill. Genetics, Commodification, and Social Justice in the Globalization Era. *Kennedy Institute of Ethics Journal* 2001; 11: 221–238; S. Holland. Contested Commodities at Both Ends of Life: Buying and Selling Gametes, Embryos, and Body Tissues. *Kennedy Institute of Ethics Journal* 2001; 11: 263–284; L. Andrews, D. Nelkin. 2001. *Body Bazaar: The Market for Human Tissue in the Biotechnology Age.* New York. Crown Publishers; M.J. Radin. 1996. *Contested Commodities.* Cambridge, MA. Harvard University Press; R. Macklin. 1996. What is Wrong with Commodification? In *New Ways of Making Babies: The Case of Egg Donation.* C.B. Cohen, ed. Bloomington. Indiana University Press: 106–121.

19. Advanced Cell Technology. Advanced Cell Technology Announces Use of Nuclear Replacement Technology for Successful Generation of Human Embryonic Stem Cells. Press Release November 12, 1998. Available at *http://www.advancedcell.com/pr_11-12-1998.html.* E. Marshall. Claim of human-cow embryo greeted with skepticism. Science 1998; 282: 1390–1391.

20. There are two lines of argument seeing major ethical problems in the use of non-human ova. The first sees the technique in itself as a transgression of an important boundary line between human and animal. The second points to a possible slippery slope from the use of this technique for the production of stem cells, to a use for reproductive purposes.

21. The literature on the ethics of reproductive cloning is extensive. A range of views can be found in a thematic issue of the *Journal of Medical Ethics* 1999; 25(2), and in a thematic issue of the *Cambridge Quarterly of Health Care Ethics* 1998; 7(2).

22. E. Check. Call for cloning ban splits UN. *Nature* 2002; 416: 3.

23. This is the approach chosen by the governments of the UK, Denmark and the Netherlands among others. For an overview of European policies in this area see: L. Matthiessen. 2001. *Survey on opinions from National Ethics Committees or similar bodies, public debate and national legislation in relation to human embryonic stem cell research and use.* Bruxelles. European Commission Research Directorate-General.

24. P.G. Wood. To what extent can the law control human cloning? *Medicine, Science & the Law,* 1999; 39: 5–10.

25. Anon. Taking stock of spin science. *Nature Biotechnology* 1998; 16: 1291.

26. Given the time needed for basic research, clinical research and regulatory approval it is unlikely that any therapy using biological materials, and based on a truly novel therapeutic approach could move from initial discovery to clinical use in 5–10 years. See also R. Lovell-Badge. The future for stem cell research. *Nature* 2001; 14: 88–91.

27. B. Albert. *Presentation to the All-Party Disablement Group* – July 25th 2000. Unpublished manuscript.

28. N. Axelsen. 2001. Commercial interests in stem cells. In *Nordic Committee on Bioethics. The Ethical Issues in Stem Cell Research.* Copenhagen. Nordic Council of Ministers: 79–80.

29. J.R. Meyer. Human embryonic stem cells and respect for life. *Journal of Medical Ethics* 2000; 26: 166–170; V. Branick, M.T. Lysaught. Stem cell research: licit or complicit? Is a medical breakthrough based on embryonic and foetal tissue compatible with Catholic teaching? *Health Progress* 1999; 80: 37–42. This kind of reasoning also seems to underlie the National Bioethics Advisory Committee report *op. cit.* note 15, although it draws the line of contentiousness between the spare embryo and the embryo produced for research.

30. Most of this debate has centred on the therapeutic use of stem cells. With regard to the "pure" scientific production of knowledge about cell biology it seems clear that each of the research programmes will produce at least some unique bits of knowledge, and that each of them must therefore be pursued if complete scientific knowledge is the goal.

31. A difference in speed of development between two research programmes is important, even if they will both eventually lead to the same goal, since any delay in implementation of stem cell therapies entail costs in term of human suffering.

32. National Bioethics Advisory Commission, *op.cit,* note 15, pp. 71–72.

33. Chief Medical Officer's Expert Group. 2001. Stem Cell Research: Medical Progress with Responsibility – A Report from the Chief Medical Officer's Expert Group Reviewing the Potential of Developments in Stem Cell Research and Cell Nuclear Replacement to Benefit Human Health. London. Department of Health, p. 40.

34. S. Holm. 2001. European and American ethical debates about stem cells – common underlying themes and some significant differences. In *Nordic Committee of Bioethics. The Ethical Issues in Stem Cell Research.* Copenhagen Nordic Council of Ministers: 35–45.

35. This might be the proper policy response even if it would lead to some delay in the development of treatments.

Dancing with the Porcupine: Rules for Governing the University–Industry Relationship

Steven Lewis, Patricia Baird, Robert G. Evans, William A. Ghali, Charles J. Wright, Elaine Gibson, and Françoise Baylis

Universities have long been involved in the creation and evaluation of pharmaceutical products. In its best form, academic participation in drug-related science both spurs innovation and, through the disinterest and skepticism that are hallmarks of the academic mission, provides a check on the premature enthusiasms of industry. In this commentary we examine the logic and behaviour of the pharmaceutical industry in pursuit of its interests and propose rules to govern university–industry partnerships that reflect the public interest.

The duty of universities is to seek truth. The duty of pharmaceutical companies is to make money for their shareholders. Drug companies that fail to do so go out of business. Universities that subordinate the disinterested search for truth to other ends lose credibility and their claim to a privileged status in society. If either abandons its fundamental mission, it ultimately fails. At times, institutional imperatives are bound to conflict.[1, 2]

Research can either serve or subvert the public interest. Its findings may advance knowledge and support useful innovation, or be filtered and twisted to support prejudices or gain commercial advantage. The capacities and integrity of researchers, and their universities, can be enhanced or corrupted in the process. Some partnerships are united by an open-minded quest for discovery; others are unholy alliances whereby researchers and universities become handmaidens of industry. Whatever ethical bed we make, we lie in.

There is abundant evidence that many such partnerships place industry imperatives above both the public interest and the fundamental ethos of the university. The evidence includes major variation in disclosure requirements,[3] insufficient protection of the right to publish in a timely fashion[4] and researchers having financial interests in companies potentially affected by the outcomes of their research.[5] The creation of the Canadian Institutes of Health Research (CIHR) and its renewed commitment to excellence and expanded capacity for innovation and discovery have created unprecedented health research opportunities in Canada. With what ethical compass will Canada chart its health research course?

The outcome will depend on 3 key players: the federal government and its agencies, the universities, and industry. The recent history of government policy is a 3-part drama. In the late 1980s the federal government concluded that increased drug research and development by the private sector in Canada would contribute to the economy. Second, multinational drug companies indicated that their expansion of research and development activities in their Canadian branches would be contingent on favourable patent protection legislation. Third, in return for extending patent protection, the government exacted a commitment from industry to invest 10% of sales in Canadian-based research.

The Medical Research Council of Canada[6] (MRC, the forerunner of the CIHR) and many faculty members and universities supported these treasures. The MRC budget declined for 3 consecutive years beginning in 1995/96 and was essentially frozen during most of the decade.[6] Elsewhere, spending on health research rose significantly, most notably in the United States, where federal funding alone doubled in real terms during the 1990s.[7] Science became more complex, expensive and competitive. To offset the severe restraints imposed on public funding of universities as part of the war on government deficits in Canada during the 1990s, researchers and universities had to look elsewhere for funding. Enter industry.

In 2000, "business enterprise," which was almost exclusively the pharmaceutical industry (although Statistics Canada does not break down the figures), accounted for about 43% of gross domestic expenditures on research and development in the health field (the amount includes $350 million from foreign sources spent on business enterprises in Canada, which we assume to be industry dollars).[8] Universities and teaching hospitals received $161 million from industry, which was more than the amount from provincial governments combined and over half the amount received from federal sources (largely the MRC-CIHR). Aside from being a major player on campus, industry exerts considerable influence on public policy by virtue of the $900 million it spends in-house on research and development.

What does industry expect for its $161 million invested in universities and teaching hospitals? Drug companies have a fiduciary duty to exploit the intellectual talent and ethical credibility of universities to advance their interests. The proximate goal is the publication of positive results of trials of new drugs, or evaluations that show that certain drugs are better than their competitors' products. The ultimate goal is sales. Negative findings often, and predictably, create an unhappy industry partner. Common sense suggests that universities must be vigilant about protecting their own, fundamentally different culture and orientation.

To date, they have not been. The new money and activity exploded onto the scene with inadequate oversight and no standardization of rules or mechanisms to resolve disputes. The results: some highly publicized aggressions,[9] tarnished institutional reputations, one-sided marriages of convenience, and who knows how much unhelpful drug therapy and increased cost.

Unsettling incidents of this nature have occurred throughout the world.[10] These are not impersonal and civil corporate disagreements; they often involve intimidating tactics by industry that profoundly affect researchers' lives and careers. Canadian cases, the details of which we do not recount for reasons of space, include the Bristol-Myers Squibb lawsuit against the Canadian Coordinating Office on Health Technology Assessment (CCOHTA) to suppress its statin report,[11] and the AstraZeneca legal threat against McMaster University researcher Anne Holbrook for her review of medications for stomach disorders (personal communication 2001). Regardless of the outcome of these cases, industry harassment consumes time and energy (and in the CCOHTA case, 13% of its budget, for legal fees) and creates unease; these are of course the intended effects.

In other cases, the financial clout of industry may influence academic behaviour more subtly, or at least appear to do so. Witness the withdrawal of an offer of employment to Dr. David Healy by the Centre for Addictions and Mental Health (CAMH) in Toronto shortly after he made a speech critical of Prozac, whose manufacturer, Eli Lilly, donated $1.55 million to the CAMH in 2000.[12–14] There is no evidence of direct involvement by Eli Lilly in this decision, but the company did withdraw corporate funding of The Hastings Centre after its journal published a series of articles critical of antidepressant prescribing practices.[15]

Such cases demonstrate yet again that, when public and private interests conflict, at least some companies will fiercely protect their shareholders' interests. If the drugs they hoped would be breakthroughs turn out to be "me-toos," they must market them at the highest possible price in order to recoup the development costs, which can exceed US$100 million. If one company's drug is the therapeutic equivalent of other companies' drugs, it is obliged to try to persuade doctors, pharmacists and the public that its drug is actually better. In this, they are identical to car manufacturers and brewers of beer.

These inevitabilities demand prudent engagement. The warrant for prudence is not that something *will* go wrong; it is simply that something *may* go wrong, and *has* gone wrong in several cases. The intimidation and lawsuits are only the tip of the iceberg. Far more prevalent and insidious is the correlation between industry funding and research that shows a positive therapeutic effect.[16] In a landmark article researchers found that industry-sponsored studies of calcium-channel antagonists are more likely to be supportive of that therapy than independently funded research.[17] Similar findings emerged from a review of economic analyses of new oncology drugs.[18] The positive skew is not dependent on such high-risk and brazen strategies as falsification of data; it is achievable by framing the questions and the design of studies to increase the probability of a positive result.

Industry funding creates an incentive to promote the positive and suppress the negative. When drug companies control publication of results or simply delay unwelcome findings, truth is partially disclosed and therefore compromised. And if researchers' laboratories and career prospects depend on renewed industry funding, their interests may begin to align with those of their paymasters. Unhappily, disinterested scholarly editorial practices often exacerbate rather than counteract this bias,[19–21] reaffirming Francis Bacon's observation that "the human intellect ... is more moved and excited by affirmatives than negatives."[19]

What is to be done? We propose the rules in Box 1 as a starting point for governing partnerships. The rules need an institutional home. One option would vest responsibility with the Association of Universities and Colleges of Canada. Health research is but a subset of all research, and the university, not its parts or affiliates, should be the institution of record. Any

---

BOX 1

Proposed rules for governing university–industry relationships

- A standard, Canada-wide contract governing university–industry relationships, enshrining the right of the academic to disclose potentially harmful clinical effects immediately, and publish freely after a modest interval.
- Guidelines to determine whether a proposed industry–university project is of sufficient intellectual originality and interest to qualify as academic activity. If the project does not qualify, it should be defined as a service or consulting contract and should be priced and managed as such.
- Mandatory filing of all university–industry agreements and contracts with the overseeing body, and registration of all clinical trials.
- Mandatory written debriefing signed by all parties at the conclusion of every university–industry agreement, to be filed with the provost or equivalent of the university and the overseeing body, with a hearings process to resolve disputes.
- A certification and rating system for industry that assesses such areas as scientific integrity, observance of contracts, commitment to intellectual freedom, degree of interference in the conduct of research and appropriateness of financial arrangements.
- A surtax levied on all university–industry contracts, the proceeds from which would help both to fund a core office and its oversight activities and to cover the costs of defending researchers against industry harassment or formal litigation as vigorously as the Canadian Medical Protective Association protects doctors against medical malpractice claims.
- The appointment of an ombudsperson to whom researchers and industry can refer concerns about partnerships.
- Participation in and endorsement of the refined and expanded set of rules based on these general principles and structures by all agencies funding health research.

tendency for the health sciences to develop ethical standards in isolation must be resisted. "Academic separatism" flies in the face of the multidisciplinary and interdisciplinary collaboration that is heavily promoted as essential to the advancement of knowledge. Even more centrally, the university must not duck its responsibility to govern activities in its well-funded peripheries, including teaching hospitals.

Is a coordinated, national approach necessary? On the basis of the evidence to date, universities and researchers cannot be expected to protect their (and by extension the public's) interests with uniform sophistication and vigour.[22] Some US commentators have proposed precisely our form of remedy.[23] In May of this year the US National Bioethics Advisory Commission called for federal legislation to create the National Office for Human Research Oversight to oversee all research involving human subjects, including the definition, disclosure, and management of conflict of interest.[24]

Not infrequently, universities encounter challenges, veiled in the language of increased accountability, to their freedom of inquiry and expression. The claim that proposed constraints would be fatal to the academic mission becomes hypocrisy if universities allow industry to define the nature of inquiry, dictate methods and shackle expression. An industry–university contract is a transaction, and our proposed rules are designed principally to protect the university's most precious commodity: intellectual integrity.

We are not asking academic researchers to forswear all interactions with industry. We are merely proposing rules for exercising due diligence to protect the essence of academic inquiry. A positive effect of the proposed rules would be voluntarily improved industry behaviour, with enlightened companies adopting honourable codes of conduct that in time may mitigate the wariness and cynicism that recent aggressions have doubtless engendered.

Some bargains are Faustian, and some horses are Trojan. Dance carefully with the porcupine, and know in advance the price of intimacy.

Acknowledgement

Dr. Ghali is supported by a Population Health Investigator Award from the Alberta Heritage Foundation for Medical Research and by a Government of Canada Research Chair in Health Services Research.

Notes

1. Press E, Washburn J. The kept university. *Atlantic Monthly* 2000; 285. Available: www.theantlantic.com/issues/2000/03/press.htm (accessed 2001 Aug 20).
2. Weatherall D. Academia and industry: increasingly uneasy bedfellows. *Lancet* 2000; 355:1574.
3. Van McCrary S, Anderson CB, Jakovljevic J, Khan T, McCullough LB, Wray NP, et al. A national survey of policies on disclosure of conflicts of interest in biomedical research. *N Engl J Med* 2000; 343:1621–6.
4. Cho MK, Shohara R, Schissel A, Rennie D. Policies on faculty conflicts of interest at US universities. *JAMA* 2000; 284:2237–8.
5. Lo B, Wolf LE, Berkeley A. Conflict-of-interest policies for investigators in clinical trials. *N Engl J Med* 2000; 343:1616–20.
6. Medical Research Council of Canada. *Report of the president 1999–2000*. Ottawa: Canadian Institutes of Health Research; 2000. Cat no MR1-2000. Available (in pdf format): www.cihr.ca/news/publications/publications/report9900_e.pdf (accessed 2001 Aug 20).
7. Meeks RL. *Federal R&D funding by budget function: fiscal years 1999–2001, special report*. Arlington (VA): National Science Foundation, Division of Science Resources Studies; 2001. Report no NSF 01-316.
8. Estimates of total expenditures on research and development in the health field in Canada, 1988 to 2000. Ottawa: Statistics Canada; 2001. Cat no. 88F0006XIE01006.
9. Hailey D. Scientific harassment by pharmaceutical companies: time to stop. CMAJ 2000; 162(2):212–3. Available: www.cma.ca/cmaj/vol-162/issue-2/0212.htm
10. Morgan S, Barer ML, Evans RG. Health economists meet the fourth tempter: drug dependency and scientific discourse. *Health Econ* 2000; 9:659–67.
11. Skolnick AA. Drug firm suit fails to halt publication of Canadian health technology report. *JAMA* 1998; 280:683–4.

12. Boseley S. Bitter pill. *Guardian Weekly* 2001; 164(22):23.

13. Hospital denies that withdrawal of MD's job offer was related to drug-company funding. *CMAJ* 2001; 164(13):1879. Available: www.cma.ca/cmaj/vol-164/issue-13/1879a.asp.

14. Lead donor Eli Lilly Canada launches education centre. In: *Foundation progress report winter 2000.* Toronto: Centre for Addiction and Mental Health; 2000. Available: www.camh.net/foundation/newsletters/foundation_news_winter2000.html (accessed 2001 Aug 20).

15. Kaebnick G. What about the report? *Hastings Cent Rep* 2001; 31(2):16–7.

16. Davidson RA. Source of funding and outcome of clinical trials. *J Gen Intern Med*, 1986; 1:155–8.

17. Stelfox HT, Chua G, O'Rourke K, Detsky AS. Conflict of interest in the debate over calcium-channel antagonists. *N Engl J Med* 1998; 332:101–6.

18. Friedberg M, Saffran B, Stinson TJ, Nelson W, Bennett CL. Evaluation of conflict of interest in economic analyses of new drugs used in oncology. *JAMA* 1999; 282:1453–7.

19. Dickersin K. The existence of publication bias and risk factors for its occurrence. *JAMA* 1990; 263:1385–9.

20. Easterbrook PJ, Berlin JA, Gopalan R, Matthews DR. Publication bias in clinical research. *Lancet* 1991; 337:867–72.

21. Naylor CD. Meta-analysis and the meta-epidemiology of clinical research. *BMJ* 1997; 315:617–9.

22. Boyd EA, Bero LA. Assessing faculty financial relationships with industry: a case study. *JAMA* 2000; 284:2209–14.

23. Hall ZA, Scott C. University-industry partnership. *Science* 2001; 591:553.

24. National Bioethics Advisory Commission. *Ethical and policy issues in research involving human participants.* Rockville (MD): The Commission; 2001 May 18. Recommendations available: http://bioethics.gov/press/finalrecomm5-18.html (accessed 2001 Aug 20).

Halushka v. University of Saskatchewan, [1965] 52 W.W.R. 608 (Sask. C.A.)

Summary prepared by Matthew Herder

Mr. Halushka learned about a study at the University of Saskatchewan from the University's employment office in late August 1961. During his initial visit with one of the researchers (Dr. Wyant), he was told that the test he would be subjected to involved a new drug that was "perfectly safe" and that "it had been conducted many times before," that electrodes would be put into his limbs and head, that an incision would be made in his arm and a catheter inserted, and that he would receive $50 for his participation. Halushka agreed to take part and signed a consent form, which purported to waive liability for the University and the researchers in the event of any "untoward effects or accidents."

Two days later, Haluska arrived at the hospital. Unbeknownst to him, the anesthetic drug to be used in the research ("fluoromar") had never been tested before. The researchers administered the fluoromar, and positioned the catheter inside Halushka's heart chambers. Shortly thereafter, the level of the anesthetic became too deep and Halushka suffered cardiac arrest. To resuscitate him, the researchers had to manually massage his heart after making a large incision in his chest.

Halushka was unconscious for four days, and was discharged ten days after waking up. Wyant paid the agreed-upon $50 fee but said it could be increased in exchange for a complete release. Halushka brought an action for trespass to the person and negligence instead. At trial, a jury found him successful on both counts, but the researchers and University appealed.

At the Court of Appeal, the primary issue concerned the validity of the consent given. The appellants argued that (1) there was no evidence before the jury capable of grounding liability because the consent was valid, and (2) the trial judge erred in characterizing the relationship between the researchers and Halushka as doctor–patient, when it was purely contractual in nature.

Justice Hall, speaking for the Court of Appeal, held against the researchers and the University, increasing the standard of disclosure for the research setting:

> There can be no exceptions to the ordinary requirements of disclosure in the case of research as there may well be in ordinary medical practice. The researcher does not have to balance the probable effect of the lack of treatment against the risk involved to the treatment itself. The example of risks being properly hidden from a patient when it is important that he should not worry can have no application in the field of research. The subject of medical experimentation is entitled to a full and frank disclosure of all the facts, probabilities and opinions which a reasonable man [sic] might be expected to consider before giving his consent. (para. 29)

Applied to the facts of this case, Wyant's description of the test as "safe" and his failure to inform Halushka that fluoromar had never been used before constituted non-disclosure. Moreover, the fact that the catheter was to be input into Halushka's heart, as opposed to simply a vein in his arm, should have been disclosed. In short, any facts that may influence the decision to consent, notwithstanding the fact that they may not pose any actual danger nor contribute to the injury ultimately sustained, should be disclosed. Furthermore, in these circumstances, and in the conduct of human research more generally, waivers, like the one Halushka had signed, will not be given effect.

Chapter 9 ISSUES IN REPRODUCTION

A Third Way

L. Wayne Sumner

The practice of abortion confronts us with two different sets of moral questions belonging to two different decision contexts. The primary context is that in which a woman chooses whether to have an abortion and a physician chooses whether to perform it; here the focus is on the moral quality of abortion itself. Because this context is one of individual decision we will call the set of moral questions which it contains the *personal* problem of abortion. The secondary context is that in which a society chooses how, or whether, to regulate abortions; here the focus is on the merits of alternative abortion policies. Because this context is one of social decision we will call the set of moral questions which it contains the *political* problem of abortion.

Although the two kinds of problem raised by abortion are distinct, they are also connected. A complete view of the morality of abortion will therefore offer connected solutions to them. In most countries in the West, public discussion of abortion has been distorted by the dominance of two such views. The liberal view, espoused by "pro-choice" groups, holds that (voluntary) abortion is always morally innocuous and (therefore) that the only acceptable abortion policy is one which treats abortion as another variety of minor elective surgery. The conservative view, espoused by "pro-life" groups, holds that abortion is always morally serious and (therefore) that the only acceptable abortion policy is one which treats abortion as another variety of homicide.

Because they define the extremities of the continuum of possible positions, and because each is sufficiently simple and forceful to be advocated by a powerful movement, these established views constitute the familiar reference points in our abortion landscape. Yet neither has managed to command the allegiance of more than a small minority of the public. For the rest of us who are unwilling to embrace either of the extreme options the problem has been the lack of a well-defined middle ground between them. In contrast to the power of the established views more moderate alternatives may appear both indistinct and indecisive.

Public distrust of the established views is well grounded: neither stands up under critical scrutiny.[1] If their demise is not to leave us without any credible view of abortion three tasks must be successfully completed. The first is to define a third way with abortion and to distinguish it from both of the views which it will supersede. The second is to give it an intuitive defense by showing that it coheres better than either of its predecessors with our considered moral judgments both on abortion itself and on closely related issues. Then, finally, the third way must be grounded in a moral theory. The first two of these tasks will be undertaken here; the more daunting theoretical challenge is confronted elsewhere.[2]

1. SPECIFICATIONS

Despite their opposition, the two established views suffer from similar defects. Collating their failures will provide us with some positive guidelines to follow in building a more satisfactory alternative. The central issue in the morality of abortion is the moral status of the fetus. Let us say that a creature has *moral standing* if, for the purpose of moral decisionmaking, it must be counted for something in its own right. To count for nothing is to have no moral standing; to count for as much as possible (as much, that is, as any creature does) is to have full moral standing. We may, for the purpose of the present discussion, make this rather vague notion more precise by adopting the rights vocabulary favored by both of the established views. We will suppose that having (some) moral standing is equivalent to having (some) right to life. The central issue in the morality of abortion is then whether fetuses have moral standing in this sense.[3]

The conservative view, and also the more naive versions of the liberal view, select a precise point (conception, birth, etc.) as the threshold of moral standing, implying that the transition from no standing to full standing occurs abruptly. In doing so they rest more weight on these sudden events than they are capable of bearing. A view that avoids this defect will allow full moral standing to be acquired gradually. It will therefore attempt to locate not a threshold point, but a threshold period or stage.

Both of the established views attribute a uniform moral status to all fetuses, regardless of their dissimilarities. Each, for example counts a newly conceived zygote for precisely as much (or as little) as a full-term fetus, despite the enormous differences between them. A view that avoids this defect will assign moral status differentially, so that the threshold stage occurs sometime during pregnancy.

A consequence of the uniform approach adopted by both of the established views is that neither can attach any significance to the development of the fetus during gestation. Yet this development is the most obvious feature of gestation. A view that avoids this defect will base the (differential) moral standing of the fetus at least in part on its level of development. It will thus assign undeveloped fetuses a moral status

akin to that of ova and spermatozoa, whereas it will assign developed fetuses a moral status akin to that of infants.

So far, then, an adequate view of the fetus must be gradual, differential, and developmental. It must also be derived from a satisfactory criterion of moral standing. Such a criterion must be general (applicable to beings other than fetuses), it must connect moral standing with the empirical properties of such beings, and it must be morally relevant. Its moral relevance is partly testable by appeal to intuition, for arbitrary or shallow criteria will be vulnerable to counter-examples. But the final test of moral relevance is grounding in a moral theory.

An adequate view of the fetus promises a morally significant division between early abortions (before the threshold stage) and late abortions (after the threshold stage). It also promises borderline cases (during the threshold state). Wherever that stage is located, abortions that precede it will be private matters, since the fetus will at that stage lack moral standing. Thus the provisions of the liberal view will apply to early abortions: they will be morally innocent (as long as the usual conditions of maternal consent, etc., are satisfied) and ought to be legally unregulated (except for rules equally applicable to all other medical procedures). Early abortion will have the same moral status as contraception.

Abortions that follow the threshold stage will be interpersonal matters, since the fetus will at that stage possess moral standing. Thus the provisions of the conservative view will apply to late abortions: they must be assessed on a case-by-case basis and they ought to be legally permitted only on appropriate grounds. Late abortions will have the same moral status as infanticide, except for the difference made by the physical connection between fetus and mother.

A third way with abortion is thus a moderate and differential view, combining elements of the liberal view for early abortion with elements of (a weakened version of) the conservative view for late abortions. The policy that a moderate view will support is a moderate policy, permissive in the early stages of pregnancy and more restrictive (though not as restrictive as conservatives think appropriate) in the later stages. So far as the personal question of the moral evaluation of particular abortions is concerned, there is no pressing need to resolve the borderline cases around the threshold stage. But a workable abortion policy cannot tolerate this vagueness and will need to establish a definite time limit beyond which the stipulated grounds will come into play. Although the precise location of the time limit will unavoidably be somewhat arbitrary, it will be defensible as long as it falls somewhere within the threshold stage. Abortion on request up to the time limit and only for cause thereafter: these are the elements of a satisfactory abortion policy.

A number of moderate views may be possible, each of them satisfying all of the foregoing constraints. A particular view will be defined by selecting (a) a criterion of moral standing, (b) the natural characteristics whose gradual acquisition during normal fetal development carries with it the acquisition of moral standing, and (c) a threshold stage. Of these three steps, the first is the crucial one, since it determines both of the others.

2. A CRITERION OF MORAL STANDING

We are assuming that for a creature to have moral standing is for it to have a right to life. Any such right imposes duties on moral agents; these duties may be either negative (not to deprive the creature of life) or positive (to support the creature's life). Possession of a right to life implies at least some immunity against attack by others, and possibly also some entitlement to the aid of others. As the duties may vary in strength, so may the corresponding rights. To have some moral standing is to have some right to life, whether or not it may be overridden by the rights of others. To have full moral standing is to have the strongest right to life possessed by anyone, the right to life of the paradigm person. Depending on one's moral theory, this right may or may not

be inviolable and indefeasible and thus may or may not impose absolute duties on others.

To which creatures should we distribute (some degree of) moral standing? On which criterion should we base this distribution? It may be easier to answer these questions if we begin with the clear case and work outward to the unclear ones. If we can determine why we ascribe full standing to the paradigm case, we may learn what to look for in other creatures when deciding whether or not to include them in the moral sphere.

The paradigm bearer of moral standing is an adult human being with normal capacities of intellect, emotion, perception, sensation, decision, action, and the like. If we think of such a person as a complex bundle of natural properties, then in principle we could employ as a criterion any of the properties common to all normal and mature members of our species. Selecting a particular property or set of properties will define a class of creatures with moral standing, namely, all (and only) those who share that property. The extension of that class will depend on how widely the property in question is distributed. Some putative criteria will be obviously frivolous and will immediately fail the tests of generality or moral relevance. But even after excluding the silly candidates, we are left with a number of serious ones. There are four that appear to be the most serious: we might attribute full moral standing to the paradigm person on the ground that he/she is (a) intrinsically valuable, (b) alive, (c) sentient, or (d) rational. An intuitive test of the adequacy of any of these candidates will involve first enumerating the class of beings to whom it will distribute moral standing and then determining whether that class either excludes creatures that upon careful reflection we believe ought to be included or includes creatures that we believe ought to be excluded. In the former case the criterion draws the boundary of the moral sphere too narrowly and fails as a necessary condition of moral standing. In the latter case the criterion draws the boundary too broadly and fails as a sufficient condition. (A given criterion may, of course, be defective in both respects.) …

A criterion of life (or teleology) is too weak, admitting classes of beings (animate and inanimate) who are not suitable loci for moral rights; being alive is necessary for having standing, but it is not sufficient. A criterion of rationality (or moral agency) is too strong, excluding classes of beings (human and nonhuman) who are suitable loci for rights; being rational is sufficient for having standing, but it is not necessary. A criterion of sentience (or consciousness) is a promising middle path between these extremes. Sentience is the capacity for feeling or affect. In its most primitive form it is the ability to experience sensations of pleasure and pain, and thus the ability to enjoy and suffer. Its more developed forms include wants, aims, and desires (and thus the ability to be satisfied and frustrated); attitudes, tastes, and values; and moods, emotions, sentiments, and passions. Consciousness is a necessary condition of sentience, for feelings are states of mind of which their owner is aware. But it is not sufficient; it is at least possible in principle for beings to be conscious (percipient, for instance, or even rational) while utterly lacking feelings. If rationality embraces a set of cognitive capacities, then sentience is rooted in a being's affective and conative life. It is in virtue of being sentient that creatures have interests, which are compounded either out of their desires or out of the experiences they find agreeable (or both). If morality has to do with the protection and promotion of interests, it is a plausible conjecture that we owe moral duties to all those beings capable of having interests. But this will include all sentient creatures.

Like rationality, and unlike life, it makes sense to think of sentience as admitting of degrees. Within any given mode, such as the perception of pain, one creature may be more or less sensitive than another. But there is a further sense in which more developed (more rational) creatures possess a higher degree of sentience. The expansion of consciousness and of intelligence opens up new ways of experiencing the world, and therefore new ways of being affected by the world. More rational beings are capable of finding either fulfillment or frustration in activities and states of affairs to which less developed creatures are, both cognitively and affectively, blind. It is in this sense of a broader and deeper sensibility that a higher being is capable of a richer, fuller, and more varied existence. The fact that sentience admits of degrees (whether of sensitivity or sensibility) enables us to employ it both as an inclusion criterion and as a comparison criterion of moral standing. The animal kingdom presents us with a hierarchy of sentience. Nonsentient beings have no moral standing; among sentient beings the more developed have greater standing than the less developed, the upper limit being occupied by the paradigm of a normal adult human being. Although sentience is the criterion of moral standing, it is also possible to explain the relevance of rationality. The evolutionary order is one of ascending intelligence. Since rationality expands a creature's interests, it is a reliable indicator of the degree of moral standing which that creature possesses. Creatures less rational than human beings do not altogether lack standing, but they do lack full standing.

An analysis of degrees of standing would require a graded right to life, in which the strength of the right varied inversely with the range of considerations capable of overriding it. The details of any such analysis will be complex and need not be worked out here. However, it seems that we are committed to extending (some) moral standing at least to all vertebrate animals, and also to counting higher animals for more than lower.[4] Thus we should expect the higher vertebrates (mammals) to merit greater protection of life than the lower (fish, reptiles, amphibia, birds) and we should also expect the higher mammals (primates, cetaceans) to merit greater protection of life than the lower (canines, felines, etc.). Crude as this division may be, it seems to accord reasonably well with most people's intuitions that in our moral reasoning paramecia and horseflies count for nothing, dogs and cats count for something, chimpanzees and dolphins count for more, and human beings count for most of all.

A criterion of sentience can thus allow for the gradual emergence of moral standing in the order of nature. It can explain why no moral issues arise (directly) in our dealings with inanimate objects, plants, and the simpler forms of animal life. It can also function as a moral guideline in our encounters with novel life forms on other planets. If the creatures we meet have interests and are capable of enjoyment and suffering, we must grant them some moral standing. We thereby constrain ourselves not to exploit them ruthlessly for our own advantage. The kind of standing that they deserve may be determined by the range and depth of their sensibility, and in ordinary circumstances this will vary with their intelligence. We should therefore recognize as equals beings who are as rational and sensitive as ourselves. The criterion also implies that if we encounter creatures who are rational but nonsentient—who utterly lack affect and desire—nothing we can do will adversely affect such creatures (in morally relevant ways). We would be entitled, for instance, to treat them as a species of organic computer. The same obviously holds for forms of artificial intelligence; in deciding whether to extend moral standing to sophisticated machines, the question (as Bentham put it) is not whether they can reason but whether they can suffer.

A criterion of sentience also requires gentle usage of the severely abnormal. Cognitive disabilities and disorders may impair a person's range of sensibility, but they do not generally reduce that person to the level of a nonsentient being. Even the grossly retarded or deranged will still be capable of some forms of enjoyment and suffering and thus will still possess (some) moral standing in their own right. This standing diminishes to the vanishing point only when sentience is entirely lost or never gained in the first place. If all affect and responsivity are absent, and if they cannot be engendered, then (but only then) are we no longer dealing with a sentient creature. This verdict accords well with the contemporary trend toward defining death in terms of the permanent loss of cerebral functioning. Although such patients are in one obvious sense still alive (their blood circulates and is oxy-genated), in the morally relevant sense they are now beyond our reach, for we can cause them neither good nor ill. A criterion of life would require us to continue treating them as beings with (full?) moral standing, whereas a criterion of rationality would withdraw that standing when reason was lost even though sensibility should remain. Again a criterion of sentience enables us to find a middle way.

Fastening upon sentience as the criterion for possession of a right to life thus opens up the possibility of a reasonable and moderate treatment of moral problems other than abortion, problems pertaining to the treatment of non-human animals, extraterrestrial life, artificial intelligence, "defective" human beings, and persons at the end of life. We need now to trace out its implications for the fetus.

3. THE MORALITY OF ABORTION

The adoption of sentience as a criterion determines the location of a threshold of moral standing. Since sentience admits of degrees, we can in principle construct a continuum ranging from fully sentient creatures at one extreme to completely nonsentient creatures at the other. The threshold of moral standing is that area of the continuum through which sentience fades into nonsentience. In phylogenesis the continuum extends from homo sapiens to the simple animals and plants, and the threshold area is the boundary between vertebrates and invertebrates. In pathology the continuum extends from the fully normal to the totally incapacitated, and the threshold area is the transition from consciousness to unconsciousness. Human ontogenesis also presents us with a continuum from adult to zygote. The threshold area will be the stage at which sentience first emerges, but where is that to be located?

A mental life is built upon a physical base. The capacity for sentience is present only when the necessary physiological structures are present. Physiology, and in particular neurophysiology, is our principal guide in locating a threshold in the phylogenetic continuum. Like a stereo system, the brain of our paradigm sentient being is a set of connected components. These components may be roughly sorted into three groups: forebrain (cerebral hemispheres, thalamus, hypothalamus, amygdala), midbrain (cerebellum), and brainstem (upper part of the spinal cord, pineal and pituitary glands). The brainstem and midbrain play no direct role in the individual's conscious life; their various parts regulate homeostasis (temperature, respiration, heartbeat, etc.), secrete hormones, make reflex connections, route nerves, coordinate motor activities, and so on. All of these functions can be carried on in the total absence of consciousness. Cognitive, perceptual, and voluntary motor functions are all localized in the forebrain, more particularly in the cerebral cortex. Sensation (pleasure/pain), emotion, and basic drives (hunger, thirst, sex, etc.) are controlled by subcortical areas in the forebrain. Although the nerves that transmit pleasure/pain impulses are routed through the cortex, their ultimate destination is the limbic system (amygdala, hypothalamus). The most primitive forms of sentience are thus possible in the absence of cortical activity.

Possession of particular neural structures cannot serve as a criterion of moral standing, for we cannot rule out encounters with sentient beings whose structures are quite different from ours. But in all of the species with which we are familiar, the components of the forebrain (or some analogues) are the minimal conditions of sentience. Thus the evolution of the forebrain serves as an indicator of the kind and degree of sentience possessed by a particular animal species. When we turn to human ontogenesis we may rely on the same indicator.

The normal gestation period for our species is 280 days from the onset of the last menstrual period to birth. This duration is usually divided into three equal trimesters of approximately thirteen weeks each. A zygote has no central nervous system of any sort. The spinal cord makes its first appearance early in the embryonic period (third week), and the major divisions between forebrain, midbrain, and brainstem are evident by the end of the eighth week. At the conclusion of the first trimester virtually all of the major neural

components can be clearly differentiated and EEG activity is detectable. The months to follow are marked chiefly by the growth and elaboration of the cerebral hemispheres, especially the cortex. The brain of a seven-month fetus is indistinguishable, at least in its gross anatomy, from that of a newborn infant. Furthermore, by the seventh month most of the neurons that the individual's brain will contain during its entire lifetime are already in existence. In the newborn the brain is closer than any other organ to its mature level of development.

There is no doubt that a newborn infant is sentient—that it feels hunger, thirst, physical pain, the pleasure of sucking, and other agreeable and disagreeable sensations. There is also no doubt that a zygote, and also an embryo, are presentient. It is difficult to locate with accuracy the stage during which feeling first emerges in fetal development. The structure of the fetal brain, including the cortex, is well laid down by the end of the second trimester. But there is reason to expect the more primitive and ancient parts of that brain to function before the rest. The needs of the fetus dictate the order of appearance of neural functions. Thus the brainstem is established and functioning first, since it is required for the regulation of heartbeat and other metabolic processes. Since the mammalian fetus develops in an enclosed and protected environment, cognition and perception are not essential for survival and their advent is delayed. It is therefore not surprising that the cortex, the most complex part of the brain and the least important to the fetus, is the last to develop to an operational level.

Simple pleasure/pain sensations would seem to occupy a medial position in this priority ranking. They are localized in a part of the brain that is more primitive than the cortex, but they could have little practical role for a being that is by and large unable either to seek pleasurable stimuli or to avoid painful ones. Behavioral evidence is by its very nature ambiguous. Before the end of the first trimester, the fetus will react to unpleasant stimuli by flinching and withdrawing. However, this reaction is probably a reflex that is entirely automatic. How are we to tell when mere reflex has crossed over into consciousness? The information we now possess does not enable us to date with accuracy the emergence of fetal sentience. Of some judgments, however, we can be reasonably confident. First-trimester fetuses are clearly not yet sentient. Third-trimester fetuses probably possess some degree of sentience, however minimal. The threshold of sentience thus appears to fall in the second trimester. More ancient and primitive than cognition, the ability to discriminate simple sensations of pleasure and pain is probably the first form of consciousness to appear in the onto-genetic order. Further, when sentience emerges it does not do so suddenly. The best we can hope for is to locate a threshold state or period in the second trimester. It is at present unclear just how far into that trimester this stage occurs.

The phylogenetic and pathological continua yield us clear cases at the extremes and unclear cases in the middle. The ontogenetic continuum does the same. Because there is no quantum leap into consciousness during fetal development, there is no clean and sharp boundary between sentient and nonsentient fetuses. There is therefore no precise point at which a fetus acquires moral standing. More and better information may enable us to locate the threshold state ever more standing. More and better information may enable us to locate the threshold stage ever more accurately, but it will never collapse that stage into a point. We are therefore inevitably confronted with a class of fetuses around the threshold stage whose sentience, and therefore whose moral status, is indeterminate....

The moral issues raised by early abortion are precisely those raised by contraception. It is for early abortions that the liberal view is appropriate. Since the fetus at this stage has no right to life, early abortion (like contraception) cannot violate its rights. But if it violates no one's rights, early abortion (like contraception) is a private act. There are of course significant differences between contraception and early abortion, since the former is generally less hazardous, less arduous, and less expensive. A woman has, there-

fore, good prudential reasons for relying on contraception as her primary means of birth control. But if she elects an early abortion, then, whatever the circumstances and whatever her reasons, she does nothing immoral.[5]

The moral issues raised by late abortion are similar to those raised by infanticide. It is for late abortions that (a weakened form of) the conservative view is appropriate. Since the fetus at this stage has a right to life, late abortion (like infanticide) may violate its rights. But if it may violate the fetus' rights, then late abortion (like infanticide) is a public act. There is, however, a morally significant difference between late abortion and infanticide. A fetus is parasitic upon a unique individual in a manner in which a newborn infant is not. That parasitic relation will justify late abortion more liberally than infanticide, for they do not occur under the same circumstances.

Since we have already explored the morality of abortion for those cases in which the fetus has moral standing, the general approach to late abortions is clear enough. Unlike the simple and uniform treatment of early abortion, only a case-by-case analysis will here suffice. We should expect a serious threat to the woman's life or health (physical or mental) to justify abortion, especially if that threat becomes apparent only late in pregnancy. We should also expect a risk of serious fetal deformity to justify abortion, again especially if that risk becomes apparent (as it usually does) only late in pregnancy. On the other hand, it should not be necessary to justify abortion on the ground that pregnancy was not consented to, since a woman will have ample opportunity to seek an abortion before the threshold stage. If a woman freely elects to continue a pregnancy past that stage, she will thereafter need a serious reason to end it.

A differential view of abortion is therefore liberal concerning early abortion and conservative (in an extended sense) concerning late abortion. The status of the borderline cases in the middle weeks of the second trimester is simply indeterminate. We cannot say of them with certainty either that the fetus has a right to life or that it does not. Therefore we also cannot say either that a liberal approach to these abortions is suitable or that a conservative treatment of them is required. What we can say is that, from the moral point of view, the earlier an abortion is performed the better. There are thus good moral reasons, as well as good prudential ones, for women not to delay their abortions....

Settling on sentience as a criterion of moral standing thus leads us to a view of the moral status of the fetus, and of the morality of abortion, which satisfies the constraints set out in Section 1. It is gradual, since it locates a threshold stage rather than a point and allows moral standing to be acquired incrementally. It is differential, since it locates the threshold state during gestation and thus distinguishes the moral status of newly conceived and full-term fetuses. It is developmental, since it grounds the acquisition of moral standing in one aspect of the normal development of the fetus. And it is moderate, since it distinguishes the moral status of early and late abortions and applies each of the established views to that range of cases for which it is appropriate.

4. AN ABORTION POLICY

A differential view of the morality of abortion leads to a differential abortion policy—one that draws a legal distinction between early and late abortions. If we work within the framework of a liberal social theory, then it is understood that the state has no right to interfere in the private transaction between a woman and her physician. No regulation of this transaction will be legitimate unless it is also legitimate for other contractual arrangements between patients and physicians. It might be quite in place for the state to require that abortions be performed by qualified (perhaps licensed) personnel in properly equipped (perhaps licensed) facilities: whether or not this is so will depend on whether the state is in general competent to regulate trade in medical skills. Both the decision to abort and the decision to use contraceptives are private ones on which a woman ought to seek medical advice and medical assistance. There is no justification

in either case for restricting access to that advice or that assistance.

An abortion policy must therefore be permissive for early abortions. There is at this stage no question of inquiring into a woman's reason for seeking an abortion. Her autonomy here is absolute; the simple desire not to have a child (or not to have one now) is sufficient. Grounds for abortion become pertinent only when we turn to late abortions. Since virtually all such abortions will result in the death of a being that has a right to life (though not all will violate that right), the state has a legitimate role to play in governing trade in abortion at this stage. Legal grounds for late abortion are a special case of conditions for justifiable homicide. As much as possible (allowing for the unique relation between mother and fetus) these grounds should authorize abortion when killing would also be justified in relevantly similar cases not involving fetuses. Two general conditions for justifiable homicide will be applicable to abortions: self-defense and euthanasia.

The usual legal grounds for abortion provided by moderate policies may be divided into four categories: (a) therapeutic (threat to maternal life or health); (b) eugenic (risk of fetal abnormality); (c) humanitarian (pregnancy due to the commission of a crime, such as rape or incest); (d) socioeconomic (poverty, family size, etc.). If a moderate treatment of late abortion is coupled (as it should be) with a permissive treatment of early ones, only the first two categories are necessary. Therapeutic grounds for abortion follow from a woman's right of self-defense. The threat, however, must be serious in two different respects: the injury in prospect must be more than trivial and the probability of its occurrence must be greater than normal. The risks generally associated with pregnancy will not here suffice. Further, there must be good medical reason not to delay until the fetus has a better chance of survival, and every effort must be made to save the fetus' life if this is possible. Thus late abortion for therapeutic reasons ought to be reserved for genuine medical emergencies in which no other course of action would qualify as proper care of the mother. In many putatively moderate policies therapeutic grounds for abortion (especially mental health clauses) are interpreted so liberally as to cover large numbers of cases that are not by any stretch of the imagination medical emergencies. This is the standard device whereby a policy moderate in principle becomes permissive in practice. Since the policy here advanced is permissive in principle (for early abortions), a strict interpretation of the therapeutic grounds for late abortions will be mandatory.

The same strictures will apply to eugenic grounds. When there is a substantial risk of some severe anomaly (rubella, spina bifida, Tay-Sachs disease, etc.), abortion may be the best course of action for the fetus. This is not obviously the case for less severe defects (Down's syndrome, dwarfism, etc.). Again there will be no justification for an interpretation of eugenic grounds so elastic that it permits abortion whenever the child is unwanted (because, say, it is the "wrong" sex). A rough rule of thumb is that late abortion for reasons of fetal abnormality is permissible only in those cases in which euthanasia for defective newborns would also be permissible. Probability will play a different role in the two kinds of case, since prenatal diagnosis of these conditions is often less certain than postnatal. But against this reason for delay we must balance the anguish of a woman carrying a fetus who may turn out at birth to be grossly deformed. Since diagnostic techniques such as ultrasound and amniocentesis cannot be employed until the second trimester, a permissive treatment of early abortions will not eliminate the need for late abortions on eugenic grounds....

There is no need for any special notice of humanitarian grounds. It is doubtful indeed whether incest ought to be a crime, except in those cases in which someone is being exploited. In any case, any woman who has become pregnant due to incestuous intercourse will have ready access to an early abortion. If she declines this opportunity and if there is no evidence of genetic abnormality, she may not simply change her mind later. The same obviously applies to

pregnancy due to rape, including statutory rape. The practical problems should be approached by providing suitable counseling.

A permissive policy for early abortions will also render socioeconomic grounds redundant. Since social constraints do not normally create an emergency for which abortion is the only solution, and since women will be able to terminate pregnancies at will in the early stages, there is no need for separate recognition of social or economic justifications for abortion.

An adequate abortion policy is thus a conjunction of a permissive policy for early abortions and a moderate policy for late abortions. The obvious remaining question is where to draw the boundary between the two classes of cases. When we are dealing with the morality of abortion, borderline fuzziness is both inevitable and tolerable. Many moral problems turn on factors that are matters of degree. Where such factors are present, we cannot avoid borderline cases whose status is unclear or indeterminate. It is a defect in a moral theory to draw sharp lines where there are none, or to treat hard cases as though they were easy. But what makes for good morals may also make for bad law. An abortion policy must be enforceable and so must divide cases as clearly as possible. A threshold stage separating early from late abortions must here give way to a cut-off point.

Since there is no threshold point in fetal development, any precise upper limit on the application of a permissive policy will be to some extent arbitrary. Clearly it must be located within the threshold period, thus sometime in the second trimester. Beyond this constraint the choice of a time limit may be made on pragmatic grounds. If a permissive policy for early abortions is to promote their autonomy, women must have time to discover that they are pregnant and to decide on a course of action. This factor will tend to push the cutoff point toward the end of the second trimester. On the other hand, earlier abortions are substantially safer and more economical of scarce medical resources than later ones. This factor will tend to pull the cutoff point toward the beginning of the second trimester. Balancing these considerations would incline one toward a time limit located sometime around the midpoint of pregnancy. But it should not be pretended that there is a unique solution to this policy problem. Differential policies may legitimately vary (within constraints) in their choice of a boundary between permissiveness and moderation....

Notes

1. I will not be defending this assessment in the present paper. For the arguments see *Abortion and Moral Theory*, chs. 2 and 3.
2. *Abortion and Moral Theory*, chs. 5 and 6.
3. The adoption of this working definition of moral standing should not be construed as a concession that rights are the appropriate category for dealing with the moral issues posed by abortion. But since both of the established views employ the rhetoric of rights, there is some point to showing how that rhetoric is equally available to a moderate view. For a generalized notion of moral standing freed from all connection with rights see *Abortion and Moral Theory*, Section 23.
4. It is unclear at present whether invertebrates are capable of feeling pain, though the discovery of endorphins (opiates manufactured by the body) even in very simple organisms suggests that they may be. If so, then we are committed to extending (some) moral standing to invertebrates as well.
5. Unless there are circumstances (such as extreme underpopulation) in which contraception would also be immoral.

Selective Termination of Pregnancy and Women's Reproductive Autonomy

Christine Overall

The development of techniques for selective termination of pregnancy has added further questions to debates about women's reproductive self-determination. The procedure is performed during the first or second trimester in some instances of multiple pregnancy, either to eliminate a fetus found through prenatal diagnosis to be handicapped or at risk of a disability, or simply to reduce the number of fetuses in the uterus. More than two hundred cases of selective termination are known to have been performed around the world.[1]

Physicians and ethicists have expressed reservations about selective termination, both with respect to its moral justification and to the formation of social policy governing access to and resource allocation for this procedure. Selective termination has been viewed as invoking a right to kill a fetus rather than to control one's body, as with abortion,[2] and some commentators have recommended restricting the procedure to pregnancies of three or more[3] and even stipulated a need for national guidelines for the procedure.[4]

Many discussions appear to assume that selective termination is primarily a matter of acting against some fetus(es) on behalf of others. For example, Diana Brahams describes the issue as follows:

> Is it ethical and legally appropriate to carry out a selective reduction of pregnancy—that is, to destroy one or more fetuses in order to give the remaining fetus or fetuses a better chance?[5]

However, this construction of the problem is radically incomplete, since it omits attention to the women—their bodies and their lives—who should be at the center of any discussion of selective termination. When Margaret Somerville, for example, expresses concern about "the right to kill a fetus who is competing with another for space," she neglects to mention that the "space" in question is the pregnant woman's uterus. In fact, selective termination vividly instantiates many of the central ethical and policy concerns that must be raised about the technological manipulation of women's reproductive capacities.

Evans and colleagues state that "the ethical issues [of selective termination] are the same in multiple pregnancies whether the cause is spontaneous conception or infertility treatment" (293). Such a claim is typical of many discussions in contemporary bioethics, which abstract specific moral and social problems from the cultural context that produced them. But the issue of selective termination of pregnancy demonstrates the necessity of examining the social and political environment in which issues in biomedical ethics arise.

Selective termination itself must be understood and evaluated with reference to its own particular context. The apparent need or demand for selective termination in fact is created and elaborated in response to prior technological interventions in women's reproductive processes, themselves the result of prevailing cultural interpretations of infertility.

Hence, it is essential to explore the significance of selective termination for women's reproductive autonomy. The issue acquires added urgency at this point in both Canada and the United States when access to and allocation of funding for abortion are the focus of renewed controversy. Although not precisely the same as abortion, selective termination is similar insofar as in both cases one or more fetuses are destroyed. They differ in that in abortion the pregnancy ends whereas in selective termination, ideally, the pregnancy continues with one or more fetuses still present. I will argue that, provided a permissive abortion policy is justified (that is, a policy that allows abortion until the end of the second trimester), a concern for women's reproductive autonomy precludes any general policy restricting access to selective termination of pregnancy, as well as clinical practices that discriminate on nonmedical grounds as to which women will be permitted to choose the procedure or how many fetuses they must retain.

A TECHNOLOGICAL FIX

In recent discussions of selective termination, women with multiple pregnancies are often represented as demanding the procedure—sometimes by threatening to abort the entire pregnancy if they are not allowed selective termination.[6]

The assumption that individual women "demand" selective termination of pregnancy places all moral responsibility for the procedure on the women themselves. However, neither the multiple pregnancies nor the "demands" for selective termination originated *ex nihilo*. An examination of their sources suggests both that moral responsibility for selective termination cannot rest solely on individual women and that the "demand" for selective termination is not just a straightforward exercise of reproductive freedom.

Deliberate societal and medical responses to the perceived problem of female infertility generate much of the demand for selective termination, which is but one result of a complex system of values and beliefs concerning fertility and infertility, maternity and children. Infertility is not merely a physical condition; it is both interpreted and evaluated within cultural contexts that help to specify the appropriate beliefs about and responses to the condition of being unable to reproduce. According to the prevailing ideology of pronatalism, women must reproduce, men must acquire offspring, and both parents should be biologically related to their offspring. A climate of acquisition and commodification encourages and reinforces the notion of child as possession. Infertility is seen as a problem for which the solution must be acquiring a child of one's own, biologically related to oneself, at almost any emotional, physical, or economic costs.[7]

The recent increase in numbers of multiple pregnancies comes largely from two steps taken in the treatment of infertility. The use of fertility drugs to prod women's bodies into ovulating and producing more than one ovum at a time results in an incidence of multiple gestation ranging from 16 to 39 percent.[8] Gamete intrafallopian transfer (GIFT) using several eggs, and in vitro fertilization (IVF) with subsequent implantation of several embryos in the woman's uterus to increase the likelihood that she will become pregnant may also result in multiple gestation. As Brahams notes, "Pregnancy rate increments are about 8 percent for each pre-embryo replaced in IVF, giving expected pregnancy rates of 8, 16, 24, and 32 percent for 1, 2, 3, and 4 pre-embyros, respectively" (1409). A "try anything" mentality is fostered by the fact that prospective IVF patients are often not adequately informed about the very low clinical success rates ("failure rates" would be a more appropriate term) of the procedure.[9] A case reported by Evans and colleagues dramatically illustrates the potential effects of these treatments: One woman's reproductive history included three cesarean sections, a tubal ligation, a tuboplasty (after which she remained infertile), in vitro fertilization with subsequent implantation of four embryos, selective termination of two of the fetuses, revelation via ultrasound that one of the remaining twins had "severe oligohydramnios and no evidence of a bladder or kidneys," spontaneous miscarriage of the abnormal twin, and intrauterine death of the remaining fetus (291).

In a commentary critical of selective termination, Angela Holder quotes Oscar Wilde's dictum: "In this world, there are only two tragedies. One is not getting what one wants, and the other is getting it" (22). But this begs the question of what is meant by saying that women "want" multiple pregnancy, or "want" selective termination of pregnancy.[10] What factors led these women to take infertility drugs and/or participate in an IVF program? How do they evaluate fertility, pregnancy, motherhood, children? How do they perceive themselves as women, as potential mothers, as infertile, and where do children fit into these visions? To what degree were they adequately informed of the likelihood that they would gestate more than one fetus? Were they provided with adequate support to enable them to clarify their own reasons and goals for seeking reproductive interventions, and to provide assistance throughout the emotionally and physically demanding aspects of the treatments? Barbara Katz Rothman's appraisal of

women who abort fetuses with genetic defects has more general applicability:

> They are the victims of a social system that fails to take collective responsibility for the needs of its members, and leaves individual women to make impossible choices. We are spared collective responsibility, because we individualize the problem. We make it the woman's own. She "chooses," and so we owe her nothing.[11]

Uncritical use of the claim that certain women "demand" selective termination implies that they are just selfish, unable to extend their caring to more than one or two infants, particularly if one has a disability. But this interpretation appears unjustified. In general, participants in IVF programs are extremely eager for a child. They are encouraged to be self-sacrificing, to be acquiescent in the manipulations the medical system requires their bodies to undergo. As John C. Hobbins notes, these women "have often already volunteered for innovative treatments and may be desperate to try another." The little evidence so far available suggests that if anything these women are, by comparison to their male partners, somewhat passive in regard to the making of reproductive decisions.[12] There is no evidence to suggest that most are not willing to assume the challenges of multiple pregnancy.

An additional cause of multiple pregnancy is the conflicting attitudes toward the embryo and fetus manifested in infertility research and clinical practice. One report suggests that multiple pregnancies resulting from IVF are generated not only because clinicians are driven by the motive to succeed—and implantation of large numbers of embryos appears to offer that prospect—but also because of "intimidation of medical practitioners by critics and authorities who insist that all fertilized eggs or pre-embryos be immediately returned to the patient."[13] Such "intimidation" does not, of course, excuse clinicians who may sacrifice their patients' well-being. Nevertheless, conservative beliefs in the necessity and inevitability of procreation and the sacredness and "personhood" of the embryo may contribute to the production of multiple pregnancies.

Thus, the technological "solutions" to some forms of female infertility create an additional problem of female hyperfertility—to which a further technological "solution" of selective termination is then offered. Women's so-called "demand" for selective termination of pregnancy is not a primordial expression of individual need, but a socially constructed response to prior medical interventions.

The debate over access to selective pregnancy termination exemplifies a classic no-win situation for women, in which medical technology generates a solution to a problem itself generated by medical technology—yet women are regarded as immoral for seeking that solution. While women have been, in part, victimized through the use of reproductive interventions that fail to respect and facilitate their reproductive autonomy, they are nevertheless unjustifiably held responsible for their attempts to cope with the outcomes of these interventions in the forms made available to them. From this perspective, selective termination is not so much an extension of women's reproductive choice as it is the extension of control over women's reproductive capacity—through the use of fertility drugs, GIFT, and IVF as "solutions" to infertility that often result, when successful, in multiple gestations; through the provision of a technology, selective termination, to respond to multiple gestation that may create much of the same ambivalence for women as is generated by abortion; and finally through the imposition of limitations on women's access to the procedure.

In decisions about selective termination, women are not simply feckless, selfish, and irresponsible. Nor are they mere victims of their social conditioning and the machinations of the medical and scientific establishments. But they must make their choices in the face of extensive socialization for maternity, a limited range of options, and sometimes inadequate information about outcomes. When women "demand" selective termination of pregnancy they are attempting to take action in response to a situation not of their own making, in the only way that seems available to them. Hence my argument is not that women are merely helpless victims and therefore must be permitted access to selective termination, but rather that it would be both socially irresponsible and unjust for a health care system that contributes to the generation of problematic multiple pregnancies to withhold access to a potential, if flawed, response to the situation.

SELECTIVE TERMINATION AND ABORTION

There is reason to believe that women's attitudes toward selective termination may be similar to their attitudes toward abortion. Although abortion is a solution to the problem of unwanted pregnancy, and the general availability of abortion accords women significant and essential reproductive freedom, it is often an occasion for ambivalence, and remains, as Caroline Whitbeck has pointed out, a "grim option" for most women.[14] Women who abort are, after all, undergoing a surgical invasion of their bodies, and some may also experience emotional distress. Moreover, for some women the death of the fetus is a source of grief, particularly when the pregnancy is wanted and the abortion is sought because of severe fetal disabilities.[15]

Comparable factors may contribute to women's reservations about selective termination of pregnancy. Those who resort to this procedure surely do not desire the invasion of their uterus, nor do they make it their aim to kill fetuses. In fact, unlike women who request abortions because their pregnancy is unwanted, most of those who seek selective termination are originally pregnant by choice. And as Evans and colleagues note, such pregnancies are "not only wanted but achieved at great psychological and economic cost after a lengthy struggle with infertility" (292).

For such women a procedure that risks the loss of all fetuses as selective termination does, may be especially troubling. The procedure is still experimental; and its short- and long-term outcomes are largely unknown. Richard C. Berkowitz and colleagues suggest that "[a]lthough the risks associated with selective reduction are known, the dearth of experience with the procedure to date makes it impossible to assess their likelihood" (1046). Further, in their report on four cases of selective termination, Evans and coworkers state that:

> [A]ny attempt to reduce the number of fetuses [is] experimental and [can] result in miscarriage, and … infection, bleeding, and other unknown risks [are] possible. If successful, the attempt could theoretically damage the remaining fetuses (290).

Note that "success" in the latter case would be seriously limited, assuming that the pregnant woman's goal is to gestate and subsequently deliver one or more healthy infants. In fact, success in this more plausible sense is fairly low.[16] As a consequence, in their study of first trimester selective termination, Berkowitz *et al.* mention the "psychological difficulty of making the decision [to undergo selective termination]," a difficulty partly resulting from "emotional bonding" with the fetuses after repeated ultrasound examinations (1046).

Thus, women undergoing selective termination, like those undergoing abortion, are choosing a grim option; they are ending the existence of one or more fetuses because the alternatives—aborting all the fetuses (and taking the risk that they will never again succeed in becoming pregnant), or attempting to maintain all the fetuses through pregnancy, delivery, and childrearing—are unacceptable, morally, medically, or practically.

THE CHALLENGES OF MULTIPLE GESTATION

Why don't women who seek selective termination simply continue their pregnancies? No matter how much it is taken for granted, the accomplishment of gestating and birthing even one child is an extraordinary event; perhaps even more praise should be given to the woman who births twins or triplets or quadruplets. Rather than setting policy limits on women who are not able or willing to gestate more than one or two fetuses, we should recognize and understand the extraordinary challenges posed by multiple pregnancies.

There are good consequentialist reasons why a woman might choose to reduce the number of fetuses she carries. For the pregnant woman, continuation of a multiple pregnancy means, Evans notes, "almost certain preterm delivery, prefaced by early and lengthy hospitalization, higher risks of pregnancy-induced hypertension, polyhydramnios, severe anemia, preeclampsia, and postpartum blood transfusions" (292).[17]

The so-called "minor discomforts" of pregnancy are increased in a multiple pregnancy, and women may suffer severe nausea and vomiting or become depressed or anxious. There is also an increased likelihood of cesarean delivery, entailing more pain and a longer recovery time after the birth.[18]

Infants born of multiple pregnancy risk "premature delivery, low infant birthweight, birth defects, and problems of infant immaturity, including physical and mental retardation."[19] Moreover, as Evans and colleagues note, there is a high likelihood that these infants "may … suffer a lengthy, costly process of dying in neonatal intensive care" (295). Thus a woman carrying more than one fetus also faces the possibility of becoming a mother to infants who will be seriously physically impaired or will die.

It is also important to count the social costs of bearing several children simultaneously, where the responsibilities, burdens, and lost opportunities occasioned by childrearing fall primarily if not exclusively upon the woman rather than upon her male partner (if any) or more equitably upon the society as a whole—particularly when the infants are disabled. A recent article on Canada's first set of "test-tube quintuplets" reported that the babies' mother, Mae Collier, changes diapers fifty times a day, and goes through twelve litres of milk a day and 150 jars of baby food a week. Her husband works full time outside of the home and "spends much of his spare time building the family's new house."[20]

Moreover, while North American culture is strongly pronatalist, it is simultaneously anti-child. One of the most prevalent myths of the West is that North Americans love and spoil their children. A sensitive examination—perhaps from the perspective of a child or a loving parent—of the conditions in which many children grow up puts the lie to this myth.[21] Children are among the most vulnerable victims of poverty and malnutrition. Subjected to physical and sexual abuse, educated in schools that more often aim for custody and confinement than growth and learning, exploited as opportunities for the mass marketing of useless and sometimes dangerous foods and toys, children, the weakest members of our society, are often the least protected. Children are virtually the last social group in North America for whom discrimination and segregation are routinely countenanced. In many residential areas, businesses, restaurants, hotels, and other "public" places, children are not welcome, and except in preschools and nurseries, there is usually little or no accommodation to their physical needs and capacities.

A society that is simultaneously pronatalist but anti-child and only minimally supportive of mothering is unlikely to welcome quintuplets and other multiples—except for their novelty—any more than it welcomes single children. The issue, then, is not just how many fetuses a woman can be required to gestate, but also how many children she can be required to raise, and under what sort of societal conditions.

To this argument it is no adequate rejoinder to say that such women should continue their pregnancies and then surrender some but not all of the infants for adoption by eager childless and infertile couples. It is one thing for a woman to have the choice of making this decision after careful thought and with full support throughout the pregnancy and afterward when the infants have been given up. Such a choice may be hard enough. It would be another matter, however, to advocate a policy that would restrict selective termination in such a way that gestating all the fetuses and surrendering some becomes a woman's only option.

First, the presence of each additional fetus places further demands on the woman's physical and emotional resources; gestating triplets or quadruplets is not just the same as gestating twins. Second, to compel a woman to continue to gestate fetuses she does not want for the sake of others who do is to treat the woman as a mere breeder, a biological machine for the production of new human beings. Finally, it would be callous indeed to ignore the emotional turmoil and pain of the woman who must gestate and deliver a baby only to surrender it to others. In the case of a multiple gestation an added distress would arise because of the necessity of somehow choosing which infant(s) to keep and which to give up.

REPRODUCTIVE RIGHTS

Within the existing social context, therefore, access to selective termination must be understood as an essential component of women's reproductive rights. But it is important to distinguish between the right to reproduce and the right not to reproduce. Entitlement to access to selective termination, like entitlement to access to abortion, falls within the right not to reproduce.[22]

Entitlement to choose how many fetuses to gestate, and of what sort, is in this context a limited and negative one. If women are entitled to choose to end their pregnancies altogether, then they are also entitled to choose how many fetuses and of what sort they will carry. If it is unjustified to deny a woman access to an abortion of all fetuses in her uterus, then it is also unjustified to deny her access to the termination of some of those fetuses. Furthermore, if abortion is legally permitted in cases where the fetus is seriously handicapped, it is inconsistent to refuse to permit the termination of one handicapped fetus in a multiple pregnancy.

One way of understanding abortion as an exercise of the right not to reproduce is to see it as the premature emptying of the uterus, or the deliberate termination of the fetus's occupancy of the womb. If a woman has an entitlement to an abortion, that is to the emptying of her uterus of all of its occupants, then there is no ground to compel her to maintain all the occupants of her uterus if she chooses to retain only some of them. While the risks of multiple pregnancy for both the fetuses and the pregnant woman increase with the number of fetuses involved, it does not follow that restrictions on selective termination for pregnancies with smaller numbers of fetuses would be justified. Legal or medical policy cannot consistently say, "you may choose whether to be pregnant, that is, whether your uterus shall be occupied, but you may not choose how many shall occupy your uterus."

More generally, if abortion of a healthy singleton pregnancy is permitted for any reason, as a matter of the woman's choice, within the first five months or so of pregnancy, it is inconsistent to refuse to permit the termination of one or more healthy fetuses in a multiple pregnancy. To say otherwise is unjustifiably to accord the fetuses a right to occupancy of the woman's uterus. It is to say that two or more human entities, at an extremely immature stage in their development, have the right to use a human person's body. But no embryo or fetus has a right to the use of a pregnant woman's body—any more than any other human being, at whatever stage of development, has a right to use another's body.[23] The absence of that right is recognized through state-sanctioned access to abortion. Fetuses do not acquire a right, either collectively or individually, to use a woman's uterus simply because there are several of them present simultaneously. Even if a woman is willingly and happily pregnant she does not surrender her entitlement to bodily self-determination, and she does not, specifically, surrender her entitlement to determine how many human entities may occupy her uterus.

Although I defend a social policy that does not set limits on access to selective termination of pregnancy, there can be no denying that the procedure may raise serious moral problems. As some persons with disabilities have pointed out, there is a special moral significance to the termination of a fetus with a disability such as Down syndrome.[24] The use of prenatal diagnosis followed by abortion or selective termination may have eugenic overtones, when the presupposition is that we can ensure only high quality babies will be born, and that "defective" fetuses can be eliminated before birth.[25] The fetus is treated as a product for which "quality control" measures are appropriate. Moreover, as amniocentesis and chorionic villus sampling reveal the sex of offspring, there is also a possibility that selective termination of pregnancy could be used, as abortion already is, to eliminate fetuses of the "wrong" sex—in most cases, that is, those that are female.[26]

These possibilities are distressing and potentially dangerous to disabled persons and to women generally. The way to deal with these and other moral reservations about selective termination is not to prohibit the procedure or to limit access to it on such grounds as fetal disability or fetal sex choice. Instead, part of the answer is to change the conditions that promote large numbers of embryos and fetuses. For example, since as Evans and colleagues astutely note, "[m]any of the currently known instances of grand multiple pregnancies should have never happened" (296), the administration of fertility drugs to induce ovulation can be carefully monitored, and for IVF and GIFT procedures, more use can be made of the natural ovulatory cycle and of cryopreservation of embryos.[27] The number of eggs implanted through GIFT and the number of embryos implanted after IVF can be limited—not by unilateral decision of the physician, but after careful consultation with the woman about the chances of multiple pregnancy and her attitudes toward it.[28] To that end, there is a need for further research on predicting the likelihood of multiple pregnancy.[29] And, given the experimental nature of selective termination, genuinely informed choice should be mandatory for prospective patients, who need to know both the short- and long-term risks and outcomes of the procedure. Acquiring this information will necessitate the "long-term follow-up of parents and children …

to assess the psychological and physical effects of fetal reduction."[30] By these means the numbers of selective terminations can be reduced, and the women who seek selective termination can be both protected and empowered.

More generally, however, we should carefully reevaluate both the pronatalist ideology and the system of treatments of infertility that constitute the context in which selective termination of pregnancy comes to seem essential. There is also a need to improve social support for parenting, and to transform the conditions that make it difficult or impossible to be the mother of triplets, quadruplets, etc. or of a baby with a severe disability. Only through the provision of committed care for children and support for women's self-determination will genuine reproductive freedom and responsibility be attained.

Acknowledgment

I would like to acknowledge the assistance of Monica Webster, Queen's University Health Sciences Library, in locating resource material for this paper.

Notes

1. Marie T. Mulcahy, Brian Roberman, and S.E. Reid, "Chorion Biopsy, Cytogenetic Diagnosis, and Selective Termination in a Twin Pregnancy at Risk of Haemophilia" (letter), *The Lancet,* 13 October 1984, 866; "Selective Fetal Reduction" (review article), *The Lancet,* 1 October 1988, 773; Dorothy Lipovenko, "Infertility Technology Forces People to Make Life and Death Choices," *The Globe and Mail,* 21 January 1989, A4.

2. "Multiple Pregnancies Create Moral Dilemma," *Kingston Whig Standard*, 21 January 1989, 3.

3. Mark I. Evans et al, "Selective First-Trimester Termination in Octuplet and Quadruplet Pregnancies: Clinical and Ethical Issues," *Obstetrics and Gynecology* 71:3, pt. 1 (1988), 289-296, at 293; Richard L. Berkowitz et al., "Selective Reduction of Multifetal Pregnancies in the First Trimester," *New England Journal of Medicine* 118:16 (1988), 1043. Berkowitz and colleagues regard even triplet pregnancies as constituting a "gray area" for physician and patient. However, it is not clear whether this hesitation is based on moral scruples in addition to the medical risks.

4. Lipovenko, "Infertility Technology."

5. Diana Brahams, "Assisted Reproduction and Selective Reduction of Pregnancy," *The Lancet,* 12 December 1987, 1409; cf. John C. Hobbins, "Selective Reduction—A Perinatal Necessity?," *New England Journal of Medicine* 318:16 (1988), 1063; Evans *et al.,* "Selective First-Trimester Termination," 295.

6. One television interviewer who talked to me about this issue described women as "forcing" doctors to provide the procedure! See also "Multiple Pregnancies Create Moral Dilemma"; Angela R. Holder and Mary Sue Henifin, "Selective Termination of Pregnancy," *Hastings Center Report* 18:1 (1988), 21–22.

7. Christine Overall, *Ethics and Human Reproduction:* A *Feminist Analysis* (Boston: Allen & Unwin, 1987), 139–56.

8. Hobbins, "Selective Reduction," 1062.

9. Gena Corea and Susan Ince, "Report of a Survey of IVF Clinics in the U.S.," in *Made to Order: The Myth of Reproductive and Genetic Progress,* Patricia Spallone and Deborah Lynn Steinberg, eds. (Oxford: Pergamon Press, 1987), 133–45.

10. Compare the ambiguity of the claim "women want it" in connection with in vitro fertilization. See Christine Crowe, "Women Want It: In Vitro Fertilization and Women's Motivations for Participation" in Spallone and Steinberg, *Made to Order*, 84–93.

11. Barbara Katz Rothman, *The Tentative Pregnancy: Prenatal Diagnosis and the Future of Motherhood* (New York: Viking, 1986), 189.

12. Judith Lorber, "In Vitro Fertilization and Gender Politics," in *Embryos, Ethics, and Women's Rights*, Elaine Hoffman Baruch, Amadeo F. D'Adamo, Jr., and Joni Seager, eds. (New York: Haworth Press, 1988), 123–26.

13. "Selective Fetal Reduction," 774.

14. Caroline Whitbeck, "The Moral Implications of Regarding Women as People: New Perspectives on Pregnancy and Personhood," in *Abortion and the Status of the Fetus*, William B. Bondeson *et al.,* eds. (Boston: Reidel, 1984), 251–52.

15. Rothman, *The Tentative Pregnancy,* 177–216. She describes abortion in the case of fetal defect as "the chosen tragedy" (180).

16. Evans *et al.* give a success rate of 50% (p. 289), while Berkowitz *et al.* give 66-2/3% (1043). Angela Holder quotes a success rate of 55% (21).

17. Cf: Berkowitz *et al.,* "Selective Reduction," 1045; and Alastair H. MacLennan, "Multiple Gestation: Clinical Characteristics and Management," in *Maternal-Fetal Medicine: Principles and Practice,* Robert K. Creasy and Robert Resnick, eds. (Philadelphia: W.B. Saunders, 2nd ed., 1989), 581–84.

18. Jose C. Scerbo, Powan Rattan, and Joan E. Drukker, "Twins and Other Multiple Gestations," in *High-Risk Pregnancy: A Team Approach,* Robert A. Knuppel and Joan E. Drukker, eds. (Philadelphia: W.B. Saunders, 1986) 347–48, 358; Martin L. Pernoll, Gerda I. Benda, and S. Gorham Babson, *Diagnosis and Management of the Fetus and Neonate at Risk: A Guide for Team Care* (St. Louis: C.V. Mosby, 5th ed, 1986), 192–93.

19. "Selective Fetal Reduction," 773.

20. Victoria Stevens, "Test-Tube Quints Celebrate First Birthday," *The Toronto Star,* 6 February 1989, A7.

21. See Letty Cottin Pogrebin, *Family Politics: Love and Power on an Intimate Frontier* (New York: McGraw-Hill, 1983), 42.

22. Overall, *Ethics and Human Reproduction,* 166–68.

23. Ibid. 76–79.

24. Adrienne Asch, "Reproductive Technology and Disability," in *Reproductive Laws for the 1990s,* Sherrill Cohen and Nadine Taub, eds. (Clifton, NJ: Humana Press, 1989), 69–117; Marsha Saxton, "Prenatal Screening and Discriminatory Attitudes About Disability," in *Embryos, Ethics, and Women's Rights,* 217–24.

25. Ruth Hubbard, "Eugenics: New Tools, Old Ideas," in *Embryos, Ethics, and Women's Rights,* 225–35.

26. Cf. Robyn Rowland, "Motherhood, Patriarchal Power, Alienation and the Issue of 'Choice' in Sex Preselection," in *Man-Made Women,* 74–87.

27. Hobbins, "Selective Reduction," 1063; "Selective Fetal Reduction," 773, 774.

28. Brahams, "Assisted Reproduction," 1409.

29. Ian Craft *et al.,* "Multiple Pregnancy, Selective Reduction, and Flexible Treatment" (letter), *The Lancet,* 5 November 1988, 1087.

30. Selective Fetal Reduction," 775.

Normalizing Reproductive Technologies and the Implications for Autonomy

Susan Sherwin

Few nations are immune to the lure of reproductive technologies. Although there are national differences in the particular types of technologies that become commonplace, and significant differences in the role of national governments in promoting or restricting each sort, most societies support development and use of at least some forms of reproductive technologies. For example, most governments have specific population targets in mind, and they encourage use of the reproductive technology that facilitates those goals. Most governments also seek to ensure a "healthier" population and value technologies that can support that goal as they understand it. Even where local cultures are inclined to be suspicious of technology generally as representative of a new form of Western imperialism, we can still generally find encouragement of some types of interventions in

reproductive processes. As various reproductive technologies take root in particular societies, they alter the reproductive experiences, opportunities, and duties of women. In this chapter I consider how the routine use of various forms of reproductive technology may affect women's autonomy.

I take the term "reproductive technology" to refer to any technological intervention in the social and biological processes of human procreation. As such, it covers such diverse activities as those associated with the prevention and interruption of pregnancy (contraception and abortion) as well as the facilitation of pregnancy through assisted conception (in vitro fertilization and its variations, artificial insemination, embryo transplants, cloning). It also includes the many activities that constitute medical surveillance and management of pregnancy and childbirth (including prenatal monitoring and diagnosis, fetal surgery and transfusions, use of electronic fetal monitors, surgical delivery) and the technology-assisted support of endangered newborns (via incubators, neonatal intensive care units, neonatal surgery). In addition, since human reproduction includes not only biological procreation but also the socialization and education of the young, reproductive activity extends throughout the period of childhood, providing many more opportunities for medical and other scientific experts to monitor and intervene in parenting practices though technological and other means. For the purposes of this chapter, I shall follow the usual convention and restrict my discussion of reproduction to the social and biological activities associated with producing babies (or preventing their birth).

Both the avoidance and the pursuit of pregnancy are now commonly construed as medical events, and, because medicine is heavily oriented toward the use of technology, they have become sites for extensive technological involvement. Indeed, throughout the industrialized world (and in many other parts of the globe), nearly all stages of pregnancy and childbirth are now inextricably found up with technological monitoring and intervention. Significantly, there is widespread social agreement that technology is a desirable resource for the pursuit of procreative goals. Although some cultures resist the attractions of reproductive technology, most have come to accept the value of at least some types of reproductive technologies; even societies that strongly distrust the impact of Western technology on traditional cultural values and practices frequently manage to accommodate certain forms of reproductive technology.[1]

In this chapter I wish to pursue the sorts of pressures that cause cultures to think that technology is inevitable. I am concerned with puzzles about the role of personal autonomy in determining appropriate medical and technological care surrounding reproduction. To understand the range of autonomy issues involved, I shall explore a variety of activities related to reproductive decisionmaking: some examples are drawn from areas where personal autonomy is clearly and explicitly restricted and others from areas where personal choice is apparently respected, although participation in the practice may seem required.

TECHNOLOGIES TO PREVENT BIRTHS

To understand how the most familiar notion of patient autonomy functions in debates about reproductive practices, I first turn to some that are highly contested in many societies. Most prominent among the reproductive technologies now subject to heated public debate in Canada and the United States are those designed to allow women the means to avoid bearing children. Abortion and, in some circles, contraception are the focus of intense political campaigns to restrict their accessibility. Anti-abortion campaigners try to defend the lives of fetuses by demanding restrictive abortion policies while pro-choice activists commonly appeal to the autonomy ideal, demanding unlimited access to abortion services by stressing women's right to choose whether or not to bear children. Most of the technology involved in preventing and terminating unwanted pregnancies is relatively commonplace and straightforward; it is legal and political policies, not technological restrictions, that often keep them out of the hands of women who might choose them. But, since abortion is classified as a medical procedure, and the most effective forms of contraception (though this may change in the United States)—the Pill, IUDs, and sterilization—still require medical action or supervision, the necessary technology is available only by action of licensed physicians; hence, women are dependent on the technical intervention—and, therefore, the sympathetic cooperation—of medical practitioners. Activists on both sides of the abortion debate understand that social and political campaigns that dissuade physicians from providing this service will interfere with women's autonomy to fully control their procreative lives.

In North America, many of those who oppose abortion also object to the use of "artificial" contraception and seek to limit its availability as well, though objection to contraception is much less common. Those who oppose contraception generally cite religious and cultural reasons to restrict personal access to any technology that separates sexual from reproductive activity. In other societies (e.g., Japan) contraception is considered more objectionable and is less accessible than abortion.[2] Although proponents of choice on abortion can be expected to support voluntary contraceptive use, many observe that contraceptive use is frequently coerced. For example, some government-sponsored population-control policies are aimed at compelling members of certain disadvantaged groups to accept permanent or long-term forms of contraception. In the United States, for instance, Latina women in New York have a rate of sterilization that is seven times higher than that of women of European descent, and there is reason to doubt that all sterilized women provided fully informed consent to the procedure.[3] In contraception, as in abortion, policies can be either coercive or permissive; that is, they can restrict women's autonomy or promote it in very explicit ways.

Although abortion and contraception are especially visible sites of political struggle, they are certainly not unique in this regard. Other very clear political battles are being waged over the uses of other sorts of technologies, such as the looming possibility of cloning human beings and contractual pregnancies. More subtle power struggles are associated with changing norms and expectations of family size, composition, and genetic links. Because the political, social, and economic significance of reproduction extend well beyond their effects on the immediate family, the impact of reproductive technologies may be felt not only by those directly involved in their use but by many others as well. As a result, many forms of reproductive technologies raise important questions of freedom and control. All are potentially subject to challenge and social conflict.

ACCEPTED TECHNOLOGIES

In the West, most public attention in regard to reproductive technologies is directed toward technologies identified as "new," namely, those concerned with assisting conception and with genetic screening and manipulation. But before exploring these headline-grabbing technologies, I want to situate them more fully in their social context—a world in which procreation is already heavily medicalized and subject to pervasive technological intervention. It is much easier to appreciate the ways in which the "new" reproductive technologies have been accepted in our society and to understand the fears many people have about their growing use if we recognize that the new reproductive technologies are not an entirely new phenomenon; rather, they represent additional steps along an already well-established continuum. The prevailing social acceptance of existing technological intervention in so many aspects of reproduction makes the treatment of infertility and the prevention of genetic defects seem familiar and appropriate. Reproduction has been widely accepted as an event requiring extensive medical involvement, so it seems "natural" to look for medical solutions to any problems that arise in this sphere.

The defining events of procreation are pregnancy and childbirth. In the developed world (and increasingly in many parts of the developing world) both events are subject to ongoing medical surveillance and control. From the initial perception of possible pregnancy, women are expected to present themselves to medical experts for certification of their pregnant state and a schedule of regular prenatal observation and advice. Physicians use technology to date the time of conception (rather than rely on a woman's estimate), monitor fetal development, evaluate routine blood tests, and perform ultrasounds ("baby's first pictures"); where deemed appropriate, they conduct various genetic tests through amniocentesis or chorionic villus sampling. During this period, medical authorities advise prospective parents on the value of genetic screening, instruct them on the changes that should be made in the woman's daily lifestyle, sexual activity, work schedules, and so on, and direct them to prenatal classes to help train them in the techniques of "natural" childbirth. Doctors interpret, evaluate, and set the standards of normalcy for the various changes associated with the different stages of pregnancy.

It is worth noting that this sort of intense surveillance is not limited to the distinctive values of North American life. In Japan, ultrasounds are "given routinely three or four times during each pregnancy and up to seven or eight times at certain institutions."[4] In China, where concern is to ensure both a lower birth rate and a "high quality" of offspring, many married women are subjected to semiannual gynecological exams and "even before marriage, some women are required to undergo examination to detect any visible structural problems with their reproductive organs and/or family history of genetic abnormalities which might lead to the birth of disabled children."[5] Medical surveillance of pregnant women and fetuses has become accepted practice throughout most of the world.

The effect of granting medical experts authority to manage pregnancies is significant. As Barbara Katz Rothman documents, such surveillance trains women to distance themselves from their pregnancies and to rely on medical interpretations of their experiences. The widely accepted emphasis on medicine's power to avert potential disaster ironically contributes to women's heightened sense of anxiety throughout their pregnancy and makes them increasingly dependent on physician reassurance. Rather than trust their own sense of well-being and excitement, most defer to medical authorities and await expert assurance of healthy outcomes before celebrating a pregnancy or allowing themselves to begin significant emotional bonding with their fetuses. In such a climate, women are well conditioned to comply with medical advice and direction about prenatal care and their own behavior.[6]

The basis of such deference is questionable, however. Although pregnancy and childbirth have become far safer events for women who are subject to technology-based prenatal care, medical monitoring and intervention are not the only factors to be credited with these improved statistics. Nontechnological measures, such as improved nutrition, fewer (and better spaced) pregnancies, more hygienic conditions, better education, and mature mothers (i.e., those past adolescence) also have helped reduce the incidence of maternal and childhood mortality and morbidity. Moreover, dependence on technology to improve maternal and fetal health may actually be quite dangerous in the developing world, if efforts are primarily geared to importing Western technological expertise and equipment instead of improving the social conditions of women.[7] Everywhere, the emphasis on technological surveillance tends to distract from the significance of social and economic conditions for the outcomes of pregnancies. In a political climate in which the basic necessities of healthy living are severely threatened for large segments of the population, concentration on the benefits of technology supports neglect of other factors, with potentially devastating consequences.

Despite the well-documented and uncontested importance of social and economic conditions for healthy pregnancies, many countries, both rich and poor, make technology the major focus of medical attention. There are several reasons for this. First, technology is profitable for those who produce it and those who deploy it; particular technologies are often aggressively marketed by companies very skilled at creating demands for their products. In addition, physicians are well trained in the use of technology, whereas most have little formal training in the relation between social conditions and health. And even if they do recognize the value of social changes, as individuals they lack the power to make such changes. Moreover, by deploying sophisticated technological instruments that provide them with data that are otherwise unavailable to women, physicians are able to establish expertise that is considered superior to a woman's intimate and unquantifiable feelings of pregnancy. Although much of the needed information can be obtained by the use of traditional technology such as stethoscopes, ultrasounds and electronic fetal monitors have vastly expanded the scope of medically mediated knowledge about the fetus in a form that fits neatly within current cultural habits of learning.

Example 1: Ultrasound

Let us look more closely, then, at these two commonplace technologies. Ultrasonography was introduced into obstetrical care in the 1960s. The technology of ultrasounds, like much of the technology used in medicine, was originally developed for military uses, in this case, the detection of submarines. When it was discovered that this visioning technique could also be used on soft tissues in the human body, medicine quickly began to explore biological uses. Once medical researchers established that ultrasounds could give them visual information about fetuses, they sought reasons to employ it; they have settled on its usefulness for dating fetal age, assessing fetal functioning, and detecting anatomical anomalies. Ultrasound is a powerfully attractive technology in a modernist culture that values visual information above all other kinds. By allowing trained personnel to gain visual access to a fetus, to record its movement and anatomical shape, ultrasounds provide medical practitioners with a highly prized "window on the womb." This visual knowledge can then be offered to the prospective parents, who are happy to have access to this new way of "getting to know" their fetus (once interpreters help them to make sense of the fuzzy images).

As Rosalind Petchesky observes, this technology serves a political purpose as well as a medical one. It "disrupt[s] the very definition, as traditionally understood, of 'inside' and 'outside' a woman's body, of pregnancy as an 'interior' experience" and "allows the fetus to be viewed and *treated* as if it were outside a woman's body."[8] Visualization helps make the existence and status of fetuses far more real to physicians and the public than anything a pregnant woman may report. When fetuses can be viewed as separate beings, they can be treated as such and pregnant women can be reduced to "uterine containers" or "fetal environments." Visual imaging allows obstetricians to treat fetuses as independent beings, existing in isolation, rather than as entities intimately connected to the women whose bodies nurture them. Or, as Rothman succinctly puts it,

"The technology that makes the baby/fetus more 'visible' renders the woman invisible."[9]

Hence, even though this technology has been well received by both patients and practitioners, and despite the fact that it sometimes plays an important role in identifying and potentially correcting certain sorts of problems in pregnancies, its effects are not all positive. As it is presently understood and used, ultrasound technology contributes to further entrenching medical control over pregnancy by increasing women's sense of dependency on scientific experts. By making frequent observation and evaluation of fetuses possible, it also makes this activity desirable, for it is now the norm in industrialized countries for pregnant women to have and to share visual images of their fetuses, along with reports of the demonstrated "health status" of the developing embryo. By now a routine part of pregnancy, the use of ultrasound has created a new set of expectations about the experience and customs of being pregnant.

It is worth reflecting on the history of this now commonplace use of a form of reproductive technology. Of particular concern is the fact that use of this technology became routine in the medical management of pregnancies despite the fact that its long-term safety for mothers and fetuses had not been established.[10] In this it follows a pattern common to many other medical interventions in pregnancy, a pattern that has sometimes led to dire results. Two notorious examples of medical treatments widely prescribed to pregnant women prior to exhaustive testing and evaluation are thalidomide and DES. In the case of thalidomide, the damaging results were almost immediately apparent: in about 15 percent of cases, women who took the drug during the first trimester gave birth to children born with limbs missing. The damage of DES use was slower to become evident, showing up only some twenty years later in the form of unusual genital cancers in some of the children whose mothers took DES during pregnancy. The tragedy of DES use is especially poignant because the drug did not even achieve the goal it was prescribed for, namely, reducing the rate of miscarriage; significantly, while it was thought to have this effect, it was widely prescribed even to women of no particular risk of miscarriage.

I do not want to be alarmist about this. Ultrasounds have been in use for decades and they do seem to be far safer than thalidomide and DES; they are certainly safer than the fetal X rays that they replace. Nonetheless, it is still too early to be certain that they involve no long-term risk. Moreover, studies by the major American regulators in the early 1980s showed "no improvement in pregnancy outcome" from routine use; in fact, the FDA specifically recommended against routine use of ultrasounds. And yet, despite unanswered questions about long-term effects and the fact that there is no clear clinical benefit, they have become a routine part of prenatal care. In fact, many centers prescribe multiple ultrasounds throughout the course of a single pregnancy. The apparent overuse of this technology has become so significant a problem that both the Canadian and American Societies for Obstetrics and Gynecology issued practice guidelines in the early 1990s, recommending ultrasounds only at eighteen to twenty weeks gestation in the hope of reducing the use of this technology at other states of pregnancy. Still, many patients and their physicians seek more frequent "looks" and find these limits hard to accept. Nor is the popularity of multiple tests confined to the West; as already noted, multiple ultrasounds are also the norm in Japan and represent the ideal in China.

Even though there is no statistical benefit in pregnancy outcomes associated with the performance of frequent ultrasounds, most women understand that their use in any particular pregnancy can still be valuable to them as individuals. Modern societies seem inevitably to constitute ablist cultures; as such, they urge women to have only "healthy" babies and they hold women accountable and responsible for the care of any child who is less than "perfect." Aware of these responsibilities, most women seek this easily available confirmation of the health of their fetuses. Prenatal surveillance provides them with both a means of improving "quality control" and, in most cases, the opportunity to obtain reassurance that all is normal. Obstetricians, for their part, fear expensive malpractice suits if they fail to detect fetal anomalies and so they are strongly motivated to recommend use of ultrasound testing. Moreover, in a modernist culture that highly prizes visual knowledge, women understandably welcome access to the visual images this technology provides; it helps them feel more intimately connected to a fetus they can "see" as well as feel. It also allows them to share with their partners, as well as with family and friends, this culturally expected way of getting to "know" their fetus, thereby increasing everyone's sense of anticipation about the coming birth.

In the ordinary sense of autonomy, the use of ultrasound would have to be said to be a matter of autonomous choice. In most nations, no laws forbid or mandate ultrasound for pregnant women. No woman is explicitly coerced by her physician or anyone else into accepting ultrasound; rather, most pregnant women are eager for the opportunity to have such exams. Still, there are questions to be asked about the degree of autonomy available to a woman regarding use of this technology. It is so commonly used and so generally valued that it is difficult for anyone to resist its use without being judged irrational and irresponsible. Now that ultrasound has become established as the normal standard of obstetrical care—despite unresolved questions about its efficacy and safety—most who are asked to decide upon its use in a particular case do not feel truly free to decline. In health matters, and especially in the realm of reproduction, in which the interests of future persons are thought to be at stake, normalization of technology places an enormous burden of proof on those who would refuse it. Hence, with each use, it becomes ever more established as part of routine prenatal care and thus helps consolidate the significant power and control that attaches to those who provide services deemed essential elements of good prenatal care, whether or not they want such power.

Example 2: Fetal Monitors

A similar story exists in the development and deployment of electronic fetal monitors. Also drawing on sonograph technology, this equipment allows medical personnel to monitor the heartbeat of a fetus throughout labor, providing a warning if fetal stress reaches dangerous levels. The technology was developed in the 1960s to provide information to assist in the management of high-risk labors (roughly 10–15 percent of cases). After an aggressive marketing campaign by the manufacturer, it was quickly taken up for use in all hospital deliveries. Fetal monitors are attractive to hospitals, for they provide more complete scientific data than earlier methods. They also reduce hospital costs, since they allow fewer staff to keep track of more patients.

Although the information they provide can be very valuable in quickly identifying problems in certain sorts of high-risk deliveries, these benefits come at a price. For one thing, this technology requires a birthing mother to remain prone and strapped to the machine, which increases her stress and discomfort. Further, the monitors distract attention away from the actual woman in labor and redirect it to machine readouts. Moreover, they support a crisis atmosphere in childbirth, which has the effect of further increasing physician control and reducing a woman's sense of her own right to control events.[11] Also, the data provided can be easily misinterpreted, appearing to signal fetal distress where none exists and unnecessarily triggering medical recommendations (sometimes demands) for surgical intervention by way of cesarean delivery, a risky procedure for both women and fetuses. In fact, once hospitals adopted these monitors for routine use, cesarean delivery rates increased by up to 50 percent.[12] Nonetheless, like ultrasounds, fetal monitors became the standard of obstetrical practice in North America long before they were subjected to controlled clinical trials to establish their efficacy and safety. When appropriate studies were finally done, some fifteen years after the introduction of this technology, no benefit could be found for their routine use. Indeed, careful clinical review suggests that better care can be achieved through alternative practices that involve a dedicated midwife attendant at each birth.[13]

The pattern represented here is common to many forms of reproductive technology: a technology that is produced to assist in a limited number of special cases becomes the standard of practice for all cases. Once available, such technology becomes subject to an overwhelming sense of technological imperative: birthing women and obstetricians face the burden of refusing (instead of requesting) their use, not feeling sufficiently confident to refuse its use in any particular case. Moreover, the environment in which this technology is employed is designed to encourage its use: in North America at least, maternity hospitals are set up to deal with deliveries that pose serious risks of complications, although this category of birth is a minority of cases seen. Procedures are followed that treat all deliveries as potentially high risk.

Under the best conditions, childbirth is an emotionally charged event; when it is conducted within a system posed for crisis, dangerous outcomes loom large and opportunities for informed personal choice are of little use to individual patients. Only careful statistical study and general practice guidelines can assist consumers and physicians in making decisions about whether or not to partake of any particular technology in such a climate. Individual patients are asked to give their informed consent to the use of technology, but since few are in a position to truly weigh relevant risks and benefits, most are not really well situated to execute autonomous choice.

Such conundrums might tempt us to romanticize the freedom of women in less industrialized nations, where use of ultrasound and fetal monitoring machinery is much less common. In general, sophisticated biomedical equipment is much less accessible in nations with low health care budgets, which is not to say that childbirth there is free of technological imperatives. As Maria De Koninck documents, international efforts to reduce maternal and infant mortality rates in very poor countries often amount to efforts to transfer the biomedical expertise and orientation developed in the West to local experts who are trained to intervene at the moment of delivery if childbirth has been designated as complicated or high risk. Although such interventions surely save some lives, they do so by focusing on problems in isolation of their causes. For example, cesarean sections are a means of saving the lives of young women who become pregnant before their pelvises have fully matured, although efforts to change social custom to postpone pregnancy until the end of adolescence would save the lives of even more women.[14] Yet in many poor countries economic pressures are forcing the age of marriage even further downward. Even in nations like the Sudan, where high-tech machinery is virtually unavailable, Western experts have transformed local birth customs and practices and introduced the values of privileging visual knowledge and favoring the comfort of medically trained birth attendants over that of the birthing women.[15] Women in many non-Western countries lack education, social status, economic independence, and recognized authority over their own lives, which means that most have very little power to influence decisions about the role of biomedicine and technology in their pregnancies and childbirth experiences. In such a climate, even the appearance of autonomy may be lacking as women struggle to situate themselves in belief and value systems that do not place much value on individual choice (especially on the part of women).

ASSISTED CONCEPTION

I have reviewed these various examples of the extent of current technology use and biomedical values in reproductive activities to clarify the context into which the so-called new reproductive technologies are being introduced. I am, finally, ready to turn to high-profile reproductive technologies, namely, efforts to assist couples experiencing infertility to procreate. Although the media tends to approach these technologies as if they are entirely distinct from current practices, I have tried to make clear that they are being developed and introduced in a cultural

milieu where many other aspects of reproduction are already subject to extensive, and virtually inescapable, technological monitoring and intervention. As a consequence, the medical community and the public are well conditioned to expect further expansion of the range of reproductive technology into new areas: it would seem very odd indeed if medical researchers were to fail to seek technological innovations to address unwanted barriers to conception.

At the same time, appreciation of the history of some existing reproductive technologies provides a basis for understanding why many feminists seem so suspicious about the possible future deployment of many of the new reproductive technologies. Even though at the moment, most new reproductive technologies are being used to treat only a minority of cases considered "high risk" or "problematic," they could become the norm for all pregnancies in the future. If that were to happen, we would again have to contend with serious questions about the degree of choice and control available to prospective parents. In reproduction, as in other areas of life, technology created to meet special needs tends to slide quickly into becoming normalized and routine for all possible cases, leaving little room for the person most directly affected to weigh its appropriateness and, perhaps, to refuse participation. Hence we must evaluate each technology for its potential impact on not only the currently targeted group of patients but all patients in the future.

Consider the technologies designed to address infertility. The most prominent of these technologies is in vitro fertilization (IVF) and its many variations. Like most reproductive technologies, new and old, IVF involves intervention in women's bodies even when the source of the problem (in this case, infertility) is associated with the male partner. In order to conduct IVF, physicians need access to gametes from both a man and a woman. It is usually a simple (technology-free) matter to collect sperm from men through masturbation. Egg collection is a much more invasive procedure, requiring careful timing (and hence frequent monitoring by ultrasound) and surgical access to the ovaries;

this involves potential risks of infection, bleeding, and damage to other organs. In fact, egg collection is such an invasive and risky procedure that the specialists involved prefer to collect several ova at once. In order to facilitate this, they begin by inducing superovulation in the woman through injection of powerful hormones (which likely increase risk of future ovarian and breast cancers). If physicians do manage to collect some viable eggs (the process often fails at this stage), the next step is to introduce those eggs to the collected sperm (in vitro) and see whether or not fertilization occurs. Physicians monitor the course of the fertilized eggs for a day or two, sometimes taking the opportunity to remove a cell from each to test for genetic anomalies. Then they either freeze or transfer the eggs that appear to be developing normally. At this point, the hope is that one transferred egg will implant in the woman's uterus and develop into a (healthy) fetus. Since approximately 80 percent of IVF attempts fail to produce a live baby at the end, physicians usually transfer a few fertilized eggs at once to increase the chances that one will continue to develop. (Three is the current norm in Canadian clinics, but it is not uncommon for clinics around the world to transfer several fertilized eggs at once in an effort to boost their pregnancy rates.) Not infrequently, these procedures result in multiple births, putting added strain on the health of both mother and fetuses.

Even though IVF technology is expensive, dangerous, disruptive, emotionally demanding, and usually unsuccessful, there is a long waiting list of anxious couples hoping to gain access to it as the preferred means of responding to infertility. Originally designed for woman with blocked fallopian tubes, it is now used for other kinds of infertility, including low sperm count in male partners.

Again, this is not a technology reserved only for rich countries. In many societies, the social pressure to reproduce is intense. Even in nations that face problems of excessive birth rates, there is significant demand for treatment of infertility. Although the plight of the infertile may easily be overlooked in countries struggling to reduce population density, there is evidence that childlessness is treated as a suspicious anomaly rather than a valued social contribution. The very practice of concentrating efforts on reducing birth rates helps to emphasize the normalcy of multiple pregnancies and renders "unnatural" the state of being childless. Hence, while China struggles to restrict all couples to a single child, those with no children face discrimination on every front; not surprisingly, many demand access to reproductive technologies.[16] And in Pemba, Tanzania, where the fertility rate is among the highest in the world and standards of living are low, there is a strong demand for technologies that can help infertile couples produce children.[17] In many less developed countries, where IVF is beyond the financial means of most, interest in reproductive assistance is probably even greater than it is in the more affluent West. In countries that focus on limiting population growth, there is a particularly strong sense that having children represents "the norm" for women, whose worth is likely to be measured in terms of their reproductive achievements.

Given the expense and risks associated with IVF, it seems unlikely that it will replace "natural" or sexual fertilization as the normal way of conceiving a child, but some practitioners have mused about a future when this will indeed become the norm for all who can afford it. They base this prediction on the fact that IVF provides the opportunity to detect genetic anomalies at the earliest possible stage of embryo development, thereby reducing the emotional and physical costs associated with late-term abortions that are required by alternative methods of genetic screening.

I do not really expect that IVF will end up becoming the preferred method of conceiving a child for couples who have nontechnological alternatives—after all, it is expensive, invasive, and risky, and there are undeniable pleasures associated with the more established, nontechnological methods. Nonetheless, in the industrialized world, IVF has already become established as a routine treatment for those who experience unwanted infertility, a sizable group now composing roughly 10 percent of the population interested in procreating. Moreover, the technology has been widely publicized with approving media coverage of "miracle" babies and happy parents, and this has contributed to a climate in which the widespread use of IVF makes most infertile couples feel a need to "try" it in their ongoing pursuit of producing a biologically related child. North American society is highly pronatalist (even if it seems rather uninterested in and even hostile to actual children). Having children is the norm for adults, and childbearing is romanticized and promoted in a multitude of ways, both explicitly and indirectly.

A few decades ago, infertility was likely to be viewed as a sad fact of life for certain couples. But the existence of IVF and numerous other fertility-enhancing technologies has made acceptance of infertility seem unnecessary and correspondingly more difficult; people are told that no one needs to accept a diagnosis of infertility as final. When success stories are reported, other couples can see the rewards of trying all available measures in the face of involuntary childlessness. Ever since this technology was first successfully used on humans, significant medical and social resources have been directed at circumventing infertility (IVF does not "cure" the condition), and these investments provide further evidence of the high level of social importance assigned to the pursuit of biological reproduction. Hence those who are involuntarily childless experience increased pressure to conform to such clearly important social expectations and do what is necessary to reproduce.

The growing use of such technologies has already become "normal" for (relatively affluent) couples experiencing infertility. The burden of proof in decisionmaking about participating in such technologies often rests with those who contemplate declining them rather than with those who seek access. Rejecting technological options tends to be especially complicated for women, since women's worth is largely defined in terms of their role as mothers. In such an environment, it is difficult for anyone to truly weigh the risks and costs of such highly prized assistance.

I do not doubt that women who pursue IVF deeply want to bear children; my worry is about a culture that demands and so readily accepts such sacrifices of its women. Moreover, when so many resources are invested in meeting the seemingly inexhaustible demand for IVF, other sorts of available responses to infertility become eclipsed. New reproductive technologies, like many of their predecessors, tend to absorb medical attention and detract from exploration of other sorts of resolutions to problems identified. Now that involuntary childlessness has been socially constructed as a medical problem, attention is shifted away from nonmedical alternatives such as acceptance of childlessness, adoption, foster parenting, change of partner, alternative family structures, and changes in lifestyle; these sorts of accommodations seem to pale in comparison to the socially privileged status of technological solutions. The priority given to technological solutions to infertility becomes even more problematic when we consider that many dollars are spent to help relatively affluent couples produce genetically related children while millions of other children are left to suffer malnutrition, abuse, and neglect. Moreover, comparably little effort is directed at the prevention of infertility (e.g., by preventing the spread of sexually transmitted diseases and becoming more proficient at diagnosing them and treating them when they occur). As in so many other areas of medicine, when technological solutions are offered, prevention seems a far less urgent priority.

CONCLUSION

What seems called for is a new interpretation of the ideal of autonomy. I suggest that we turn to a concept of relational autonomy that is intended to supplant the prevailing individualistic conception of autonomy and address some of the puzzles we have identified. Where the traditional conception envisions the individual as existing separate from and independent of society, a relational ideal recognizes the essential complexity of the relation between persons and their culture. It is rooted in a relational concept of the self which recognizes that selves are social beings significantly shaped within a web of interconnected social and political relationships. In relational theory, individuals are understood to engage in the events constitutive of identity and autonomy (e.g., defining, questioning, revising, and pursuing projects) within a configuration of relationships, both interpersonal and political. Thus autonomy is recognized as a capacity that can be enhanced (or repressed) by one's social position (e.g., the degree of internalized oppression one experiences).[18]

A conception of relational autonomy helps explain why the expression of an informed preference is not an adequate measure of autonomous choice, for it makes visible the ways in which social norms often condition preferences and also make alternative choices inconceivable. It helps us see the political dimensions of circumstances where decisions may at first appear to be primarily matters of personal choice. In so doing, this concept helps explain why personal preference is not an adequate measure of autonomy. Within the context of reproductive technologies, an ideal of relational autonomy reveals the importance of evaluating the political climate in which reproductive choices are made before determining whether or not some reproductive decision is autonomous.

For many of the forms of reproductive technology reviewed in this chapter, important social programs have been developed and promoted in the West as if they were merely opportunities for the exercise of individual choice. Use of patient autonomy language and the implementation of informed consent procedures foster the sense that we are simply dealing with private decision-making. As a society, however, we are currently engaged in a process of transforming reproductive activities and setting new norms of reproductive behavior that individuals may soon be in no position to resist. In a context of medicalized procreation, the appearance of personal choice may well become more illusionary than real.

In nations that are less committed to the value of individual freedom and autonomy than Canada or the United States, practices aimed at controlling the "quality" of offspring may be so forcefully imposed that even the illusion of private choice is absent. Women are always caught within social forces that constitute public policy about the ways in which their reproductive functions are best pursued. Although there is often apparent space for them to make some choices within those structures (such as whether to seek assistance from biomedical or traditional caregivers), their choices are inevitably structured by the prevailing value system and the rewards and punishments it provides for the results of their reproductive practices. Typically, women everywhere make pragmatic choices within the governing frameworks that adapt (rather than docilely obey) dominant values and expectations. Whereas they may negotiate some space for alternative values and exercise agency in the way in which they interpret the dominant values, their choices generally reflect and often support the existing power structures.[19]

Therefore, simply observing that women choose to use a technology is not a sufficient test to determine that they are exercising autonomy in a given aspect of reproductive practice sphere. Moreover, once a technology becomes routine, its very familiarity can undermine a woman's realistic chance of refusing its use. Hence, we must be very careful to evaluate each technology that is introduced and not consider the issue settled by data on how frequently women use that form of technology. Only by questioning and examining the goals and achievements of each particular technology will we be able to tell if it is something that should become routine in the reproductive lives of women. To date, that step has largely been missing in the implementation of many reproductive technologies. We cannot afford to omit this level of discussion in the future because the emerging new technologies promise to have an even greater impact on the shape of every society than have those in the past. Nor can we afford to let ourselves be so absorbed by the glitter and promise of technology as to forget that nontechnological programs will always be essential elements of healthy reproductive practices. Adopting a nuanced, contextualized, politicized understanding of autonomy as relational can help guide these necessary, but difficult, discussions.

Notes

Earlier versions of this essay were read at the University of Manitoba and the University of King's College. I am grateful for the thoughtful comments received on both occasions. Barbara Parish was particularly helpful in responding to the earliest drafts. The final draft was prepared at the Bellagio International Study and Conference Center.

1. Margaret Lock and Patricia A. Kaufert, eds., *Pragmatic Women and Body Politics* (Cambridge: Cambridge University Press, 1998).
2. In Japan, for example, the Pill did not become legally available until 1999. Apparently there is concern about the health risks of artificial hormones and social worries that a truly reliable contraceptive would encourage promiscuity among both men and women. (Margaret Lock, "Perfecting Society: Reproductive Technologies, Genetic Testing, and the Planned Family in Japan," in *Pragmatic Women*, pp. 206–239.) More cynical commentators ascribe the long resistance to the power of a large gynecological lobby dependent on the fees they receive for performing abortions.
3. Iris Lopez, "An Ethnography of the Medicalization of Puerto Rican Women's Reproduction," in *Pragmatic Women*, pp. 240–259.
4. Margaret Lock, "Perfecting Society," in *Pragmatic Women*, p. 228.
5. Lisa Handwerker, "The Consequences of Modernity for Childless Women in China: Medicalization and Resistance," in *Pragmatic Women*, pp. 178–205.
6. Barbara Katz Rothman, *The Tentative Pregnancy: Prenatal Diagnosis and the Future of Motherhood* (New York: Viking, 1986), p. 86.
7. Maria De Koninck, "Reflections on the Transfer of 'Progress': The Case of reproduction," in The

Feminist Health Care Ethics Research Network, *The Politics of Women's Health: Exploring Agency and Autonomy* (Philadelphia: Temple University Press, 1998), pp. 150–177.
8. Rosalind Pollack Petchesky, "Foetal Images: The Power of Visual Culture in the Politics of Reproduction," in Michelle Stanworth, ed., *Reproductive Technologies: Gender, Motherhood, and Medicine* (Minneapolis: University of Minnesota Press, 1987), p. 65.
9. Rothman, *Tentative Pregnancy,* p. 113.
10. Murray Enkin, Mark J. N. C. Keirse, and Iain Chalmers, *A Guide to Effective Care in Pregnancy and Childbirth* (Oxford: Oxford University Press, 1989).
11. As Enkin, Keirse, and Chalmers observe, "Use of continuous electronic monitoring changes the delivery room into an intensive care unit…. The presence of a monitor may also change the relationships between the woman and her partner on the one hand, and the woman, midwife, and doctor on the other" (*Guide to Effective Care*, p. 198).
12. Judith Kunisch, "Electronic Fetal Monitors: Marketing Forces and the Resulting Controversy," in Kathryn Strother Ratcliff, ed., *Healing Technology: Feminist Perspectives* (Ann Arbor: University of Michigan Pres, 1989), p. 54.
13. Enkin, Keirse, and Chalmers, *Guide to Effective Care.*
14. De Koninck, "Reflections," pp. 150–177.
15. Janice Boddy, "Remembering Amal: On Birth and the British in Northern Sudan," in *Pragmatic Women*, pp. 28–59.
16. Handwerker, "Consequences of Modernity," pp. 178–205.
17. Karina Kielmann, "Barren Ground: Contesting Identities of Barren Women in Pemba, Tanzania," in *Pragmatic Women*, pp. 127–163.
18. Susan Sherwin, "A Relational Approach to Autonomy in Health Care," in *Politics of Women's Health*, pp. 19–47.
19. Lock and Kaufert, *Pragmatic Women.*

Judicial Intervention in Pregnancy and Birth

Royal Commission on New Reproductive Technologies

The use of legislation and court decisions to control a pregnant woman's behaviour in situations where a fetus is thought to be at risk—that is, judicial intervention in pregnancy and birth—provides an example of how technological developments can raise new ethical issues for society. The increasing incidence of judicial intervention has occurred in part because recent technological and medical developments have contributed to the ability to visualize, and hence to conceptualize, the fetus as an entity separate from the pregnant woman.

Technology, by enabling us to "see" the fetus, in particular through clearer and more detailed ultrasound images, provides a graphic depiction of the fetus that was previously not possible. Other medical technologies have reinforced this impression among medical practitioners and in society generally: prenatal diagnosis contributes to the perception of the fetus as a separate being with a specific medical condition that can be detected before birth; the ability to sustain newborns of lower and lower birth weight outside the womb changes perceptions of a fetus at the same stage of development *in utero;* and the emerging capacity to perform fetal surgery for certain conditions reinforces the view of the fetus as a separate patient. This new way of conceptualizing the fetus is even apparent in popular media images and illustrations portraying the fetus as an isolated entity suspended in an unidentifiable medium— seldom acknowledging the presence of the pregnant woman's body, without which the fetus cannot exist....

Changing ideas about the fetus, fostered by technological development, have the potential for both positive and negative consequences. On the positive side, for example, society has become increasingly aware of the effects on the health of the fetus of nutrition and tobacco and alcohol use during pregnancy. Information gained through prenatal diagnosis can allow fetuses with certain anomalies to be treated at birth, and, in much rarer cases, treatment prenatally can lead to the birth of a healthier child.

At the same time, society must be aware of the ethical and legal difficulties inherent in regarding the fetus as a patient who is separate from the pregnant woman. Considering the interests of the fetus in isolation from those of the woman has the potential to establish adversary relationships that, at their extreme, can lead to efforts to force the pregnant woman to act in the interests of this "separate patient." This may mean that a woman's right not to be subject to unwanted interference with her physical integrity is taken away from her, with serious implications not just for that woman, but for all women who become pregnant.

Judicial intervention tends to occur when the ethic of care has broken down—situations that the Commission seeks to prevent. What should society do to protect the fetus? Should it empower the courts to over-ride a pregnant woman's refusal of health care? Should it enact legislation of some kind? Or are other measures more appropriate? In the next few pages we consider the issues raised by judicial intervention in pregnancy and birth. We outline the views of Canadians and discuss the issues from both a legal and an ethical perspective, with a view to reaching conclusions and recommendations that reinforce or re-establish the ethic of care in such cases.

JUDICIAL INTERVENTION DEFINED

Our mandate directed us to examine "judicial interventions during gestation and birth." This examination involved considering how legislation and court decisions are or may be used to control a pregnant woman's behaviour. Such judicial intervention usually occurs when a woman is believed to be endangering the fetus she is carrying by refusing medical treatment believed necessary for fetal health, by abusing drugs or alcohol, or by engaging in behaviour such as prostitution. The matter is typically brought before the courts by a children's aid society, a health care facility, or, in some cases, a physician.

Judicial interventions during gestation and birth can take several forms. Canadian courts, for example, have ordered pregnant women to refrain from specified behaviours and to undergo certain medical procedures considered necessary for the health of the fetus.... U.S. courts have issued similar directives, ordering women to engage or not to engage in certain behaviours during pregnancy, to undergo Caesarian section and other medical treatment, and to be incarcerated until they had given birth.

Few cases have reached the courts in Canada, because the women most likely to encounter this situation are often in no position to resist and therefore they comply with the wishes of a physician or child welfare authority. An examination of the cases that have been reported shows that the women most likely to be subjected to judicial intervention are disproportionately poor, Aboriginal, or members of a racial or ethnic minority—all factors that influence their capacity to resist intervention. Whether overt discrimination is at work or whether the life circumstances of these women are such that their behaviour during pregnancy is more likely to come under scrutiny is difficult to disentangle.

Judicial intervention is an issue for all women in Canada, however, regardless of socioeconomic status, because its implications go beyond the consequences for an individual woman; it is an issue for women more generally if becoming pregnant means that they waive the constitutional protections afforded other citizens....

THE ETHICAL VIEW

The Commission's position on judicial intervention in pregnancy and birth ... relies primarily on our ethical stance and guiding principles, which we have applied throughout our report and in our recommendations. Although many legal and constitutional arguments can be made, our conclusions with respect to judicial intervention rest largely on our ethical reasoning. In our view, it is ethically (as well as legally) wrong to suggest that pregnant women's rights to make decisions about their medical care and treatment should be changed or lessened because they are pregnant.

Consistent with the ethic of care—which is concerned with preventing conflicts instead of trying to resolve them after they arise—we begin by asking questions about how to ensure the best possible prenatal health and the maximum degree of well-being for both the pregnant woman and the fetus. Regardless of whether a fetus is a "person" with "rights," it is clear that the interests of the fetus are worthy of protection: what transpires before birth—the behaviour of the woman during pregnancy, the provision of medical treatment to her and to the fetus—can seriously affect the health and well-being of the child that is eventually born. Society therefore has an interest in promoting the prenatal health and well-being of the fetus and of the woman carrying it.

From the woman's perspective, however, considering the interests of her fetus separately from her own has the potential to create adversary situations with negative consequences for her autonomy and bodily integrity, for her relationship with her partner, and for her relationship with her physician. Judicial intervention is bound to precipitate crisis and conflict, instead of preventing them through support and care. It also ignores the basic components of women's fundamental human rights—the right to bodily integrity, and the right to equality, privacy, and dignity. Importantly, as we will see, such measures are also unlikely to be effective and may not in fact protect the fetus.

If we impose a legal obligation upon a woman to care for her fetus—even if it were possible to legislate a caring and nurturing relationship—the potential for curtailing women's choices and behaviour becomes staggering. The kinds of substances and activities that could pose a danger to the fetus are many, varied, and increasing: cigarettes, alcohol, drugs (both legal and illegal), environmental pollutants, strenuous exercise, saunas, and inadequate nutrition. As scientific knowledge develops, the list is becoming longer. Many women's management of pregnancy could be subject to challenge and scrutiny, and pregnancy could become the source of potential liability suits against women who failed to comply with certain standards of behaviour. In some cases, fearing a less-than-perfect outcome, a pregnant woman might feel compelled to seek abortion instead of care.

Moreover, the threat of judicial intervention could have significant negative effects on fetal and maternal health. If women knew that they could be confined against their will, forced to submit to medical treatment, or charged with criminal offences, they might well avoid seeking medical care. Unfortunately, those who might avoid seeking care would likely be those who need it most—for example, women who are dependent on drugs or alcohol. As a result, health problems would escape detection and treatment—precisely the opposite effect sought by those who would use judicial means to intervene.

The resort to judicial intervention also has serious implications for the relationship between a pregnant woman and her physician. If the physician is perceived to be potentially coercive instead of a caregiver, the woman might begin to withhold information or stop seeking prenatal care, with detrimental consequences for her health and that of the fetus. These dangers are recognized by many professional associations of physicians. Moreover, experience with judicial intervention has shown the uncertainties inherent in diagnosis and treatment; in several cases of judicial intervention, the medical treatment deemed essential by the courts later turned out not to have been necessary, For example, a woman who went into

hiding in defiance of a court order to undergo a Caesarian section later gave birth vaginally to a healthy child. Thus, medical and judicial judgements—even those made with the best of intentions—can be mistaken. In addition, the very limited time frame within which most such decisions must be made and acted upon makes the process of judicial intervention unlikely to lead to fully considered, principled, or constitutional conclusions.

Finally, judicial intervention both emerges from and reinforces a social perception of the role of women in reproduction that instrumentalizes them and devalues their humanity and individuality. At the core of the impulse toward judicial intervention in pregnancy and birth is the view that pregnant women are the means to an end—the birth of healthy children. To the extent that judicial intervention reinforces the notion that a pregnant woman's role is only to carry and deliver a healthy child, it denies her existence as an autonomous individual with legal and constitutional rights and is dangerous to the rights and autonomy of all women.

In summary, judicial intervention offers no satisfactory answer to ensuring the well-being of the fetus: it precipitates crisis and conflict, it ignores women's fundamental constitutional and human rights, it contributes to an instumentalized view of their role in reproduction—with adverse consequences for women individually and as a group—and, most important, it is not effective in achieving its goal of protecting fetal well-being.

Society cannot care for a fetus, in the absence of the pregnant woman's cooperation, without taking control of the woman herself. The physical relationship between the fetus and the pregnant woman and the dependency of the fetus on the pregnant woman for sustenance make this impossible. By forcing medical intervention, society would be requiring pregnant women to do something that is asked of no other individual: to undergo medical treatment for the benefit of another. Even a living child has no right to force a parent to undergo medical procedures for the child's benefit, however morally compelling the case might be. This infringement of bodily autonomy and physical integrity is not justified on any grounds.

This imperative will not change even as research pushes the boundaries of what can be done to treat a fetus *in utero*. For example, if and when surgery on a fetus moves beyond the research stage for a range of conditions, there may be increasing pressure on pregnant women to consent to such procedures. Whether these techniques remain experimental or move into the realm of accepted practice, they must be offered only in the context of the ethical and legal considerations set out in this chapter—that is, in the context of the pregnant woman's autonomy and with her informed consent, based on full knowledge of the nature and risks of the proposed treatment.

AN APPROACH BASED ON SUPPORT AND CARE

If we reject judicial intervention in pregnancy and birth on moral, practical, and legal grounds, we must return to the question of how to ensure the health and well-being of the fetus and the pregnant woman. How should society respond to a situation where a woman is not caring for her fetus or engaging in behaviour that may harm it? In the Commission's view, the answer lies in examining the reasons for that behaviour and seeking solutions that address them.

Some of the situations that give rise to attempts at judicial intervention are among the most difficult and tragic imaginable. The potential for harm is evident; the dangers to a fetus of alcohol abuse, drug addiction, or sexually transmitted diseases are real and potentially devastating. These situations are all the more distressing because the caring and nurturing assumed to be inherent in the relationship between woman and fetus appear to be absent.

Although many cases involving refusal to follow medical advice or to accept surgical or other medical treatment have involved drug or alcohol abuse, a woman's reasons for choosing a particular course of action may include her socioeconomic circumstances, her educational level, her religious convictions, her cultural beliefs, her fears, or other deeply held values or personal beliefs. Of relevance in this regard is the fact that most of the women who have been subject to judicial intervention to date have been Aboriginal women and women of colour.

Whatever the circumstances, judicial intervention does not provide a solution, because it does nothing to address the circumstances that bring about attempts to intervene or to create the social conditions and support that help to ensure a successful pregnancy and healthy outcome for both the woman and the child.

In reaching this conclusion, Commissioners are acutely aware of the tragic nature of some of the situations that give rise to efforts to intervene in a pregnancy. As members of the helping professions, physicians and child welfare workers face situations that call on their basic human instinct to help where possible—an impulse that is rightly very difficult to resist because it is so fundamental to who they are and the job they do. The decision to respect a woman's autonomy and physical integrity and not to intervene must surely be one of the most difficult decisions any human being would ever be called upon to make. That is why the Commissioners' decision in this matter was reached through long and careful deliberation and consideration of the issues from all sides. We made this decision not because harm to a fetus is acceptable or even tolerable, but because the dangers posed by judicial intervention far outweigh any benefits that a given individual intervention might yield.

In line with the ethic of care, we believe that the best approach is to seek ways to ensure that the needs of both the woman and the fetus are met—in other words, to prevent a situation developing in which child welfare, medical, or other authorities might consider judicial intervention appropriate or necessary. The ethic of care offers a means of avoiding the conflicts inherent in judicial intervention by promoting two fundamental values: respect for the rights and autonomy of the pregnant woman and concern for the health and well-being of the fetus. The best way to accomplish this is not by compelling pregnant women to behave in certain ways, but by providing a supportive and caring environment in which they can make informed decisions and choose from among realistic options before and during pregnancy.

The situations that lead to judicial intervention are inherently distressing because of the commitment we, as a society and as individuals, have to respect human life and dignity—the life and dignity of the pregnant woman, expressed through her autonomy, and that of the fetus, as a potential person. Judicial intervention sacrifices the human dignity and rights of one for the potential well-being of the other. Taking the alternative route of care and assistance means that the human life and dignity of both woman and fetus are respected—and it may even accomplish what legislation or court decisions cannot: establish a caring and nurturing relationship.

Clearly, the vast majority of women will act in a way they believe to be in the best interests of their fetus. The best way to promote prenatal health is therefore to provide the information and support necessary to enable pregnant women to make healthy choices for the well-being of themselves and their fetuses and informing them—in non-coercive, non-judgemental ways—about the implications of their decisions. This includes providing safe and accessible contraception and abortion services; offering accessible and culturally appropriate prenatal care and social services to pregnant women; counselling pregnant women about healthy lifestyles and ensuring they have the means to make these choices, including financial assistance where necessary; and providing information, outreach, and supports in the forms pregnant women need to make informed choices and realistic decisions about care and treatment, particularly for addictions.

The Canadian Bar Association pointed out, in its brief to the Commission, that recourse to judicial intervention should be seen as a failure—a failure to provide policies and programs that sustain a woman's right to manage her pregnancy and to support her decisions with

appropriate services and resources in the community. By itself, prohibiting judicial intervention does not fulfil our responsibility as a society to promote the health and well-being of pregnant women. Meeting this responsibility also requires appropriate programs, services, and outreach designed specifically to support pregnant women who are in the difficult circumstances we have outlined. This is not the case at present. In fact, overall, the behaviour that attracts judicial intervention may be less threatening to fetal and neonatal health than the well-documented effects of poverty on a much larger number of pregnancies.

As we discuss in Chapter 14, a variety of appropriately designed supportive programs for pregnant women can at the same time help to ensure the well-being of the fetus. In particular, with respect to pregnant women who endanger the health of their fetuses by using alcohol or drugs, the Board of Trustees of the American Medical Association has recommended that "[p]regnant substance abusers should be provided with rehabilitative treatment appropriate to their specific physiological and psychological needs." Similar conclusions have been reached by this Commission and by others studying the problem of drug use during pregnancy. What is required is ready access to facilities and services that provide outreach, counselling, and treatment designed specifically for pregnant women that are appropriate to their needs.

CONCLUSION AND RECOMMENDATIONS

In summary, trying to use the law and the courts to protect fetal health can only be counterproductive. Such laws may, on the surface, have appeal, because we all support the goal of the well-being of the fetus, and enacting them may appear to be a logical extension of society's interest in the health of the fetus. But there is nothing in our experience to demonstrate that such laws work in practice. Indeed, there is strong evidence to the contrary, particularly because the instruments available to the courts—forcing action under penalty of fines or incarceration—are brutally blunt and patently unsuited to the goal of promoting anyone's health or well-being. Clearly, if protecting the fetus is the goal, other methods are needed.

A societal interest in pregnancy and birth—to maximize the chances for the birth of a healthy child—is a goal Commissioners strongly endorse; it is an important and worthy goal. But our examination of the legal, ethical, and social implications of judicial intervention leads to the inescapable conclusion that judicial intervention is neither an acceptable nor an effective method of achieving that goal. Because the woman's consent and cooperation are needed to ensure a positive outcome for the fetus, it follows that the most effective way of caring for the fetus is through appropriate support and caring for the pregnant woman. The Commission therefore recommends that

> 273. Judicial intervention in pregnancy and birth not be permissible. Specifically, the Commission recommends that
>
> (a) medical treatment never be imposed upon a pregnant woman against her wishes;
>
> (b) the criminal law, or any other law, never be used to confine or imprison a pregnant woman in the interests of her fetus;
>
> (c) the conduct of a pregnant woman in relation to her fetus not be criminalized;
>
> (d) child welfare or other legislation never be used to control a woman's behaviour during pregnancy or birth; and
>
> (e) civil liability never be imposed upon a woman for harm done to her fetus during pregnancy.

> 274. Unwanted medical treatment and other interferences, or threatened interferences, with the physical autonomy of pregnant women be recognized explicitly under the Criminal Code as criminal assault.

and that

> 275. All provinces/territories ensure that they have in place
>
> (a) information and education programs directed to pregnant women so that they do not inadvertently put a fetus at risk;
>
> (b) outreach and culturally appropriate support services for pregnant women and young women in potentially vulnerable groups; and
>
> (c) counselling, rehabilitation, outreach, and support services designed specifically to meet the needs of pregnant women with drug/alcohol addictions.

In conclusion, it is the Commission's view that almost all pregnant women will take steps to maximize their chances of a healthy birth if they have ready access to the information, prenatal care, social services, and income support necessary to do so. In the Commission's view, extending care to the fetus by giving the pregnant woman the support she needs provides the best hope for enhancing the health and well-being of both the fetus and the woman carrying it.

General Sources

Rodgers, S. "Juridical Interference with Gestation and Birth." In *Research Volumes of the Royal Commission on New Reproductive Technologies*, 1993.

Annex: Judicial Intervention in Pregnancy

Suzanne Rozell Scorsone

The role of law is largely to protect the rights of individuals, and, in cases of conflict, to balance those rights. Where there is a question of legal intervention, then, there are two related questions. What is the evil which the law is to remedy, and does any given remedy create more problems than did the original evil itself? The possible evils we must consider exist at a minimum of two levels. The more obvious is the individual level, as between the life-long harm to a fetus and the limitation of a woman's autonomy. The second is the societal, as between the potential effects of judicial intervention in pregnancy on the collective status and autonomy of women and, by contradistinction, the potential effects on both equality and the nature of the rule of law arising from the absolute preclusion of such intervention.

Judicial intervention in pregnancy is a question which only arises because of situations which are tragic in the conflicts which they embody. In this I am in full accord with my fellow Commissioners. No matter what the disposition of an individual case, there will be results which one wishes had not occurred. To intervene means to save the child at the cost of coercing an unwilling woman into surgery or close supervision or imprisonment to control her harmful behaviour. Not to intervene means to leave the woman free to act in any way whatever at the cost of accepting preventable but almost certain harm, handicap, or death for her child. One cannot regard any resolution of the question without ambivalence.

The questions which must be resolved are many and complex. I do not believe that there has been sufficient reflection on them, by Canadian society as a whole or by the relevant expert disciplines, to warrant any categorical statements by this Commission on the most humane and consti-tutionally consistent approach. The arguments adduced here will have to suffice for the present, as the Decima survey done for this Commission did not ask the Canadian public their views on this question, confining itself to new reproductive technologies per se. Given the importance of its broad implications, this is a question on which the views of Canadians should be actively and representatively sought before any legislative change is even contemplated.

My task here is not to resolve the issue but to raise questions as to whether there are not other, still greater evils which arise if we hold that a woman must not or cannot ever, in principle, have her autonomy limited in these ways. Unless we are certain—and I am one among many who are not—we should not take premature action to alter the existing legislative and other protective structures.

THE DILEMMA

As presented to us, judicial intervention in pregnancy seems chiefly to arise under two sets of circumstances, those of harmful lifestyle at any point in pregnancy or those of medical emergency, usually at the point of birth. Intervention in the first set of circumstances, in the rare instances in which it occurs, takes the form of measures to alter the substance abuse or other harmful behaviour, whether by mandatory supervision, treatment or incarceration. Intervention in the second set would chiefly take the form of court-ordered Caesarian sections. There has been discussion of court-enforced surgery to correct a disorder in the fetus *in utero*, but this seems to be a hypothetical concern rather than a concrete situation. A related question is that of whether a woman would be liable for civil damages or would be subject to criminal charges for damage done to the fetus after the child is born.

I am in full agreement with my colleague Commissioners that the question of judicial intervention in pregnancy arises when the ethic of care has broken down, and that our primary concern must be to provide such social, educational, economic, and medical supports to pregnant women that such conflicts may be avoided. Most pregnancies are models of the ethic of care in action, first on the part of women, and with their partners, relatives, friends, and societal institutions providing all possible support.

A lapse in this manifesting of care does, however, sometimes occur. Our task, then, is to find a way to deal with something that everyone wishes had not happened. The ethic of care has broken down and we are faced, unavoidably, with a conflict of rights which an appeal to mutual and universal care will not resolve.

The fetus is vulnerable, and is certainly in no position to help herself or himself. One question, then, is whether the woman should be obliged to give the help, obliged, that is, to follow the principles of care for the vulnerable and respect for life, or whether her autonomy is of such prior importance as to be sacrosanct, even in a case in which most people would choose otherwise and would wish that she, too, would choose otherwise. A second question is what the broader implications of either conclusion would be.

THE COURTS AND THE DEFENCE OF ACTUAL CONSENT AND AUTONOMY

The recommendation that judicial intervention in pregnancy not be permissible assumes that the courts would necessarily be oppressive and coercive in overriding a woman's consent. Yet we must consider the possibility that in some cases the courts, in mandating treatment, could be acting in defence of a woman's best interests, actual intent and consent, and thus her authentic autonomy, against the coercion she experiences from some other factor in her life, such as severe drug addiction.

The only practical mode of determining whether this is or is not so is to carry out the examination of the particular case. It follows,

then, that judicial review and possible intervention would have to remain a possibility in order to determine what the exercise of her best interests, intent, consent, and hence actual autonomy would be and to mandate measures which would enable it. Precluding judicial intervention in pregnancy, then, could in some cases militate against the very autonomy which the Commission report wishes to protect.

I agree that in general a woman's refusal to consent to treatment should not be overridden; this is not because she is a woman but because she is a human being. Since the one patient is inside the other, he or she can only be reached by intervention in the body or the behaviour of the non-consenting other. We do not force a person to undergo invasive treatment for the sole benefit of another (as in living donation of a kidney), even when the other would die without the intervention. Nor do we force those of sound mind to accept medical treatment for themselves, even if we consider their judgement to be in error, or when non-treatment is likely to result in their death.

The principle of the requirement of consent would seem to mean that in general a pregnant woman ought not to be coerced into treatment against her will. The Commission report, however, appears to assume exceptionless, perpetual and unambivalent, unambiguous, consistent, and rational choice on the part of the woman. In some cases as they actually occur in practice there may be doubt as to the competence and hence the nature of the consent of an individual woman. This may be so if she is drug-impaired or in a state of drug withdrawal which would cause her to say or do anything to get a fresh supply, whatever her deeper intent for her fetus might be. Perhaps a clinician is faced with a woman whose statements of intent are shifting because of some emotional state or panic, or because of some form of lack of capacity to understand that treatment is the only mode of bringing about the outcome she has explicitly said she wants, the birth of a healthy baby.

There may, therefore, be a question as to what her most fundamental choice actually is. Is she acting as a rational, choosing adult, having decided that drug ingestion is more important to her than the welfare of her fetus? It seems that the Commission report predicates its interpretation of autonomy only on this assumption. Or does she in fact intend good for her fetus but is being coerced at one irrational moment by the urgency and desperation of her drug withdrawal to say and do things which in another, rational moment, she would not wish to say or do? In such cases it may be that some form of objective assessment of her intent is necessary, not only in the child's interests but in her own. Would a court be coercing her, or would it be protecting her from coercion?

The weighing of consent or refusal of consent on the part of a woman under conditions of medical emergency and distress is not as straightforward as it might be were she deciding calmly over a period of weeks on whether or not to donate a kidney. The consent or refusal of a woman chronically under the influence of alcohol or drugs is similarly difficult to determine. If we as a society are ambivalent about such situations, it is highly likely that any given woman in that position would be far more so.

Society recognizes that diminished competence diminishes the capacity for informed consent. Our own Commission concludes that informed consent must go beyond mere acceptance to informed choice, which seems to me to presuppose not only full information, and awareness of alternatives and implications, but also sufficient rational capacity to choose. At what point does some state of impairment or incoherence or panic or incapacity so diminish competence that a disinterested party must become involved?

Our society accepts the principle that, while the mentally ill should in general be hospitalized only with their consent, well-founded fear that a person will harm himself or herself or someone else can warrant committal. Because of the human consequences of either a narrow or a broad interpretation of that harm, the point at which this principle would apply is the subject of ongoing debate, or indeed struggle. The principle itself, however, is accepted and there is clear recognition that the dilemma is real. The question must arise whether severe drug addiction resulting in incoherence or uncontrollable compulsion is sufficiently parallel to or cognate with severe mental illness in some respects that similar approaches are appropriate.

The Commission report asserts that "the use of mental health legislation to commit or treat a pregnant woman against her will, even where the language of the statute appears to be applicable, would clearly offend Charter principles," but it does not give any reason why this should be so. One would assume, rather, that mental health legislation is applicable to both sexes, and is not suspensible solely because a person is female or because she is pregnant. If a woman is not mentally competent to determine the nature of her own consistent choice or her own best interest, even prior to consideration of the welfare of another, help may be needed as in many other instances of grave impairment.

The Commission report seems, indeed, to contradict itself on this point. It states that the "legal consequence of being found mentally incompetent is the appointment of a legal guardian to make decisions on one's behalf." Precisely. This requires judicial intervention, whether a person is pregnant or not, and even if the best interest of the woman were considered the primary or even the sole consideration. It may well be that treatment or behaviour which would protect the fetus would also be in her best interest with respect to her own health, were she found, under the principles of mental health legislation, likely to do herself severe and irretrievable harm. It would certainly be in her best interest with respect to her future life of responsibility for the care and custody of a child who could, were there to be the action of a guardian or some other modality of treatment, be born without handicaps burdensome, not only to the child, but to the woman.

It is in the face of these dilemmas that the application of ethical principles, social analysis, medical diagnosis and therapy, and the role of the courts come to overlap.

The courts are a disinterested forum with accepted legitimacy in our society for the resolution of what will necessarily be grave doubts, ambiguities, and conflicts. Any other body, such as an ethics committee, or another individual, such as an ombudsman or even a mediating social worker, designated to take responsibility for these conflicts will rapidly find themselves exercising what amount to quasi-judicial functions. Yet the mandates of such bodies and persons are not, in fact, judicial; ambiguities may remain and time-limited emergency conditions may compound the urgency of finding a resolution. The final forum in our society is, and must be, the courts.

WOMEN AS AN AGGREGATE

Arguments opposing judicial review in individual cases on grounds of a posited effect on the collective status of women or on the autonomy of all individual women seem to me to have serious internal contradictions, and to leave insufficient room for sensitivity to these specific individual women's interests and situations.

The assumption appears to be that no claim should exist which might limit the autonomy of any woman. This has many political, constitutional, and other implications.

The individuals, women and children, who are caught in these tragic situations are not being treated in these arguments as ends in themselves but more a secondary means to a separate and arguably unrelated political end, an end concerning which the individual women in these conflicts may have no—or some other—personal awareness or commitment. It is they, the individual women, however, who will be left with the care of the handicapped child, or with the bereavement, which follows non-intervention.

Judicial intervention in rare instances of grave circumstances does not in any way reinforce "the notion that a pregnant woman's role is *only* [emphasis mine] to carry and deliver a healthy child" or for that reason deny "her existence as an autonomous individual with legal and constitutional rights," hence being "dangerous to the rights and autonomy of all women." Every person has a multiplicity of often overlapping roles. To define any person in

terms of only one of them—or to posit, as the Commission report does, that unspecified other people define and may be further encouraged to define all members of a group in terms of only one of them—is reductionist. Indeed I know of no group anywhere on any contemporary political or philosophical spectrum which claims that the delivering of a healthy child is a woman's— or a pregnant woman's—only role. When the subject is raised, the notion is universally condemned. It is hence a red herring, however politically potent the slogan.

Women and men both, as adult human beings, have formal and informal rights and responsibilities arising from each of the roles they undertake. This may be, to take just a few of the more commonly experienced examples, as employer, employee, spouse, friend, contractor, contractee, parent, child, and, yes, gestating woman. Gestation toward the goal of delivering a healthy child is not the only role a pregnant woman has, as any woman who has been pregnant and any other person who has lived or worked with a pregnant woman knows. It is, nonetheless, one of the roles she does have, and the responsibilities which go with it exist as the responsibilities which arise from any other of her roles exist.

It is certainly true, as the Commission report points out, that a caring and nurturing relationship cannot be legislated. Society does, however, quite routinely legislate the minimum fulfilment of the formal responsibilities and obligations of various social roles, including those, such as the parent–child or the marital role, which are best generated and supported by the informal and strong bonds of affect, caring, and commitment. This is because it is often upon the fulfilment of social roles that the essential welfare of others depends.

If, as must be the case, women are to be deemed equal, women must be deemed to have the full responsibilities which accompany full rights. We expect every adult to act responsibly with respect to the roles they freely undertake, and with respect to the persons to whom they have undertaken both the rights and the obligations which characterize those roles. To expect that pregnant women act as responsibly as we expect every other adult to act is to uphold and defend the rights of women as competent, free, and full participants in society. It is the negation or the waiving of those responsibilities which, in my view, would be "dangerous to the rights and autonomy of all women."

Those who argue against judicial intervention in pregnancy in order to protect or advance a gender-based, aggregate, absolute autonomy may be viewed, particularly if they are themselves women, as being in a conflict of interest. Whatever resolution is reached by society with respect to these situations, it should be primarily for the welfare of the principals, the specific woman and the specific child. It should not be in aid of positions on any other issue, or in aid of the separate and different interests of the members of any larger group.

Many of those who subscribe to the collective status argument would never intend to use individuals as means to an end; this nonetheless seems to me to be the other side of the collective status coin. The issue of judicial intervention in pregnancy should not be caught in, or be treated as a strategic element in, a larger and distinct political struggle, however important and worthy some of the issues in that struggle may be.

Such arguments may, moreover, by placing women either or both above or beneath the law, be ultimately counterproductive to furthering the equality of men and women within our common humanity. This, as I shall suggest, would be a far greater evil than would a continued wrestling with these agonizing conflicts on a case-by-case basis.

RESPONSIBILITY, EQUALITY, AND THE CONSTITUTION

We must deal with the question of a woman's accountability for her actions. The case of judicial intervention in pregnancy is different from that of abortion, in that the child is to be born and, if surviving, he or she will have to live with whatever the consequences of the conflict turn out to be. Fetal alcohol syndrome, brain damage

from oxygen deprivation at the time of birth, and the results of being born with cocaine or heroin addiction are among the more common of such consequences.

Again, we must deal with this question not only in pragmatic terms but in principle. There can be no doubt that the inconvenience or loss of mobility or other effects experienced by a woman of mandatory but temporary care or treatment would be far less severe than the effects of an entire lifetime of mental and/or physical handicap on the child who is to be born. This is a very important question of proportion. On the practical level, however, were women to be systematically threatened with lawsuits or criminal penalties when their addictions or choices had damaged their children, some pregnant women might well, as the Commission report rightly points out, avoid medical care for themselves and for their children, or perhaps abort out of fear of sanctions. This would obviously be counterproductive from the perspective of the good of the fetus along with that of the mother.

The concerns expressed in the Commission report that "the potential for curtailing women's choices and behaviour becomes staggering" and that many women's pregnancies could become "subject to challenge and scrutiny" nonetheless seem to me to be alarmist. It would be not only repugnant and totalitarian but simply impossible to set up some sort of science-fictional infrastructure to enforce the compliance of every woman who did not seek adequate prenatal care or who did not follow her doctor's advice. Equally repugnant and bureaucratically impossible would be the assessment of every newborn for possibly matrigenic (parallel to iatrogenic) damage, and the resultant laying of charges. A significant segment of the literature on the subject paints just such bizarre scenarios representing judicial intervention in pregnancy as the harbinger of some total and coercive (male) medico-governmental dictatorship over women.

The painting of such extremes, however, or rather the setting up of such straw men, tends to obscure the rather more prosaic but far more probable scenarios in the instances one finds on the ground. Specific children are born severely damaged in ways which were entirely preventable and which were entirely within the responsibility of the mother. Once the children are born there is no question that they are legal persons. Laws exist which allow them to sue for damage done—or to inherit—through events which occurred before they were born, so long as they are subsequently born alive. It would probably be imprudent, counterproductive, and impracticable to sue women for the developmental and other handicaps children may suffer because of what their mothers did while they were *en ventre sa mère.* Yet we may ask whether women are not responsible in principle, and therefore what the implications of the question itself are for the status of women before the law.

The Commission report says that pregnant women "are no different from any other responsible individual; to treat pregnant women differently from other women and men, or to impose a different standard of behaviour on them, is neither morally nor legally defensible." It should be clear by this point that I agree. Where we disagree is on the application. Autonomy is a necessary good, but it is not an absolute. All of us have, as the report says, the right to make our own choices, but rights necessarily entail responsibilities; where our choices may or do harm others, our choices are, in fact, limited, and we are held accountable, whatever our gender. It is the suspension of that accountability with respect to pregnant women which would constitute the setting of a different (and lower) standard of behaviour.

An employer who chooses to employ people in his or her factory or office is responsible before the law to provide them with a safe environment. If one of them is injured in some way for which the employer is responsible, the injured person can sue or the employer may be charged with offences related to negligence, up to and including negligent homicide.

A woman, unless she has been raped, has in some measure willed her pregnancy, at least to the degree that she consensually participated in the sexual union which initiated it. If family plan-

ning was not used, she participated in that choice also. Is she not to be deemed responsible for the environment she provides the one who is there at her initiative, even as the employer is responsible for the environment he or she provides for the employee who is there at his or her initiative? A householder who is liable for injury suffered by a person on his or her hazardously maintained property provides yet another parallel.

To some it may appear that a woman should not be held responsible in a manner parallel to the responsibility of an employer or a householder. Yet let us look at the questions raised by such an exemption. It seems to me that the rationale would have to be that a woman is either above or beneath the law on grounds of gender and pregnancy, assertions which one may question.

If the argument is that a woman must not be held responsible because she is a woman and it is her choice, this seems to me to imply that a woman is above the ordinary application of the law because she is a woman. I have not yet seen a clear, let alone persuasive, argument as to why this should be true.

Be it granted, only a woman can become pregnant, as only a man can produce sperm. Neither fact is discriminatory; they are simply an empirically observable given, a function of the highly adaptive, population-variability-maintaining sexual dimorphism that human beings share with most organisms above the evolutionary level of the worm. Granted, too, given the unique human capacity for awareness and, with that, the development of the philosophy and ethics of social and legal responsibility, that there may therefore be modes of exercise of responsibility which are possible only for a woman, as there are other modes of exercise of responsibility which are possible only for a man.

The standard of behaviour, however, is the same. While one *ought* to act in accord with the principles of benevolence and care, that is in ways which are supportive of and helpful to others, at a minimum one is free to act as one wills so long as one acts in ways which do not harm others. As only a woman can, by her own drug abuse or other actions, severely handicap someone for life, only a man can rape. That only one gender can do one or the other form of harm does not make accountability for either discriminatory. The single standard of behaviour pertains to both. The difference in culpability has to do with the probable social circumstances of such a woman and the physiological and psychological burden of addiction, as compared with the improbability of any credible mitigating factors in rape. The difference, however, has to do with an independent assessment of the capacity of the individual to choose not to do harm, and hence an assessment of competence; it has nothing to do with gender discrimination.

If the argument is that any woman in this sort of situation is vulnerable, has arrived in her unfortunate situation for reasons utterly beyond her control, and ought not to be burdened with the ordinary application of the law, this seems to imply that she is beneath the law because she is incapable of the responsible, rational choice which underpins all adult participation in the society as framed by the law, again because she is a woman. It appears to me that a blanket application of this so all cases involving all women would be to return women to the patronizing and disenfranchising protections once offered to "women, children, and the insane."

That all persons are to be assumed mentally and morally competent and capable in the absence of evidence to the contrary is essential to their full, adult participation in a democracy. Placing this in doubt with respect to women as a group rather than with respect to particular individual women appears to me to be highly counterproductive.

The argument from aggregate seems to suppose that if any woman is judged incompetent, all women are by extension judged incompetent. Conversely, it seems to suppose that if all women are to be viewed as full legal and moral persons, every woman must be assumed under any and all circumstances to be wise, objective, and rational (and right "for her") in everything she does.

I would not make the assumption that if women are not deemed universally competent,

they are condemned to being deemed universally incompetent as a class or group. They are individuals. Most would fall into the rational, decision-competent, responsible category, at least most of the time, not because they are women but because they are adult human beings. Some individual women, like some individual men, however, do have diminished responsibility which is due to temporarily, chronically, or permanently impaired judgement. If this is so in individual cases, then the question of the protections and treatments—and the controls—which ordinarily apply to those of seriously impaired capacity must arise. Otherwise, freedom requires that women, adults indistinguishable from men on that ground, are assumed to be competent, and hence both responsible and accountable.

We must, as women, beware of overusing arguments claiming protections and privileges on grounds that we will otherwise be victims. Victims are victims because they are weaker than those seen as victimizing them. The unspoken correlate of such arguments is that women are, in fact, the weaker vessel, and that we cannot stand on our own taking full responsibility for our actions. It is *because* I see women and men as equal that I cannot accept arguments from collective victimization. Some individual women are victims as some individual men are victims, and protections must be constructed accordingly. Arguments for protections and exemptions from responsibility on grounds of what amounts to a collective victim status, however, negate and undermine the collective and individual equality of women.

STATE INTEREST IN THE FETUS

The question of the personhood of the fetus is irrelevant to that of judicial intervention in pregnancy. By extension so, too, is the question of the treatment of the fetus as a separate patient, although in my view it is no more than a recognition of reality, whatever rights that patient may or may not be deemed under the law to have.

Even were the fetus to be recognized as a full person before the law, the ordinary protections of one person, the woman, against medical intervention or confinement for the sole benefit of another would still exist. If they apply with respect to aid to those already born and physically independent of the prospective donor, they will certainly apply with respect to aid to those located physically within another.

The Commission report raises the fact that the fetus has not been recognized to have the independent legal or constitutional rights of a person under the law. The woman is seen from this perspective by the report as having no legal obligation to undergo intervention since there is, in effect, no rights-endowed legal person whom she has an obligation not to harm. The report goes on to say that no third party can "volunteer to defend the 'rights' of a being that has no legal existence."

Many questions are raised by this approach.

The Supreme Court of Canada, in the Morgentaler decision, recognized a state interest in the fetus. The decision of the Court and the opinions of all but one Justice made no distinction between levels of advancement. Instances of judicial intervention in pregnancy have in any case for the most part arisen in later pregnancy.

Since such a state interest in the fetus does exist, one wonders what meaning it would have were that interest not to be of any force or effect even when a child is about to be born or is viable and the removal of the mother's access to drugs or alcohol or so very routine a medical procedure as a Caesarian section would be sufficient to save his or her life and health. If an interest exists it must have application in some set of circumstances. If that interest were not applicable in these extreme circumstances it would be applicable in no conceivable circumstances which involved a conflict with the woman carrying the child.

Since the Morgentaler case focussed on abortion, which does indeed involve a conflict between the mother and the child *en ventre sa mère,* it is precisely in the welfare of the fetus in the event of some measure of conflict with the mother herself that the Court saw the state to have an interest, rather than in some conflict with another party, such as some individual committing assault on the mother or some corporate entity polluting the available drinking water with teratogenic effects on the fetus.

To argue, then, that a woman in principle has the unlimited right to endanger her fetus in any way she wishes at any stage before birth and that no third party, which would include the state, can defend the fetus is to argue that the Court, in finding a state interest in the fetus, had enunciated an absurdity, which I doubt.

THE QUESTION OF CRIMINALIZATION

I do not see sufficient reason for the recommendation that unwanted medical treatment and other interferences or threatened interferences with the physical autonomy of pregnant women be recognized explicitly under the *Criminal Code* as criminal assault. Making an action an offence under the *Criminal Code* implies that the action is unequivocally and clearly repugnant to the Canadian body politic, so much so that other remedies are neither sufficient to control it nor capable of a sufficient degree of symbolic censure. One must ask, then, whether all intervention in pregnancy fulfils those conditions.

First, as I have argued above, intervention in pregnancy under some very limited circumstances is not unequivocally repugnant to all members of Canadian society on either the symbolic or the practical level. Second, it appears to me that intervention in pregnancy can be and now is effectively controlled by more moderate and gender-neutral means. Third, there are internal difficulties with the recommendation itself.

One would assume that what is being suggested is that intervention without benefit of judicial warrant be criminalized. Judicial intervention itself could not, of course, be criminalized, since a judge cannot be charged or penalized for decisions he or she makes on the bench. To seek sanctions against judges for reaching particular decisions would strike at the roots of the independence of the judiciary and hence of the rule of law.

That a person has the right to refuse invasive treatment or detention by a physician or other professional is accepted both in ethics and in law. Protections already exist. The Commission has been told that the main remedy in the case of non-consensual medical intervention is in the form of *tort* law, claims of civil damages when suit is brought by the claimant. Malpractice is a parallel instance. One may ask whether the criminal sanctions with respect to assault would also already apply. They may; if so, their focus is the protection of persons, not of women as a separate group.

It is unclear to me why intervention in pregnancy would be more heinous than any other sort of medical or social/ psychological intervention without consent. If it is at the same level of seriousness, then I do not see why it should be singled out so that a different and more severe set of sanctions should apply. Non-consensual intervention in a situation which is by definition confined to women is not more invasive than intervention in others which could occur in both men and women, such as kidney failure or removal of bone marrow for transplantation. An argument that confinement of or surgery on women is more serious than confinement or surgery which pertains to both sexes would be discriminatory; such an argument would privilege women on grounds of their sex and hence deny equality. I therefore cannot see justification for making the offence and the sanctions different in kind from those pertaining to all medical procedures or other interventions.

Even the criminalization of intervention in pregnancy would not remove the possibility of judicial intervention. In judicial intervention, it is the judge, not the physician or other professional, who is the prime actor, mandating the actions of others. A judge can authorize police to search premises or to seize property—or remove children—for sufficient cause. A judge can also authorize detention for certain grave reasons. These activities, without such authorization, would be criminal. Criminalization of medical and other forms of intervention would therefore affect only the activities of doctors or other professionals acting on their own, not judicial review and intervention itself. If the present

sanctions are adequate deterrents to professionals' acting on their own, and if judicial intervention can take place whatever the sanctions, I can see no practical effect of a new measure of criminalization.

Nor does the number of instances of judicially mandated intervention in pregnancy seem to present sufficient concrete cause for concern. The small handful of cases which have come to appeal in Canada, and the fact that they have often been overturned, would seem to suggest that the present system is functioning to discourage judicial intervention in pregnancy. If the present system seems to be producing the outcomes desired by the Commission report, and if there is no evidence of an epidemic of such interventions, let alone of interventions for less than grave cause, I do not see any practical reason for an escalation of sanctions or for altering the judicial modes by which decisions are reached.

I grant that the workings of the Canadian judicial system may be imperfect, as the workings of any system are imperfect. If, however, we were to assume that all courts would make oppressive, biased, or erroneous decisions, and that women require protection from them by removing from the courts the capacity to review and decide such questions, we cast into doubt the entire system our society has created for the resolution of disputes and harm-causing ambiguity with no viable replacement.

Nor is the argument from the claim that medical or judicial judgements may err, citing one selected case, convincing. To take the possibility of error as an argument for never acting upon expert advice under any circumstances whatever is an extreme which would paralyze all social action. Our own report in another place has made the point that all of medicine carries some level of risk. Physicians offer expertise, not omniscience. The same is true of judges. In this they are like all human beings; beyond this they bear the same heavy responsibility as all those in positions of particular social trust.

On these questions as in all others within the body politic, within medicine and within the social services, evidence must be examined, prudence and caution exercised, but some degree of uncertainty is simply a reality of the human condition. It does not absolve us as a society, or the judges who act as the arbiters for our society under grave circumstances, of the responsibility to weigh what can be known of fact, expert advice, and concern, to take care that any intervention will avoid doing serious or disproportionate harm to any party, and then to make decisions. Argument that those delegated by society should absent themselves entirely from doing so because of the possibility of error would be, were this accepted in principle and universally applied, to abdicate all active and governmental or custodial forms of human social responsibility. If it would be absurd to apply it universally, one may question the applicability of the argument to this one field.

It appears to me to be more reasonable to accept that judicial review may, in very rare and serious cases and with all due caution and attention to interests and evidence, take place at the time the question arises, before the decision on whether or not to take action is made. It should, however, be very clear that the ordinary protections against non-consensual intervention apply in cases of pregnancy as in all others.

SOCIAL CONTEXT

A woman's social context can certainly dispose toward the sorts of conflict we are considering, so it is largely through the social context that we as a society can seek to prevent them.

It seems that the majority of cases in which these conflicts arise are associated with poverty. It has been alleged by some (and is implied as a distinct possibility in the text of the Commission report) that the high proportion of cases of judicial intervention in pregnancy which involve the poor and members of visible minorities is due to racism and class discrimination in the medical and judicial systems. This is easy enough to assert, and carries a potent political impact. We as a Commission have not, however, been given a fully documented social analysis of such cases,

including adequate evidence corroborating bias. We have not seen, for instance, a retrospective random or universal sample study of judicial decisions rendered to middle-class/working-class as compared with poor women, or white and visible minority women. I would not, as a social scientist, say that such bias has been demonstrated. There may well be individual judges whose outlook is biased; this must be dealt with on that individual level. The remedy, however, is neither a restructuring of the jurisdiction of the courts nor an attribution of bias to the entire judicial system.

Applying Occam's razor, looking for the simplest explanation for the available data, it is more probable that it is poverty which is the root cause. Poverty is associated with the low levels of education and consequent low awareness of the importance of prenatal care, the low recourse to the health care system, the fear of complex, high-tech procedures, and the alienation and addictions which tend to foster these conflicts. While in Canada the majority of poor women are not members of visible minorities, minority women are over-represented among the poor for their proportion in the general population, an inequity which must be remedied on its own terms. It is not necessary to assume—or to imply—that all doctors and judges who have mandated supervision or treatment for poor women are biased.

There is, moreover, no evidence that any causal relationship should even be suggested between the "religious convictions … cultural beliefs … or other deeply held values or personal beliefs" of Aboriginal women and women of colour on the one hand and cases of judicial intervention in pregnancy related to the "refusal to accept surgical or other medical treatment or to follow medical advice" on the other.

First, there are no grounds on which to make such a collective connection. Aboriginal women and women of colour come from highly diverse social, ethnic, religious, and other traditions, since their ancestors were born in lands spanning not only the wide expanse of Canada but the globe itself. If there are groups who do hold refusal of medical treatment and advice as a value, we have not had evidence of it brought before us. Even if a specific group or groups did hold such a view, however, it could not be generalized to all Aboriginal women or women of colour. Each group and individual should be able to speak for themselves in this regard.

Second, we have had no concrete instances brought before us of judicial review or intervention in a case of refusal on principle or on grounds of culture, deeply held personal values, or belief. It is certainly hypothetically possible that instances of such refusal might arise, parallel to the refusal of Jehovah's Witnesses to accept blood transfusions or of Christian Scientists to seek various sorts of medical technology. There may also be some women who wish to give birth within a "women's circle," with a group-chosen "wise woman" or unlicensed midwife rather than a medically credentialled practitioner. It may be that the defence of such latter groups against feared requirements of professional medical supervision is related to some significant segment of the feminist concerns which dominate discussion of this issue. No cases of judicial intervention on grounds of culture-based values or principle, however, whatever the ethnic or other context of the woman, appeared in the evidence with which we have been presented.

Third, as the report acknowledges, cases of judicial intervention in pregnancy usually involve abuse of drugs, alcohol, or both. Still others involve often-related activities such as prostitution. Both substance abuse and prostitution carry a serious risk of violence and disease (such as AIDS, the toxic effects of cocaine, or the effects of alcohol on the brain) which damage and can kill both mother and child. Alcohol and drug addiction or prostitution are not part of the "cultural values" or "religious beliefs" of any Aboriginal or other visible minority groups, whatever the enmeshment of those dysfunctional behaviours with social conditions.

The testimony we as a Commission heard from Native groups emphasized the great and positive cosmic value placed on women and on their bearing and bringing forth of life as part of the work of the Creator. Many other groups hold equally positive views of the importance of a woman's nurturance of her child, including before birth. Many Aboriginal and other ethnocultural groups are engaged in movements to revitalize aspects of their traditional cultures, bringing them to bear on their contemporary lives by integrating today's realities with a strong sense of identity, dignity, and values arising from centuries of experience understood through elements of their own tradition. One of the many purposes of this revitalization is to heal individuals affected by precisely those same sorts of behaviour which give rise to judicial review. Women, whatever their culture or ethnic background, do not "choose a particular course of action," refusing treatment or refusing to follow medical advice which would divert them from engaging in the substance abuse and prostitution which have in actual cases drawn the scrutiny of the courts, on grounds of their "deeply held values or personal beliefs."

The ethnic or cultural origin of a woman is therefore not a root factor in her behaviour in any case of judicial intervention in pregnancy of which I am aware. The courts have not scrutinized cases where rejection was based on principle, and those cases in which the courts have intervened have concerned dysfunctional behaviour unrelated to and indeed antithetical to the cultural, religious, and other beliefs of all women, including Aboriginal women and women of colour. If some Aboriginal or visible minority women have been among the tiny handful of Canadian cases of judicial intervention in pregnancy, it is due to disproportionate rates of marginalization and poverty, not to the cultural or religious beliefs or values of the groups from which these specific women come.

I would agree with the Commission report that judicial intervention does not change the circumstances that bring about the attempts to intervene, or at least it does not change them directly. That the Commission report would object to judicial intervention in pregnancy on those grounds seems to me to be somewhat inconsistent, however. That an approach may not cure a problem, only circumventing it and changing its practical outcome, seems elsewhere to be presented in this report as acceptable and constructive. Circumvention and outcome alteration are, after all, precisely the modality of several of the approaches to infertility which this Commission accepts, with due safeguards. The social context is, of course, very different, but the logical structure of the approach is the same.

I would disagree, moreover, with the report's view that intervention provides no solution. Any solution of such cases will probably be imperfect—indeed, non-intervention is itself concerned with avoidance of engagement, not with offering a solution of any sort. The very point, however, of those rare instances in which intervention is appropriate is to "create the social conditions and support that help to ensure a successful pregnancy and health outcome for both the woman and the child."

For example, a woman required to reside for a period of time in a treatment centre, well-fed, with access to counselling, peer support, and referral to services to upgrade her education and prospects of employment, and free of the ready availability of the substances to which she is addicted (and which may elsewhere be pressed upon her by her companions) has precisely those social conditions and supports conducive to a "healthy outcome," if this is taken to mean the withdrawal of the woman from drug dependency, her reception of other forms of prenatal and perinatal care, and the absence of mental and/or other permanent disabilities in the child. The supports would indeed be temporary; the woman could later return to a dysfunctional pattern of life if she chose to. Yet there would be concrete benefits, not only to the child but to the woman. The child would not have been harmed; that particular systemically devastating source of harm would have been avoided and, for that child at least, could not recur. The woman herself would have been given the opportunity, the supports and the access to resources to choose to make a definitive and permanent change in her mode of life toward social and economic independence; she would also herself benefit from the fact that the child for whom she would have maternal responsibility and care would be unimpaired by the multiple severe disabilities which are the reason for the concern which gives rise to judicial intervention.

Middle-class and working-class women of all races and cultures in this country tend to have had knowledge of and relatively ready access to prenatal care, and to have been sufficiently aware of the need to avoid substance abuse and other harmful behaviour, particularly during pregnancy, that they would have been unlikely to have come to a judge's attention in the first place. If poverty is associated with the root conditions for much of the tragedy and conflict in society, the fact that the poor are those whose consequence-ridden turmoil comes before judges is precisely what one would expect.

The effective remedy to the problem, then, would lie in combatting poverty, not in removing the capacity of judges to review and adjudicate the conflicts of the poor.

PREVENTION

If, then, we seek to avoid these conflicts, the place to start is in outreach to women in low-income and any other vulnerable groups. There are many possible strategies, many or all of which could be used in concert. They dovetail with the concerns which have emerged over and over again in our work as a Commission.

Family life education is the first point of prevention, transmitting a strong awareness of responsibility, of pregnancy, and of prenatal care and birth long before a girl or woman becomes pregnant.

Outreach to women (and men) with substance addictions is already a priority, but more is needed. In a sense, any social and economic and job training program which gives people hope and a means of building a constructive life is, directly or indirectly, contributing to primary prevention of addictions and to rehabilitation of those who have been addicted.

If many poor women do not receive adequate prenatal care, even in this society in which care is universally offered, perhaps innovative strategies to reach them should be attempted. Public health departments are already engaged in much work of this kind. Public health consultations should be encouraged with a random sample of poor women from all groups at risk, with public health personnel, with anthropologists and sociologists, and with community groups; such consultations could perhaps give rise to new or improved ways of bringing mobile prenatal care, combined where appropriate with addiction treatment, in their own settings, cultures, and languages, to women who do not spontaneously seek out care in large hospital institutions or in stationary private medical offices.

Programs of this type would be helpful, not only to those who would be at risk of conflicts which could come to the point of judicial examination, but to all women at reproductive risk of any kind. They complement efforts to prevent or control STDs, to avoid adverse outcomes of pregnancy from any cause, and to further maternal and child care.

It is probable that no program can eliminate all situations of conflict. The principles we have discussed will, in rare instances, have to be brought into play. Judicial interventions in pregnancy and birth are nonetheless already very few: if, in our overall support for women, we can answer most needs before they reach the point of conflict, judicial review and intervention in pregnancy can in large degree be avoided.

CONCLUSION

The judiciary provides the final forum with the broadest scope and accepted legitimacy for the assessment and resolution of otherwise irresolvable dilemmas. For the hard cases which we are discussing, there is no superior mode of seeking, with the full range of testimony and expert advice, the real intent, consent, and interests of the individual woman, even if these are placed prior to the recognized, affirmed, and supported interests of the child within her. Some nightmarishly vast system of supervision of every pregnant woman would obviously be both repugnant and opera-

tionally impossible. It does not follow that rare cases cannot exist in which judicial intervention would be feasible, appropriate, and reasonable.

The unvaried assumption that a woman, because she is one of the class of women, must always be deemed to be fully and unambivalently certain at each given moment of what she intends and of its full implications, isolated from the context of her other expressions of intent, could well leave many individual women with the consequences having been allowed by default to abandon a positive intent under conditions of impairment or some other transitory state. So too would an assumption that, for broader reasons of the collective interests of women, even if a woman is not fully competent she must be treated as though she is. The same would be true of the opposite assumption that a woman, because she is a woman, should be taken solely at her word in such a moment, because she is so constrained by victimization, circumstance, and addiction that she is not responsible for the results of her actions and that those consequences, therefore, do not matter.

The women in such cases would then be left, not only with sorrow and guilt, but with a handicapped child. It is these women, not their doctors, not the members of hospital bioethics committees, nor yet the members of this Commission, who would have the burden of caring for their damaged children for what could be a lifetime, a burden which would be only partly alleviated by services provided by the state or by turning the children over for full-time state institutional care. The children would be left with those handicaps, not just as a burden, but as an overriding reality of life.

No system can guarantee that this would never occur. Only the availability of the objectivity of judicial assessment in cases of manifest ambivalence or impairment, however, will allow flexibility and sensitivity to individual women and their situations. If the wellbeing of a woman and the wellbeing, health, and very life of a child depend upon that sensitivity, the absolutization of an approach which would preclude it would seem to me to be a deeply inadequate response.

Moreover, many of the arguments or recommendations against judicial intervention in pregnancy or for the imposition of criminal sanctions distinct from the ordinary, non-gender-related sanctions against nonconsensual intervention are premised on assumptions which are, in my view, at odds with the fundamental principles of human equality and of full participation, irrespective of gender, in a free and democratic society. To accept them would ultimately be counterproductive for women and for children, and also for men. By identifying rights, protections, and interests with membership in a group, such as the aggregate of women, rather than with universal human identity, responsibilities, and protections, it would raise questions about the constitutional structures which underlie our polity itself, with implications which have yet to be examined.

For all these reasons, I see grave difficulties with, and would generally wish to discourage, overriding a woman's refusal of consent to surgical or behavioural intervention in pregnancy. Like my fellow Commissioners, I see every effort at prevention before these tragic situations arise as being the most constructive mode of approach. For both ethical and constitutional reasons, however, I see neither the absolute preclusion of judicial intervention in pregnancy nor the imposition of new sanctions distinguishing the protections of women from those of men as being justified....

Notes

1. *The Toronto Star,* Friday, August 20, 1993, p. A3.
2. Expert Interdisciplinary Advisory Committee on Sexually Transmitted Diseases in Children and Youth (EIAC-STD) and the Federal /Provincial/ Territorial Working Group on Adolescent Reproductive Health: Guidelines for Sexual Health Education, Principle 3, Guidelines. Segment 6. (Pagination varies by printed format.)
3. Ibid.: Principle 2, First Paragraph.
4. Ibid,: Principle 2, Second and Third Paragraphs.
5. King, Alan J.C. et al.: *Canada Youth and AIDS Study;* Queen's University at Kingston, pp. 83, 85.
6. Barnes, Alan: "Fewer Metro girls sexually active, 3-city poll finds"; *The Toronto Star,* Tuesday, November 24, 1992.
7. King, op. cit.: pp. 18, 32–34.
8. Santin, Sylvia, Gen. Ed.: *Fully Alive;* Maxwell Macmillan Canada, Don Mills, Ontario, 1988–1992.
9. *Catechisme de L'Église Catholique:* (Français) Mame-Librairie Éditrice Vaticane, Paris. 1992. Sections 2357-9, p. 480: (Latin) Libreria Editrice Vaticana, Citta del Vaticano, 1992.

R. v. Morgentaler, [1988] 1 S.C.R. 30

Summary prepared by Martina Munden

The *Criminal Code of Canada* set out procedures respecting abortions. Under section 251, a woman wishing to obtain an abortion had to receive a certificate from a therapeutic abortion committee at an accredited or approved hospital prior to a physician performing the abortion. These committees had the authority to issue a certificate stating that, in the opinion of a majority of the committee, the continuation of the pregnancy would be likely to endanger the pregnant woman's life or health. Once the certificate was given to a qualified medical practitioner, the practitioner was permitted to perform an abortion without either the physician or woman being subject to criminal liability. Failure of the woman to receive the medical approval for the abortion meant that the abortion was a criminal offence for both the woman and the physician who provided the abortion. The therapeutic abortion committee would only provide a certificate when the s. 251 criteria were complied with, that being, a woman's life or health was endangered by the pregnancy.

The physicians in this case had set up a clinic to perform abortions upon women who had not obtained a certificate from a therapeutic abortion committee of an accredited hospital as required by s. 251. The physicians had also made statements questioning the wisdom of Canadian abortion laws, asserting that a woman had an unfettered right to choose whether an abortion was appropriate in her individual circumstances. The physicians were charged with illegally performing an abortion. The physicians argued that s. 251 was contrary to the *Canadian Charter of Rights and Freedoms*.

By a five to two majority, the Supreme Court of Canada held that the provisions of s. 251 infringed the right to life, liberty, and security of the person as guaranteed by s. 7 of the *Charter*.

The majority also held that s. 251 was not a reasonable limitation on the infringed right and thus was not justified under s. 1 of the *Charter*.

Chief Justice Dickson (for himself and Justice Lamer as he then was) held that state interference with bodily integrity and serious state-imposed psychological stress, at least in the criminal law context, constitutes a breach of security of the person. The Chief Justice held that forcing a woman by threat of criminal sanctions to carry a fetus to term unless she met certain criteria unrelated to her own priorities and aspirations was a profound interference with a woman's body and thus an infringement of security of the person. He stated:

> At the most basic physical and emotional level, every pregnant woman is told by the section [s. 251] that she cannot submit to a generally safe medical procedure that might be of clear benefit to her unless she meets criteria entirely unrelated to her own priorities and aspirations. Not only does the removal of decision-making power threaten women in a physical sense; the indecision of not knowing whether an abortion will be granted inflicts physical and an emotional stress. Section 251 clearly interferes with a woman's bodily integrity in both a physical and an emotional sense. Forcing a woman, by threat of criminal sanction, to carry a foetus to term unless she meets certain criteria unrelated to her own priorities and aspirations is a profound interference with a woman's body and thus a violation of security of the person. Section 251, therefore, is required by the *Charter* to comport with the principles of fundamental justice.

Chief Justice Dickson also outlined the problems with the procedures stipulated in s. 251. Some of the problems noted were: criteria of danger to life or health were applied unevenly across Canada, with some committees requiring additional criteria; some hospitals had no committee set up or the committee existed in name only; many communities had no hospital of the size and kind that met the requirements for being an approved hospital; the mechanisms for decision making caused a certain amount of delay for women who were successful in meeting the criteria and this delay could have profound consequences for the women's physical and emotional well-being. Chief Justice Dickson then found that the combined effect of these procedures was a further breach of security of the person.

Chief Justice Dickson then considered whether these breaches of security of the person were in accordance with the principles of fundamental justice (the second step in any s. 7 analysis). He held that "one of the basic tenets of the criminal justice system is that when parliament creates a defence to a criminal charge, the defence should not be illusory or so difficult to attain as to be practically illusory." While noting that Parliament must be given room to design appropriate administrative and procedural structures for bringing into operation a particular defence to criminal liability, Chief Justice Dickson stated that where "that structure is 'so manifestly unfair, having regard to the decisions it is called upon to make, as to violate the principles of *fundamental* justice' that structure must be struck down." He noted that the problems women encountered in attempting to obtain an abortion were created by the structure that Parliament had put in place. Chief Justice Dickson found that the structure in s. 251—the system regulating access to therapeutic abortions—was manifestly unfair. He concluded that the procedures created in s. 251 for obtaining a therapeutic abortion did not comport with the principles of fundamental justice and therefore infringed s. 7 of the *Charter*.

In determining whether the infringement of s. 7 could be saved by s. 1 of the *Charter*, Chief Justice Dickson noted that s. 1 could be used to save the legislative provision only if the party seeking to uphold the provision could demonstrate that the objective was of sufficient importance to warrant overriding a constitutionally protected right or freedom and that the means chosen in overriding the right or freedom were reasonable and demonstrably justified in a free and democratic society. This second aspect ensures that legislative means are proportional to the legislative ends.

Chief Justice Dickson stated that the SCC's job was evaluating the particular balance struck by Parliament in s. 251 as it related to the priorities and aspirations of pregnant women and the government's interest in the protection of the fetus. He noted that Parliament itself had stated in s. 251 that the "life or health" of pregnant women was paramount. He found that the protection of the interests of pregnant women was a valid governmental objective where life and health could be jeopardized by criminal sanctions and that the protection of fetal interests by Parliament was also a valid governmental objective. Thus the balancing of those interests, with the lives and health of women a major factor, was clearly an important governmental objective. He concluded that "the objective of s. 251 as a whole, namely, to balance the competing interests identified by Parliament was sufficiently important to meet the requirements of the first part of the s. 1 inquiry."

However, with respect to the proportionality aspect of the s. 1 analysis, Chief Justice Dickson found that the means used to advance the legislative objectives did not meet the requirement of proportionality. He noted that the procedures and administrative structures created by s. 251 were often arbitrary and unfair; the procedures established to implement the policy of s. 251 impaired the s. 7 rights far more than was necessary because they held out an illusory defence to many women who would prima facie qualify. Therefore, the restrictive abortion law in the *Criminal Code* could not be saved by s. 1 of the *Charter* and it was struck down. It has never been replaced by Parliament.

Justices Beetz, Estey, and Wilson also wrote decisions in this case. They all agreed that s. 251

of the *Criminal Code* violated s. 7 of the *Charter*, that it could not be saved by s. 1 of the *Charter*, and, therefore, that it should be struck down. However, they offered different reasons for their conclusions.

Significantly, the SCC did not engage in a discussion of whether the fetus is a person or individual within the meaning of "every one" referred to in the *Charter*.

Winnipeg Child and Family Services (Northwest Area) v. G.(D.F.) [1997] 3 S.C.R. 925

Summary prepared by Maegen Giltrow

Ms. G was five months pregnant and suffered an addiction to glue sniffing. Because glue sniffing can damage the nervous system of a developing fetus, Ms. G, on the recommendation of a children's aid worker, had sought to enter a residential treatment facility. Unfortunately, there was initially no space available for her. On the day space did become available, Ms. G was intoxicated, and refused to go. The Director of Child and Family Services sought and received an order of the court that Ms. G be detained at the Health Sciences Centre until the birth of her child. The order was stayed two days later, and D.F.G. voluntarily remained at the Health Sciences Centre until she was discharged. She stopped sniffing glue and bore an apparently healthy child.

Despite the resolution of the facts of this particular case, the legal question remained before the Supreme Court of Canada (SCC): "assuming evidence that a mother is acting in a way that may harm her unborn child, does a judge, at the behest of the state, have the power to order the mother to be taken into custody for the purpose of rectifying her conduct?" The majority of the SCC held that the legal answer to this question must address both detention and a concomitant power to order treatment upon the mother, in order for the detention to have any purpose. The dissent addressed only detention, holding that once a woman was detained, she would remain free to reject all suggested medical treatment.

For the judge to have the authority in question, the power of the court must reside in one of two legal places. The first possibility lies in tort law, through which an injunction might be granted to detain the pregnant woman in order to prevent harm to her fetus. The second possibility is that the power of the court to protect children under its *parens patriae* jurisdiction be extended to protect fetuses.

Each of these possibilities was rejected by the majority for the same fundamental reason: the law recognizes only the rights of the born person. This principle is enshrined particularly in the "live birth rule." The majority and the dissent differed in particular on the foundations of the "live birth rule" and the validity of these foundations. While the dissent insisted that there is no defensible difference between a born and unborn child, and that the rule should be dismissed as an anachronistic rule of evidence, the majority maintained that the distinction is a contemporary and substantive legal one, not to be diminished by biological argument.

The majority offered several reasons to maintain the legal distinction. First, the life of the fetus and that of the pregnant woman are so intimately connected that they must legally be treated as one. The SCC pointed out that the liberty of the mother is intricately bound to her fetus, and to develop an antagonistic dichotomy between mother and fetus, where the fetus has the power of the state behind it, would deprive mothers control of their own bodies and the power to make autonomous choices. It would also usurp women's fundamental rights to bodily integrity, equality, privacy, and dignity.

Second, were the courts to allow intrusions upon the mother in cases where her lifestyle was found to be a risk to the fetus, there would be no clear line (both in evidence and in principle) between offensive and allowable behaviour on the part of the woman.

Third, the majority took issue with the suggestion that the state's intervention would be in response to the mother's "choice" to risk harm to her fetus. "[L]ifestyle 'choices' like alcohol consumption, drug abuse, and poor nutrition may be the products of circumstance and illness rather than free choice capable of effective deterrence by the legal sanction of tort."

Fourth, imposing a duty of care in relation to lifestyle choices of pregnant women would increase the level of outside scrutiny upon them, and could result in harm rather than benefit to not only the mother, but the fetus as well. There is, the SCC said, no evidence that a tort duty would decrease the incidence of substance-abused children; in fact, the evidence suggests that the duty might have negative effects on the health of children.

Finally, extending the law to provide for the detention of pregnant women whose lifestyles may pose risks to their fetuses would extend the law in ways far too radical to be the domain of the courts. The only current means by which the state can detain people is under criminal law, or under mental health legislation when a person has been declared incompetent.

The majority of the SCC rejected extending the court's *parens patriae* jurisdiction to allow for the confinement of pregnant women for reasons similar to those by which they dismissed any such power under tort law. In particular, the SCC noted that extending the power of the state to protect fetuses would be an invasion of the liberty of pregnant women of a different order than that associated with the current power. That is, under the current *parens patriae* power, the state constrains the liberty of parents only in so far as

to affect their liberty in making decisions on behalf of their children. However, if the jurisdiction of the courts were to be extended to the protection of fetuses, the liberty of a pregnant woman would be impinged in relation to her ability to make decisions for herself—such as, for instance, where to live and what medical treatments to undergo, including whether to undergo a cesarian section delivery. The majority held that an intrusion of this magnitude directly on the rights of women was not one that could be authorized in the first instance by the courts, but was, rather, a question for the legislature.

Despite the reasons offered by the majority, the dissent wrote that it "seems fundamentally unfair and inexplicable for this Court to hold that a foetus, upon live birth, can sue for damages to recompense injuries suffered in utero, yet have no ability to obtain a remedy preventing that damage from occurring in the first place."

The dissent held that the state has an enforceable interest in protecting the rights of fetuses, despite the fact that the rights of the pregnant woman would necessarily be impinged by this interest. It held, however, that this was justified by the fact that the pregnant woman could choose not to carry the child to term, and to have an abortion instead. That is, once a woman chooses to become a mother (that is, does not choose to have an abortion), held the dissent, she forfeits her liberty rights to the state's interest in protecting her fetus.

Contrary to the substantive reasons the majority cited underlying the "born alive rule" and treating mother and fetus as one, the dissent held that the rule is a legal anachronism that had arisen originally for evidentiary reasons, and not substantive ones. Now that we have medical technology that can show us "that a foetus is alive and has been or will be injured by the conduct of another," we should, the minority held, do away with the rule. The dissent wrote with a confidence in medical technology's ability to "know" the fetus not shared by the majority. Nor was the majority willing to use whatever knowledge medical technology is capable of securing at any point in time against pregnant mothers.

While the majority did not hold that in fact mother and fetus are one, and that their body and interests are in fact the same, it held that in law, they are indeed one. The majority left open that mother and fetus could be split into two legal entities, not by the courts, but by legislatures. The dissent responded to the majority's unwillingness to engage the "slippery slope" of state intervention by saying that this reluctance should not be used as a principled bar to granting an injunction in this case. The facts in this case had, however, resolved themselves; what the dissent sought was, in fact, a principle in law by which the rights of the mother would necessarily suffer at the hands of the state's interest in her fetus.

Chapter 10 ISSUES IN GENETICS

Prenatal Genetic Testing and Screening: Constructing Needs and Reinforcing Inequities

Abby Lippman

PRENATAL DIAGNOSIS: A TECHNICAL AND A SOCIAL CONSTRUCTION

Of all applied genetic activities, prenatal diagnosis is probably most familiar to the general population and is also the most used. Prenatal diagnosis refers to all the technologies currently in use or under development to determine the physi(ologi)cal condition of a fetus before birth. Until recently, prenatal diagnosis usually meant amniocentesis,[1] a second trimester procedure routinely available for women over a certain age (usually thirty-five years in North America),[2] for Down syndrome detection. Amniocentesis is also used in selected circumstances where the identification of specific fetal genetic disorders is possible.[3] Now, in addition to amniocentesis, there are chorionic villus sampling (CVS)[4] tests that screen maternal blood samples to detect a fetus with a neural tube defect or Down syndrome, and ultrasound screening.[5] Despite professional guidelines to the contrary,[6] ultrasound screening is performed routinely in North America on almost every pregnant woman appearing for prenatal care early enough in pregnancy. And although ultrasound is not usually labeled as "prenatal diagnosis," it not only belongs under this rubric but was, I suggest, the first form of prenatal diagnosis for which informed consent is not obtained.[7]

Expansion of prenatal diagnosis techniques, ever widening lists of identifiable conditions and susceptibilities, changes in the timing of testing and the populations in which testing is occurring, and expanding professional definitions of what should be diagnosed *in utero*, attest to this technology's role in the process of geneticization.[8] But these operational characteristics alone circumscribe only some aspects of prenatal diagnosis. Prenatal diagnosis as a social activity is becoming an element in our culture and this aspect, which has had minimal attention, will be examined in depth.

A. Prenatal Diagnosis and the Discourse of Reassurance

Contemporary stories about prenatal diagnosis contain several themes, but these generally reflect either of two somewhat different models.[9] In the "public health" model, prenatal diagnosis is presented as a way to reduce the frequency of selected birth defects.[10] In the other, which I will call the "reproductive autonomy" model, prenatal diagnosis is presented as a means of giving women information to expand their reproductive choices.[11] Unfortunately, neither model fully captures the essence of prenatal diagnosis. In addition, neither acknowledges the internal tension, revealed in the coexistence of quite contradictory constructions of testing that may be equally valid: 1) as an assembly line approach to the products of conception, separating out those we wish to discontinue;[12] 2) as a way to give women control over their pregnancies, respecting (increasing) their autonomy to choose the kinds of children they will bear;[13] or 3) as a means of reassuring women that enhances their experience of pregnancy.[14]

The dominant theme throughout the biomedical literature, as well as some feminist commentary, emphasizes the last two of these constructions.[15] A major variation on this theme suggests, further, that through the use of prenatal diagnosis women can avoid the family distress and suffering associated with the unpredicted birth of babies with genetic disorders or congenital malformations, thus preventing disability while enhancing the experience of pregnancy.[16] Not unlike the approach used to justify caesarean sections,[17] prenatal diagnosis is constructed as a way of avoiding "disaster."

The language of control, choice, and reassurance certainly makes prenatal diagnosis appear attractive. But while this discourse may be successful as a marketing strategy,[18] it relates a limited and highly selected story about prenatal diagnosis. Notwithstanding that even the most critical would probably agree prenatal diagnosis *can be* selectively reassuring[19] (for the vast majority of women who will learn that the fetus does not have Down syndrome or some other serious diagnosable disorder), this story alone is too simplistic. It does not take account of why reassurance is sought, how risk groups are generated and how eligibility for obtaining this kind of reassurance is determined. Whatever else, prenatal diagnosis *is* a means of separating fetuses we wish to develop from those we wish to discontinue. Prenatal diagnosis does approach children as consumer objects subject to quality control.

This is implicit in the general assumption that induced abortion will follow the diagnosis of fetal abnormality.[20] This assumption is reinforced by the rapid acceptance of CVS, which allows prenatal diagnosis to be carried out earlier and earlier in pregnancy when termination of a fetus found to be "affected" is taken for granted as less problematic.[21] The generally unquestioned assumption that pre-implantation diagnosis is better than prenatal diagnosis also undermines a monotonic reassurance rhetoric.[22] With pre-implantation (embryo) diagnosis, the selection objective is clear: only those embryos thought to be "normal" will be transferred and allowed to continue to develop.[23] Thus, embryo destruction is equated with induced abortion.[24] …

B. Constructing the "Need" for Prenatal Diagnosis

While reassurance has been constructed to justify health professionals' offers of prenatal diagnosis, genetic testing and screening have also been presented in the same biomedical literature as responses to the "needs" of pregnant women. They are seen as something they "choose." What does it mean, however, to "need" prenatal diagnosis, to "choose" to be tested?[25] Once again, a closer look at what appear to be obvious terms may illuminate some otherwise hidden aspects of geneticization and the prenatal diagnosis stories told in its voice.

We must first identify the concept of need as itself a problem and acknowledge that needs do not have intrinsic reality. Rather, needs are socially constructed and culture bound, grounded in current history, dependent on context, and, therefore, not universal.

With respect to prenatal diagnosis, "need" seems to have been conceptualized predominantly in terms of changes in capabilities for fetal diagnoses: women only come to "need" prenatal diagnosis after the test for some disorder has been developed. Moreover, the disorders to be sought are chosen exclusively by geneticists.[26] In addition, posing a "need" for testing to reduce the probability a woman will give birth to a child with some detectable characteristic rests on assumptions about the value of information, about which characteristics are or are not of value, and about which risks should or should not be taken. These assumptions reflect almost exclusively a white, middle-class perspective.[27]

This conceptualization of need is propelled by several features of contemporary childbearing.[28] First, given North American culture, where major responsibility for family health care in general, for the fetus she carries and for the child she births, is still allocated to a woman,[29] it is generally assumed that she must do all that is recommended or available to foster her child's health. At its extreme, this represents the pregnant woman as obligated to produce a healthy child. Prenatal diagnosis, as it is usually presented, falls into this category of behaviors recommended to pregnant women who would exercise their responsibilities as caregivers.[30] Consequently, to the extent that she is expected generally to do everything possible for the fetus/child, a woman may come to "need" prenatal diagnosis, and take testing for granted. Moreover, since an expert usually offers testing, and careseekers are habituated to follow through with tests ordered by physicians,[31] it is hardly surprising that they will perceive a need to be tested.[32] With prenatal diagnosis presented as a "way to avoid birth defects," to refuse testing, or perceive no need for it, becomes more difficult than to proceed with it.[33] This technology perversely creates a burden of not doing enough, a burden incurred when the technology is *not* used.[34]

A second feature, related to the first, is that women generally, and pregnant women specifically, are bombarded with behavioral directives[35] that are at least as likely to foster a sense of incompetence as to nourish a feeling of control.[36] ...

Third, prenatal diagnosis will necessarily be perceived as a "need" in a context, such as ours, that automatically labels pregnant women thirty-five years and over a "high risk" group.[37] ...

Fourth, as prenatal diagnosis becomes more and more routine for women thirty-five years and older in North America, the risks it seems to avoid (the birth of a child with Down syndrome) appear to be more ominous,[38] although the frequency of Down syndrome has not changed....

Fifth, on the collective level, prenatal diagnosis is generally presented as a response to the public health "need" to reduce unacceptably high levels of perinatal mortality and morbidity associated with perceived increases in "genetic" disorders. This reduction is of a special kind, in that prenatal diagnosis does not *prevent* the disease, as is usually claimed.[39] ...

"Needs" for prenatal diagnosis are being created simultaneously with refinements and extensions of testing techniques themselves.[40] In popular discourse—and with geneticists gener-

ally silent witnesses—genetic variations are being increasingly defined not just as problems, but, I suggest, as problems for which there is, or will be, a medical/technical solution. With but slight slippage these "problems" come to be seen as *requiring* a medical solution. This again hides the extent to which even "genetic" disease is a social/psychological experience as much as it is a biomedical one.[41] This process is likely to accelerate as gene mapping enlarges the numbers of individuals declared eligible for genetic testing and screening. Given the extent of human variation, the possibilities for constructing "needs" are enormous.

C. Prenatal Diagnosis and the Social Control of Abortion and Pregnancy

The third element in the prenatal discourse that I will consider here stems from the often told story that testing is an option that increases women's reproductive choices and control. This claim has had much attention in the literature and I will examine it only with respect to how some features of prenatal diagnosis do increase control, but allocate it to someone other than a pregnant woman herself. This is most apparent in the context of abortion.[42]

Without doubt, prenatal diagnosis has (re)defined the grounds for abortion[43]—who is justified in having a pregnancy terminated and why—and is a clear expression of the social control[44] inherent in this most powerful example of geneticization. Geneticists and their obstetrician colleagues are deciding which fetuses are healthy, what healthy means, and who should be born, thus gaining power over decisions to continue or terminate pregnancies that pregnant women themselves may not always be permitted to make.

To the extent that specialists' knowledge determines who uses prenatal diagnosis and for what reasons, geneticists determine conditions that will be marginalized, objects of treatment, or grounds for abortion.[45] Prenatal diagnosis is thus revealed as a biopolitical as well as a biomedical activity.[46] For example, an abortion may only be "legal" in some countries if the fetus has some recognized disorder,[47] and the justifying disorder only becomes "recognizable" because geneticists first decide to screen for it. Fuhrmann suggests that in Europe, in fact, geneticists significantly influenced legislators establishing limits within which abortion would be at all permissible, by arguing that access to abortion be maintained through a gestational age that reflected when results from amniocentesis might be available.[48] One wonders where limits might have been placed had first trimester chorionic villus sampling been available *before* amniocentesis? Would they have been more restrictive?...

V. CONCLUSION

... Prenatal testing and screening ... are most often presented as ways to decrease disease, to spare families the pain of having a disabled child, and to enhance women's choice. The best-selling stories about them speak of reassurance, choice, and control. As has also been suggested, this discourse presents a child born with some disorder requiring medical or surgical care as (exhibiting) a "failure."[49] This failed pregnancy theme is reinforced in counseling provided to these families when counselors emphasize how most fetuses with an abnormality abort spontaneously during pregnancy, are "naturally selected," as it were, and how prenatal testing is merely an improvement on nature.

Just as there are several ways to construe reassurance, choice, and control, the birth of a child with a structural malformation or other problem, "genetic" or otherwise, can be presented in other than biomedical terms. Is the story claiming that the pregnancy has malfunctioned (by not spontaneously aborting),[50] resulting in a baby with a malformation, any "truer" than the story suggesting that *society* has malfunctioned because it cannot accommodate the disabled in its midst?[51] Social conditions are as enabling or disabling as biological conditions. Why are biological variations that create differences between individuals seen as preventable or avoidable while social conditions that create similar distinctions are likely to be perceived as intractable givens?[52]

While "many people don't believe society has an obligation to adjust to the disabled individual,"[53] there is nothing inherent in malformation that makes this so. Consequently, arguing that social changes are "needed" to enable those with malformations to have rich lives is not an inherently less appropriate approach. Actually, it may be more appropriate, since malformation, a biomedical phenomenon, requires a social translation to become a "problem." Expanding prenatal diagnostic services may circumvent but will not solve the "problem" of birth defects; they focus on disability, not on society's discriminatory practices.[54] They can, at best, make only a limited contribution to help women have offspring free of disabilities, despite recent articles proposing prenatal diagnosis and abortion as ways to "improve" infant mortality and morbidity statistics.[55] Thus, as sociopolitical decisions about the place of genetic testing and screening in the health care system are made, it will be important to consider how problems are named and constructed so that we don't mistakenly assume the story told in the loudest voice is the only one—or that the "best seller" is best.

Unarguably, illness and disability *are* "hard" (difficult) issues,[56] and no one wants to add to the unnecessary suffering of any individual. But being "hard" neither makes illness or disability totally negative experiences,[57] nor does it mean they must all be eliminated or otherwise managed exclusively within the medical system. Women's desire for children without disability warrants complete public and private support. The question is how to provide this support in a way that does no harm....

When amniocentesis was introduced, abortion subsequent to a diagnosis of fetal abnormality was presented as a temporary necessity until treatment for the detected condition could be devised.[58] Advocates assumed that this would soon be forthcoming. With time, however, the gap between characterization and treatment of disease has widened.[59] New information from efforts at gene mapping will certainly increase the ability to detect, diagnose, and screen, but not to treat. A human gene map will identify variations in DNA patterns. Genes that "cause" specific disease, as

well as those associated with increased susceptibility to specific disorders, will be found.
Simultaneously, prenatal screening and testing are
evolving in a context where a "genetic approach"
to public health is gaining great favor.[60] All the
variations that will be mapped can become targets
of prenatal testing. Which targets will be selected
in the quest for improved public health? And who
will determine that they have been reached? Given
the extraordinary degree of genetic variability
within groups of people, what does "genetic
health" actually mean—and does it matter?…

Notes

1. In amniocentesis, a hollow needle is inserted through
a woman's abdomen and into the amniotic sac in
order to remove a small sample of the fluid that sur-
rounds the developing fetus. The procedure is usually preceded by an ultrasound examination to
document the age of the fetus and its location so that
an appropriate site for insertion of the amniocentesis
needle can be chosen. The fluid that is removed—
amniotic fluid—contains cells from the fetus that,
if allowed to divide in the laboratory, can then be
analyzed. In particular, one can count the number of
chromosomes in the cells, determine fetal sex and
carry out biochemical and specific genetic analyses
on these cells. Amniocentesis is performed at about
sixteen to twenty weeks' gestation, the second
trimester of pregnancy: before this time not enough
fluid or enough cells are available. Once a fluid
sample has been obtained, there is a further three to
four week wait for the analyses to be completed and
results to be available, since it takes this long to
grow a sufficient number of cells for study. Thus, if a
fetus is found to be affected with the condition for
which testing was done and the woman chooses to
abort the pregnancy, the abortion is not induced until
about the twentieth week, which is halfway through
the pregnancy. *See* E. Nightingale & M. Goodman,
Before Birth: Prenatal Testing for Genetic
Disease 32–35 (1990) [hereinafter Before Birth].
Recent technical developments that allow diagnoses
to be made following amplification of the genetic
materials in a single cell can shorten considerably
the time needed to obtain results. *See infra* note 4
and accompanying text.
2. *See infra* note 37 and accompanying text for a discussion of the social, rather than biological, bases
for categorizing women over 35 as "at risk."

3. Over 150 "single gene" disorders can now be
detected, and testing may be carried out for
women who have a documented family history of
one of these or who are otherwise known to be at
increased risk. Testing is not carried out for these
disorders without specific indications. *See generally* Antonarakis, *Diagnosis of Genetic Disorders
at the DNA Level*, 320 New Eng. J. Med. 153
(1989) (reviewing recent progress in identifying
single gene disorders).
4. In chorionic villus sampling (CVS), a small tube
(catheter) is inserted through the vagina and cervix.
It is then advanced, under ultrasound guidance,
until it reaches the placenta, from which a small
amount of tissue (chorionic villi) is removed. Some
obstetricians now obtain a sample through a needle
inserted into the abdomen instead. Any chromosomal or biochemical disorder can, in theory, be
diagnosed with tissues obtained by CVS, because
the cells of the fetus and placenta (which are
formed from chorionic villi) are genetically the
same. *See* Vekemans & Perry, *Cytogenic Analysis
of Chorionic Villi: A Technical Assessment*, 72
Hum. Genetics 307 (1986). This procedure was
first used successfully in China as early as 1975 to
determine fetal sex. Tietung Hosp. Dep't of
Obstetrics & Gynecology, *Fetal Sex Prediction by
Sex Chromatin of Chorionic Villi Cells During
Early Pregnancy*, 1 Chinese Med. J. 117 (1975).
CVS can be done as early as eight or nine weeks
after a woman's last menstrual period and, while
the results of tests carried out on the placental
tissue can be available within hours, a two or three
day waiting period is usually required. *See* Before
Birth, *supra* note 1, at 35–36. If a woman chooses
to abort the pregnancy following CVS, the abortion
can be carried out in the first trimester. Finally,
CVS does not appear more likely to cause a spontaneous abortion than amniocentesis. Canadian
Collaborative CVS – Amniocentesis Clinical Trial
Group. *Multicentre Randomised Clinical Trial of
Chorion Villus Sampling and Amniocentesis*, 1
Lancet 1, 4 (1989).
5. During an ultrasound examination, high frequency
sound waves are projected into the uterus; the
sound waves that are reflected back are resolved
visually to allow one to "see" the fetus on a
television-like display screen. A. Oakley, The
Captured Womb: A History of the Medical
Care of Pregnant Women 155–68 (1984).
6. See Before Birth, *supra* note 1, at 31–32. A consensus development conference in the United States
recently recommended reserving the use of ultra-

sound for pregnancies that may require it for specific medical reasons. PUB. HEALTH SERV., U.S. DEP'T OF HEALTH & HUM. SERVS., CONSENSUS DEVELOPMENT CONFERENCE: DIAGNOSTIC ULTRASOUND IMAGING IN PREGNANCY 11 (National Inst. Of Health Publications No. 667, 1984). This recommendation is clearly not being followed and, at present, in many major North American teaching hospitals, almost all pregnant women are referred for two "routine" ultrasound examinations—one before the twentieth week and one in the third trimester—for purposes of dating the pregnancy, even though the benefits of such a policy have not been established. Even more frequent scans are considered routine in France. As a specific tool for prenatal diagnosis, ultrasound can be used to identify certain malformations such as neural tube defects, cleft lip, or limb shortening in fetuses known to be at risk for one of the abnormalities. It can also be used to identify fetal sex. Most subtle malformations will not be identified when ultrasound is applied routinely on a non-diagnostic basis, however; the detailed examination that would be necessary requires more than the time that is usually allowed (or the machinery that is employed) when the primary goal is pregnancy dating. Nevertheless, some fetal problems can be diagnosed and their recognition may influence subsequent decisions about how pregnancy is managed.

7. *See* Chervenak, McCullough & Chervenak, *Prenatal Informed Consent for Somogram.* 161 AM. J. OBSTETRICS & GYNECOLOGY 857, 860 (1989); Lippman, *Access to Prenatal Screening: Who Decides?* 1 CANADIAN J. WOMEN L. 434 (1986) [hereinafter *Who Decides?*]. Chervenak and colleagues have recently called attention to the issue of informed consent for ultrasound, but their conclusions are troublesome. They consider the pregnant woman "the patient's fiduciary," the "patient" to them being the fetus. Chervenak, McCullough & Chervenak, *supra,* at 858. This suggests that the consent process they propose will be coercive. It is also worth noting that ultrasound is no longer the only genetic technology applied without prior consent. Screening for carriers of hemoglobin disorders, for example, is also done unbeknownst to the individuals being tested in certain jurisdictions. *See* Rowley, Loader, Sutera & Walden, *Do Pregnant Women Benefit from Hemoglobinopathy Carrier Detection?* 565 ANNALS N.Y. ACADEMY SCIENCES 152, 153 (1989) [hereinafter Rowley]. These authors noted that consent for sickle cell and other hemoglo-

binopathies was not obtained because: "Consent for screening was not routinely sought; providers agreed that obtaining timely informed consent required counseling approaching that to be provided to identified carriers and many providers declined to participate if they had to obtain it." Rowley, *supra,* at 153.

8. *See generally Who Decides?*, *supra* note 7, at 434.

9. *Id.*

10. *See, e.g.,* Kolker, *Advances in Prenatal Diagnosis: Social-psychological and Policy Issues,* 5 INT'L J. TECH. ASSESSMENT HEALTH CARE 601 (1989); see also Dalgaard & Norby, *Autosomal Dominant Polycystic Kidney Disease in the 1980s,* 36 CLINICAL GENETICS 320, 324 (1989) (placing importance on "selective reproduction prevention").

11. *See* PRESIDENT'S COMM'N FOR THE STUDY OF ETHICAL PROBLEMS IN MEDICAL AND BIOMEDICAL AND BEHAVIORAL RESEARCH, SCREENING AND COUNSELING FOR GENETIC CONDITIONS: THE ETHICAL, SOCIAL, AND LEGAL IMPLICATIONS OF GENETIC SCREENING, COUNSELING, AND EDUCATION PROGRAMS 55 (1983) [hereinafter PRESIDENT'S COMM'N]. ("In sum, the fundamental value of genetic screening and counseling is their ability to enhance the opportunities for the individual to obtain information about their personal health and childbearing risks and to make autonomous and noncoerced choices based on that information.")

12. *See* B. Rothman, RECREATING MOTHERHOOD: IDEOLOGY AND TECHNOLOGY IN A PATRIARCHAL SOCIETY 21 (1989) (describing the "commodification of life, towards treating people and parts of people … as commodities…. We work hard, some of us, at making the perfect product, what one of the doctors in the childbirth movement calls a 'blue ribbon baby.' "). *See also* Ewing, *Australian Perspectives on Embryo Experimentation: An Update,* 3 ISSUES REPRODUCTIVE & GENETIC ENGINEERING 119 (1990); Rothman, *The Decision to Have or Not to Have Amniocentesis for Prenatal Diagnosis,* in CHILDBIRTH IN AMERICA: ANTHROPOLOGICAL PERSPECTIVES 92, 92–98 (K. Michelson Ed. 1998) [hereinafter CHILDBIRTH IN AMERICA].

13. See Hill, *Your Morality or Mine? An Inquiry into the Ethics of Human Reproduction,* 154 AM. J. OBSTETRICS & GYNECOLOGY 1173, 1178–80 (1986).

14. *See generally* Royal College of Physicians of London, PRENATAL DIAGNOSIS AND GENETIC SCREENING: COMMUNITY AND SERVICE IMPLICATIONS (1989).

15. *See, e.g.,* WOMEN'S RIGHTS LITIGATION CLINIC, REPRODUCTIVE LAWS FOR THE 1990s: A BRIEFING

HANDBOOK (1987); *Who Decides?, supra* note 7, at 438.

16. McDonough, *Congenital Disability and Medical Research: The Development of Amniocentesis,* 16 WOMEN & HEALTH 137, 143–44 (1990). McDonough notes that three rationales for amniocentesis emerged from her survey: "The procedure offered those at risk the possibility of 'health' … [it] provided parents with reassurance and avoided abortion … [and it] prevent[ed] disease and disability." *Id.*

17. *See e.g.,* McClain, *Perceived Risk and Choice of Childbirth Service,* 17 SOC. SCI. & MED. 1857, 1862 (1983).

18. There is no evidence that control, autonomy, and reassurance are actually enhanced and not merely assumed to occur. In fact, there have been very few in-depth studies in this area, and the conclusions of these investigations seem to vary with the orientation of the investigator. Studies reported in the social science and feminist literature suggest that prenatal diagnosis removes control; studies reported in the biomedical literature are interpreted to show how reassurance is provided. For an overview of these studies, see Lippman, *Research Studies in Applied Human Genetics: A Quantitative Analysis and Critical Review (Biomedical) Literature,* to be published in AM. J. MED. GENETICS (1991). Much more ethnographic work in this area is required.

19. *See infra* text accompanying notes 48–51 [in original] for a reconstruction of the notion of reassurance.

20. *See supra* notes 12–13 and accompanying text.

21. This issue is discussed in A. Lippman, Led Astray by Genetic Maps (speech given, Ottawa, Canada, 1991). Treatment, often said to be a goal of early identification of affected fetuses, becomes even less likely with CVS. Pharmaceutical companies will not be motivated to invest in developing treatments for conditions that "need not occur." Rarely will they base business decisions on their social worth rather than on their financial value. This situation contains elements of an unusual conflict. Increasingly, geneticists are promising to have treatments available for a wide range of disorders and, for some conditions, therapeutic developments have occurred which make them far more benign than previously. The promises, and the available examples, are likely to be sufficiently persuasive that women "at-risk" may either make use of prenatal diagnosis less frequently or see less reason to abort an affected fetus than today. Yet, at the same time, the very availability of prenatal

diagnosis and abortion may be seen as justifications for *not* investing in the further development of these therapies that parents will have been led to expect. *Cf.* Varekamp, Suurmeijer, Bröcker-Vriends, Van Dijck, Smit, Rosendaal & Briët, *Carrier Testing and Prenatal Diagnosis for Hemophilia: Experiences and Attitudes of 549 Potential and Obligate Carriers,* 37 AM. J. MED. GENETICS 147, 153 (1990) [hereinafter Varekamp] (noting decrease in hemophilia screening as treatment capabilities increased).

22. *See* Bell, *Prenatal Diagnosis: Current Status and Future Trends*, in HUMAN GENETIC INFORMATION: SCIENCE, LAW & ETHICS 1836 (Ciba Foundation Series 1990). *See also* Kolker, *supra* note 10, at 612 (prevention is "clearly cheaper than providing services for those with genetic disorders"); Modell, *Cystic Fibrosis Screening and Community Genetics,* 27 J. MED. GEN. 475, 476 (1990) ("undesirable [diseases] may be all but eradicated"); Dalgaard & Norby, *supra* note 10, at 323–24 ("access to selective reproductive prevention" is important).

23. S. Wymelenberg, SCIENCE AND BABIES: PRIVATE DECISIONS, PUBLIC DILEMMAS 130 (1990).

24. In fact, some consider the combined procedures of *in vitro* fertilization and embryo diagnosis to be "ethically better" than prenatal diagnosis for detecting problems because it "avoids" abortion. *See* Michael & Buckle, *Screening for Genetic Disorders: Therapeutic Abortion and IVF*, 16 J. MED. ETHICS 43 (1990). *But see* J. Testart, LE MONDE DIPLOMATIQUE 24 (1990) (suggesting that it is the very need to consider abortion ["de terribles responsabilités"] that is perhaps the best safeguard against ordinary eugenics ["l'eugenisme ordinaire"]).

25. While those in need are identified explicitly as (certain) pregnant women, it is worth noting that clinical geneticists, themselves, have a need for this technology, too. For instance, when a child is born with a malformation, geneticists likely feel most "helpful" when prenatal diagnosis, a technological palliative for the pains of etiologic ignorance, can be offered. Saying that the malformation is not likely to happen again, given the usually low empiric recurrence risks associated with most of these problems, is not nearly as comforting for genetic counselors as is offering *in utero* detection. Counselors "need" this technique for the satisfactory performance of their jobs no less than they believe a family "needs" prenatal diagnosis to prevent the birth of a second affected child.

26. *See* Lippman, *Prenatal Diagnosis: Reproductive Choice? Reproductive Control?* [hereinafter

Reproductive Choice?], in THE FUTURE OF HUMAN REPRODUCTION 182, 187 (C. Overall ed. 1989) [hereinafter THE FUTURE OF HUMAN REPRODUCTION] (consideration of prenatal diagnosis as a professional resource).

27. *See* Nsiah-Jefferson, *Reproductive Laws, Women of Color and Low Income Women* in REPRODUCTIVE LAWS FOR THE 1990s 17, 17–58 (S. Cohen & N. Taub eds. 1988) [hereinafter REPRODUCTIVE LAWS FOR THE 1990s] (discussing potential areas of cultural conflict in genetic counseling).

28. There is an extensive literature on "medicalization" in general and on the medicalization of pregnancy and childbirth *per se* in which this discussion is rooted and from which it derives guidance. *See, e.g.,* A. Oakley, *supra* note 5, at 275. ("The medicalization of everyday life is a phenomenon described in many radical and liberal critiques of medicine."); *id* at 276 ("For both birth and death normal signs have become neon lights flagging risks which demand and validate medical intervention."); Raymond, *Feminist Ethics, Ecology, and Vision*, in TEST-TUBE WOMEN 427, 427–37 (R. Arditti, R. Klein & S. Minden eds. 1984) [hereinafter TEST-TUBE WOMEN]; I. Zola, *Healthism and Disabling Medicalization*, in I. Illich, I. Zola, J. McKnight, J. Caplan & H. Shaiken, DISABLING PROFESSIONS 41 (1977); Zola, *In the Name of Health and Illness: On Some Socio-Political Consequences of Medical Influence,* 9 SOC. SCI. & MED. 83, 85–87 (1975) (noting that control by medical value not achieved through political means but by "medicalization"); Zola, *Medicine as an Institution of Social Control*, 20 SOCIOLOGY REV. 487 (1972); *see also* Lewin, *By Design: Reproductive Strategies and the Meaning of Motherhood*, in SEXUAL POLITICS OR REPRODUCTION 123, 123–38 (H. Homans ed. 1985) [hereinafter THE SEXUAL POLITICS OF REPRODUCTION] (women "must adapt" to "motherhood" but can also approach it as "active strategists").

29. See Oakley, *Smoking in Pregnancy: Smokescreen or Risk Factor? Towards a Materialist Analysis,* 11 SOCIOLOGY HEALTH & ILLNESS 311 (1989).

30. See Farrant, *supra* note 50 [in original], at 96; Oakley *supra* note 29, at 311.

31. *See* R. Hatcher & H. Thompson, SATISFACTION WITH OBSTETRICAL CARE AMONG CANADIAN WOMEN (Health Servs. Res. Unit, Department of Community Health, Queen's Univ., Kingston, Ontario 1987) (results of a survey showing pregnant women's reluctance to question medical authority).

32. *See* Lippman, *supra* note 26, at 182. Physicians may pressure women into being tested, even using false

information to do so. Marteau, Kidd, Cook, Michie, Johnston, Slack & Shaw, *Perceived Risk not Actual Risk Predicts Uptake of Amniocentesis,* 96 BRIT. J. OBSTETRICS & GYNAECOLOGY 739 (1989).

33. See Hubbard & Henifin, *Genetic Screening of Prospective Parents and of Workers: Some Scientific and Social Issues,* 15 INT'L J. HEALTH SERVS. 231 (1985); Rothman, *The Meaning of Choice in Reproductive Technology,* in TEST-TUBE WOMEN, *supra* note 28, at 23. I have previously discussed the "burden" of decisionmaking in the context of genetic counseling and a similar "burden" would seem to exist here. See Lippman-Hand & Fraser, *Genetic Counseling I: Parents' Perceptions of Uncertainty,* 4 AM. J. MED. GENETICS 51, 5863 (1979) [hereinafter *Genetic Counseling I*]; Lippman-Hand & Fraser, *Genetic Counseling II: Making Reproductive Choices,* 4 AM. J. MED. GENETICS 73 (1978) [hereinafter *Genetic Counseling II*]. This theme is present in contemporary literature as demonstrated by Goldstein's reference to the "momentous decision" that childbearing now involves. R. Goldstein, THE MIND-BODY PROBLEM 200 (1983). Hubbard and Henifin, in fact, identify a "new Catch-22" wherein participating in a genetic screening program may lead to a person's being identified as a "genetic deviant," but failure to participate (or to abort a fetus diagnosed with a disorder *in utero*) may lead to her being labeled as a "social deviant." Hubbard & Henifin, *supra.* At 231–48.

34. The degree of this burden is demonstrated by the frequency with which women queried about their reasons for having prenatal diagnosis say that they "had no choice." Sjögren & Uddenberg, *Decision Making During the Prenatal Procedure,* 8 PRENATAL DIAGNOSIS 263 (1988). *See* Kirejczyk, *A Question of Meaning? Controversies About the NRT's in the Netherlands,* 3 ISSUES REPRODUCTIVE & GENETIC ENGINEERING 23 (1990) (individuals often accept a medical technique because of fear that they might later regret not having done so); *see also* A. Finger, PAST DUE: A STORY OF DISABILITY, PREGNANCY AND BIRTH (1990); Beck-Gernsheim, *From the Pill to Test-Tube Babies: New Options, New Pressures in Reproductive Behavior,* in HEALING TECHNOLOGY: FEMINIST PERSPECTIVES 23 (1988) [hereinafter HEALING TECHNOLOGY]; Rapp, *Moral Pioneers: Women, Men and Fetuses in a Frontier of Reproductive Technology,* 13 WOMEN & HEALTH 101 (1987).

35. B. Rothman, *supra* note 12, at 92–97. Women are expected to behave in accordance with norms set

up by those in power. *See* Rodgers, *Pregnancy as Justifications for Loss of Judicial Autonomy*, in THE FUTURE OF HUMAN REPRODUCTION, *supra* note 26, at 174.

36. *See e.g.,* Fleischer, *Ready for Any Sacrifice? Women in IVF Programmes*, 3 ISSUES REPRODUCTIVE & GENETIC ENGINEERING 1 (1990) (referring to a "code of good conduct" pregnant women ought to follow); *see also* M. De Koninck & F. Saillant, ESSAI SUR LA SANTÉ DES FEMMES (Conseil du Statut de la femme 1981); A. Quéniart, LE CORPS PARADOXAL: REGARDS DE FEMMES SUR LA MATERNITÉ (1988); Simkin, *Childbearing in Social Context*, 15 WOMEN & HEALTH 5 (1989) (all discussing the ideology of risk and behavioral expectations in pregnancy).

37. *See* Fuhrmann, *Impact, Logistics and Prospects of Traditional Prenatal Diagnosis*, 36 CLINICAL GENETICS 378, 380 (1988). This categorization is more a cultural than biological creation. *See* Bourret, *Le temps, l'espace en Génétique: Intervention Médicale et Géographique Sociale du gène*, 6 SCIENCES SOCIALES ET SANTÉ 171 (1988); A. Lippman, The Geneticization of Health and Illness: Implications for Social Practice (manuscript in preparation based on presentation at National Ass'n for Science, Tech. & Soc'y, Washington, D.C., Feb. 2, 1991). It reflects prevailing ideas about the kinds of children women should have and when the probability for them is or is not diminished. *See* Finkelstein, *Biomedicine and Technocratic Power*, HASTINGS CENTER REP. 1990, at 13, 14–16; *see also infra* note 43 for a discussion of the role of genetics in creating these ideas. Age has thus become more than an event, a birthday; it has been redefined as a marker, a risk, although nothing inherent in it makes it so. *See* Fuhrmann, *supra.* at 380 (35 is the crucial age in North America); J. Moatti, J. Lanoë, C. LeGalés, H. Gardent, C. Julian & S. Aymé, Economic Assessment of Prenatal Diagnosis in France (unpublished manuscript presented at Joint Meeting of European Health Economic Societies, Barcelona, Spain. Sept. 21–23, 1989) (age 38 in France); Sjögren & Uddenberg, *supra* note 34, at 263 (age 37 in Sweden). This age marker may even serve to stigmatize the "older" woman. *See* Hubbard & Henifin, *supra* note 33, at 238 (1985). Further discussion of the arbitrariness of age 35 as a criterion for access to prenatal diagnosis can be found in *Who Decides?, supra* note 7, at 434; Vekemans & Lippman, *Letter to the Editor: Eligibility Criteria for Anmiocentesis*, 17 AM. J. MED. GENETICS 531 (1986).

38. This may be an example of what Tversky and Kahnemann have called the "availability" heuristic. Tversky & Kahneman, *Availability: A Heuristic for Judging Frequency and Probability,* 5 COGNITIVE PSYCHOLOGY 207 (1973). That is, having become familiar through constant reference to it and to prenatal diagnosis, Down syndrome may be perceived by the general population as "worse" and as more frequent than it is statistically.

39. *See, e.g.* Modell, *Cystic Fibrosis Screening and Community Genetics*, 27 J. MED. GENETICS 475 ("Cystic fibrosis ... is fast becoming preventable ... [because] [t]he gene in which mutation can lead to CF ... has recently been identified.... [This creates] an imminent need to set up population screening for CF carriers.").

40. These techniques are likely to be driven by financial considerations of the pharmaceutical companies developing them. *See, e.g.,* D. Nelkin & L. Tancredi, DANGEROUS DIAGNOSTICS: THE SOCIAL POWER OF BIOLOGICAL INFORMATION 33–36 (1989); A. Lippman, *supra* note 21; *cf.* Note, *Patents for Critical Pharmaceuticals: The AZT Case*, 17 AM. J.L. & MED. 145 (1991) (analyzing the validity of pharmaceutical companies' claims that without a federally granted monopoly, they would not have the incentive to research and develop orphan drugs).

41. *See* Shiloh, Waisbren & Levy, *A Psychosocial Model of a Medical Problem: Maternal PKU*, 10 J. PRIMARY PREVENTION 51 (1989).

42. For thorough analyses of the question of women's control, see generally Rapp, *Chromosomes and Communication: The Discourse of Genetic Counseling.* 2 MED. ANTHROPOLOGY Q. 143 (1988).

43. In fact, the availability of amniocentesis "influenced legislation so that the upper limit of gestational age for legally tolerated termination of pregnancy was adjusted to the requirements of second trimester prenatal diagnosis in several countries." Fuhrmann, *supra* note 37, at 378. Evidently, geneticists can accomplish what women's groups cannot: a revisioning of abortion.

44. The term "social control" is used in accord with its original use to embrace "the widest range of influence and regulation imposed by society upon the individual." D. Gordon, *Clinical Science and Clinical Expertise: Changing Boundaries Between Art and Science in Medicine*, in BIOMEDICINE EXAMINED 257 (M. Lock & D. Gordon eds. 1988).

45. *Reproductive Choice? supra* note 26, at 187–192.

46. Finkelstein, *Biomedicine and Technocratic Power,* HASTINGS CENTER REP. 1990, at 14–16.

47. Fetal abnormality as grounds for abortion is of fairly recent vintage, having first become "legal" in the United States in 1967 in response to a rubella epidemic. The Canadian Medical Association gave its approval the same year. Beck, *Eugenic Abortion: An Ethical Critique*, 143 CANADIAN MED. ASS'N J. 181, 181–84 (1990). Today, members of the general population as well as physicians regularly and strongly agree that fetal abnormality is a justification for abortion. *See* Annas, *The Supreme Court, Privacy and Abortion*, 321 NEW ENG. J. MED. 1200 (1989); Breslau, *Abortion of Defective Fetuses: Attitudes of Mothers of Congenitally Impaired Children*, 49 J. MARRIAGE FAMILY 839 (1987); Varekamp, *supra* note 21, at 147.

48. *See* Fuhrmann, *supra* note 37, at 383–84. A recent example of the use of genetics to set social policy in this area is the position taken by the American Society of Human Genetics with respect to possible restrictions on abortion under consideration in various parts of the United States. This professional group has proposed as model legislation that any pregnant female whose pregnancy has not reached the point of viability and who has been informed by a licensed or certified health care professional that her fetus (or fetuses) is/are likely to have a serious genetic or congenital disorder shall have the right, among other options, to choose to terminate her pregnancy. This right shall extend to situations where the female is at significantly increased risk for bearing a child with a serious disorder for which precise prenatal diagnosis is not available. Letter from Phillip J. Riley to the author. The merits for/against this position aside, it certainly demonstrates how geneticists seek to influence the resolution of fundamentally political, legal (and ethical) problems.

49. Dunstan, *Screening for Fetal and Genetic Abnormality: Social and Ethical Issues,* 25 J. MED. GENETICS 290 (1988).

50. Dunstan thus sees genetic screening and "selective abortion" as a "rationalized adjunct to natural processes" in which "defective products" (babies) are "discard[ed] spontaneously." *Id.* at 292.

51. For a full development of these ideas, see Asch, *Reproductive Technology and Disability*, in REPRODUCTIVE LAWS FOR THE 1990s, *supra* note 27, at 69; Asch & Fine, *Shared Dreams: A Left Perspective on Disability Rights and Reproductive Rights*, in WOMEN WITH DISABILITIES 197 (M. Fine & A. Asch eds. 1988).

52. There would seem to be similar assumptions beneath the transformation of problems with dirty workplaces into problems with women workers who may become pregnant. *See, e.g.,* Bertin, *Women's Health and Women's Rights: Reproductive Health Hazards in the Workplace*, in HEALING TECHNOLOGY, *supra* note 34, at 289, 297 (advocating legislation requiring safe workplaces and prohibiting sterility requirements); Woolhandler & Himmelstein, *Ideology in Medical Science: Class in the Cliinic,* 28 SOC. SCI. & MED. 1205 (1989).

53. Levin, *International Perspectives on Treatment Choice in Neonatal Intensive Care Units,* 30 SOC. SCI. & MED. 901, 903 (1990) (citation omitted).

54. For a further discussion on this, see McDonough, *supra* note 16, at 149.

55. Powell-Griner & Woolbright, *Trends in Infant Deaths from Congenital Anomalies: Results from England and Wales, Scotland, Sweden and the United States,* 19 INT'L. J. EPIDEMIOLOGY 391, 397 (1990) (probable that level of infant mortality will be influenced by prenatal screening and selective abortion); Saari-Kemppainen, Karjalainen, Ylostalo & Heinonen, *Ultrasound Screening and Prenatal Mortality: Controlled Trial of Systematic One-Stage Screening in Pregnancy*, 336 LANCET 387, 391 (1990) (Researchers of ultrasound screening in Helsinki, Finland concluded that "[t]he decrease in perinatal mortality of about half in this trial can be explained mainly by the detection of major fetal anomalies by ultrasound screening and the subsequent termination of these pregnancies.").

56. Lippman, *Genetics and Public Health: Means, Goals and Justices,* to be published in AM. J. HUM. GENETICS (1991). *See* A. Finger, *supra* note 34; P. Kaufert, The Production of Medical Knowledge: Genes, Embryos and Public Policy (paper presented at *Gender, Science and Medicine II* conference, Toronto, Ontario, Nov. 2, 1990). Moreover, illness and disability are *hard* (i.e., difficult) issues partly because society defines them as such, in its decisions about how (not) to allocate resources to deal with them. Unfortunately, since resources are always "scarce," the programs or projects that do (not) get supported will merely be those which policymakers choose (not) to fund. No specific choice is inherent in the limited budgets available, although the requirement that choices be made is. In choosing how to deal with health problems, budget limitations may sometimes be secondary to limitations in our visions about what to do. And, in choosing how to approach (even) "hard" issues, genetic prevention is but one possibility.

57. Asch, *Reproductive Technology and Disability,*
    supra note 51, at 70.

58. See Friedmann, *Opinion: the Human Genome*
    Project—Some Implications of Extensive "Reverse
    Genetic" Medicine, 46 AM. J. HUM. GENETICS 407,
    412 (1990).

59. *Id.* at 411.

60. Lippman, Messing & Mayer, *Is Genome mapping*
    the Way to Improve Canadians' Health?
    81 CANADIAN J. PUB. HEALTH 397 (1990).

A Critique of Some Feminist Challenges to Prenatal Diagnosis

Dorothy C. Wertz and John C. Fletcher

INTRODUCTION: THE NEW CRITICS OF PRENATAL DIAGNOSIS

In earlier years, most opposition to prenatal diagnosis came from religious groups opposed to abortion.[1] Recently, however, the strongest arguments against widespread use of prenatal diagnostic procedures have come from some feminists[2-4] and some advocates for people with disabilities.[5, 6] Although these critics do not represent the entire range of the feminist or disability rights movements, they have provided fuel for political moves that would limit use of prenatal diagnosis and other reproductive technologies, especially in parts of Europe. Since these arguments have important implications for public policy, it is important to examine them carefully. The arguments run as follows: Women are being coerced into having prenatal diagnosis by their doctors and by the culture. There is a "technological imperative" to have prenatal diagnosis simply because it exists. Women feel guilty if they do not use it. Many feel that they "have no choice" about having prenatal diagnosis or aborting a fetus with a genetic condition.[3] Both women and their doctors are pawns of larger economic, class, and patriarchal forces.[2, 7, 8] Their actions are determined by social class interests and by society's rejection of persons with disabilities. Medicine and the biotechnology industry are using prenatal diagnosis to exploit women for professional and monetary gain.

According to the critics, prenatal diagnosis has become a "search and destroy mission"[9] to eliminate fetuses with disabilities. This amounts to discrimination before birth and will lead to reduced benefits for people with disabilities. Society may decide that it is easier and cheaper to prevent their births than it is to care for them. In siding with persons who have been "victimized," many feminists have felt a contradiction between empowerment of people with disabilities and selective abortion of fetuses with disabilities.[2, 3, 5–8, 10–15] Prenatal diagnosis could become a eugenic program comparable with those used in Nazi Germany to eliminate those with "lives not worth living." Individual choices in prenatal diagnosis have social consequences and are therefore eugenic. By aborting fetuses with certain characteristics, women and families are labeling certain kinds of persons as not worthy of life. Assuming that most individuals make similar choices, that these choices will be influenced by prevailing economic and social standards, and that prenatal diagnosis will become routine in most pregnancies, we will sooner or later arrive at a eugenic society. Although all critics defend women's right to abortion, including abortions for genetic disorders or fetal malformations, some regard abortion after prenatal diagnosis as more ethically problematic than abortion of a healthy fetus for even the most "frivolous" reason.[3–6, 11, 16, 18] If a woman does not want to be pregnant at all, so be it. But to not want to continue a pregnancy after unfavorable findings from prenatal diagnosis is to commit a eugenic act.

In sum, according to the critics, the world is *not* better off for having prenatal diagnosis available. Some women may experience genuine relief at avoiding the burden of caring for a child with a disability, but most women experience only increased anxiety and the burden of unwanted decision-making. Some critics claim that most women would not terminate pregnancies after unfavorable prenatal diagnostic findings if they had a real choice, namely the choice of raising the child in a supportive and accepting society. According to this argument, all disability, including mental retardation, is socially constructed and can be overcome.

These arguments should not be regarded as typical of all feminists. There are sound reasons to believe that most feminists, especially those interested in equal rights in employment, support the use of prenatal diagnosis.[19, 20] Nor do all activists for disability rights oppose prenatal diagnosis. Patient organizations for people with genetic conditions usually tacitly support prenatal diagnosis or keep an open mind on the issue. They are often reluctant, however, to discuss openly the possibility of aborting fetuses who may be similar to their own living children. Some well-known advocates for people with disabilities also believe in keeping an open mind, although they believe that women should consider carefully and compassionately before terminating for conditions such as blindness or deafness whose effects can be overcome. They also believe that women should be free to make individual decisions about what kinds of children they are able and willing to raise.[5]

It is important to reply to the critics' arguments for two reasons. First, political actions often have unintended consequences. Feminist criticisms of prenatal diagnosis have provided fuel for religious groups and others who wish to ban abortion. Second, the critics' arguments have touched upon areas that give many women a deep unease—social coercion, definitions of normalcy, and class distinctions in access to medical care, to name a few. Many arguments have at least partial validity. In what follows, we examine feminist criticisms of prenatal diagnosis.

RESPONSES TO THE CRITICS
The Social Context of Choice

Some feminists have claimed that women say they "have no choice" about having prenatal diagnosis, implying that they have been pressured into it.[3] Yet when asked in surveys or interviews, most women say that they had a free choice, without interference from their partners, family, or doctors.[21, 30] Both statements may be true, depending upon the meaning of "choice." If choice is the absence of legal coercion or coercion by partner or family, clearly women have a choice. There is no evidence of direct coercion by doctors, as some have alleged.[31] If choice is interpreted in the broader context of economic and social realities, however, many women may feel that the possible alternative to prenatal diagnosis—raising a child with a disability—is so unattractive that it does not present a real choice. In the liberal tradition or in socialism, freedom of choice means the practical ability to act upon one's decision.[32, 33] ...

In a sense, prenatal diagnosis is an extension of earlier methods to ensure a "better quality" baby. It belongs alongside other methods, such as the cesarean sections that now account for about one fourth of births in the United States and that are performed largely to protect the baby's intellectual potential. Few women have rejected these methods as long as they appeared to produce superior, or at least healthy, babies. Fewer still decided to give birth outside hospitals, where they could avoid use of high technology. Despite the plethora of books on natural birth, independent (lay) midwifery, birthing centers, and homebirth, most women continue to give birth in hospitals. Perhaps 1% of North American women give birth at home.[35] Most women fear that something could go wrong for the baby if they give birth in the absence of high technology, despite considerable evidence that home is as safe as hospital for low-risk women and newborns.[34] Perhaps there is an analogy here with choices about prenatal diagnosis. The choice exists, but the possibility of having a child with a severe birth defect, if the birth could have been prevented, weighs so heavily on women's minds that it is as if they had no choice.

Yet women's stated beliefs that they had a choice are more than "false consciousness." The fact that about 7% in both the United Kingdom[36] and in California[37] have refused maternal serum α-fetoprotein (MSAFP, an indicator of possible spina bifida in the fetus) screening or prenatal diagnosis on moral grounds, even when tests are offered free of charge under national or state health-care systems, suggests that some women are in fact making choices, instead of acting as the puppets of larger social forces.

The history of prenatal diagnosis also points to women's active and personal choices. In contrast to other areas of experimentation in the history of obstetrics, where poor women especially were exploited as research subjects,[34, 38, 39] the history of prenatal diagnosis suggests that women actively encouraged research in this area. Women who participated in the early experiments with amniocentesis tended to be white, middle-class, well-educated, and vocal, characteristics that encouraged physicians to pursue this line of research with more vigor than they might have otherwise.[40] The actions of individual women, such as Dolores Becker, in suing physicians for not offering prenatal diagnosis have ensured that it became a routine part of obstetrical practice.[40–42] The women (and their husbands) who initiated these suits were not acting as the pawns of social class interests. Many would have sued even if there were optimum social supports for their children, because social support still does not provide them with the child for which they had hoped.

It is extremely difficult, if not impossible, for women to choose to reject technologies approved by the obstetrical profession. Once tests are offered, to reject them is a rejection of modern faith in science and also a rejection of modern beliefs that women should do everything possible for the health of the future child. Women may have more choice about prenatal diagnosis, however, than about most other childbirth technologies, largely because they are not confined to a hospital at the time of testing and because there is strong religious and cultural support in many groups for carrying a child with a disability to term.

Effects of Disability on Women's Lives

If the economic and social cost of a healthy child is greater to women than ever before, on account of women's entry into the workforce, the cost of a child with a disability is enormous. The irony is that women who have invested heavily in their education or careers and who have postponed childbearing until their late thirties or early forties face the highest risks for having children with chromosomal abnormalities. These are the women who have the most to lose, economically and socially. Most of the care for children with disabilities falls on the mother.[43–45] Not only must she give up much of her paid employment, but she must often adopt motherhood as her primary self-identification. In a world where many women now identify themselves as workers, to identify oneself first as a mother places a woman in a position of relative isolation. Furthermore, she may be a mother for the rest of her life. Medicine has greatly extended the lives of people with disabilities, so that most people with retardation now live a nearly normal lifespan. It is not uncommon for parents in their eighties to be caring for children with Down syndrome who are in their fifties.[46, 47] When the elderly parents die, care usually falls on the siblings.[48] Some siblings have expressed resentment at the extra attention given to the affected person and their own corresponding neglect in childhood.[48–50]

Most people with mental retardation, perhaps 80%, live at home under the care of parents or relatives.[51, 52] This has always been the case. Historically, the majority of people with retardation or developmental disabilities have always lived with their families. Institutions were for those who had no families, or who were violent or profoundly retarded (and almost half of those with profound retardation lived at home). Society has never provided either institutional care or in-home care for most persons with mental disabilities. In 1967, the peak year for institutionalization in the United States, 197,000 persons with mental retardation or developmental disabilities were institutionalized, out of an estimated one to two million. In 1990, 82,000 were institutionalized. Cost-saving is not the only reason for deinstitutionalization. Many child psychologists have argued that children with retardation or developmental disorders are more likely to develop their full potential at home under the care of their parents, than in an institutional setting. It is now virtually impossible for parents in many areas to place a newborn or infant in an institution no matter how severe the retardation. In-home care, even occasional respite care, is difficult to obtain. Under these conditions, the choice of not having prenatal diagnosis appears to be no choice at all, unless a woman is opposed to abortion under most conditions.[53] For pregnant women who will be single parents, as is the case for 22% of white women, 34% of Hispanic women, and 59% of African-American women, the prospect of raising a child with a disability may be even more distressing.[54, 55]

Much of the literature on effects of prenatal diagnosis on attitudes toward people with disabilities regards all disabilities as a generic class and treats them as if equal.[2, 3, 5, 6, 17, 18, 56–60] This is not a realistic approach. Most physical and some mental disabilities can be overcome with social support and changes in the physical environment.[61] Some mental and neurologic disabilities, however, require lifetime care and overwhelm the parents' lives. Such disabilities may never be overcome even with massive economic and social support. Although increased support is necessary in the interests of social justice, it may not present an alternative to prenatal diagnosis and selective abortion in all cases. The

writings of parents of children with disabilities present a mixed message. Although generally intended to inspire by presenting triumphs over adversity, many of these biographies describe the immense effort and sacrifice on the part of the parents.[62–66] There is no clear outcome that might be labeled "joy."[67] Instead, many parents write as if the grieving process that began at the child's birth continues throughout the child's life, as a never ending sense of loss.[68, 69] Parents' accounts represent after-the-fact, largely successful, attempts at coping. Those whose children have mental retardation or behavioral problems have described the immense difficulty of daily life. We do not know what these parents might have done if they had had a choice. Probably many would prefer not to think about the possibility, because to negate the birth of a child like theirs is to devalue both their child and their own coping efforts.

It is impossible to return to a pretechnological state in which women do not have to face the possibility of prenatal diagnosis and abortion. Although some feminists imply that such a return to nature would be desirable,[4] medicine has so transformed nature that we can no longer refer to "what nature intended" as a guide for either prenatal or postnatal decisions. In childbirth, North Americans lost the sense of nature sometime in the nineteenth century.[34] We must face the fact that we live in a technological age that women themselves helped to bring about.[40, 70]

Parents have always made choices—often negative ones—about infants with disabilities; for centuries Europeans exposed or abandoned such newborns, usually placing them where they would *not* be found by kindly passersby.[71] The Catholic Church made no effort to eradicate this custom. Many of these infants would have died anyway before modern medicine. Although some modern writers have argued in favor of allowing or even helping newborns with severe disabilities to die,[72, 75] legal or hospital regulations, together with the urge of perinatologists to save life, effectively prevent this. It is no longer possible for parents to decide whether to have a lifesaving operation on a newborn with mental retardation;

in most cases, the hospital will overrule the parents and proceed with the operation.[74, 75]

For most parents, choices are now limited to the preconception or prebirth period. Having foreclosed choices that once existed postnatally, medicine now offers new choices prenatally. The increase in use of prenatal diagnosis in Canada,[75–77] Denmark,[78] Germany,[79] the United Kingdom,[36, 80, 81] and the United States[82–86] suggests rapid uptake of the new technologies. Women who have had amniocentesis and have aborted fetuses with Down syndrome write of their relief at being able to avoid becoming mothers of severely disabled children.[87–92] Even though the decision was often difficult and psychologically stressful, these women believe that prenatal diagnosis freed them to go on with their lives, to continue their careers, and to have healthy children. While sensitive to the need to provide adequate supports for those with disabilities, they believe that prenatal diagnosis will continue to offer the best alternative for many women carrying fetuses with serious mental retardation.[29, 30, 90–92]

Women could, of course, decide to carry the child to term and place it for adoption, but few do so even though there are waiting lists of people willing to adopt children with Down syndrome. (Adoption is less likely for infants with profound mental retardation or likelihood of death within the first few years.) Most parents apparently consider giving up a child with a disability for adoption as the most socially "deviant" course of action that they could take. Many doctors do not even mention this possibility. If there is a choice that parents feel they really do not have, that choice is probably giving up their baby for adoption, an alternative which receives little social support.

"The Exploitation of Women"

Exploitation is not the same as coercion. As Feinberg has pointed out, exploitation can exist in the absence of coercion, as long as one party benefits disproportionately from an interaction.[93] Critics argue that the new reproductive technologies exploit women and aggrandize the medical–scientific establishment or the biotechnology industry. At the extreme, some critics claim that *all* modern technology is a manipulative patriarchal plot against women, or a form of "quality control" that ensures that children meet men's specifications.[94–102] …

Another reason why critics label prenatal diagnosis as exploitative is that it is big business for the companies that manufacture the equipment and conduct the tests. Commercialization creates laboratory capacity. It then becomes necessary to increase consumer demand in order to keep the laboratory working at capacity. Laboratory capacity in the United States has increased to the point that the original recommendations of government bodies[103] or professional organizations[104, 107] about maternal age, which were recognized at the time as arbitrary, have been relaxed. The majority of geneticists would perform prenatal diagnosis for any anxious woman, even without indications of age or family history. In 1985, 78% of United States geneticists would perform prenatal diagnosis for an anxious woman of 25 with no medical or genetic indications for its use, and an additional 11% would offer a referral.[106] More women (76%) than men (61%) geneticists would perform prenatal diagnosis for anxiety alone. Most believed that they were alleviating anxiety. Socially speaking, they were opening the door to making prenatal diagnosis a routine procedure in prenatal care. Most pregnant women are anxious. Not all tests are invasive or risky. The so-called "triple test" (α-fetoprotein, estriol, and human chorionic gonadotropin) is a blood test that poses no risk. It was applied to women in 1992 and may become routine. It serves to determine which women should have amniocentesis. Having proceeded as far as a "positive" blood test that indicates possible bad news, many women will find it difficult to decline further testing.

This is what critics mean by exploitation. The biotechnology industry is making large sums of money, and women are having more tests, which become more difficult to refuse. That most women probably welcome the tests does not change the facts of commercialization.

Prenatal diagnosis is already one of the most frequently used procedures in prenatal care[106, 107] and could become routine in most pregnancies.

Is Prenatal Diagnosis a Eugenic Program?

The underlying concern of those who criticize prenatal diagnosis is often summarized in the word *eugenics.* Most modern authors associate eugenics with Nazi programs to eradicate Jews, Gypsies, and other "inferior" groups.[108–112] Historians of the eugenics movements in Canada,[113–114] the United States,[115, 116] Germany,[117] France,[118] and the United Kingdom[119] remind us that genetics has served corrupt political and social ends.

Eugenics has many meanings, so many, in fact, that the Commission of the European Communities has omitted it from its revised human genome proposal (1989) as lacking precision.[120] According to Paul's excellent review,[33] the various definitions of eugenics include the following dichotomies: (1) intention versus effect, (2) science versus social policy, (3) coercion versus voluntary choice, and (4) individual versus social responsibility. The following paragraphs outline Paul's argument.

Intention versus effect. If eugenics means intentions, it does not apply to most abortions following prenatal diagnosis, because women do not abort with the intent of improving the gene pool.[121, 122] If eugenics applies to unintended effects of individual decisions, however, prenatal diagnosis and selective abortions could be considered eugenic.[123] Duster believes that individual, private decisions are a "backdoor to eugenics," because their collective results will affect the genetic makeup of the entire population.[124] According to this view, the majority of individuals and families will make similar decisions, because they subscribe to a unified ideal of human health and perfection. The sharp reduction in incidence of certain birth defects, such as Tay-Sachs in the United States and spina bifida or thalassemia in the United Kingdom, suggests that families are making what amount to eugenic decisions in regard to these disorders, which most people regard as serious. For less serious disorders, however, it is less likely that individual decisions will have a eugenic effect in a pluralistic society. Individuals and diverse social groups usually have a wide variety of ideas about what constitutes health, unless they are given biased information.

Science versus social policy. Originally, eugenics was defined as a science rather than social policy. Francis Galton, who originally coined the term in 1883, described eugenics as "the science of improvement of the human race germ plasm through better breeding."[125] A few modern definitions follow Galton.[126] Most definitions, however, assume interference with a natural process. The agents of change may be individuals or families rather than (or in addition to) the state or other social institutions. The collective results of individual actions may be unanticipated by or even abhorrent to the individuals who made these decisions. Families will choose the kind of children they want, and the result will be a form of "homemade" eugenics in the absence of direct social policy.[124] It is exactly this kind of eugenics that gives feminists fear.[2–4, 7, 8, 95–99, 127–129] They point out that (1) individual decisions are not always truly individual, but occur in a social context that may alter or limit choice,[3] and (2) the collective results of individual decisions may lead to social policies that discriminate against the minority who make different decisions and especially against persons with disabilities.[2] This kind of "eugenic discrimination" could be particularly invidious in a democratic society where it could occur by virtue of majority vote (or at least majority action) rather than by authoritarian decree.

Coercion versus voluntary choice. Many people define eugenics as including coercion and/or social goals. For example, Holtzman defines eugenics as "any effort to interfere with an individual's procreative choices in order to attain a societal goal."[130] What people are most likely to find objectionable in eugenics is not the goal, but the coercive means of achieving it. To this way of thinking, policies and practices designed to improve the health of the population cannot be eugenic unless coercive. Yet the history of the eugenics movement, especially in the

United Kingdom, points to many noncoercive approaches that were considered as eugenic.[131]

Individual versus social responsibility. Individual versus social responsibility is another dichotomy in definitions of eugenics. Actions may be defined as eugenic if their intentions are social (such as preventing the costs to society of raising children with disabilities) and as not eugenic if their intentions are to promote informed choices by individuals. One reason why eugenics has such a negative connotation is that all eugenicists, whether radical, liberal, or conservative, including Francis Galton,[125] Madison Grant,[132] George Bernard Shaw,[133] Bertrand Russell,[134] and Jane Clapperton,[135] believed that individual desires must be sacrificed to the public good. Even John Stuart Mill, who believed in the widest possible scope of individual choice, thought that the state should take responsibility in regard to reproduction. Urging "responsible parenthood," he argued, "to undertake this responsibility—to bestow a life which may be either a curse or a blessing—unless the being on whom it is to be bestowed will have at least the ordinary chances of a desirable existence, is a crime against that being."[133] Echoing Mill's statement, Hungarian obstetrician and geneticist Andrew Czeizel argues that children have a "right to be born healthy" and that the state has the moral and legal responsibility to ensure their healthy birth.[134] Czeizel is the last geneticist to advocate this kind of eugenics openly, but others may tacitly support this view. Feminist critics of new reproductive technologies are uneasy with statements such as Mill's and Czeizel's. They reject interference with women's choices, but are at the same time uncomfortable with both the existence and the social outcomes of these choices.[136]

The Goals of Counseling: Eugenics or Informed Choice?

Most genetic counseling around the world would be considered noneugenic today, because 99 to 100% of counselors strive to be nondirective and to "help individuals/couples achieve their parenting goals," and to "help individuals/couples understand their options and the present state of medical knowledge so they can make informed decisions.[55, 137–140] Counselors claim to "tell patients that decisions, especially reproductive ones, are theirs alone and refuse to make any for them" (92%); they also claim to "support any decisions patients make" (94%).[105, 138–139] It is not only the nondirectiveness, but the individual and family focus of genetic counseling that places it outside most definitions of eugenics.

As Kevles points out, however, in his concluding chapter "The New Eugenics," during the 1960s, the shift of counseling from concern with improving the welfare of the population to improving the welfare of individuals and families took place partly for political reasons.[115] Many of the early post-World War II geneticists in Canada and the United States sincerely believed in improving the biological quality of the population but rejected any association with the eugenics movement.[33, 141] In order to pursue their objectives in politically acceptable ways, they focused on voluntary, individual decision-making. Sheldon Reed coined the term *genetic counseling* in 1947 to replace the earlier terms *genetic advice* or *genetic hygiene,* which sounded too directive.[142] Kevles believes that this shift in ethos to place the needs and rights of individuals and families above the welfare of the population or gene pool marked a decisive break with the past and that the so-called "new eugenics" is beneficial, because it is devoted to the interests of individuals rather than society.

Ludmerer and others believe that there was no shift in ethos and that the goals of the eugenics movement entered medicine, unpretentiously, through genetic counseling.[116, 143] The majority of geneticists in Canada (68%), the United Kingdom (71%), the United States (78%), France (81%), and 15 other nations (74%) still believe that the eugenic goal of "improvement of the general health and vigor of the population" is important.[105, 139] A smaller majority in Canada (51%) and substantial percents in the United Kingdom (48%), the United States (47%), France (50%), and 15 other nations (54%) believe that another goal of Kevles' "old" eugenics, namely "reduction in the number of carriers of genetic disorders in the population," is an important goal of counseling.[105] Most (97%) in the United States and 18 other nations (98%) believe that "the prevention of disease or abnormality" is an important goal of counseling.

Labelling a technology "eugenic" does little to clarify the issues. In view of its multitudinous and sometimes contradictory meanings, the word should perhaps be dropped from discussions of prenatal diagnosis altogether. There remains the problem of defining what it is that people fear when they use the word eugenics. The basic fears appear to be (1) coercion into having prenatal diagnosis and abortion; (2) exploitation of women for the benefit of medical or social institutions; (3) excesses or misuses of prenatal diagnosis for "frivolous" purposes such as sex selection; (4) discrimination against people with disabilities, especially if their births could have been prevented. Underlying this final fear is a sense that there may be a deep undercurrent of eugenic thinking in the public, sometimes voiced as a belief that "some people should not have children." ...

In the future, differential uses of prenatal diagnosis and selective abortion by different social groups could lead to an unbalanced distribution of genetic disorders among social classes. In this event, many will look down on the lower classes because they do not use prenatal diagnosis and continue to have children with mental retardation.

Effects of Prenatal Diagnosis on Societal Attitudes toward People with Disabilities

Many people fear that increased use of prenatal diagnosis will shift social resources away from people with disabilities.[2-6, 36, 79, 145-149] Most disabilities, however, are not genetic in origin. They result from accidents, aging, viral or bacterial diseases, birth traumas, acts of violence, or environmental exposures. Genetics does not even account for the majority of severe mental retardation. Altogether, chromosomal disorders (e.g., Down syndrome), single-gene disorders (e.g., Tay-Sachs, fragile-X syndrome), and developmental malformation syndromes (e.g., neural tube defects) account for about 40%

of individuals with an intelligence quotient under 50.[150] Accidents at birth, prematurity, low birthweight, environmental or substance exposures, and unknown factors account for the remaining 60%. Genetic disorders do account for substantial numbers of deaths at early ages, including perhaps 20% of all infant deaths. They are second only to prematurity and birth injuries as causes of perinatal mortality. They are estimated as the second leading cause of death in children between the ages of one and four years and the fourth leading cause in individuals between the ages of 15 and 24 years,[103, 150] behind accidents, suicide, and homicide.[144] Nevertheless, genetic disorders are never *the* leading cause of death or disability. Many fetal malformations, including some congenital heart defects, cannot be diagnosed prenatally. Even disorders that can be diagnosed prenatally, such as Tay-Sachs, will not be tested for in low-risk groups and will continue to appear. Other disorders, such as neurofibromatosis, have a high rate of new mutations. This means that disability will always be with us, regardless of what we do with prenatal diagnosis. Society needs to be prepared to offer support to people with disabilities. Even if every pregnancy underwent chromosomal prenatal diagnosis and testing for neural tube defects (an unlikely event, given the negative risk–benefit ratio for younger women) and every woman agreed to abortion (also an unlikely event), society would still have children with birth defects of genetic origin from unsuspected inborn errors of metabolism, new mutations, heart defects, and so on. The majority of birth defects, however, would still originate from prematurity, low birthweight, and environmental exposure, as is the case now.[151] This argues for preventive measures that aim at the social and environmental causes of birth defects. There is no reason why social and economic programs cannot go hand-in-hand with public education about genetics and use of prenatal diagnosis, if desired. There is also no reason why prevention of disabilities—through adequate maternal nutrition, prenatal care, prevention of substance abuse or physical abuse, and prenatal diagnosis—must be at cross-purposes to support for living people with disabilities. It is illogical to argue that support for people with disabilities will be reduced if there are fewer such persons, or that support will be increased if more children with disabilities are born.

It appears unlikely that society will have fewer people with disabilities in the future. As society ages, we can expect more, rather than fewer, people with disabilities of all types, including mental disabilities. It is therefore important to increase, rather than to contemplate decreasing, supports for people with disabilities.

However, those who are concerned about the effects of prenatal diagnosis on attitudes toward disabilities have some legitimate fears. Sooner or later, as health-care budgets are rationed … the taxpayers may decide that they do not wish to provide extraordinary support for a child with very limited potential if the birth could have been prevented. This is not to say that the majority of people lack all sympathy for those with disabilities or that this is the beginning of a Nazi extermination program. When treatment is not effective, however, and the state underwrites the cost of care, at some point there must be a limit to the amount expended, so that funds can go to patients whose treatment may be successful…. If a woman has prenatal diagnosis and then decides to carry to term a baby with a serious and costly problem that cannot be treated successfully, she may indeed face social opprobrium.[152, 153] (She could, of course, have refused prenatal diagnosis, but may still be considered socially irresponsible for doing so.) …

CONCLUSION

Some feminist criticisms of prenatal diagnosis are well taken. Some women do feel social pressure to have prenatal diagnosis: many women find the "choice" of bearing and raising a child with a disability so unattractive under present conditions that it appears tantamount to no choice at all.

Differential use of prenatal diagnosis by different social groups could have a divisive effect on society's views about disability. Increasing fragmentation in American society could lead to reductions in services for those with disabilities. Commercial laboratories do profit from prenatal diagnosis and some have sought to expand its use for social, rather than strictly medical, indications. There are hidden arguments in public health programs, including genetics, that shift attention away from social and cultural causes of ill health or definitions of ill health. Goals of "prevention of disease" or cost–benefit arguments may be at odds with goals of genetic counseling that stress "helping individuals come to decisions that are best for them." Finally, there are abuses, notably for sex selection.

On the other hand, people always have *some* choice. Sartre characterized the excuse "I have no other choice" as "bad faith." Most women believe they have a choice and some refuse prenatal diagnosis. There is no evidence of coercion by doctors. Women have collaborated actively in encouraging the spread of prenatal diagnosis. Discouraging women from having prenatal diagnosis will not necessarily increase benefits for people with disabilities. The reverse is more likely. An increase in the number of affected children would most likely mean that each individual would receive less, rather than more support. Comparing prenatal diagnosis with coercive eugenic programs or with the death camps does nothing to help either women or people with disabilities. Instead, this line of argument leads only to backlash from anti-abortionists who would like to see women return to traditional—subordinate—roles.

In all, the evidence is that (1) women exercise choice in regard to prenatal diagnosis; (2) there are social pressures to use prenatal diagnosis in a "technological culture," just as there are pressures to give birth in hospitals and to use other birth technologies; (3) women probably have more power over choices about prenatal diagnosis than they do over other technologies used in birth; (4) most women, including most who consider themselves feminists, seem relieved to be able to make the choices implied in prenatal diagnosis; (5) many of the ethical problems in prenatal diagnosis arise from inequalities in our health-care system rather than from the technology itself; and (6) prenatal diagnosis is not a eugenic program.

Acknowledgment

Dr. Wertz thanks the Royal Commission on New Reproductive Technologies, Canada, and the Ethical, Legal, and Social Issues Program of the National Center for Human Genome Research (NIH).

Notes

1. Fletcher JC, Wertz DC. Ethics and prenatal diagnosis: Problems, positions, and proposed guidelines. In: Milunsky A, ed. *Genetic disorders and the fetus*. Baltimore: Johns Hopkins University Press, l992, in press.

2. Hubbard R. *The politics of women's biology*. New Brunswick, NJ: Rutgers University Press, 1990.

3. Lippman A. Prenatal genetic testing and screening: constructing needs and reinforcing inequities. *Am J Law Med* 1991a; 17:15–50.

4. Rothman BK. *The tentative pregnancy: prenatal diagnosis and the future of motherhood*. New York: Norton, 1986.

5. Asch A. Reproductive technology and disability. In: Cohen S, Taub N, eds. *Reproductive laws for the 1990s*. Clifton, NJ: Humana Press, 1989:69–127.

6. Saxton M. Prenatal screening and discriminatory attitudes about disability. In: Baruch EH, D'Adamo AF, Seager J. eds. *Embryos, ethics, and human rights: Exploring the new reproductive technologies*. New York: Harrington Park Press, 1987b:217–224.

7. Hubbard R. Prenatal diagnosis and eugenic ideology. *Women's Stud Int Forum* 1985; 8:567–576.

8. Hubbard R. Eugenics: new tools, old ideas. *Women & Health* 1987; 13:225.

9. Schaeffer FA, Koop CE. *What ever happened to the human race?* Old Tappan, NJ: Revell, 1979.

10. Henifin MS, Hubbard R, Norsigian J. Prenatal screening. In: Cohen S, Taub N, eds. *Reproductive laws for the 1990s*. Clifton, NJ: Humana Press, 1989:155–184.

11. Rothman BK. *Recreating motherhood: Ideology and technology in a patriarchal society*. New York: Norton, 1989.

12. Wexler NS. The oracle of DNA. In: Rowland LP, Wood DS, Schon EA, Dimauro S, eds. *Molecular Genetics and Diseases of the Brain, Nerve, and Muscle*. New York: Oxford University Press, 1989:429–442.

13. Zola IK. Medicine as an institution of social control. *Sociological Review*, 1972; 20:487–504.

14. Zola IK. In the name of health and illness: On some socio-political consequences of medical influence. *Soc Sci & Med* 1975; 83:85–87.

15. Zola IK. Healthism and disabling professions. In: Illich I, Zola IK, McKnight J, Caplan J, Shaiken H, eds. *Disabling professions*. London: Calder & Boyars, 1977.

16. Hubbard R, Henifin S. Genetic screening of prospective parents and workers: Some scientific and social issues. *Int'l J Health Services* 1985; 15:231.

17. Kaplan D. Prenatal screening and its impact on persons with disabilities. *Fetal Diagnosis and Therapy*. November 1992, in press.

18. Saxton M. Prenatal screening and discriminatory attitudes about disability. *Genewatch* Jan/Feb 1987a:8–11.

19. Luker K. *Abortion and the politics of motherhood*. Berkeley: University of California Press, 1984.

20. Lasker JN, Borg S. *In search of parenthood: Coping with infertility and high-tech conception*. Boston: Beacon Press, 1987.

21. Sjögren B, Uddenberg N. Decision making during the prenatal diagnostic procedure: a questionnaire and interview study of 211 women participating in prenatal diagnosis. *Prenat Diagn* 1988; 8(4):263–273.

22. Swerts A. Impacts of genetic counseling and prenatal diagnosis for neural tube defects. In: Evers-Kiebooms G, Cassiman JJ, Van den Berghe H, D'Ydewelle G, eds. Genetic risk, risk perception, and decision-making. *Birth Defects* 1987; XXII(2):61–83.

23. Frets PG, Niermeijer M. Reproductive planning after genetic counselling: a perspective from the last decade. *Clin Genet* 1990; 38:295–306.

24. Ever-Kiebooms G. Decision making in Huntington's disease and cystic fibrosis. *Birth Defects: Original Article Series* 1987; 23(2):115–149.

25. Evers-Kiebooms G, Denayer L, Van den Berghe H. A child with cystic fibrosis: 2. Subsequent family planning decisions, reproduction, and use of prenatal diagnosis. *Clin Genet* 1990; 37:207–215.

26. Adler NE, Keyes S, Robertson P. Psychological issues in new reproductive technologies: Pregnancy including technology and diagnostic screening. In: Rodin J, Collins A, eds. *Women and*

new reproductive technologies: Medical, psychosocial, legal and ethical dilemmas. Hillsdale, NJ: Lawrence Erlbaum Associates, Publishers, 1991:111.

27. Rapp R. The power of positive diagnosis: Medical and maternal desicourses on amniocentesis. In: Michaelson KL, ed. *Childbirth in America: Anthropological perspectives.* South Hadley, MA: Bergin & Garvey, 1988a:103–116.

28. Rapp R. Constructing amniocentesis: Medical and maternal voices. In: Ginsburg F. Tsing A, eds. *Uncertain terms: Negotiating gender in America.* Boston: Beacon Press, 1990.

29. Rapp R. Chromosomes and communication: The discourse of genetic counseling. *Med Anth Quart* 1988b; 2(2):143–157.

30. Rapp R. Reproduction and gender hierarchy: Amniocentesis in contemporary America. In: Miller B, ed. *Sex and gender hierarchies.* Chicago: University of Chicago Press, 1991.

31. Clarke A. Is non-directive genetic counselling possible? *Lancet* Oct. 19, 1991; 338:998–1001.

32. Green TH. Liberal legislation and the freedom of contract. In: Nettleship RL ed. *Works of Thomas Hill Green.* Reprint of 1889 ed. Krauss reprint 1968.

33. Paul DB. Eugenic anxieties and social realities. *Social Research* October 1992, in press.

34. Wertz RW, Wertz DC. *Lying-in: A history of childbirth in America,* expanded edition. New Haven, CT: Yale University Press, 1989.

35. Pearse WH. Parturition: Places and priorities. *Am J Pub Hlth* 1987; 177:923–924.

36. Harris R, Wertz DC. Ethics and medical genetics in the United Kingdom. In: Wertz DC, Fletcher JC, eds. *Ethics and human genetics: A cross-cultural perspective.* Heidelberg: Springer Verlag, 1989:388–418.

37. Richwald GA, Clark RD, Crandall B et al. Cost and acceptance of MSAFP screening in public prenatal clinics. *Am J Hum Genet* 1990; 47(suppl):A291.

38. Oakley A. *Women confined: Towards a sociology of childbirth.* Oxford. UK: Martin Robertson, 1980.

39. Oakley A. *The captured womb: A history of the medical care of pregnant women.* Oxford, UK: Basil Blackwell, 1984.

40. Cowan RS. A history of prenatal diagnosis. *Fetal Diagnosis and Therapy.* 1993; 8(Suppl. 1).

41. Andrews LB. *Medical genetics: A legal frontier.* Chicago: American Bar Foundation, 1987.

42. Elias S. Annas GJ. *Reproductive genetics and the law.* Chicago: Yearbook Publishers, 1987.

43. Byrne EA, Cunningham CC. The effects of mentally handicapped children on families: A conceptual review. *J Child Psychol & Psychiat* 1985; 26:847–864.

44. Thompson L, Walker AJ. Gender in families: Women and men in marriage, work, and parenthood. *J Marr Fam* 1989; 51:845–871.

45. Marcenko MD, Meyers JC. Mothers of children with developmental disabilities: Who shares the burden? *Fam Relat* 1991; 40:186–190.

46. Krauss MW, Seltzer MM. Coping strategies of older mothers of adults with retardation: A lifespan developmental perspective. In: Turnbull AP, Patterson J, Behr SK, Murphy DL, Marquis J, Blue-Banning M, eds. *Cognitive coping research in developmental disabilities.* Baltimore: Paul H. Brookes, 1992, in press.

47. Janicki MP, Wisniewski HM, eds. *Aging and developmental disabilities: Issues and approaches.* Baltimore: Paul H Brookes, 1985.

48. Seltzer MM, Krauss MW. Sibling relationships of persons with mental retardation in adulthood. In: Stoneman Z, Berman P, eds. *Siblings of individuals with mental retardation, physical disabilities, and chronic illness.* Baltimore: Paul H Brookes, 1992, in press.

49. Lobato D. Siblings of handicapped children: A review. *J Autism & Dev Disord* 1983; 13:347–364.

50. Drotar P, Crawford P. Psychological adaptation of siblings of chronically ill children: Research and practice implications. *Dev & Behavioral Pediatrics* 1985; 6:355–362.

51. Fujuira GT, Garza J, Braddock D. *National survey of family support in developmental disabilities.* Mimeo, IL: University of Illinois at Chicago, 1989.

52. Meyers CE. Borthwick SA, Eyman RK. Place of residence by age, ethnicity, and level of retardation of the mentally retarded/developmentally disabled population of California. *Am J Mental Deficiency* 1985; 90:266–270.

53. Petchesky R. Giving women a real choice. *Nation* 1990; 250:732.

54. United States Bureau of the Census. *Single parents and their children.* Washington: U.S. Government Printing Office, 1990.

55. United States National Center for Health Statistics. *Wanted and unwanted childbearing in the U.S.: 1973–1988.* Washington: U.S. Government Printing Office, 1990.

56. Kaplan D. Disability rights perspectives on reproductive technologies and public policy. In: Cohen S, Taub N, eds. *Reproductive laws for the 1990s.* Clifton, NJ: Humana Press, 1989:241–248.

57. Degener T. Debates across social movements on reproductive technologies, genetic engineering, and eugenics. In: Duncan B, Woods DE, eds. *Ethical issues in disability and rehabilitation.* World Rehabilitation Fund. New York: Printing Production Services, 1989:73.

58. Degener T. Female self-determination between feminist claims and "voluntary" eugenics, between "rights" and ethics. *Issues in Reproductive and Genetic Engineering* 1990; (3):87.

59. Finger A. Claiming all of our babies: Reproductive rights and disabilities. In: Arditti R, Klein RD, Minden S, eds. *Test-tube women: What future for motherhood?* London: Pandora Press, 1984.

60. Finger A. *Past due: A story of disability, pregnancy, and birth.* Seattle, WA: Seal Press, 1990.

61. Carrier JG. *Learning disability: Social class and the construction of inequality in American education.* Westport, CT: Greenwood Press, 1986.

62. Dorris M. *The broken cord.* New York: Harper & Row, 1989.

63. DeFord F. *Alex: The life of a child.* New York: New American Library, 1984.

64. Forecki M. *Speak to me.* Washington, DC: Gallaudet University Press, 1985.

65. Fraiberg A, Fraiberg L. *Insights from the blind: Comparative studies of blind and sighted infants.* New York: New American Library, 1979.

66. Spradley TS, Spradley JP. *Deaf like me.* Washington. DC: Gallaudet University Press, 1985.

67. Retsinas J. The impact of prenatal technology upon attitudes toward disabled infants. In: Wertz DC, ed. *Research in the Sociology of Health Care* 1991; 9:75–104.

68. Wikler L, Waso M, Hatfield E. Chronic sorrow revisited: Parent vs. professional depiction of the adjustment of parents of mentally retarded children. *Am J Orthopsychiatry* 1981; 5:63–70.

69. Simons R. *After the tears: Parents talk about raising a child with a disability.* New York: Harcourt Brace, 1987.

70. McDonough P. Congenital disability and medical research: The development of amniocentesis. *Women and Health* 1990; 16(3–4):137–153.

71. Boswell J. *The kindness of strangers: The abandonment of children in western Europe from late antiquity to the Renaissance.* New York: Pantheon Books, 1988.

72. Glover J. *What sort of people should there be?* New York: Penguin Books, 1984.

73. Kuhse H, Singer P. *Should the baby live? The problem of handicapped infants.* London: Oxford University Press, 1985.

74. Fletcher JC. *Coping with genetic disorders: A guide for clergy and parents.* San Francisco: Harper & Row, 1982.

75. Guillemin JH, Holmstrom LL. *Mixed blessings: Intensive care for newborns.* Oxford: Oxford University Press, 1986.

76. Hunter AG, Thompson D, Speevak M. Midtrimester genetic amniocentesis in Eastern Ontario: A review from 1970 to 1985. *J Med Genet* 1987; 24:335–343.

77. Roy DJ, Hall JG. Ethics and medical genetics in Canada. In: Wertz DC, Fletcher JC, eds. *Ethics and human genetics: A cross-cultural perspective.* Heidelberg: Springer-Verlag, 1989:119–140.

78. Therkelsen AJ, Bolund L, Mortensen V. Ethics and medical genetics in Denmark. In: Wertz DC, Fletcher JC, eds. *Ethics and human genetics: A cross-cultural perspective.* Heidelberg: Springer-Verlag, 1989:141–155.

79. Schroeder-Kurth TM, Huebner J. Ethics and medical genetics in the Federal Republic of Germany. In: Wertz DC, Fletcher JC, eds. *Ethics and human genetics: A cross-cultural perspective.* Heidelberg: Springer-Verlag, 1989:156–175.

80. Farrant W. Who's for amniocentesis? The politics of prenatal Screening. In: Homans H, ed. *The sexual politics of reproduction.* Aldershot, Hants. UK: Gower Publishing, 1985:96–122.

81. Terzian E, Boreham J, Cuckle HS, Walk NJ. A survey of diagnostic amniocentesis in Oxford from 1974 to 1981. *Prenat Diagn* 1985; 5:401–414.

82. Mulvihill JJ, Walters L, Wertz DC. Ethics and medical genetics in the United States of America. In: Wertz DC, Fletcher JC, eds. *Ethics and human genetics: A cross-cultural perspective.* Heidelberg: Springer-Verlag, 1989:419–456.

83. Hook EB, Chambers GM. Estimated rates of Down syndrome in live births by one year maternal age intervals for mothers aged 20–49 in a New York State study—implications of the risk figures for genetic counseling and cost benefit analysis of prenatal diagnosis programs. In: Bergsma D, Lowry RB, eds. *Numerical taxonomy of birth defects and polygenic disorders.* New York: Alan R Liss, 1972.

84. Hook EB, Schreinemachers DM. Trends in utilization of prenatal cytogenctic diagnosis by New York State residents in 1979 and 1980. *Am J Publ Hlth* 1983; 73(2):198–202.

85. Adams MM, Finley S, Hansen H, et al. Utilization of prenatal diagnosis in women > 35 years, United States, 1977–78. *Am J Obstel Gynecol* 1981; 139:673.

86. Marion JP. Acceptance of amniocentesis by low-income patients in an urban hospital. *Am J Obstet Gynecol* 1980; 130:11–15.

87. Anonymous. When risk factors have little meaning. *Br Med J* 1989; 299:1599–1600.

88. Hodge SE. Waiting for the amniocentesis. *New Engl J Med* 1989; 320:63–64.

89. Green R (pseud). Letter to a genetic counselor. *J Genetic Counseling* 1992; 1:55–70.

90. Rapp R. XYLO: A true story. In: Arditti R, Klein RD, Minden S, eds. *Test-tube women: What future for motherhood?* London: Pandora Press, 1984:313–328.

91. Brown J (pseud). The choice. *JAMA* 1989; 262:2735.

92. Eichholz A. Amniocentesis: The experience of invasion and the ambivalence of foreknowledge. In: Offerman-Zuckerberg J, ed. *Gender in transition: A new frontier.* New York: Plenum, 1989:173–177.

93. Feinberg J. Noncoercive exploitation. In: Sartorius R, ed. *Paternalism.* Minneapolis: University of Minnesota Press. 1990:201–236.

94. Rothschild J. ed. *Machina ex dea: Feminist perspectives on technology.* New York: Pergamon Press, 1983.

95. Spallone P. *Beyond conception: The new politics of reproduction.* Granby, MA: Bergin & Garvey, 1989.

96. Spallone P, Steinberg DL. *Made to order: The myth of reproductive and genetic progress.* New York: Pergamon Press, 1987.

97. Corea G. *The mother machine: Reproductive technologies from artificial insemination to artificial wombs.* New York: Harper & Row, 1985.

98. Arditti R, Klein RD, Minden S, eds. *Test-tube women: What future for motherhood?* London: Pandora Press, 1984.

99. Rothman BK. *In labor: Women and power in the birthplace.* New York: W W Norton, 1982.

100. Whitbeck C. Theories of sex difference. *Philosophical Forum* 1973; 5(1,2):54–80.

101. Whitbeck C. The moral implications of regarding women as people: New perspectives on pregnancy and personhood. In: Bondeson WB, ed. *Abortion and the status of the fetus.* Boston: D Reidel, 1984:251–252.

102. Atwood M. *The handmaid's tale.* Boston: Houghton Mifflin, 1986.

103. United States Department of Health, Education, and Welfare. Antenatal diagnosis. April 1979. NIH Pub. No. 79-1973. Washington, DC, U.S. Government Printing Office, April 1979.

104. Canadian College of Medical Geneticists. *Professional and ethical guidelines.* Ottawa: CCMG, 1986.

105. Wertz DC. The 19-nation survey: Genetics and ethics around the world. In: Wertz DC, Fletcher JC, eds. *Ethics and human genetics: A cross-cultural perspective.* Heidelberg: Springer-Verlag, 1989a:1–79.

106. Nightingale EO, Goodman M. *Before birth: Prenatal testing for genetic disease.* Cambridge, MA: Harvard University Press, 1990.

107. Blatt RJR. *Prenatal tests.* New York: Vintage Books, 1988.

108. Chorover SL. *From genesis to genocide.* Cambridge. MA: Massachusetts Institute of Technology Press, 1979.

109. Lifton RJ. *The Nazi doctors.* New York: Basic Books, 1986.

110. Luria S. Human genome program (letter). *Science* October 13, 1989; 246:873.

111. Mueller-Hill B. *Murderous science: Elimination by scientific selection of Jews, gypsies, and others, Germany 1933–1945.* Oxford, UK: Oxford University Press, 1988.

112. Proctor RN. *Racial hygiene: Medicine under the Nazis.* Cambridge, MA: Harvard University Press, 1988.

113. McLaren A. *Our own master race: Eugenics in Canada 1885–1945.* Toronto, Ontario: McClelland & Stewart, 1990.

114. McLaren A, McLaren AT. *The bedroom and the state: The changing practices and politics of contraception and abortion in Canada, 1880–1980.* Toronto, Ontario: McClelland and Stewart, 1986.

115. Kevles DJ. *In the name of eugenics: Genetics and the uses of human heredity.* New York: Knopf, 1985.

116. Ludmerer KM. *Genetics and American society.* Baltimore: Johns Hopkins University Press, 1972.

117. Adams M, ed. *The wellborn science: Eugenics in Germany, France, Brazil and Russia.* New York: Oxford University Press, 1990.

118. Schneider WH. *Quality and quantity: The quest for biological regeneration in twentieth-century France.* Cambridge, UK: Cambridge University Press, 1990.

119. Soloway RA. *Demography and degeneration: Eugenics and the declining birthrate in twentieth-century Britain.* Chapel Hill: University of North Carolina Press, 1990.

120. Commission of the European Communities. Modified proposal for a Council decision adopting a specific research and technological development in the field of health: Human genome analysis (1990 to 1991). Official Journal of the European Communities, CB-CO89-485-EN-C. Brussels November, 13, 1989:3.

121. Carlson EA. *Human genetics*. Lexington, MA: DC. Heath, 1984, glossary V.

122. Carlson EA. Ramifications of genetics. *Science* April 25, 1986; 232:531–532.

123. Wright R. Achilles' helix. *The New Republic* July 9 & 16, 1990:21–31.

124. Duster T. *Backdoor to eugenics*. New York: Routledge, 1990.

125. Galton F. *Inquiries into the human faculty and its development*. London, 1883.

126. Haller MH. *Eugenics: Hereditarian attitudes in American thought*. New Brunswick, NJ: Rutgers University Press, 1984:ix.

127. Holmes HB, Hoskins BB, Gross M, eds. *The custom-made child? Women-centered perspectives*. Clifton, NJ: Humana Press, 1981.

128. Holmes HB, Hoskins BB, Gross M, eds. *Birth control and controlling birth*. Clifton, NJ: Humana Press, 1980.

129. Rodin J, Collins A. eds. *Women and new reproductive technologies*. Hillsdale, NJ: Lawrence Erlbaum, 1991.

130. Holtzman NA. *Proceed with caution: Predicting genetic risks in the recombinant DNA era*. Baltimore: Johns Hopkins University Press, 1989.

131. Hogben L. *Genetic principles in medicine and social science*. London 1931:207.

132. Grant M. *The passing of the great race*. New York 1916:14–45.

133. Shaw GB. *Sociological papers*. London 1905:74–75.

134. Russell B. Eugenics. In: Russell B, ed. *Marriage and morals*. New York: Liveright, 1970:255–273.

135. Clapperton J. *Scientific meliorism*. London 1885:10.

136. Fox-Genovese E. *Feminism without illusions*. Chapel Hill: University of North Carolina Press, 1991.

137. Fraser FC. Genetic counseling. *Am J Hum Genet* 1974; 26:636–659.

138. Sorenson JR, Swazey JP, Scotch NA. *Reproductive pasts, reproductive futures: Genetic counselling and its effectiveness*. New York: Alan R Liss, 1981.

139. Wertz DC, Fletcher JC. Attitudes of genetic counselors: A multinational survey. *Am J Hum Genet* 1986; 42(4):592–600.

140. Wertz DC, Fletcher JC. Ethical decision-making in medical genetics: Women as patients and practitioners in 18 nations. In: Ratcliff KS et al, eds. *Healing technology: Feminist perspectives*. Ann Arbor: University of Michigan Press, 1989b:221–241.

141. Sorenson JR. Genetic counseling: Values that have mattered. In: Annas GJ, Elias S, eds. *Gene mapping: Using law and ethics as guides*. New York: Oxford University Press, 1992:203–211.

142. Reed SC. A short history of genetic counseling. *Soc Biol* 1974; 21:332–339.

143. Kessler S. Psychological aspects of genetic counseling. VII. Thoughts on directiveness. *J Genetic Counseling* 1992; 1:9–18.

144. United States Department of Health and Human Services, National Center for Health Statistics. Health USA 1990. Washington, DC: U.S. Government Printing Office, 1991.

145. King's Fund Forum. King's Fund Forum consensus statement: Screening for fetal and genetic abnormality. *Br Med J* 1987; 295:1551–1553.

146. Holder AR, Henifin MS. Selective termination of pregnancy. *Hastings Center Rep* 1988; 18(1):21–22.

147. Hull RT, Nelson JA, Gartner LA. Ethical issues in prenatal therapies. In: Humber JM, Almeder RF, eds. *Biomedical Ethics Reviews*. Clifton, NJ: Humana Press, 1984:225–249.

148. Johnson SR, Elkins TE. Ethical issues in prenatal diagnosis. *Clin Obstet Gynecol* 1988; 31:408.

149. Motulsky A, Murray J. Will prenatal diagnosis with selective abortion affect society's attitude toward the handicapped? In: Berg K. Tranøy KE, eds. *Research ethics*. New York: Alan R Liss, 1983.

150. NICHD. Antenatal diagnosis: Report of a consensus development conference. Washington. DC: DHEW, 1979, Pub. No. (NIH) 79–173.

151. Yankauer A. What infant mortality tells us. *Am J Pub Health* 1990; 80:653.

152. Billings P, Kohn M, DeCuevas M, Beckwith J, Alper J, Natowicz M. Discrimination as a consequence of genetic screening. *Am J Hum Genet* 1992; 50:476–482.

153. Natowicz MR, Aiper JK, Alper JS. Genetic discrimination and the law. *Am J Hum Genet* 1992; 50(3):465–475.

Patenting of Genetic Material:
Are the Benefits to Society Being Realized?

Donald J. Willison and Stuart M. MacLeod

Patents represent a contract between an inventor and society. By granting time-limited market exclusivity, patents create the potential for inventors to generate high returns on successful innovations. In exchange, the inventor provides a complete description of the invention so that others may build on the technology to create improvements or other breakthrough discoveries. Patent protection of intellectual property is particularly important to inventors in the biotechnology field because of the relatively high fixed cost of research and the ease with which discoveries may be copied. By attracting investment capital for research, patent protection increases the pace of innovation, thus benefiting society.

To qualify for a patent, the invention must be deemed useful, novel and not obvious. The utility criterion requires that a clear application is known. Novelty means that the invention has not been described before in the literature. The criterion of non-obviousness demands creativity on the part of the inventor. For example, the courts in the United Kingdom have ruled, on the grounds of obviousness, that Pfizer's patent on the use of the entire drug class of phosphodiesterase-5 inhibitors for erectile dysfunction was invalid because the knowledge was already in the public domain when the patent was issued.[1]

Although contentious in principle, patenting of life forms is now well established in law. The landmark case identifying the patentability of life forms occurred in 1980, when the US Supreme Court ruled in a 5–4 decision that the genetic modification of a bacterium to break down oil spills was consistent with "a new composition of matter" as defined in the Patent Act of 1793.[2] This decision did not directly address the patentability of genes; however, the courts eventually reasoned that, if whole organisms were patentable, then their components would also be eligible for patent protection. Subsequently, the patenting of isolated gene sequences (but not the human genome) was permitted by the American and European patent offices, provided the applicant could demonstrate utility of the gene sequence. The Canadian Intellectual Property Office has recognized the patentability of isolated genetic sequences, and the status of patents for higher life forms (e.g., the Harvard oncomouse) is currently before the Supreme Court.[3] The Canadian Biotechnology Advisory Committee has recently recommended that higher life forms (i.e., plants, seeds and nonhuman animals) that meet the criteria of utility, novelty and non-obviousness be patentable, subject to certain restrictions.[4]

A wave of new diagnostic and therapeutic inventions is coming to market, based on innovations in genomics and proteomics. Development has been funded in large part through private capital, stimulated by the patenting of genetic materials. As gene-based tests and therapies come to market, practising physicians have an important professional role to play in interpreting the growing debate for their patients and for the general public. Consider the case of Myriad Genetics Laboratories (Myriad) involving the *BRCA1* and *BRCA2* gene patents.

In June 2001 Myriad declared that hospitals in several provinces were violating its patent on a test of genetic susceptibility to breast cancer. Myriad demanded that all testing be conducted in its laboratory in the United States at a cost of about US$2500, almost 5 times what is currently being charged.[5] Although other provinces either stopped using the test or quietly went on as usual, in September 2001 the Ontario government announced that it would challenge private companies' rights to patent genes and to control, and profit from, diagnostic and medical treatments using the patent.[6] To date, Ontario continues to defy Myriad's patent claim[7] and has taken steps toward charting a path that balances societal and commercial interests in the area of genomics.

Genetic patents were intended to benefit society through more rapid access to innovations that would improve the health and well being of society. In this article we review key issues in the patenting of genetic materials and ask whether the intended benefits from patenting of genetic material are actually occurring.

CONCERNS OVER PATENTING OF GENETIC MATERIAL

Effects on the Biotechnology Sector

Patenting of genetic material has created a huge market for private investment capital. Indeed, private investment in biotechnology has become an important aspect of Canadian science and industrial policy, supporting Canada's goal of leadership in the information economy.[8, 9] The race to decipher the human genome probably finished ahead of schedule because of the entry of private sector funds. How, though, has the patenting of basic discoveries affected the research process and the resulting innovations produced?

Research Process. In a survey of over 2100 life scientists, about 20% of respondents reported delays in publication of 6 months or more to allow for patent application, to protect their scientific lead, to slow dissemination of undesired results, to allow time for patent negotiation or to resolve disputes over ownership of intellectual property.[10] Engagement in academic–industry research partnerships and commercialization of university research were significantly associated with publication delays. In another survey, 47% of geneticists who asked other faculty for additional information, data or materials

regarding published research reported denial of at least 1 request in the preceding 3 years.[11] In 28% of cases, respondents were unable to replicate published research as a direct result of this refusal to share information. The rate of denial of requests for data was equivalent to that reported by non-geneticists. However, geneticists were more likely to report that the withholding of data impeded progress of their research (58% v. 38% respectively). Thirty-five percent of geneticists felt that data sharing had decreased during the past decade.

Innovations. There are 2 types of innovation: breakthrough discoveries and those that improve on existing technology by creating either a better product or a cheaper product of equivalent quality.

Breakthrough discoveries. Privatization of new tests or therapies can go astray when too many owners hold rights to discoveries.[12] Before 1980, basic discoveries, such as the H_2-receptor responsible for gastric acid secretion, were considered to be in the public domain. (These basic discoveries are often called "upstream discoveries.") Only the specific tests or therapies that harnessed this basic knowledge, such as H_2-receptor antagonists, were patented. (These tests and therapies are commonly called "downstream applications.") Currently, patentable upstream discoveries include genes, gene sequences, gene fragments or expressed sequence tags, the proteins expressed by these genes and single nucleotide polymorphisms, commonly used in researching genetic diseases. Although the patenting of upstream discoveries has stimulated a huge influx of private investment capital, inventors of downstream applications are likely to cross the boundaries of several patents, necessitating the "stacking" of royalties to patent holders. This could reduce the value of all patents, vastly increase legal costs and actually inhibit innovation. Indeed, Barton[13] noted a 70% increase between 1986 and 1994 in the number of intellectual property lawyers employed per dollar spent on research and development.

Discoveries that improve on an innovation.
An excessively broad patent—particularly on an upstream discovery—might block or place severe constraints on the ability of others to develop new tests or therapies that build on the patented invention. This is one of the criticisms directed at Myriad Genetics by Institut Curie and the French government concerning their patent on the *BRCA1* gene.[14]

Effects on Society

Research Focus. In general, genetic patenting issues mirror those associated with commercialization of research. Effort is placed disproportionately on discoveries that would maximize profits to the inventor, by targeting large, potentially lucrative markets, rather than on discoveries that would maximize benefit to society. This exacerbates existing disparities in the availability of treatments across socioeconomic and ethnic groups within countries and between developed and developing countries.[15] In addition, research into genetic "solutions" may overshadow research into the roles of less glamorous but important contributors to disease prevention. For example, modifiable behavioural factors, such as obesity, inactivity and smoking, account for over 70% of the cases of stroke and colon cancer, over 80% of coronary artery disease and over 90% of adult-onset diabetes.[16] Ignoring these targets of innovation will result in a narrower and more costly range of solutions than might otherwise occur.

Market Control. High licensing fees and royalties may constrain the number of laboratories prepared to provide a particular test. For example, Merz and colleagues[17] found that 30% of laboratories testing for hemochromatosis ceased to develop or provide the test once the patent holder began enforcing its patent. Access to tests is thus reduced, and an environment is created wherein patent holders dictate the conditions under which tests will be performed.[18]

Even more constraining is the refusal to license a product to other laboratories. Although Myriad Laboratories cites quality control as its reason for refusing to license out its *BRCA1* and *BRCA2* tests, this practice also provides Myriad with an expanding exclusive database for researching and patenting new mutations in the 2 genes, potentially extending for years the company's monopoly in this area.

Consumption. Society has limited funds to distribute between health care and other social benefits. The socially optimal amount to be spent on any one therapy takes into account that, beyond a certain point, greater health benefits may be achieved by investing elsewhere. By contrast, the patent holder seeks to maximize sales of its invention. This induces pressures to broaden the pool of patients considered eligible for a test or therapy beyond that which is socially optimal. For example, if one compares Myriad Genetics' indications for its *BRCA* tests with those recommended by an independent academic body, one finds that the latter excludes women without a family history of breast or ovarian cancer, whereas Myriad's guidelines include these lower risk women.[19]

One may argue that individuals deemed ineligible for a particular test or treatment within the public health care system should be allowed to purchase these out-of-pocket. However, this ignores the induced costs to the public system in follow-up to the genetic test itself—costs that may quickly exceed that of the test.[20] Without controls on direct-to-consumer marketing similar to those in place in Canada for pharmaceutical products, potential over-consumption is likely to be exacerbated.

POLICY IMPLICATIONS

The evidence suggests several areas in which patenting of genetic materials may actually be slowing innovation through delayed publications, increased secrecy, increased transaction costs due to royalty stacking, and excessively broad patents. Researchers themselves will generate some solutions, such as the SNP Consortium—a collaboration of several pharmaceutical firms and the UK Wellcome Trust—that places the commonly used single nucleotide polymorphisms (SNPs) in the public domain.[21]

However, there is now no clear delineation between patentable discoveries and those in the public domain. Other solutions may come from regulators. For example, the US Patent Office has recently suggested the use of patent pools, which are a form of cross-licensing agreement between patent holders, allowing for the sharing of technologies in a common field.[22]

The need for patent reform is generally recognized.[23–25] Ontario's report on genetics, testing and gene patenting[26] recommends tightening the existing interpretation of Canada's Patent Act as it relates to biological materials, and it recommends amendments to the act to:

- narrow the scope of gene patents;
- create clear exemptions for experimental and noncommercial clinical use of a patented invention;
- introduce a morality clause, the basis on which a patent may be challenged;
- make provision for a separate ethics review panel;
- create a faster, less expensive dispute-resolution mechanism; and
- permit compulsory licensing of genetic diagnostic and screening tests, giving government authority to require the patent holder to license the test to another firm, under reasonable conditions.

Although necessary, these patent reforms do not address the bias toward producing products that will maximize a return on investment. Federal and provincial governments must ensure adequate, continued funding for research that does not have commercial potential—for example, lifestyle and environmental contributors to health and well being.

CONCLUSION

A handful of large biotechnology enterprises is emerging from existing small and medium-sized biotechnology firms. As this occurs, it is important that adequate mechanisms be in place to limit the potential for abuse of monopoly power. Federal leadership is needed to clarify interpre-

tation of current patent laws. Ultimately, however, Canada must work in concert with other nations on fundamental reform of these laws to fit societal needs for both innovation and affordable access to these innovations. This effort will require engagement with all stakeholders, including the medical community and the general public. The national and provincial medical associations have important roles to play as advocates for both patients and physicians to ensure that workable and sustainable approaches are found.

Acknowledgements

We thank Steve Morgan for his helpful comments on an earlier draft of this article.

Notes

1. Viagra patent invalid, says UK court. *Scrip* 2002; 2716(Jan 30):6.
2. Crespi RS. An analysis of moral issues affecting patenting inventions in the life sciences: a European perspective. *Sci Eng Ethics* 2000; 6(2):157–80.
3. Gold R. Building a better patent law. *Globe and Mail* [Toronto] 2002 May 17; Sect A:7.
4. *Patenting of higher life forms and related issues. Report to the Government of Canada Biotechnology Ministerial Coordinating Committee.* Ottawa: Canadian Biotechnology Advisory Committee; June 2002. Available: www.cbac-cccb.ca/documents/en/ E980_IC_IntelProp.pdf (accessed 2002 July 5).
5. Mallan C. Gene test for cancer won't stop. *Toronto Star* 2001 Sep 20; Sect A:3.
6. Mackie R. Harris battles firm over gene patenting. *Globe and Mail* [Toronto] 2001 Sep 20; Sect A:14.
7. Eggertson L. Ontario defies US firm's genetic patent, continues cancer screening. *CMAJ* 2002; 166(4):494.
8. Innovation. In: *The speech from the Throne to open the first session of the 37th Parliament of Canada.* Ottawa: Office of the Prime Minister; 2001. Available: www.sft-ddt.gc.ca/sft-ddt/03_e.htm (accessed 2002 July 5).
9. *Achieving excellence: investing in people, knowledge and opportunity. Canada's innovation strategy.* Ottawa: Industry Canada; 2002. Cat no

C2-596/2001-1E-1N2. Available: www.innovation-strategy.gc.ca (accessed 2002 July 8).

10. Blumenthal D, Campbell EG, Anderson MS, Causino N, Louis KS. Withholding research results in academic life science. Evidence from a national survey of faculty. *JAMA* 1997; 277(15):1224–8.

11. Campbell EG, Clarridge BR, Gokhale M, Birenbaum L, Hilgartner S, Holtzman NA, et al. Data withholding in academic genetics: evidence from a national survey. *JAMA* 2002; 287(4):473–80.

12. Heller MA, Eisenberg RS. Can patents deter innovation? The anticommons in biomedical reserach. *Science* 1998; 280:698–701.

13. Barton JH. Reforming the patent system. *Science* 2000; 287:1933–4.

14. Shulman S. Owning the future: doctors without patents. *Technol Rev* 2001; 104(10):33.

15. Singer PA, Daar AS. Harnessing genomics and biotechnology to improve global health equity. *Science* 2001; 294:87–9.

16. Willett WC. Balancing life-style and genomics research for disease prevention. *Science* 2002; 296(5568):695–8.

17. Merz JF, Kriss AG, Leonard DG, Cho MK. Diagnostic testing fails the test. *Nature* 2002; 415:577–9.

18. Merz JF. Disease gene patents: overcoming unethical constraints on clinical laboratory medicine. *Clin Chem* 1999; 45(3):324–30.

19. Caulfield TA, Gold ER. Genetic testing, ethical concerns, and the role of patent law. *Clin Genet* 2000; 57:370–5.

20. Miller F, Hurley J, Morgan S, Goeree R, Collins P, Blackhouse G, et al. *Predictive genetic tests and health care costs: final report prepared for the Ontario Ministry of Health and Long-Term Care*. Toronto: Ontario Ministry of Health and Long-Term Care; 2002.

21. Sachidanandam R, Weissman D, Schmidt SC, Kakol JM, Stein LD, Marth G, et al. A map of human genome sequence variation containing 1.42 million single nucleotide polymorphisms. *Nature* 2001; 409(6822):928–33.

22. Clark J, Piccolo J, Stanton B, Tyson K, Critharis M, Kunin S. *Patent pools: a solution to the problem of access in biotechnology patents?* Washington: US Patent and Trademark Office; 2000.

23. Thurow LC. Needed: a new system of intellectual property rights. *Harv Bus Rev* 1997; 75(5):95–103.

24. Mooney PR. *The impetus for and potential of alternative mechanisms for the protection of biotechnological innovations.* Prepared for the Canadian Biotechnology Advisory Committee, Project Steering Committee on Intellectual Property and the Patenting of Higher Life Forms; 2001. Available (pdf format): www.cbac-cccb.ca/documents/en/AltMechanisms_Mooney.pdf (accessed 2002 July 5).

25. Gold ER. Moving the gene patent debate forward. *Nat Biotechnol* 2000; 18(12):1319–20.

26. Ontario Provincial Advisory Committee on New Predictive Genetic Technologies. *Genetics, testing and gene patenting: charting new territory in healthcare*. Toronto: Ministry of Health and Long-Term Care; 2002.

Will Genetics be Used Wisely?

Patricia Baird

We have seen remarkable progress in genetics over the last several decades. The DNA code has been elucidated, specific genes can now be identified, sequenced, manipulated and put into other organisms. A molecular genetic approach has led to greater understanding of numerous specific disease pathways in individuals, and recombinant DNA is used to produce several kinds of therapeutically useful molecules such as hormones or vaccines. The Human Genome Project is progressing rapidly, and it is a rare week that the media do not announce that one or more genes related to some disease has been identified.

As a consequence, a widely shared view is that the sequencing of the human genome will tell us just which genes cause diseases—cancer, arthritis, heart disease or mental illness, for example. Then, in light of that information we will design and customize new drugs for individuals, and in the longer term, even re-engineer the genes in question. This scenario for the future is shaping the way in which a great deal of research money is being spent by governments and by industry. But is this scenario in fact likely?

This article provides a realistic assessment of what genetic knowledge is likely to contribute to the health of the population in the next few decades. It addresses the overly naïve interpretation often put on genetic research findings in our society and explores the potentially unfortunate implications that this could have for health and social policies.

In evaluating what we can realistically expect from a genetic approach, the article starts by examining data on the frequency of various categories of illness.

DETERMINANTS OF HUMAN HEALTH AND DISEASE

One can think of illnesses as being on a continuum—at one end of the spectrum having a particular gene makes it impossible for the individual to live and function normally in the usual range of available environments; at the other end, the noxious or traumatic effect of an environmental circumstance is such that no usually occurring human genotype could function normally. Illnesses at either of the two ends of the spectrum are fairly rare. An example at one end would be a single gene disorder such as Tay-Sachs disease, an example at the other end of the spectrum would be exposure to a high dose of electricity.

Population studies show that single gene caused diseases—those at one end of this spectrum—are relatively rare. For example, in a study of over a million consecutive live-born individuals followed to age 25 years in British Columbia, we found that single gene disorders occurred in only 3.6 per 1000 individuals.[1] The vast majority of illnesses in humans are the result of complex interactions, over time, between their genetic constitutions and such aspects as how they are nurtured in childhood, what they eat, whether they smoke, whether they have a satisfying job, have a reasonable income

and whether they feel valued. The evidence is overwhelming that the determinants of the common chronic diseases of modern life are complex, interrelated, act over time and are embedded in a social context.

A clear indication that genetic components of disease causation do not predominate in populations is that we have seen striking changes in population frequency of the most important diseases, over time spans far too short for any change in genetic constitution of that population. For example, without changing the genome, during the 20th century, life expectancy has risen over 30 years in developed countries.

Other indicators of the importance of the environment for most serious diseases are the dozens of migrant studies showing massive changes in frequency of diseases such as breast cancer, heart disease or colon cancer within a generation or two of migration from low incidence settings to high incidence settings.[2] Genetic differences cannot provide the explanation for these dramatic changes—the gene pool in the migrant population could not change that quickly, suggesting that environmental factors are at play here.

Additional evidence of the role of nongenetic factors in common diseases is that in any given country's population these diseases show a very strong socio-economic gradient. Many studies, in many countries, over many years, show very strong correlations of death rates with measures of social status.[3] This is particularly well illustrated in a study of more than 10,000 British civil servants, who have now been followed for more than 25 years. Even in this cohort—all of whom are in stable employment and relatively well off—the effect is large: there is a three- to four-fold difference in the age standardized mortality from the top to the bottom of four categories of employment. It is noteworthy that the gradient occurs all the way up—the top people do a little better than those just near the top—which means the environmental effect is not poverty or deprivation-driven. It remains even after identified risk factors such as cholesterol level, blood pressure, smoking, etc., are controlled for.[4] This social gradient for disease distribution is seen for many different diseases and in many studies. It occurs for all cause mortality as well as for heart disease and cancer. So whatever the environmental influence is, it has had an effect on many pathways to disease.

The stepwise nature of this environmental determinant of disease is shown in a particularly striking study of Canadian data on half a million males categorized by earned incomes between ages 45 and 65.[5] The more you earned, the less likely you are to die early…. The effect is large—if the mortality of the bottom 80 percent was the same as the average of the top 20 percent, it would have the same impact as eliminating all cancer deaths.

Hypertension in black people provides another example of the important effects of environment. Thirty-five percent of African-Americans suffer from hypertension, and this is attributed by many to an intrinsic genetic racial difference. But if you look at the incidence of hypertension in blacks in different settings—West Africa, the Caribbean, rural and urban United States—the incidence of hypertension goes from low to high.[6] This evidence suggests that hypertension may largely be a disease of modern life and of the current circumstances African-Americans live in. Given these geographic differences in incidence in genetically similar populations, a genetic explanation is not sufficient to account for the high rates of hypertension seen in black Americans.

The point is that the most widespread, serious diseases of modern life seem to be very sensitive to the environment—both physical, nutritional and social/psychological.[7] Genetic differences are probably involved to some extent in many cases but usually other factors are important. Some of these environmental effects are reversible and potentially preventable.

Research that helps [us] understand how social forces act on individuals to affect their biological processes and change their disease risk is essential if we are to improve the health of the public and address the burden of illness….

SIMPLE SOLUTIONS MAY NOT WORK FOR COMPLEX PROBLEMS

Purely genetic manipulations likely could benefit those at very high risk for largely genetic reasons—for example, single gene conditions such as Huntington Disease, familial hypercholesterolemia or the small fraction of common diseases due to monogenic pathways. But the conditions from which *most* people suffer in their adult years will require us to consider both genetic and environmental components and how these interact if we are going to understand them. There will be benefits eventually from using the new genetics to better understand disease processes and intervening in specific subgroups with a given disease, and benefits in tailoring medications for people who are ill but metabolize medication in different ways. However, the multiplicity of routes to the chronic common disease end-points of adulthood, and the complexity of interacting factors over time on the way, make it unlikely there will be widely applicable "genetic magic bullet" solutions for these diseases. Genetically based approaches to diagnosis and treatment will have to be tailored to individual variation, and it is doubtful that this will be practical or cost effective. The ubiquitous nature of codetermination of most health ill-effects means that it is unrealistic to expect that genetic interventions alone will be sufficient to make us all healthier.[8]

There is also another barrier. There is an implicit assumption in the genetic approach that people identified as having risk genotypes will follow some on-going strategy (usually taking medication) to decrease their risk. This is unlikely, given what we know about the way people actually behave. One reviewer of the compliance literature estimates that on average only a third of patients follow physicians' directions, and persistence in taking long-term medication of various kinds, for illnesses which are already present, is approximately 50 percent.[9] Compliance for years with a "preventive" regime of medication in the absence of illness is likely to be low.

EXAMPLES OF UNWISE USE OF GENETICS

Are there straws in the wind to tell us how we are likely to handle our new capacities in genetics? A couple of instances suggest we should be more aware of the need to use genetic approaches cautiously. The first of these is breast cancer.

The discovery of the BRCA1 and 2 genes in recent years has led to many requests for testing by women and their physicians. A recent survey of 340 women in a primary care practice in the United States showed almost two thirds thought physicians should offer breast cancer gene testing to all women, not just those with a family history.[10] It has constituted a substantial additional workload for the health care system, in terms of assessing women's risk, counseling them appropriately and testing those who can genuinely benefit. Is this a cost-effective way to use resources to reduce the incidence of breast cancer? Evidence is already emerging to suggest that it is not. For one thing, early estimates of the proportion of all breast cancers that occurred in carriers of these two genes were too high. It is now believed to be less than five percent, although it is slightly higher among cases under age 35. Early estimates of the frequency of these genes in the general population have been mitigated by the finding that BRCA1, for example, occurs in only 12 per 10,000 women in North America. Another factor limiting potential impact is that even among proven, multi-case BRCA1 carrier families, only 43 percent of women invited for testing participate fully and want their test results.

The point is not that BRCA1 and 2 or similar gene testing has no place in the rational and compassionate management of breast cancer risk among high-risk families, but rather it is a question of balance. Widespread, unrestricted population use of these tests is what is of concern. Inappropriate overuse is likely if the anxiety of low-risk women is capitalized on by commercially oriented testing labs. Such widespread use, rather than the appropriate use of the tests in women with legitimate family history risk markers, is what is of concern from the point of view of evidence-based medicine and the public's health. In short, there is much potential for both harm and wasted health care resources, and little promise of net health benefits, if overly enthusiastic utilization of such technology occurs in the wider population.

A second example of the need to use genetics carefully is in the area of pre-implantation diagnosis. If [in] vitro fertilization is carried out, the early embryo is accessible for genetic testing before it implants. A cell may be taken from the cluster of cells making it up and genetic probes used to identify particular genes, or the chromosomes may be examined. Only those embryos without an identified "undesirable" genotype may then be transferred to the woman's uterus.

The number of instances where it is appropriate to offer pre-implantation diagnosis is extremely small.[11] It is relevant only for people at identified high risk for a specific single gene or chromosomal genetic disease and who are unwilling to have prenatal diagnosis. In spite of this, private clinics providing this technology can be expected to market and promote it. The more services they provide, the more successful they are. In 1997, a Toronto private fertility clinic offered, for a fee of about $8,000 per cycle of treatment, to screen embryos for risk of "genetic disease" before implantation. It offered pre-implantation diagnosis to the public for 27 "genetic" diseases—some of which had little correspondence between having a particular gene and the disease—for example, breast cancer. The clinician involved said "This is the beginning of the end of genetic disease" and added that the roster of diseases the clinic would identify could grow dramatically over time, and this should have "the same impact antibiotics did to bacterial disease."

This kind of promotion and hyperbole markets the technology as "quality control for parents" and is likely to lead to inappropriate overuse. The public may not readily understand that having a particular gene does not necessarily lead to having its "related" disease.

Letting such genetic testing develop "ad hoc" is not a recipe for ensuring that it will be provided in a way that is beneficial. Most people would like to have healthy children, and the marketing of this technology could play into that goal in an exploitive and misleading way. If it is going to bring health benefits, pre-implantation testing should only be offered in programs with clear protocols, with demonstrated benefit, demonstrable expertise and resources for counseling and follow-up.

These are just two examples of the need for responsible use and some accountability in how genetics is applied in the treatment of human illness.

REASONS A GENETIC APPROACH TO ILL HEALTH MAY BE PUSHED

Several factors, in Western societies in particular, may lead to unwise overuse of a genetic approach to human illness.

Pharmaceutical/biotechnology companies: A great deal of money and a large industry are involved in supplying technology for genetic testing and identification and in producing therapeutic agents based on a molecular genetic understanding. Companies investing in genetic/biotechnology research have an obligation to shareholders to market and promote the use of a genetic approach to disease. The more it is used, the more commercially successful they are. In the process, they are likely to divert attention (and possibly funding) from exploration of other determinants of health. Biotechnology companies in the United States raised $8 billion a year annually during the period 1994 to 1996, and that figure has increased since then. The major U.S. pharmaceutical companies spend 24 percent of their income on marketing; their sales people make 30 million visits a year to doctors' offices to market their products. Entrepreneurs in the industry are quite naturally looking for a large market. A very large market potential would be predictive diagnostic DNA tests done on a large proportion of the healthy population to assess their "risk" status. Companies interested

in predictive diagnostic DNA tests are also likely to be the ones who are developing drug interventions to prevent or treat the disease to be predicted. Policy makers and health care payers need to bear in mind the influence of the biotechnical/pharmaceutical industry when deciding the appropriate place for these technologies in their funding priorities. They should require demonstration of cost-effective benefit and lack of harm before funding them.

Media portrayal of disease causation: Another factor contributing to the increased focus on genetics is overly simplistic media portrayals of disease causation. Genetic accounts of the cause of disease are common in the media, and this is facilitated because its explanatory model is resonant with the "body as machine" explanatory model which underlies the most prevalent understanding of the body/self relationship in developed countries. It is also a simple message that is easier to capture in today's short media formats.

Scientists in biomedical disciplines also play a role in the focus on genetics. The Human Genome Project is the largest "Big Science" project outside physics/engineering, with over 100 laboratories participating, and well over U.S. $3 billion in expenditures involved. Molecular geneticists in academia have increasing ties with biotechnological companies. This means that the opinions of academic researchers with investments in biotechnological firms or with appointments on boards or as consultants cannot necessarily be accepted as objective. This situation has not been sufficiently taken into account or disclosed in publications. The blurring of academia with industry means we have lost a societal resource—a body of independent scientists without commercial affiliation—that can provide more objective input and opinion when society has to deal with choices posed by developing genetic technologies.

Governments: In the rush to a new knowledge-based economy, governments have often facilitated genetic technology transfer from academia to industry without necessarily taking into account the long-term, broader consequences and implications, or the need for balance. They have not supported to the same degree the exploration of other avenues to decrease disease incidence. One kind of worthwhile research has crowded out another. The promotion of partnerships with industry at universities and granting councils means that public funds are redirected by the joint venture. Research projects having public-good content but not likely to generate a saleable product lose out in this milieu. The pendulum may have swung too far in this area.

Service providers and laboratories: Both laboratories and service providers have incentives to offer more genetic tests as these become available. The motivation is not necessarily financial—when researchers have developed a new genetic test or technological capability, they do not want to hear there is no need for it. They are expected to provide answers to individuals' questions about health risks, and genetics is their field. Having had to deal with single gene and chromosomal disorders in their work, they tend to underestimate the non-genetic components related to complex diseases.

Some decision makers and some sectors of the public: Lastly but as important, genetic explanations are attractive to those who do not want to deal with complex social and economic determinants of health. Framing most ill health as genetic and promoting individual genetic or pharmacologic solutions push the problem back to the individual. In this way, awkward questions on social and health policies, or inappropriate workplace organization, can be avoided.

When decisions are being made about what role genetic approaches should have in health policies and health care for the population, we need to bear in mind that these forces will tend to promote overuse. There is a danger that a good balance between a genetic, individualized approach, and social, collective approaches to achieving a healthy population will not be found. Although such a balance is in the diffuse public interest, it is in the concentrated interest of the sectors outlined above to overemphasize genetic

factors. We can expect lobbying to steer things in this direction; there is already a move to direct marketing of genetic testing to the public, framed in the rhetoric of freedom to choose.[12]

There will be instances where elucidating a disease pathway or differences in drug metabolism will enable better therapy, and I am not advocating that we stop pursuing these. The individual clinical view underlies medical training and biomedical science and provides a framework for the treatment of sick individuals. I am advocating that it is in the public interest to extend this framework to recognize and explore other important influences on health. A balance in funding research on what leads to most ill health is needed. Other kinds of questions need to be asked as well as genetic ones.

CONSEQUENCES OF NEGLECTING NON-GENETIC INFLUENCES ON DISEASE

What are the consequences of neglecting non-genetic determinants of health? If we neglect environmental aspects in our assessment of the extent to which illness can be avoided or mitigated, we will not identify environmental factors that can be changed. These may be more or at least as effective at avoiding disease as the use of biologic/pharmaceutic products. The approach of genetic identification as well as modern risk-factor epidemiology have focused almost exclusively on finding the individual correlates of disease. Yet there are important determinants of health that are not based on the individual, and that are completely left out of consideration by this approach, for example, air pollution, inadequate child care policies, stressful working conditions or availability of healthy food.

Focusing on the individual who is ill, rather than on the social, economic and environmental factors which may have interacted with genetic variation in people to arrive at this outcome in some, leads to different social policies to produce health. If causes of ill health are defined as genetic, innate and simply unfolding, then social supports, good early nurturing, narrowing economic gaps and appropriate workplace organization are less likely to be underwritten by society. Given the critical importance of these factors, this will be detrimental to health.

WHAT CAN WE DO TO ENSURE THE WISE USE OF GENETICS?

Regulations: Currently no legislation prevents a company from selling what it claims to be predictive genetic tests for hundreds of different diseases, marketing them intensively to physicians and the public. If genetic testing is not simply just another market commodity, regulation is needed. But regulation to ensure appropriate use will only occur if the public understands why it is needed. The public needs to be street-proofed. Simplistic perceptions that "genes cause disease" lead to a population of consumers ripe for marketing of gene-based diagnostics and products.

Increased public awareness is desirable but currently there is no clear structure in Canada where public concern can be focused to bring about regulation. Decisions about how genetic technologies should be used involve not only medical, but ethical and social aspects. This article has not explored uses of genetics such as prenatal sex selection, genetic alteration for enhancement or reproductive cloning. Any policy-making body relating to the application of genetics should include people from different sectors and with differing experience. Such a body would allow public concern and input to be channelled, so that the public interest could be a counter-weight to the market in helping ensure that genetic knowledge is used in a non-exploitive way.

Equitable access: As well as regulation, there is another side to the coin. Equitable access to those uses of genetics that are effective and beneficial should be incorporated in health care delivery systems. If there is to be equitable access to beneficial genetic services, these must be included in health care systems that provide care for all, regardless of ability to pay. Not just testing but counselling and interpretation should be covered so that individuals may make informed choices. It is impossible to avoid issues of distributive jus-

tice, and proven beneficial genetic services should be considered in priority setting by policy makers responsible for health care.

The increasing ability to detect genes related to common complexly determined disorders is a major cause for concern. Before large-scale genetic testing or preventive treatment are offered to healthy people, there should be requirements to have data demonstrating benefit and that harms are unlikely to occur, and that safeguards against these are in place.

SUMMING UP

We are at an exciting time in genetics. There have been remarkable advances in our knowledge, and there will be real and undoubted benefits from a carefully considered application of genetic knowledge in the future. Steady progress in understanding will allow us in some specific instances to ameliorate particular disease processes or use medication more effectively. However, policy makers should view new and expanded expenditures in the area of genetic testing/therapy with the opportunity cost in mind, a healthy scepticism, and an evaluation of who is advocating such expenditures and whether they are the ones who will gain. Genetics is only part of the story, and it is important to evaluate genetic components to disease causation within a larger frame.

The continuing challenge for researchers will be to examine specific genetic, environmental and social effects acting over time, and then put the pieces back together in a big picture. Social processes, psychological and biological pathways and genetic endowment interact in myriad ways to result in disease. No one doubts that an important pathway to health is through the mind. But to carry out studies that document *how* different nurturing experiences and social or work circumstances affect health outcomes is not easy. Genetic and environmental explanations are not competing alternatives—for most diseases expression of genetic endowment depends in a complex way on their environment.

To focus too strongly on the genetic strand of the web of causation, although profitable for some, does not address other important determinants and could lead us to miss opportunities and neglect dimensions essential to health. Because some sources in our society push for a genetic approach to ill health, we are at risk of overusing genetics with resultant expensive harm. But if we take a measured approach, putting genetics into a broader context, we will avoid the dashed expectations and consequent backlash from overselling, and be able to bring benefit in a responsible way.

Notes

Parts of this article are drawn from a longer discussion paper entitled "Genetic Technologies and Achieving Health for Populations," *International Journal of Health Services*, Vol. 30, no. 2 (2000), pp. 407-424.

1. P.A. Baird, T.W. Anderson, H. Newcombe and R.B. Lowry. "Genetic Disorders in Children and Young Adults: A Population Study," *American Journal of Human Genetics*, Vol. 42, (1988), pp. 677–693.

2. M.G. Marmot *et al.* "Epidemiologic Studies of Coronary Heart Disease and Stroke in Japanese Men Living in Japan, Hawaii and California: Prevalence of Coronary and Hypertension Heart Disease and Associated Risk Factors," *American Journal of Epidemiology*, Vol. 102 (1975), pp. 514–525.

3. R.G. Evans, M.L. Barer and T.R. Marmor (eds.), *Why are Some People Healthy and Others Not?* (New York: Aldine de Gruyter, 1994).

4. M. Marmot, "Multi-Level Approaches to Understanding Social Determinants," in Berkman and Kawachi (eds.), *Social Epidemiology* (New York: Oxford University Press, 2000), pp. 350–357.

5. M. Wolfson, G. Rowe, J.G. Gentleman and M. Tomiak, "Career Earnings and Death: A Longitudinal Analysis of Older Canadian Men,"
Journal of Gerontology: Social Sciences, Vol. 48, no. 4 (1993), pp. S167–179.

6. R.S. Cooper, C.N. Rotimi and R. Ward, "The Puzzle of Hypertension in African-Americans," *Scientific American* (February 1999), pp. 56–63.

7. R.G. Wilkinson, *Unhealthy Societies* (London and New York: Routledge, 1996).

8. N.A. Holtzman and T.M. Marteau, "Will Genetics Revolutionize Medicine?," *New England Journal of Medicine*, Vol. 343, no. 2 (2000), pp. 141–144.

9. Marshall H. Becker, "Patient Adherence to Prescribed Therapies," *Medical Care*, Vol. 23, no. 5 (May 1985), pp. 539–555.

10. A.W. Helmes, D.J. Bowen and J. Bengel, "Report on the Second National Conference on Genetics and Public Health. Genetic Testing for Breast Cancer: An Issue of Money," *Community Genetics*, Vol. 2, no. 2–3 (1999), p. 124.

11. This is because most diseases are not determined by single gene or chromosome abnormalities. Further, because you need to know what condition to test for, it is only appropriate to offer pre-implantation diagnosis where a couple has already been identified as at increased risk for having a child with a particular serious single gene or chromosomal disorder. Usually the identification will have been made because of a previous affected child. Such couples already have the option of pre-natal genetic diagnosis. Diagnosis during pregnancy is far less costly, more accurate and has fewer health risks for the woman, so the proportion of couples where it is appropriate to offer pre-implantation diagnosis is small.

12. Spending on direct-to-consumer advertising in the United States totaled $1.5 billion from March 1998 to March 1999. This was a 16 percent growth rate. http://www.straightgoods.com

Human Cloning: Three Mistakes and an Alternative

Françoise Baylis

I. HUMAN CLONING: THREE MISTAKES AND AN ALTERNATIVE[1]

Human cloning by somatic cell nuclear transfer is arguably the most exciting and at the same time foreboding technological–biological development of our times. Specifically, the prospect of cloning humans using nuclear transfer technology challenges our understanding of ourselves (i.e., what it is to be human), and our place in the world. When we reproduce by sexual intercourse we do not reproduce ourselves, what we reproduce or perpetuate is our own kind. Significantly, our kind is one that reproduces by recombining genes. In marked contrast, with nuclear substitution there is no recombination of the genes. We do not reproduce our kind, rather we reproduce, or more precisely, replicate ourselves.[2] Thus, the cloning of humans theoretically makes possible an important departure from species-typical functioning—one deserving of critical attention.

The term "cloning" properly applies to any procedure that produces a genetic replica of a cell or organism. In the literature on cloning humans, the term frequently refers to two distinct technologies used to create whole beings: embryo splitting (also referred to as twinning and blastomere separation) and somatic cell nuclear transfer. In late 1993, Jerry Hall and colleagues at George Washington University reported their success with cloning human polyploid embryos. The technique they developed involved blastomere separation at the two-cell to eight-cell stage, and transfer to an artificial zona pellucida for continued growth into separate but identical embryos (Hall et al., 1993). Seventeen chromosomally abnormal human embryos were divided, and 48 developing embryos were obtained. A few years later, in February 1997,

Ian Wilmut and colleagues at the Roslin Institute announced the existence of Dolly, the cloned sheep (Wilmut, Schnieke, McWhir, Kind, & Campbell, 1997). The nucleus of a cell from a six-year-old sheep was removed, transferred to an unfertilized enucleated egg, and encouraged to develop. Two hundred and twenty-seven embryos were reconstructed; Dolly was the only success. With the birth of Dolly (the first mammalian clone), the idea that humans might eventually be cloned by somatic cell nuclear transfer seized the public imagination and renewed the debate on the ethics of cloning people. Since then several other species have been cloned from adult somatic cells including mice, cows, the rhesus monkey and transgenic pigs (Kato et al., 1998; Onishi et al., 2000; PPL, 2000; Wakayama et al., 1998; Wells, Misica, & Territ, 1999; Wolf, Meng, Ouhibi, & Zelinski-Wooten, 1999). As regards the cloning of humans, in 1999 there was an unconfirmed report of human cloning from somatic cells by South Korean scientists (Watts & Morris, 1999). Then, in November 2001, Advanced Cell Technology (ACT) reported that it had cloned human embryos as a possible future source of stem cells for regenerative medicine (Cibelli et al., 2001).

Prior to the birth announcement of Dolly, and subsequent scientific and technological developments involving non-human animals, a number of countries had laws banning human cloning (Bonnicksen, 1995). As the prospect of human cloning appeared to draw nearer, however, additional committee reports, policy documents and legislation were issued specifically condemning human *reproductive*[3] cloning, where cloning technology is used to create whole beings. For example, in 1997, the Fiftieth World Health Assembly adopted the following resolution: "cloning for the replication of human individuals is ethically unacceptable and contrary to human dignity and integrity" (WHO, 1997). In the same year, the US National Bioethics Advisory Commission (NBAC) concluded that "it is morally unacceptable ... to attempt to create a child using somatic cell nuclear transfer cloning," (NBAC, 1997, p. 106) and President Clinton enacted the NBAC recommendation to extend the moratorium on the use of federal funding for such research for five years. Under President Bush, the US House of Representatives passed a bill in July 2001 that would make it a federal crime to clone humans either to produce children or to create embryos for research purposes (the US Senate has yet to vote on the bill). Meanwhile, in the UK, it is legal to clone human embryos for research purposes (Human Fertilisation, 2001), but the use of cloning for human reproduction is prohibited. And, closer to home, the Canadian government is poised to introduce legislation in 2002 that would prohibit the cloning of humans for either research or reproductive purposes (Health Canada, 2001).

For some, these policy statements and legislative prohibitions are an important first step in precluding the further development of human cloning to replicate individuals. For others, these initiatives are at most useful temporizing maneuvers to preclude the trivial and misguided uses of cloning technology. Proponents of this latter view believe that the cloning of whole beings is inevitable. The underlying reasoning is as follows: (1) cloning humans represents an irresistible scientific and technological challenge which means that some research group(s) somewhere will develop the technology, and this effort will be defended on the grounds of freedom of scientific inquiry; (2) the commitment, in some jurisdictions, to free enterprise and personal choice, coupled with the burgeoning support for the compassionate use of cloning technology to assist certain infertile couples, means that the technology (once developed and shown to be reasonably safe and effective) will be "for sale"; and (3) once the technology is for sale, there will be eager customers.

The likely development and possible future use of cloning technology to create individuals raises important ethical questions about the common good and the integrity of the human species. These questions require timely and careful reflection. As Hans Jonas wrote more than twenty-five years ago: "Since no less than the very nature and image of man [sic] are at issue, prudence becomes itself our first ethical duty, and hypothetical reasoning our first responsibility" (Jonas, 1974, p. 141). In this spirit, the reader's attention is drawn to some of the more pervasive and egregious mistakes with the current debate on the ethics of cloning humans using nuclear transfer technology.

II. A FIRST MISTAKE

A first mistake with the public debate on the ethics of cloning humans is our apparent comfort with a discourse that lulls us into complacency about a technology that represents a fundamental challenge to our understanding of ourselves and the species to which we belong. Consider, for example, the following summary caricatures of potentially complex arguments against the cloning of humans as unnatural, as "playing God," as contrary to human dignity.

A. Cloning Humans is Unnatural

According to some, cloning humans is "contrary to nature". While the splitting of human embryos does occur in nature, spaced twinning (using both embryo splitting and freezing), and somatic cell nuclear transfer do not. Further, while asexual reproduction does occur in nature, it is unnatural for the species Homo Sapiens which practices sexual reproduction.

This argument against cloning humans presumes an understanding of nature as a primordial structure that is independent of, and authoritative with respect to, all other possible structures (for example, social structures). There are two common responses to this argument. One response posits a specific understanding of "human nature" that encompasses the desire for knowledge and the capacity for self-transformation. In this view, our nature includes mastering ourselves and choosing our own destiny (i.e., making plans for our own nature). Another response side-steps the debate about the scope and meaning of human nature and asks somewhat facetiously: "So what? So are all sorts of other interventions that we happily accept."

B. Cloning Humans is "Playing God"

Warnings against "playing God" have been interpreted in multiple ways. What is common to these interpretations "is the idea that there is a natural order or structure, perhaps divinely ordained, and that proposals to exceed the limits which this natural order defines should be rejected out of hand—or at least considered very carefully" (Grey, 1998). In its religious applications, the phrase "playing God" alludes to God's omniscience and omnipotence and serves to identify acts or decisions outside the realm of legitimate human activity. Some of the religious interpretations of the phrase "playing God" are helpfully summarized in the NBAC report, *Cloning Human Beings*:

> Human beings should not probe the fundamental secrets or mysteries of life, which belong to God. Human beings lack the authority to make certain decisions about the beginning or ending of life. Such decisions are reserved to divine sovereignty. Human beings are fallible and also tend to evaluate actions according to their narrow, partial, and frequently self-interested perspectives. Human beings do not have the knowledge, especially knowledge of outcomes of actions attributed to divine omniscience. Human beings do not have the power to control the outcomes of actions or processes that is a mark of divine omnipotence. (NBAC, 1997, pp. 42–43)

In response, some argue that God expects us to use our reason, imagination, and freedom to improve our quality of life. In this view, human beings are created co-creators and human action

is an expression of divine will (Hefner, 1998). An alternative response to the "playing God" argument against cloning is that in a pluralistic society, discussions about the ethics of cloning humans should not be constrained by a particular conception of God as "the creator" (Silver, 1998, p. 172). More generally, others suggest that accusations of "playing God" sometimes operate as rhetorical devices that ultimately obfuscate rather than clarify discussion (Grey, 1998).

C. Cloning Humans is Contrary to Human Dignity

This admonition against cloning humans rests, in part, on the Kantian view that persons should be treated as ends in themselves (Kahn, 1997). In this view, cloning humans is morally wrong because typically clones are created exclusively as a means for benefitting another. For example, clones may be created solely to satisfy an interest in having a biologically related child, to replace a dying or deceased loved one or to serve as an organ or tissue donor.

In response, some insist that this argument against cloning is flawed insofar as it ignores the fact that typically there are multiple motives and reasons for procreating (whether by cloning or sexual relations), and that clones would never be created exclusively as a means to another's end. Others grant that some clones likely will be treated *as mere means,* but they argue that this problem is not unique to cloning since persons who conceive "in the usual way" sometimes also act instrumentally as, for example, when persons reproduce to save a failing marriage, to prove their virility, to continue their genetic line, or to have someone to care for them in their old age. Still others insist that it is a matter for debate whether human embryos fall within the scope of the Kantian categorical imperative (given their contested moral status) and, more generally, they argue that Kant's principle is sufficiently vague and open to selective interpretation as not to be very helpful (Harris, 1997).

These three arguments against cloning humans are "familiar" in that they rehearse old arguments against novel technologies. To be precise, versions of these arguments have been elaborated previously, for example, against the introduction of the contraceptive pill, the development of organ transplantation and the use of life-extending technologies. The pattern that has emerged is one of initial condemnation, followed by ambivalence, questioning and limited use, followed in turn by a change in public perceptions, advocacy and *finally* widespread acceptance. For those who are mindful of this pattern, there is a sense of *deja-vu* with the debate about cloning humans, and there is the expectation that both the debate and practice will evolve in a similar manner.

Another cluster of familiar arguments against cloning humans focus on the possible/probable harmful consequences of the technology for society and for the individuals thus created. These arguments are worn because although the objections raised are unique to cloning technology, they do little more than reiterate concerns identified years ago when the prospect of cloning humans was pure science fiction. Consider, for example, the claim that cloning technology will be used purposely to create inferior beings to do boring and menial work (think, for example, of the "Deltas" of *Brave New World).* Or, consider the claim that cloning technology will be abused by power-hungry authoritative regimes to more effectively oppress others (think, for example, of *The Boys from Brazil).* As well, there is the claim that human cloning violates the clone's right to a unique genetic identity, and the clone's right to an open future—that is, a future with a reasonable range of opportunities (Brock, 1997).

Typically, responses to these sorts of arguments begin with a basic lesson on the science of cloning in an effort to correct mistaken views about the science and about genetic determinism. For example, it is explained that individuals cloned by nuclear transfer technology are not really identical to one another, though they may be very similar. This is because genes are not constant, they mutate. As well, there can be important differences in gene expression. Added to this is the fact that a fraction (0.05%)

of the human genome comes from mitochondrial genes contributed by the egg so that with cloning by somatic cell nuclear transfer, the clonant and the clone cannot be genetically identical unless they have the same maternal lineage. At the same time, it is also explained that identity is shaped by environmental as well as genetic factors: "genes do not *determine* in tight detail how a creature turns out ... [they] merely propose possibilities. It is the environment that shapes the final outcome" (Wilmut, Campbell, & Tudge, 2000, pp. 302–303). For example, with cloning by somatic nuclear cell transfer, the clonant and the clone will have developed in different uterine environments. As well, they will be born years apart and thus be subject to different environmental choices and influences.

In addition to this introductory lesson, there are the usual responses to the specific concerns about societal harm. The most common of these express significant confidence in our ability to ensure that cloning technology will not be abused, but rather will be developed and practiced under controlled conditions (i.e., within appropriate professional, regulatory and legislative constraints). And as for the concerns about potential harm to individuals, it is noted that conventional identical twins are natural clones and they are not psychologically harmed by their lack of genetic uniqueness. This claim is morally relevant since genomic clones would be more different from each other than conventional identical twins. Further, it is argued that the concern about parents coercing their clones' development and subverting their independence by structuring the scope of their experiences and opportunities is not a unique feature of human cloning. This is also a risk for conventionally conceived children whose parents' hopes for their children quickly become expectations.

In my view, all of the arguments against cloning humans identified above and the typical rejoinders are not particularly interesting or challenging. Consistent with this view is Daniel Callahan's recent conclusion, based on his review of the cloning debate from the early 1970s to the present, that "[n]o arguments have been advanced this time that were not anticipated and discussed in the 1970s" (Callahan, 1998, p. 141). Interestingly, on this basis, Callahan credits bioethicists writing in the early 1970s—in particular, Paul Ramsey, Hans Jonas and Leon Kass—with remarkable prescience. But isn't this hubris on the part of bioethics? Shouldn't the fact that no new arguments have been introduced in the post-Dolly era be cause for concern, not congratulations? Others suggest that our imagination has stagnated even longer—that the issues currently addressed in the debate about cloning humans are no different from those that concerned Aldous Huxley in the 1930s when he originally published *Brave New World,* his fictional account of a cloned "utopia". How is it that greater knowledge of the science and a better understanding of the technological possibilities has not introduced new ethical questions or concerns, has not sparked the moral imagination? Are we to believe those who insist that "there are no new ethical issues in relation to the current hysteria over cloning" (Wolpert, 1999, p. 282)?

III. A SECOND MISTAKE

A second mistake with the current debate on the ethics of cloning humans—a mistake informed, in part, by a fear of eugenics—is that much of the discussion remains at the level of the personal, as though the *raison d'etre* of the technology were to address individual needs and wants. This perspective is clearly evident in discussions about the motives for pursuing human cloning (Robertson, 1998).

It has been suggested, for example, that some couples may want to use cloning technology because it is the only way to have a child that is biologically related to each of the partners. This might include: infertile couples where both have no gametes (where the male partner could provide the somatic cell and the female partner could provide the enucleated oocyte); women undergoing *in vitro* fertilization (IVF) with too few oocytes who might benefit from embryo splitting; and lesbian couples (where one partner could provide the somatic cell and

the other could provide the enucleated oocyte) (Baird, 1999). Others possibly interested in human cloning are couples at high risk of having a child with a serious genetic disease. Cloning could also be used to satisfy a wish to re-create a deceased loved one; the usual example given is of parents who want to re-create a dying or deceased child. There may also be those who would use cloning technology to get a compatible organ or tissue donor for themselves or their offspring. Finally, there may be individuals who for reasons of "curiosity, vanity, the wish for personal power, or an undoubtedly misguided desire for immortality" (Wilmut et al., 2000, p. 306) want a genetic replica of themselves.

One consequence of the unrelenting focus on the personal is the perception of human cloning as a bi-generational issue. Human clones are described as "spaced twins," "later-born identical twins," " 'delayed' genetic twins," and the "ultimate single-parent child." As well, the dominant image for human cloning is one of mass production with multiple images of the identical phenotype—"xeroxed human beings" and "carbon-copied humans"—not the traditional pedigree chart or family tree with missing or unusual linkages. Cloning is thus portrayed as horizontal multiplication, not as vertical, multigenerational replication.

With attention focused on the present and the next generation, priority is given to concerns about possible medical and psychological harms to future children and fundamental questions about what it means to be human are set aside. Notably, this dominant perspective is highly compatible with contemporary silence on the possible uses of human cloning to pursue public health or broader societal goals.

When the possibility of cloning humans was discussed in the 1960s, there was considerable speculation about the potential societal benefits of human cloning. One suggestion was to clone individuals with a high pain threshold or resistance to radiation (Haldane, 1963, pp. 353, 355). Another suggestion was to clone individuals skilled at certain jobs, for example, soldiers (Fletcher, 1971, p. 779). Today, the examples have changed and the focus is on cloning specific persons of extraordinary talent such as Beethoven or Einstein. As well, there is particular attention to the potential societal harms of human cloning resulting from the replication of persons with undesirable traits—the most common example being Hitler. In response to such fanciful claims, scientists have been successful in labeling most speculation about the eugenic applications of human cloning as "stupid talk" that obscures the real scientific issues (Butler & Wadman, 1997). To avoid the charge of "stupid talk" serious academics dutifully focus on the "more immediate and realistic possibilities" and abdicate their responsibility to engage in hypothetical reasoning.

IV. A THIRD MISTAKE

A third mistake with the current debate on the ethics of cloning humans is that it wrongly focuses much of the discussion on reproductive issues and reproductive freedom. Physicians and researchers, for example, justify human cloning as an aid for infertile couples and an aid in pre-implantation diagnosis. They also frequently note that cloning technology promotes procreative autonomy.

Among those who view cloning as a form of assisted conception are those who believe that the principle of reproductive freedom entrenches the right to reproduce by any means chosen. Dan Brock, for example, maintains that the right to reproductive freedom presumptively includes the right to select the means of reproduction that best serve one's interests and needs, including human cloning (Brock, 1997). Some even go so far as to argue that, in the United States at least, this is a constitutionally protected right. John Robertson, for example, maintains that "[t]he right of married and arguably even unmarried persons to procreate is a fundamental constitutional right that cannot be restricted unless clearly necessary to protect compelling state interests" (Robertson, 1994, p. 13). In his view, cloning appears to fall within this fundamental freedom. At the other extreme are those who insist that human cloning is intrinsically wrong. George Annas, for example, counters that reproductive rights are not absolute and that cloning by somatic cell nuclear transfer is sufficiently different from other means of reproduction as not to be considered constitutionally protected (Annas, 1997). The Vatican insists that "human beings have a right to be 'born in a human way, and not in a laboratory'" (Butler & Wadman, 1997, p. 8).

Between these extremes are those who maintain that cloning humans should be prohibited for the time being because of potential medical and psychological harms to future clones (including harms arising from possible commodification). Only when human cloning is shown to be reasonably safe and effective might it become available to further reproductive goals, subject to appropriate constraints aimed at preventing possible abuses.[4] For example, a distinction might be drawn between frivolous reasons for cloning such as vanity, and "legitimate" socio-medical reasons for cloning such as allowing persons with otherwise untreatable infertility to have a biologically related child.

The cloning of humans, however, ought not to be construed narrowly as a reproductive technology. While it is certainly the case that cloning technology likely will be provided by those who currently work in, or are affiliated with, IVF clinics, it is a serious mistake to believe that cloning is just another means of assisted reproduction. As George Annas writes, cloning "represents a difference in kind, not in degree in the way that humans continue the species" (Annas, 1997, p. 80). With reproduction by means of sexual intercourse, each offspring (except for identical twins, triplets, or rarely even quadruplets) has a unique genetic make-up that is a combination of genes from his or her biological parents. Assisted reproductive technologies preserve this feature of human reproduction. In marked contrast, human cloning by somatic cell nuclear transfer not only separates reproduction from sexual relations, it also separates reproduction from recombination, as there is no reshuffling of the genes. Unlike current assisted reproductive technologies, therefore, this type of human cloning transgresses species norms. The ethics of transgressing species norms, though widely discussed in the literature on xenotransplantation, is not central to discussions about human cloning; instead, autonomy (procreative liberty), utility and safety appear to be the predominant concerns.

Attempts to map the cloning debate onto the debate about reproductive freedom is not surprising since the domain of reproductive ethics is reasonably familiar territory. There is, for instance, much material in the bioethics literature on autonomy and reproductive choice on the one hand, and the sanctity of human life and the concept of family on the other. In comparison, there is little on transgenerational justice that spans more than one or two generations, and still less on the notion of species integrity that is not about the creation of transgenic animals—these issues merit careful consideration.

V. AN ALTERNATIVE

The way in which any discourse is framed informs (if not determines) the issues identified, the questions asked, the interpretations offered and the range of responses advocated. The common view of cloning technology as a reproductive technology thus explains the current interest in rights (both reproductive rights and property rights), personal autonomy, informed consent, family privacy, safety and potential harms to children. According to the NBAC, for example, "The unique and distinctive ethical issues raised by the use of somatic cell nuclear transfer to create children relate to, for example, serious safety concerns, individuality, family integrity, and treating children as objects" (NBAC, 1997, pp. 3-4). To be sure, these are important issues. There are, however, other equally important issues that are not identified, much less debated, with the current analytical framework. To correct this, an alternative framework is recommended where human cloning is also viewed as an individual and a species enhancement technology—a mechanism for

environmental and biological improvements on a scale never before possible.

Humans have always sought to enhance their own and their children's physical, intellectual, emotional and moral capacities with a view to improving health and increasing the prospects for happiness and "success". Common contemporary enhancements include: vaccines to enhance the immune response to specific diseases; good nutrition to enhance physical development; sound education to enhance intellectual, social and other abilities; music lessons to enhance manual dexterity and mathematical ability; dance lessons and gymnastics to enhance balance and posture; sports training (and/or steroids) to enhance athletic ability, build muscle mass and strength; and cosmetic surgery to enhance physical appearance. With adults the use of these enhancements is generally a matter of personal choice. With children, some of these enhancements are legally and morally required (e.g., vaccinations and basic education), others are optional (e.g., music lessons and cosmetic surgery). Elective enhancements are generally used at the discretion of parents, with or without consultation with the child, and based on their assessment of their child's abilities and interests. Significantly, parents may choose enhancements that will expand the range of opportunities for their child, or they may choose enhancements that will considerably narrow the range of opportunities because of a very limited focus on select talents that are not widely adaptable.

With the cloning of whole beings, parental efforts at enhancing children's capacities will intensify because of the available knowledge regarding the child's genetic structure. The cloning of humans thus will not simply be about having children but about having a unique opportunity to improve on a desired specimen (e.g., a clone of oneself or a loved one) by investing in enhanced genes and/or enhanced environments in order to increase/accentuate desired traits and/or to modify/eliminate negative traits. Consider the following scenario. A talented concert violinist chooses to clone herself using her egg (enucleated oocyte), her nucleus (somatic cell) and her uterus to achieve near perfect cloning. Like all parents, she wants her child to have a "better" life. This motivates her to embark on a unique enhancement project made possible by her decision to reproduce asexually. She does not want her daughter to suffer the disappointments she has known and is thus intent on enhancing her child's talent for creating (her understanding of) beautiful music. With germline gene transfer, the violinist hopes to improve her clone's dexterity, hearing and memory. To be sure, attempts at genetically enhancing these traits will be difficult (if not ultimately impossible) because many genes affect these abilities and each of these genes may affect multiple body systems. Nonetheless, the violinist is willing to experiment. Also, persuaded that a little melancholy (sweet sorrow) will add a creative edge to her clone's music, she agrees to altering the genes responsible for the production of serotonin. When her child is a toddler, the environmental enhancement begins in earnest.

The violinist teaches her clone special exercises to improve the genetically improved dexterity and memory. As well, there is the drug regimen to alter the serotonin levels, the Stradivarius and the Juilliard School music lessons that her own parents could not afford to give her until she reached her mid-teens. In these ways the violinist hopes that her child—a genetic replica of herself—will have a better future.

As illustrated above, with cloning by somatic cell nuclear transfer the parent (i.e., clonant) has intimate knowledge of the child's (i.e., clone's) future possibilities because of their shared genotype. This unique foreknowledge necessarily influences (possibly skews) the enhancements chosen, and this is not because of misguided views about genetic determinism. Our genes do not determine who we are, but they clearly do suggest certain possibilities and set certain boundaries. Foreknowledge of these possibilities and boundaries, which becomes possible with cloning technology, will influence the genetic, surgical, pharmaceutical and other medical enhancements that will be pursued in order to improve the clone's form. In turn, these biolog-ical enhancements may influence behaviour. For example, a physical change can alter/improve an individual's psychological and social dispositions. As well, this unique foreknowledge will influence the choice of social, cultural, ecological, physical and other environments to which the clone will be exposed in an effort to further improve performance. In this way, human cloning technology to produce a genetic replica of a person whose potential is known makes possible a unique and complex kind of biological and environmental enhancement.

To be sure, any cloning experiment ultimately may fail to achieve its objective. For example, the violinist's clone may become a disgruntled clerk at an airport car rental. Nonetheless, the point remains. Cloning (at least of those who have lived a reasonable life span) is not simply about reproduction. Rather, it is very much about "getting it right" (avoiding the errors of a previous generation), on the basis of unique advance knowledge about which genetic and environmental factors might benefit from enhancement.

If we now move the discussion from the means of enhancement to the goals of enhancement, an important difference emerges between the goals of *intentional individual enhancement* and the goals of *intentional species enhancement.* With the intentional biological and environmental enhancement of individual human beings, the goals are typically to promote health, happiness, and "success". In turn, these will be the *de facto* goals of inadvertent species enhancement—a phenomenon that will occur over time, as enhancements made at the individual level are passed on to subsequent generations (with or without further alterations), and as the environment of which these individuals are an integral part continues to evolve. In marked contrast, with *intentional species enhancement,* where changes are not merely the inadvertent cumulative long-term side-effect of idiosyncratic changes at the individual level, more communal goals can be pursued such as the survival of the species, the elimination of misery and an improvement in the quality of life.

For example, in the not-too-distant future, if pollution and overpopulation were to cause our environment to deteriorate so significantly that our survival on the planet were threatened, the cloning of humans might be an important element of a survival strategy for the species. Individuals with certain biological traits conducive to survival in this emerging inhospitable environment could be cloned (and possibly genetically enhanced) while at the same time efforts were made to stabilize the deteriorating environment. In this way, it would be possible to enhance the species in a single generation and thereby increase the probability of survival.

From the perspective of some, however, a more immediate threat to our survival and the cause of considerable misery is "our limited capacity for altruism, and for the imaginative sympathy it depends on" (Glover, 1984, p. 181). Jonathan Glover suggests, for example, that although war may appear to be the result of particular economic, social and political arrangements, our failure to eliminate war suggests that psychological changes may be required in addition to political and social reforms. In this view, species enhancement using both genetic and environmental methods may be necessary to overcome certain emotional and imaginative limitations. This might involve direct genetic intervention to ensure that genes we value, such as those that contribute to our capacity for altruism and human sympathy, survive through cloning and are genetically and environmentally enhanced.

Finally, a less dramatic reason for pursuing biological species enhancement would be to improve our quality of life perhaps by enhancing our intellectual capacities. We can, for example, imagine a time in the remote future when we will have exhausted our capacity to understand our world: "Just as calculus is too much for a dog's brain to grasp, so some parts of physics might turn out to be too difficult for us as we are" (Glover, 1984, p. 180). At that time, "[b]ecause our growing understanding of the world is so central a part of why it is good to be human," we may want to select from among us a number of good specimens for replication and genetic enhancement in order that we might transcend our intellectual limitations (Glover, 1984, p. 180). Before any such hypothetical need should arise, however, we can perhaps more easily imagine a world in which the increasing abilities of machines are fast outpacing those of humans. In response to this threat, humans might want to genetically enhance their cognitive skills by cloning good specimens to be genetically engineered in order to acquire new and increasingly sophisticated judgment, decision-making, and adaptation skills.

In addition to the obvious genetic planning that cloning technology makes possible for the species, it is important to stress the interesting possibilities for environmental species enhancement. The cloning of humans provides us with a unique opportunity to study the nature/nurture question on a grand scale. For the first time, it would be possible to hold constant one element of this dyad and, in so doing, to learn how best to cultivate/nurture desirable traits. Leaving aside, for the sake of argument, questions of research ethics, the same "gene bundles" could be exposed to different social, environmental and generational influences so that we might better understand human development and evolution. In an ideal world, this knowledge could then be used to improve our quality of life—to modify our political and economic systems, to alter our educational programs and to introduce social changes that would nurture the traits we value for ourselves and subsequent generations.

In closing, the benefit of regarding the cloning of humans as an enhancement technology is twofold. The first benefit is that this perspective will shed a new light on questions that are already the subject of intense debate. Among these questions: What are the moral costs of human cloning? What obligations do we have to subsequent generations who will be subject to an unprecedented measure of control from preceding generations? How are these obligations to be weighed against obligations to those who are living? What about issues of social justice? While many live in poverty and lack basic health care, can we responsibly devote energy and resources to the project of cloning humans? Is human cloning necessary? If so, necessary for what? Is human cloning progressive? If so, progressive towards what end? Is it efficient? If so, effecting what? Is it good for the species, for the individual clonant, for the individual clone, or is it good for its own sake? Answers to these questions will differ significantly depending upon the framework for analysis—whether one considers cloning to be a reproductive and/or an enhancement technology.

The second benefit of considering the cloning of humans as an enhancement technology is that this perspective will bring into sharp focus a range of novel questions that merit thoughtful reflection. For example: With the cloning of humans are we bound to embrace "volitional evolution" whereby we intentionally intervene in the shaping of human purpose? Would volitional evolution result in a domestication of the species? What is the value of diversity? What is the value of homogeneity? What social norms regarding race, gender and appearance might (inadvertently or intentionally) be entrenched with cloning technology? While undeniably offensive in its eugenic implications, in the long term, would homogenization of the species be a cure for such social and political ills as racism, sexism, classism, homophobia and so on, or would any initiative of this kind only serve to exacerbate existing prejudices?

As well, another cluster of questions might stem from an understanding of human cloning as the modern equivalent to reincarnation. This perspective might refashion our understanding of such concepts as "a life span" and "a life plan". For example, given the belief that reincarnation is a mechanism that allows individuals to improve upon themselves over time, in our modern production-oriented society would there develop an expectation that persons should avail themselves of cloning technology for the express purpose of improving upon the prior incarnation? What would be the end-point? Would it be

culturally informed or socially stipulated? What would be the social, political and moral responses to this new eugenics?

When the cloning of humans is considered solely as a reproductive technology, the questions listed above garner hardly any serious attention. Instead we concentrate on questions about possible harms to children and personal choice: "Is a clone any worse off than a 'normal' but unwanted child? Is Steve, who wants to clone himself, any more egotistical than Saul, who wants to conceive naturally, though his children will have a 25 percent chance of getting Tay-Sachs disease? And if cloning should be outlawed because it may undermine family values, should we outlaw divorce as well?" (Bilger, 1997, p. 19). In marked contrast, when the cloning of humans is considered an individual or species enhancement technology, broader societal and species-type questions outside the protected realm of personal and reproductive autonomy are "front and center".

Thus, it is salient to understand that the current debate on the ethics of cloning humans with its predominant focus on autonomy (individuals' rights, desires and choices) is profoundly unsatisfactory and lacking in imagination. This debate is sustained and remains sustainable, however, because it occurs in a social context sympathetic to the claim that "the principles of personal liberty and personal fortune are the primary determinants of what individuals are allowed and able to do" (Silver, 1997, p. 9). As a result, the debate about cloning humans stagnates at the level of the personal; it never really moves beyond the framework of private relationships and reproductive choice. Thus, profound value questions are set aside and potentially dramatic societal and species consequences arising from the use of cloning technology are inappropriately downplayed or exaggerated. Only in recognizing the individual and species enhancement dimensions of cloning technology can we begin to recognize the broader issues and grapple with the threat/opportunity that cloning humans represents. For all of us.

Notes

1. The research for this paper was supported by grants from the Social Sciences and Humanities Research Council of Canada and from Dalhousie University. This is a revised version of the *Dr. John P. Maclean Memorial Lecture, Department of Internal Medicine, University of Manitoba,* Winnipeg, Manitoba, April 1999, that was also presented at the Second Annual *International Bioethics Retreat,* Florence, Italy, October 1999.
2. I owe the distinction between "reproducing our kind" and "reproducing ourselves" to Ford Doolittle, Dalhousie University.
3. In the literature a distinction is drawn between *reproductive* cloning, where the aim is to reproduce whole beings, and *therapeutic* cloning, where the aim is to reproduce cell lines for the treatment of disease or disability.
4. The Report of the National Bioethics Advisory Commission would appear to fall in this general category. See National Bioethics Advisory Commission (1997). The Executive Summary (1997) of this report is reprinted in the *Hastings Center Report,* 27(3), 7–9.

References

Annas, G.J. (1997). Human cloning. *ABA Journal,* 83, 80–81.

Baird, P.A. (1999). Cloning of animals and humans: What should the policy response be? *Perspectives in Biology and Medicine,* 42(2), 179–194.

Bilger, B. (1997, September/October). Cell block. *The Sciences,* 17–19.

Bonnicksen, A.L. (1995). Ethical and policy issues in human embryos twinning. *Cambridge Quarterly of Healthcare Ethics,* 4(3), 268–284.

Brock, D. (1997). Cloning human beings: An assessment of the ethical issues pro and con. In: National Bioethics Advisory Commission. *Cloning human beings: Report and recommendations of the National Bioethics Advisory Commission, Volume II Commissioned Papers.* Rockville, Maryland.

Butler, D., & Wadman, M. (1997). Calls for cloning ban sell science short. *Nature,* 386, 8.

Callahan, D. (1998). Cloning: Then and now. *Cambridge Quarterly of Healthcare Ethics,* 7(2), 141–144.

Cibelli, J.B., Kiessling, A.A., Cunniff, K., Richards, C., Lanza, R.P., & West, M. (2001). Somatic cell nuclear transfer in humans: Pronuclear and early embryonic development. *E-biomed: The Journal of Regenerative Medicine,* 2, 25–31.

Fletcher, J. (1971). Ethical aspects of genetic controls. *New England Journal of Medicine,* 285, 776–783.

Glover, J. (1984). *What sort of people should there be?* Great Britain: Richard Clay (The Chaucer Press) Ltd.

Grey, W. (1998). Playing God. *Encyclopedia of applied ethics* (Vol. 3). USA: Academic Press.

Haldane, J.B.S. (1963). Biological possibilities for the human species in the next ten thousand years. In: G.E.D. Wolstenhome (Ed.), *Man and his future* (pp. 337–361). London: Churchill.

Hall, J.L., Engel, D., Gindoff, P.R., Motto, G.L., & Stillman, R.I. (1993). Experimental cloning of human polyploid embryos using an artificial zona pellucida. *The American Fertility Society, Co jointly With the Canadian Fertility and Andrology Society. Program Supplement* [Abstract of the Scientific and Oral Poster Sessions, Abstract 0-001S1].

Harris, J. (1997). 'Goodbye Dolly?' The ethics of human cloning. *Journal of Medical Ethics,* 23, 353–360.

Health Canada. (2001). *Draft Legislation on Assisted Human Reproduction.* http://www.hc-sc.gc.ca/English/reproduction/legislation.pdf.

Hefner, P. (1998). Cloning as quintessential human act. In: M. Ruse (Ed.), *Philosophy of biology* (pp. 352–256). Amherst, New York: Prometheus Books.

Human Fertilisation and Embryology (Research Purposes) Regulations. (2001). Statutory Instrument 2001 No. 188. http://www.legislation.hmso.gov.uk/si/si2001/20010188.htm.

Jonas, H. (1974). Biological engineering—a preview. In: H. Jonas (Ed.), *Philosophical essays: From ancient creed to technological man* (pp. 141–167). Englewood Cliffs, NJ: Prentice Hall.

Kahn, A. (1997). Clone mammals … clone man. *Nature, 386,* 119.

Kato, Y., Tani, T., Sotomaru, Y., Kurokawa, K., Kato, J., Doguchi, H., Yasue, H., & Tsunoda, Y. (1998). Eight calves cloned from somatic cells of a single adult. *Science, 282,* 2095–2098.

National Bioethics Advisory Commission (NBAC). (1997). *Cloning human beings: Report and recommendations of the National Bioethics Advisory Commission.* Rockville, MD: National Bioethics Advisory Commission.

Onishi, A., Iwamoto, M., Akita, T., Mikawa, S., Takeda, K., Awata, T., Hanada, H., & Perry, A.C.F. (2000). Pig cloning by microinjection of fetal fibroblast nuclei. *Science, 289,* 1188–1190.

PPL Therapeutics plc. (2000). *PPL produces world's first cloned pigs.* Press release March 5, http://www.ppl-therapeutics.com.

Robertson, J. (1994). The question of human cloning. *Hastings Center Report, 24*(2), 6–14.

Robertson, J. (1998). Human cloning and the challenge of regulation. *New England Journal of Medicine, 339*(2), 119–122.

Silver, L.M. (1997). *Remaking Eden: Cloning and beyond in a brave new world.* New York: Avon Books.

Silver, L.M. (1998). Cloning, ethics, and religion. *Cambridge Quarterly of Healthcare Ethics, 7*(2), 168–172.

Wakayama, T., Perry, A.C., Zuccotti, M., Johnson, K.R., & Yanagimachi, R. (1998). Full-term development of mice from enucleated oocytes injected with cumulus cell nuclei. *Nature, 394,* 369–374.

Watts, J., & Morris, K. (1999). Human cloning trial met with outrage and scepticism. *The Lancet, 353,* 43.

Wells, D.N., Misica, P.M., & Territ, H.R. (1999). Production of cloned calves following nuclear transfer with cultured adult mural granulosa cells. *Biology of Reproduction, 60,* 996–1005.

Wilmut, I., Schnieke, A.E., McWhir, J., Kind, A.J., & Campbell, K.H.S. (1997). Viable offspring derived from fetal and adult mammalian cells. *Nature, 385,* 810–812.

Wilmut, I., Campbell, K., & Tudge, C. (2000) *The second creation: The age of biological control by the scientists that cloned Dolly.* London, England: Headline.

Wolf, D.P., Meng, L., Ouhibi, N., & Zelinski-Wooten, M. (1999). Nuclear transfer in the rhesus monkey: Practical and basic implications. *Biology of Reproduction, 60,* 199–204.

Wolpert, L. (1999). Is science dangerous? *Nature, 398,* 281–282.

World Health Organization. (1997, May 14). *Cloning in human reproduction.* Fiftieth World Health Assembly. WHA50.37 Supplementary agenda item. Geneva.

The Inevitability of Genetic Enhancement Technologies

Françoise Baylis and Jason Scott Robert

INTRODUCTION

For some, the development and use of any technology to enhance human capacities and traits is laudable—likely to improve the human condition.[1] For others, the development and use of all but a narrow set of environmental enhancements (such as education) is deeply problematic.[2] Between these extremes are those who are not so much concerned with the technical means of enhancement—that is, whether the alterations are sought by environmental, surgical, pharmacological or genetic means—but rather who are worried about the nature of the alterations sought—that is, whether the enhancement technology will be used (alone or in combination) to make physical, intellectual, psychological or moral alterations to the self.[3] In the category of *physical enhancements* there might be a range of alterations aimed at improving size, increasing muscle mass, reducing sleep dependence, increasing endurance, decelerating aging, altering skin colour, or changing gender. *Intellectual enhancement*s might include alterations aimed at improving memory and cognitive ability, promoting multi-dimensional thinking, and increasing imagination. *Psychological enhancements* might include efforts to improve sociability, reduce shyness, and instil confidence. And, *moral enhancements* could seek to control violent behaviour, encourage kindness, and promote the capacity for sympathy. Some of these types of enhancements are considered worthy of pursuit, while others are thought to be of questionable value.

Moreover, for some individuals the worry is not with the technical means of enhancement or with the human characteristics to be enhanced, but rather with the underlying motivation(s). In very general terms, enhancements may be sought for a variety of reasons: to be in fashion; to improve performance; to gain a competitive advantage; to secure and exercise power; to promote and protect health and well-being; to increase the lifespan; to assuage or even overcome existential angst; or to meet the demands of justice.[4] And, depending upon the underlying motivation, the resulting alterations may be conservative (i.e., used to normalize the self), liberal (i.e., used to liberate the self), or radical (i.e., used to fashion a self that effectively challenges others' conception of oneself).[5] From the perspective of some theorists, not all of these reasons for seeking to enhance human capacities and traits are equally meritorious.

With this rough taxonomy of means, objects, and motivations in mind, we turn our attention to genetic enhancement technologies in particular. For our purposes, a *genetic enhancement technology* is any technology that directly alters the expression of genes that are already present in humans, or that involves the addition of genes that have not previously appeared within the human population (including plant, animal, or custom-designed genes), for the purpose of human physical, intellectual, psychological, or moral improvement. This includes somatic cell nuclear transfer (SCNT) technology, somatic and germ line gene transfer technology, cosmetic gene insertion, cosmetic stem cell transfer, and the creation of human-to-human and animal-to-human chimeras, as well as animal-to-human hybrids. We contend that attempts to develop and use such technologies are inevitable. While the argument offered here might be developed and applied more broadly to encompass additional or even all new forms of (bio)technology, we restrict our attention, and so the scope of our claim, to genetic enhancement technologies as defined above.

To be sure, not all of the envisioned genetic enhancements will come to pass. The complexities of organismal development[6] are such that some of the genetic tinkering imagined and promoted by enhancement enthusiasts will prove to be impossible.[7] This fact is irrelevant to our argument, however. What matters to our argument is that *despite* the likely failure of particular genetic enhancements, there are some among us who will *inevitably attempt* to engineer the human genome[8] for the purpose of improving *Homo sapiens*. And, to our surprise (and perhaps our disgust or delight) some will succeed.

… We explore various reasons for the inevitability of genetic enhancement technologies, and conclude that accepting the inevitability of genetic enhancement will spur us to profitably redirect ethical energy to the all-important tasks of ensuring that the process of attempting genetic enhancement is morally acceptable, and that successfully developed genetic enhancements are used in a socially responsible manner. In this way we hope to guard against a defeatist interpretation of our inevitability claim, while simultaneously opening moral space for a more productive dialogue.[9]

ESCHEWING BOUNDARIES: SUPPORT FOR GENETIC ENHANCEMENT TECHNOLOGIES

Some insist that the pursuit of all enhancement technologies is not just ethically permissible, but also a moral imperative for humans,[10] and that specific objections to the development and use of genetic enhancement technologies are wrong-headed. Among the proponents of this view are those who maintain that humans are sorely imperfect, and so humans should do whatever can be done to augment human traits and capacities. In many respects, however, this suggestion is less an argument than a manifesto.[11] What we take to be the standard argument in support of genetic enhancement technologies must be reconstructed; abstracted, it runs as follows: (1) *Enhancing* human capacities and traits is a worthy ideal, as evidenced by the general social commitment to education, medicine, and welfare; (2) *genetically* enhancing human capacities and traits—for example, somatic cell nuclear transfer (i.e., cloning) for the purpose of replicating and improving upon a desired specimen,[12] and cosmetic stem cell transfer to supplement the functioning of normal genes—represents but one end of a continuum of enhancement technologies to pursue the goal of enhancing human capacities and traits; (3) if the *goal* of genetic enhancement is the same as the (laudable) goal of generic enhancement, then the *means* of enhancement do not matter morally; (4) the goal of genetic enhancement is in fact the same as the goal of generic enhancement, and so is itself laudable; therefore, (5) genetic enhancement technologies should be developed and their use promoted and supported.

While the first premise seems unassailable, and the conclusion does indeed follow from the premises taken together, premises (2–4) deserve further scrutiny. The second and fourth premises are the subject of many of the objections outlined below. The third premise is the subject of the final objection surveyed.

ESPOUSING LIMITS: OBJECTIONS TO GENETIC ENHANCEMENT TECHNOLOGIES

Current objections to genetic enhancement technologies are many and varied. Though some of the arguments to be discussed below have been treated in considerably more detail by others,[13] it will become evident that sketching them here is necessary to our programmatic endeavour to change the subject and tenor of ethical debates about genetic enhancements. In our view, the objections to genetic enhancement technologies cluster around the following themes: (i) the technologies are intrinsically wrong; (ii) whether the technologies are effective or not, there likely will be negative biological consequences; (iii) if the technologies are effective and their use is widespread, this will result in harmful social consequences; and (iv) the means of achieving laudable ends are not all equally morally meritorious....[14]

1. *Transgression of divine laws.* There are two major thrusts to the argument against genetic enhancement technologies as 'playing God.' The first focuses on God's omniscience. The claim is that the requisite knowledge and capacities to plan for the physical, intellectual, psychological and moral well-being of distant future generations is beyond the grasp of humans. On this view, volitional evolution—the intentional genetic shaping of human purpose—should remain beyond human reach. It is sheer hubris for anyone to attempt to directly manipulate the human genetic structure, for only God can know (and accordingly plan for) the future of the species. The second major thrust of the argument against 'playing God' focuses on God's omnipotence. The claim is that the planned (hoped for) use of genetic enhancement technologies aimed at creating or modifying life is an unwarranted, unwise and profoundly immoral attempt to usurp God's power.[15]

2. *Transgression of natural laws.* According to some, the use of genetic enhancement tech-

nologies is unnatural for at least two reasons: it is contrary to the natural course of events; and it is contrary to human nature. The putatively unnatural features of genetic enhancement technologies are objectionable from the perspective of those who believe that the natural order has intrinsic value, independently of human valuers. On this view, nature deserves respect; this respect sets limits on human intervention; and these limits preclude the use of genetic enhancement technologies. Despite a wide range of opinion on the nature of human nature,[16] and against the historically prevalent view that humans are by nature meant to master nature,[17] the second, related objection is that as humans are part of nature, rather than separate from nature, the essence of humans is to nurture and protect the natural world, not to dominate it through, for instance, genetic engineering.

3. *Introduction of an unacceptable risk of harm.* There is considerable speculation about the possible negative biological consequences of the introduction and use of genetic enhancement technologies. The possibility of error, and the potential for serious correlative physical, psychological and other harms to individuals, are typical objections to enhancement technologies especially during their early research phases. These objections are particularly significant in the case of genetic enhancement technologies where: (i) any error may be irreversible; (ii) the underlying risk of harm is unknown and unknowable; and (iii) the direct consequences of any error will be borne by many in addition to the individual who may be enhanced, particularly if the error is perpetuated into future generations.

4. *Introduction of a threat to genetic diversity.* It is said that genetic enhancement technologies will have a deleterious impact on the genetic variability characteristic of the human gene pool. Though it is widely recognized that there is no real prospect of eliminating genetic diversity altogether,[18] some argue that even small changes could lead to serious harm.[19] One possible reason for concern is that scientists know so little about gene function in organismal development, and not much more about development above the level of the genes....

5. *Introduction of a threat to our common genetic heritage.* The United Nations Educational, Scientific, and Cultural Organization adopted a *Universal Declaration on the Human Genome and Human Rights* in 1997. In Article 1 of that document, UNESCO declared that 'the human genome underlies the fundamental unity of all members of the human family, as well as the recognition of the inherent dignity and diversity of each of its members.'[20] If the human genome represents humanity's common heritage ... then this heritage may be seriously threatened by genetic enhancements. Some believe that there is the distinct possibility that with the genetic enhancement of successive generations—by altering the expression of genes that are already present or adding new genes that have not previously appeared in humans—a segment of society will engineer itself out of the species *Homo sapiens*. Already those who worry about the possibility of radical transformation jest about the creation of a new species—*Homo Glaxo Wellcomus*.[21]

6. *Paradoxical counterproductivity.* In liberal democratic societies, at least, decisions about the use of genetic enhancement technologies are thought to be a private matter. This view is mistaken, however, insofar as there would be enormous social ramifications to the millions of individual decisions to use genetic enhancement technologies. Consider, for example, the potentially devastating social impact of a genetic technology to alter the aging process and extend

life. If it were possible to genetically opti-
mise human biology to be resistant to disease and the ravages of old age, and the
middle classes in economically advanced
industrialised countries availed themselves
of this technology for themselves and their
children, enormous social problems would
result from ever-increasing population
density,[22] not to mention ever-increasing
healthcare spending for a population that is
(by global standards and at least for now)
very healthy.[23] This is an instance of what
Ivan Illich refers to as 'paradoxical counter-
productivity,' the process by which an institution or technology, in its normal course of
operation, paradoxically subverts the very
purpose it was intended to serve.[24] …
[A] genetically enhanced human species, by
threatening to overwhelm existing social
institutions and practices, may become,
paradoxically, disabled.[25] Consider, for
example, the elective use of genetic
enhancement technologies to increase
height with the aim of securing competitive
advantage. Particular social and economic
advantages may be accessible only to tall
people; but there are of course height limits
beyond which being tall would in fact be
disadvantageous. As Dan Brock notes,
'to be nine feet tall would on balance be
harmful in nearly any human society
because our social world is constructed for
persons whose height rarely reaches beyond
seven feet. One would literally become, in a
physical respect, unfit for human company.'[26] Now, if everyone were to be nine
feet tall, the expected competitive advantage
would dissipate; and if instead the social
world were to be reconstituted so as to
accommodate those who are nine feet tall (if
not everyone were), then the competitive
advantage would be a result of social, rather
than genetic, enhancement.

7. *A misuse of social resources.* Considerable
time, money and talent typically are
required for the development of new technologies. When these technologies respond
to a widespread need (or even the needs of a
very deserving few), and there is the political will to ensure their just distribution, one
may legitimately conclude that financial and
human resources have been invested wisely.
This is not the case, however, when the new
technologies address the perceived needs of
an affluent minority and serve to entrench
existing power relations. In these instances,
there are likely huge opportunity costs as
other needed social and health objectives
are not pursued.[27]

8. *A widening of the gap between the 'haves'
and the 'have-nots'.* The first genetic
enhancements available, and quite possibly
the only ones, will likely be physical and
intellectual enhancements. These enhancements will initially be very expensive and
only the rich (and powerful) will be able to
gain access. As with other advanced technologies (such as computers and elec-
tronics), however, in time the cost of these
enhancements should decrease. Even so, in
all likelihood the technologies will still only
be available to the middle classes, and only
in some countries. A potential problem with
this is that the widespread use of these technologies by those who can afford them will
accentuate both the vagaries of the natural
lottery as well as socio-economic differences.[28] The idea that humans are all created equal is a useful political fiction
helping to establish solidarity amongst
humans and to undergird social commitment to a principle of equality of opportunity, namely that despite the differences
between individuals, each individual should
have the opportunity to strive for success
(however defined). Mehlman notes that,
'in the worst case scenario, unequal access
to genetic enhancement will divide society
into the enhanced and the un-enhanced.'[29]
He argues that this split would critically
threaten the basis of the principle of equality
of opportunity by freezing prospects of
upward social mobility. Shenk, citing
Thomas Jefferson's observation that 'the

mass of mankind has not been born with saddles on their backs, nor a favored few booted and spurred, ready to ride them,' worries that we simply cannot be confident in either the truth or the rhetorical power of those words in future.[30] More globally, Silver notes that:

> … the social advantage that wealthy societies currently maintain could be converted into a genetic advantage. And the already wide gap between wealthy and poor nations could widen further and further with each generation until all common heritage is gone. A severed humanity could very well be the ultimate legacy of unfettered global capitalism.[31]

The claim, then, is that use of genetic enhancement technologies will increase the gap between the haves and have-nots, unmask the myth of social equality, and result in significant social disruptions both within and between societies.

9. *Promotion of social conformity and homogeneity.* While genetic enhancement technologies are commonly thought to be liberating, they can be very constraining. Experience shows that enhancement technologies are often used to reinforce inappropriate social roles, prejudices and stereotypes as people seek to advantage themselves or their children relative to others. Consider, for example, cosmetic surgery for women to achieve their ideal(ised) shape, for individuals of Japanese descent to 'Westernize' their eyes, and for individuals of Jewish heritage to alter their 'Jewish' noses. These sorts of physical enhancements promote a harmful conception of normality and hide the fact that such norms are socially and culturally constructed. This problem can only be exacerbated with genetically based physical and intellectual enhancements.[32]

10. *Undermining free choice.* Many are familiar with the aphorism 'more is not always better.' In this context, the point is that 'more options' does not mean necessarily 'more choice.' While the use of genetic enhancement technologies can be described as empowering, as when rational individuals autonomously choose to avail themselves of the technologies,[33] the fact remains that choice is always constrained by context. If the context includes the widespread use of a particular enhancement technology, personal freedom may be seriously threatened as people feel obliged to avail themselves of the technology. For example, if a significant minority of people freely choose to genetically alter their children's ability to produce growth hormone and the average height shifts upward, it will be extremely difficult, if not impossible, for parents to freely choose not to provide their child with this genetic enhancement. There will be strong social pressure to conform, as there already is in the case of prenatal diagnosis;[34] concerning genetic enhancements, parents may well feel the need to conform just to compete.[35]

11. *The means matter morally.* While some would suggest that enhancement technologies from education to germ-line engineering exist on a continuum and are of a piece in promoting a single goal—the laudable augmentation of human capacities and traits—it is not clear that the end justifies the use of any and all possible means. Consider that particular means may be valuable in themselves (because edifying, or taxing, or demanding persistence)—independently of the overarching end—and not merely instrumentally (as means to that pre-specified end, no matter how valuable). The idea is that the experience of accomplishment (the means by which accomplishment is achieved) could itself be valuable, and not just the accomplishment (the end) alone: value is not exclusively consequential. Moreover, different means target different variables, and alternative means may well have different opportunity costs and collateral consequences—some of which will have a moral dimension—independently of shared ends. The

objection is, thus, that it is inappropriate to pretend that genetic enhancement technologies are just 'more of the same' and so are therefore ethically unproblematic.[36]

TO STEER, BUT NOT TO STOP

Not all of the ethical objections described above will be persuasive for everyone, and some will persuade no one…. In our view, however, the concerns raised about the negative social consequences can be developed most persuasively, as can the worry about paradoxical counter-productivity and the notion that means matter morally….

These objections, [properly elaborated and] taken together, would seem to provide ample good reason to forsake the development and use of genetic enhancement technologies. There is no evidence as yet, however, that these arguments in particular, or any other arguments, *however well developed*, will suffice to stop the refinement and use of genetic enhancement technologies. As it happens, contemporary Western democracies have no experience with permanently halting the development and use of any enhancement technology on ethical grounds.

The typical response to the development and use of enhancement technologies involves a complex mix of outright 'condemnation' and what might be described as 'passive-aggressive resignation.' Policy statements and legislative or regulatory prohibitions are introduced with full knowledge (and acceptance) of the fact that these 'barriers' will not be entirely effective. The overarching pragmatic goal is not to stop the development and use of a specific technology, but rather to slow and possibly to steer basic and applied research. Examples in this category include the use of performance enhancement drugs, the use of psychedelic drugs and the current effort to clone a human being.

… In each of these instances, prohibitions have been, and continue to be, introduced with the putative goal of stopping the deleterious activity, knowing that in practice, the prohibitions are at most containment initiatives or speed bumps.

We fully anticipate that a similar pattern of response will prevail with the development and use of human genetic enhancement technologies. If so, we can further anticipate the following progression: 'initial condemnation, followed by ambivalence, questioning and limited use, followed in turn by a change in public perceptions, advocacy and widespread acceptance.'[37] Examples of enhancement technologies where the progression from 'condemnation' to 'widespread acceptance' are evident include cosmetic surgery, organ transplantation and gender reassignment. Though initially criticised, these alterations to the self are now either commonplace or well on their way to being so considered.

In anticipation of this sequela, we are driven to ask: why do arguments underscoring probable, unsavoury and unethical consequences have such a limited prospect of stopping the development and use of enhancement technologies, the potential for benefit notwithstanding? More precisely, *why is the development and use of genetic enhancement technologies inevitable?* As will become evident in what follows, by 'inevitability' we do not mean to invoke either a technological imperative or a slippery slope, but rather something more akin to 'resilient to (moral) argument and resultant from particular conceptions of contemporary humanity.'[38]

THE INEVITABILITY THESIS

According to some, genetic enhancement technologies are inevitable—and welcome—because they promise to secure health, success, wealth and happiness, especially for the presently disadvantaged…. [D]espite its popularity, this hypothesis surely strains one's credulity. Ours is not a kind, caring, compassionate world, but rather a capitalist, heedlessly liberal, curiosity-driven, competition-infused world in which some are intent on controlling the human evolutionary story.

Genetic enhancement technologies are inevitable because so many of us are crass capitalists, eager to embrace biocapitalism.[39] In economically advanced industrialised countries, ours is a corporate world where there is a shared commitment to capitalism, privatisation and a market-driven global economy. In this world, marked by globalisation, free markets and consumer choice, there is no enhancement technology that is too dangerous, or too transgressive, for it not to be pursued. Unrestrained consumerism is good and if this results in a free-market eugenic meritocracy, so be it.

In this worldview, only commercial viability (marketability and profitability) matters. If a genetic enhancement technology can be developed and sold (at a profit), it will be made and marketed (and not necessarily in that order). Particular nation-states can try to prohibit the development of the technology, but ultimately are unlikely to be successful. One reason, explored by Gardner, is that once any nation-state endorses human genetic enhancement as a way to gain an industrial-commercial edge, other nation-states will be forced to follow suit.[40] A second reason concerns not nation-states but multinational corporations. The state's authority and power have been seriously eroded by globalisation. Multinationals are widely recognised as more powerful than elected governments and thus, not surprisingly, their commercial interests prevail.[41] Whether at the level of nation-states or multinational industries, ethical concerns are easily swept aside when there is (serious) money to be made.

This mercantile account of the modern world is critically incomplete, however—not least because very many of us aim to transcend crass capitalism. So, eagerness to embrace biocapitalism cannot completely explain the inevitability of genetic enhancement technologies.

Genetic enhancement technologies are inevitable because heedless liberalism is rampant. Leon Kass observes that prohibitionists are struggling 'against the general liberal prejudice that it is wrong to stop people doing something.'[42] Jeffrey Kahn similarly notes the (perhaps uniquely) American reticence to prohibit certain types of research and development because of the prevailing attitude that 'capitalistic acts between consenting adults are none of its business.'[43] Within states, the liberal reduc-tion of the ethical complexities of genetic enhancement technologies to the sacred paradigm of individual free choice virtually guarantees the inevitability of the technologies; meanwhile, more globally, the liberal reluctance to move beyond this paradigm engenders a more general attitude of cultural relativism whereby there is neither the imperative nor the opportunity to deem some activities as just plain wrong.

Such a political diagnosis of the modern world is also seriously incomplete, however—not least because it invokes an unfair caricature of liberalism and fails to appreciate the complexities of political life both nationally and globally. So heedless liberalism is also unable to completely account for the inevitability of genetic enhancement technologies.[44]

Genetic enhancement technologies are inevitable because humans are naturally inquisitive (and tinkering) beings. Ours is a curiosity-driven, knowledge-based world that is fascinated with technology and in which the guiding mantra is 'if it can be done, it will be done, and so we should do it first.' In this world, the quest for knowledge for knowledge's sake is an all-consuming passion; understanding ourselves, unravelling the mystery of our existence, is our Holy Grail. Add to this our love of technology, and the inevitability of embracing genetic enhancement technology becomes evident. With research on genetic manipulation there is the prospect 'to improve our understanding of the most complex and compelling phenomenon ever observed—the life process. We cannot be expected to deny ourselves this knowledge.'[45] Nor can we be expected to restrain ourselves from harnessing and applying this knowledge.

A key feature of this worldview is the belief that scientific knowledge is value-free and yet immensely valuable.... In this view, while knowledge can be used to pursue less than praiseworthy technological interventions, this is not sufficient reason to halt the quest for scientific knowledge and understanding. If there are concerns about the misuse of knowledge in the development of a particular technology, then these should appropriately be directed to the eventual application of the technology, not hinder the search for purest scientific knowledge.

Again, some would argue that this view of the world is seriously flawed, not least because scientific knowledge, like all knowledge, is value-laden.[46] Moreover, the distinction between (basic) scientific knowledge and (applied) technology does not withstand critical scrutiny. While some would want to restrict or forbid genetic engineering in humans, it must be remembered 'that it would be difficult to separate … knowledge of molecular genetics from the know-how that manipulates the chromosome.'[47]

This account of the inevitability of genetic enhancement technologies is therefore also incomplete, as the pursuit of knowledge is bound up with social and political (and economic) factors. A worldview according to which knowledge is neutral and can be sought for its own sake, is impoverished and so cannot completely explain the inevitability of genetic enhancement technologies.

Genetic enhancement technologies are inevitable because humans are competitive beings, always looking for new and challenging opportunities to maximize personal, social and economic advantage. Competition is (and has been) a valued human activity not only in itself but also instrumentally—competition promotes the drive to succeed and thus fosters improvement. In work, in sport, in reproduction, (and in other contexts as well), competition is both encouraged and rewarded. Humans have, throughout the ages, repeatedly shown themselves to be competitive beings driven to succeed (and/or to exceed), and willing to use most any means available to achieve the desired end.

In this view, there can be no doubt that genetic enhancement technologies will be among the means used to secure competitive or positional advantage. To be sure, this use of genetic enhancement technologies may be unfair (as when the genetic enhancements are available only to a small elite) or it may be self-defeating (as when the genetic enhancements are universally available and electively used by all so that no relative advantage is gained).[48] No matter. The point

remains that genetic enhancement technologies will be used (by some or all) in attempts to gain a competitive advantage either by strengthening a particular capacity needed to pursue a specific life goal (increased height for the aspiring basketball player, or increased dexterity for the budding pianist), or by strengthening a range of capacities likely to increase one's ability to effectively pursue and master a range of options.

This worldview is flawed, however, in its narrow account of the human drive to compete and succeed. As Dan Brock astutely notes, and as we make clear above regarding means mattering morally, 'sometimes a valued human activity is defined in part by the means it employs, not just by the ends at which it aims.'[49] While competition is a valued human activity, this is, in large measure, because of the way it engages our physical, intellectual and other capacities. For many of us it is not only about winning, but also about how the game is played. In large part this explains the ban on the use of performance enhancement drugs in Olympic competition. On this view, achieving success in the workplace or elsewhere by means of genetic enhancement would hardly be worth the candle. As such, our competitive spirit alone cannot account for the inevitability of genetic enhancement technologies.

In sum, a common flaw with each of these characterisations of the modern world—characterisations of worldviews—is that they are one-dimensional: based either in simplistic economic, political, scientific, or sociological terms. The inevitability of genetic enhancement technologies demands a more encompassing, multi-dimensional diagnosis.

Genetic enhancement technologies are inevitable because the future is ours for the shaping. Ours is a dynamic world in which change is a constant, characterised historically by a variety of cultural revolutions (in language development, agriculture, political organization, physical technologies and, now, biotechnologies) each of which has significantly shaped the human species.[50] Given the economic, political, scientific and sociological realities sketched above, some firmly believe that the time has come for humans to shape our own destiny and to direct the course of evolution. Genetic enhancement technologies are seen as our most powerful tool for this purpose.

In previous times, humans saw themselves as beings created in the image of a divine God, later as products of natural selection and more recently as bundles of selfish genes shaped by selection.[51] Now some see humans as self-transforming beings capable of, and intent on, refashioning ourselves in our own image of what we should be.[52] In this worldview there are and should be no restrictions—financial, moral, epistemic, biological—on what is possible.

This worldview would appear to rest on a particular understanding of human purpose. Following Maslow,[53] what distinguishes humans is the drive toward self-actualization—the desire to realize human potentialities. For generations, increasing percentages of the population in many countries have not had to strive to meet lower-order physiological and safety needs. A direct consequence of this is that some humans have been able to direct their energies to the pursuit of higher order needs, the ultimate goal being to satisfy their desire to realise themselves to the fullest. These individuals have tested their physical, intellectual, emotional and moral limits seeking to learn, for example, what are the limits of the human body? What are the limits of the human mind? What are the limits to human suffering? What are the limits to human evil? These limits have been tested in sport, in business, in play, in war and in love—not with the hope of actually identifying any limits, but rather with the evolutionary goal of transcending all possible limits.

As needed, some among these few have avidly pursued physical, intellectual, psychological and moral enhancements. Now the option of pursuing these enhancements using genetic technologies is on the horizon and keenly awaited....

Here we offer an *avant garde* sketch of human nature. Humans are indeed imperfect creatures, but imperfection is not a necessary condition for humanness. Humans are not merely inquisitive or competitive; rather, we posit that the essential characteristics of humanness are *perfectibility* and the biosocial drive to pursue perfection. These essential characteristics are neither merely naturally present nor culturally driven, but rather biosocially overdetermined. We are on the cusp of what may prove to be our final evolutionary stage.

CONCLUSION

To summarise, there are good reasons to believe that attempts to develop and use genetic enhancement technologies are fraught with moral peril. Nevertheless, in our view, their development and use are inevitable, not simply because of capitalist forces (though these are by no means inconsequential), or because of heedless liberalism (which surely plays a role), or because of a natural desire for knowledge (which is also a significant consideration), or because of a natural or fostered desire to outperform (which, too, is partly explanatory), but also because this is our destiny chosen by those among us who are intent on achieving self-actualisation by controlling the human evolutionary story.

In closing, we maintain that accepting the inevitability of genetic enhancement technologies is an important and necessary step forward in the ethical debate about the development and use of such technologies. We need to change the lens through which we perceive, and therefore approach, the prospect of enhancing humans genetically. In recognizing the futility of trying to stop these technologies, we can usefully direct our energies to a systematic analysis of the appropriate scope of their use. The goal of such a project would be to influence how the technologies will be developed, and the individual, social, cultural, political, economic, ecological and evolutionary ends the technologies should serve. It is to these tasks that bioethical attention must now fully turn.

Acknowledgements

The research for this paper was supported by grants from the Social Sciences and Humanities Research Council of

Canada, Dalhousie University, and the Canadian Institutes of Health Research (to FB), and from the Canadian Institutes of Health Research and Associated Medical Services, Inc. (to JSR). We are grateful to John MacMillan and other members of the Strategic Research Network on Enhancement Technologies and Human Identity, as well as several anonymous referees, for detailed comments on a draft; we are also grateful to members of the Department of Bioethics at Dalhousie University, and to participants at the Fifth World Congress (2000) of the *International Association of Bioethics*, London, UK, and the 2001 meeting of the *Society for Social Studies of Science*, Cambridge MA, for lively discussion of early versions of this article.

Notes

1. See, for instance: B. Stableford. 1984. *Future Man.* New York. Crown; and A Sandberg. (n.d.). Genetic Modifications. Available online at: *http://www.aleph.se/Trans/Individual/Body/genes.html* (accessed 7 February, 2002).

2. For instance: L.J. Kass. 1985. *Toward a More Natural Science: Biology and Human Affairs.* New York. Free Press; and L.J. Kass. The Wisdom of Repugnance. *New Republic* 1997; 216: 17–27.

3. L. Walters & J.G. Palmer. 1997. *The Ethics of Human Gene Therapy.* New York. Oxford University Press.

4. Generally, see: E. Parens, ed. 1999. *Enhancing Human Traits: Ethical and Social Implications.* Washington. Georgetown University Press. For considerations of justice specifically, see, for instance: N. Holtug, Does Justice Require Genetic Enhancements? *Journal of Medical Ethics* 1999; 25: 137–143; and A. Buchanan, D.W. Brock, N. Daniels & D. Wikler. 2000. *From Chance to Choice: Genetics and Justice.* New York. Cambridge University Press.

5. A.D. Dreger, personal communication.

6. J.S. Robert. Interpreting the Homeobox: Metaphors of Gene Action and Activation in Evolution and Development. *Evolution & Development* 2001; 3: 287–295.

7. J.W. Gordon. Genetic Enhancement in Humans. *Science* 1999; 283: 2023–2024.

8. A caveat about *the* human genome: at the genetic level, humans differ from each other by 1/10 of 1%, but it is not the case that there is some "one" genome shared by all humans that is 99.9% identical. There is no single human genome representative of all humans, for genetic variation is the

norm. See: A.L. Tauber & S. Sarkar. The Human Genome Project: Has Blind Reductionism Gone Too Far? *Perspectives in Biology and Medicine* 1992; 35: 220–235, at 228; see also E.A. Lloyd. 1994. Normality and Variation: The Human Genome Project and the Ideal Human Type. In *Are Genes Us? The Social Consequences of the New Genetics.* C.F. Cranor, ed. New Brunswick, N.J. Rutgers University Press: 99–112; and J.S. Robert. Illich, Education, and the Human Genome Project: Reflections on Paradoxical Counterproductivity. *Bulletin of Science, Technology, and Society* 1998; 18: 228–239, at 229–230.

9. In a broad discussion of genetic engineering, Heta Häyry has warned against a particular kind of defeatist pessimism, one that we avoid here. That attitude 'cynically assumes that nothing can be done,' and that 'the total prohibition of gene-splicing activities is the only way to save humankind from the slippery slope to which mad scientists and big corporations are leading us.' Such pessimism may be self-fulfilling, in the sense that 'ordinary citizens' may decide not even to bother attempting to influence the development and use of genetic engineering technologies. Our inevitability claim, as will become evident below, is a different sort of claim altogether; it does not rest on slippery-slope foundations, and its objective is rather to spur attention to the question of how best to mediate the consequences of the development of genetic enhancement technologies. See H Häyry. 1994. How to Assess the Consequences of Genetic Engineering? In *Ethics and Biotechnology.* A. Dyson & J. Harris, eds. New York. Routledge: 144–156, at 152. See also note 38, below.

10. Sandberg, *op. cit.* note 1.

11. Stableford, *op. cit.* note 1; see also hints in this direction offered by Joseph Rosen in: L. Slater. Dr. Daedalus: A Radical Plastic Surgeon Wants to Give You Wings. *Harper's Magazine* 2001; July:57–67.

12. F. Baylis. Human Cloning: Three Mistakes and an Alternative. *Journal of Medicine and Philosophy* 2002; 27: 319–337.

13. See, for instance: J. Glover. 1984. *What Sort of People Should There Be? Genetic Engineering, Brain Control and Their Impact on Our Future World.* New York. Penguin Books; J. Harris. 1992. *Wonderwoman and Superman: The Ethics of Human Biotechnology.* Oxford. Oxford University Press; D. Heyd. 1992. *Genethics: Moral Issues in the Creation of People.* Berkeley. University of

California Press; J. Wood-Harper. 1994. Manipulation of the Germ Line: Towards Elimination of Major Infectious Diseases? In *Ethics and Biotechnology*, *op. cit.* note 9, pp. 121–143; P. Kitcher. 1996. *The Lives to Come: The Genetic Revolution and Human Possibilities.* New York. Simon & Schuster; Walters and Palmer, *op. cit.* note 3, especially Chapter 4; and M-W. Ho. 1999. *Genetic Engineering: Dream or Nightmare?* 2nd edition. New York. Continuum.

14. Nils Holtug has noted that intuitive worries about human gene therapy are generally of the slippery slope variety and, moreover, he has argued that such slippery slope arguments can generally be overcome in the context of human gene therapy. We have thus striven to avoid explicit slippery slope objections to genetic enhancement technologies (though some of the objections may be reconstructed in slippery slope terms). See N. Holtug. Human Gene Therapy: Down the Slippery Slope? *Bioethics* 1993; 7: 402–419. See also note 38, below.

15. P. Ramsey. 1970. *Fabricated Man: The Ethics of Genetic Control.* New Haven. Yale University Press; N. Messer. Human Cloning and Genetic Manipulation: Some Theological and Ethical Issues. *Studies in Christian Ethics* 1999; 12:1–16.

16. R. Trigg. 1988. *Ideas of Human Nature: An Historical Introduction.* Oxford. Basil Blackwell.

17. As documented in: C. Merchant. 1989. *The Death of Nature: Women, Ecology, and the Scientific Revolution.* New York. Harper and Row.

18. G.E. Pence. 1998. *Who's Afraid of Human Cloning?* Lanham, MD. Rowman and Littlefield: 129–131.

19. D.T. Suzuki & P. Knudtson. 1990. *Genethics: The Ethics of Engineering Life.* Revised edition. Toronto. Stoddart.

20. UNESCO. 11 November, 1997. *Universal Declaration on the Human Genome and Human Rights.* 29th Session of the General Conference. Paris. Available online at: *http://unesdoc.unesco.org/images/0010/001096/109687eb.pdf* (accessed 7 February 2002); see also C. Byk. A Map to a New Treasure Island: The Human Genome and the Concept of Common Heritage. *Journal of Medicine and Philosophy* 1998; 23: 234–246.

21. Anonymous. Editorial: The Big Test. *New Republic* 2001; 223. Of course, it is worth emphasising again that there is no such thing in nature as *the* human genome, given the predominance of genetic variability; moreover, there is no such thing in nature as the *human* genome, given that humans share significant DNA sequences with virtually all extant and extinct creatures from apes to amoebae.

22. J. Harris. Intimations of Immortality. *Science* 2000; 288: 59.

23. D. Callahan. 1999. *False Hopes: Overcoming the Obstacles to a Sustainable, Affordable Medicine.* New Brunswick, NJ. Rutgers University Press.

24. Robert. *op. cit.* note 8, p. 229; see also: I. Illich. 1978. *Toward a History of Needs.* Berkeley. Heyday: 35, 117; and I. Illich. Disabling Professions, I.K. Illich, I.K. Zolal, J. McKnight, J. Caplan, H. Shaiken, eds. 1977. *Disabling Professions.* New York. Marion Boyars: 11–39, at pp. 28–31.

25. On 'detrimental enhancements,' see: D. Shickle. Are 'Genetic Enhancements' Really Enhancements? *Cambridge Quarterly of Healthcare Ethics* 2000; 9: 342–352, at 344–345.

26. D.W. Brock. 1998. Enhancements of Human Function: Some Distinctions for Policymakers. In *Enhancing Human Traits*, *op. cit.* note 4, pp. 48–69, at 59.

27. See, for instance: A. Lippman. Led (Astray) by Genetic Maps: The Cartography of the Human Genome and Health Care. *Social Science and Medicine* 1992; 35: 1469–76.

28. M.H. Shapiro. The Impact of Genetic Enhancement on Equality. *Wake Forest Law Review* 1999; 34: 561–637; L.M. Silver. 1997. *Remaking Eden: Cloning and Beyond in a Brave New World.* New York. Avon Books.

29. M.J. Mehlman. How Will We Regulate Genetic Enhancement? *Wake Forest Law Review* 1999; 34: 671–714, at 687.

30. D. Shenk. Biocapitalism: What Price the Genetic Revolution? *Harper's* 1997; December: 37–45, at 45.

31. L.M. Silver. 9 November, 1999. Reprogenetics: How Do a Scientist's Own Ethical Deliberations Enter into the Process? Paper presented at the conference *Humans and Genetic Engineering in the New Millenium—How Are We Going to Get 'Genethics' Just in Time?* Available online at: *http://www.etiskraad.dk/publikationer/genethics/ren.htm#kap02* (accessed 7 February 2002).

32. See, for instance: S. Bordo. 1998. *Braveheart, Babe,* and the Contemporary Body. In *Enhancing Human Traits: Ethical and Social Implications,* *op. cit.* note 4, pp. 189–221; M.O. Little. 1998. Cosmetic Surgery, Suspect Norms, and the Ethics of Complicity. In *Enhancing Human Traits, op. cit.* note 4, pp. 162–176.

33. K. Davis. 1995. *Reshaping the Female Body: The Dilemma of Cosmetic Surgery.* New York. Routledge.

34. B. Duden. 1993. *Disembodying Women: Perspectives on Pregnancy and the Unborn.* Translation by Lee Hoinacki. Cambridge. Harvard University Press; see also: Robert, *op. cit.* note 4; and J.S. Robert. Moral Truthfulness in Genetic Counseling. *Business and Professional Ethics Journal* 1998; 17: 73–93.

35. W. Gardner. Can Human Genetic Enhancement Be Prohibited? *Journal of Medicine and Philosophy* 1995; 20: 65–84.

36. Brock, *op. cit.* note 26; see also R. Cole-Turner. 1998. Do Means Matter? In *Enhancing Human Traits op. cit.* note 4, pp. 151–161; E. Parens. Is Better Always Good? The Enhancement Project. *Hastings Center Report* 1998; 28: S1–S15; S. Goering. Gene Therapies and the Pursuit of a Better Human. *Cambridge Quarterly of Healthcare Ethics* 2000; 9: 330–341; and Shickle, *op. cit.* note 25.

37. Baylis, *op. cit.* note 12.

38. An anonymous reviewer suggested that we expand on our notion of inevitability, especially to distinguish it from other arguments for inevitability. There is, for instance, a large literature on slippery slope arguments for inevitability, ably summarised in Holtug *op. cit.* note 14. Holtug follows W. van der Burg (The Slippery Slope Argument. *Ethics* 1999; 102: 42–65) in distinguishing between logical and empirical versions of the slippery slope argument. Some commentators would, of course, respond to our question ('why is the development and use of genetic enhancement technologies inevitable?') by invoking an argument to the effect that no line (or no principled line) can be drawn to prevent particular enhancements once genetic enhancement technologies have been developed (a logical slippery slope argument), or to the effect that the mere possibility of developing a technology leads to the development of that technology, and further that the mere existence of a technology leads to its inevitable use (and, possibly, abuse) (the technological imperative—an empirical slippery slope argument). It should be evident that our notion of inevitability is not of the slippery slope variety—in fact, we are not certain that there is anything at the bottom of the slope toward which to slip! Rather, we interpret inevitability in the sense of political immunity to moral criticism, on the basis of common views of the nature of humans and/in the contemporary world. This is, of course, an empirical claim; we hope to be shown to be wrong (and if we are wrong, then, ironically, our aim will have been accomplished). But it is not a pessimistic claim in the sense objected to by Häyry; and it is not a slippery slope claim in any of the senses addressed by Holtug.

39. As cited in Shenk, *op. cit.* note 30, p. 41.

40. Gardner, *op. cit.* note 37.

41. See, for instance, R. Sandbrook. Neoliberalism's False Promise. *Literary Review of Canada* 2000; 8.8: 20–24.

42. As cited in Anonymous. The Politics of Genes: America's Next Ethical War. *Economist* 2001; 14 April: 21–24, at 21.

43. Ibid. p. 22.

44. We make this claim with some hesitation, inasmuch as Buchanan *et al.*, in *From Chance to Choice* (*op. cit.* note 4), offer a sophisticated defense of liberalism generative of the result that genetic enhancements should in principle be permissible (subject to the satisfaction of particular requirements of justice).

45. Gordon, *op. cit.* note 7, p. 2024.

46. See, for instance: H. Longino. 1990. *Science as Social Knowledge.* Princeton. Princeton University Press; L. Code. 1991. *What Can She Know? Feminist Theory and the Construction of Knowledge.* Ithaca. Cornell University Press; and R. Campbell. 1998. *Illusions of Paradox: A Feminist Epistemology Naturalized.* Lanham, MD. Rowman & Littlefield.

47. B. Allen. Forbidding Knowledge. *Monist* 1996; 79: 294–310, at 307–308.

48. Brock, *op. cit.* note 26, p. 60.

49. Ibid. p. 58.

50. J. Lederberg. 1963. Biological Future of Man. In *Man and His Future.* G.E.W. Wolstenholme, ed. Toronto. Little, Brown and Company: 263–273, at 269.

51. R. Dawkins. 1976. *The Selfish Gene.* Oxford. Oxford University Press.

52. Stableford, *op. cit.* note 1; Sandberg, *op. cit.* note 1; and Slater, *op. cit.* note 11.

53. A.H. Maslow. 1954. *Motivation and Personality.* New York. Harper.

Chapter 11 END OF LIFE ISSUES

The Problem with Futility

Robert D. Truog, Allan S. Brett, and Joel Frader

"Futility" is one of the newest additions to the lexicon of bioethics. Physicians, ethicists, and members of the media are increasingly concerned about patients and families who insist on receiving life-sustaining treatment that others judge to be futile. A clear understanding of futility has proved to be elusive, however. Many clinicians view futility the way one judge viewed pornography: they may not be able to define it, but they know it when they see it.[1]

The notion of futile medical treatment may go back to the time of Hippocrates, who allegedly advised physicians "to refuse to treat those who are overmastered by their diseases, realizing that in such cases medicine is powerless."[2] More recently, the concept has appeared frequently in court decisions and policy statements.[3–6] The so-called Baby Doe law exempts physicians from providing treatment that would be "virtually futile."[7] The Council on Ethical and Judicial Affairs of the American Medical Association (AMA) recently concluded that physicians have no obligation to obtain consent for a do-not-resuscitate (DNR) order when cardiopulmonary resuscitation (CPR) is deemed futile.[8] The fact that this concept has appeared in law and policy may seem to indicate that it is clearly understood and widely accepted. In reality, however, the notion of futility hides many deep and serious ambiguities that threaten its legitimacy as a rationale for limiting treatment.

PARADIGMS OF FUTILITY

Contemporary discussions of futility have centered primarily on cases involving patients in a persistent vegetative state and those involving the use of CPR. A third type of case, involving organ-replacement technology, has received little attention but is helpful to our understanding of futility.

Futility and the Persistent Vegetative State

The first type of scenario involving the question of futility is represented by the recent Minnesota case of Helga Wanglie.[9] Mrs. Wanglie was an 86-year-old woman who had been dependent on mechanical ventilation and in a persistent vegetative state for more than a year. Her husband insisted that she believed in maintaining life at all cost, and that "when she was ready to go … the good Lord would call her."[10] Her physicians, on the other hand, believed that the continued use of mechanical ventilation and intensive care was futile. When attempts to transfer her elsewhere failed, they sought to have a court appoint an independent conservator with responsibility for making medical decisions on her behalf. The judge denied this petition and reaffirmed the authority of her husband as legal surrogate. Three days later, Mrs. Wanglie died.

Cases like that of Mrs. Wanglie seldom reach the courts, but they are probably not rare. A similar case involving a child with severe brain damage was concluded with a settlement favorable to the family before a judicial decision.[11]

Futility in Cases Involving CPR

The second prototypical scenario involves the use of DNR orders. Although the techniques of CPR were originally intended only for use after acute, reversible cardiac arrests, the current practice is to use CPR in all situations unless there is a direct order to the contrary. Since cardiac arrest is the final event in all terminal illness, everyone is eventually a candidate for this medical procedure. DNR orders were developed to spare patients from aggressive attempts at revival when imminent death is anticipated and inevitable. Nevertheless, patients or families sometimes request CPR even when care givers believe such attempts would be futile. Some have argued that in these circumstances a physician should be able to enact a DNR order without the consent of the patient or family.[12–14]

Futility and Organ-Replacement Technology

Although the bioethical debate over the question of futility has been most concerned with cases involving CPR and the treatment of patients in a persistent vegetative state, a third type of futility-related judgment has gone essentially unchallenged. It involves the increasingly large number of interventions that could possibly prolong the life of virtually any dying patient. For example, extracorporeal membrane oxygenation can replace heart and lung function for up to several weeks. Physicians now use this intervention when they expect organ systems eventually to recover or while they await organs for transplantation. However, it could prolong the life of almost anyone with cardiorespiratory failure, reversible or not. Patients thus kept alive may remain conscious and capable of communicating. Care givers do not now offer this therapy to terminally ill patients, presumably because it would be futile. This judgment has gone largely unchallenged, yet it is not obvious why a clinician's unilateral decision not to use "futile" extracorporeal membrane oxygenation is inherently different from a decision not to use "futile"

CPR or "futile" intensive care. If all three treatments can be characterized as objectively futile, then unilateral decisions not to offer them should be equally justified.

As it is used in these three cases, the concept of futility obscures many ambiguities and assumptions. These can be usefully grouped into two categories: problems of value and problems of probability.

FUTILITY AND VALUES

It is meaningless simply to say that an intervention is futile; one must always ask, "Futile in relation to what?" The medical literature provides many examples in which the importance of identifying the goals of treatment has not been fully appreciated. The effectiveness of CPR, for example, is often discussed in terms of whether patients who require the procedure can survive long enough to be discharged from the hospital.[15] This definition of success usually implies that short-term survival is a goal not worth pursuing. Patients or family members may value the additional hours of life differently, however. Indeed, physicians and other care givers have repeatedly been shown to be poor judges of patients' preferences with regard to intensive care.[16–18]

Schneiderman and colleagues have argued that treatments that merely preserve permanent unconsciousness or that cannot end dependence on intensive medical care should be considered futile.[19] Although society may eventually endorse decisions to override the previously expressed wishes of patients or the desires of surrogates who demand such treatments, it does not follow that the treatments are futile. Mr. Wanglie would have rejected this conclusion, and there is no reason to dismiss his view out of hand. The decision that certain goals are not worth pursuing is best seen as involving a conflict of values rather than a question of futility.

Certainly in this context, the plurality of values in our society makes agreement on the concept of futility difficult if not impossible. Several groups have therefore attempted to arrive at a value-free understanding of the concept.[20, 21] The most promising candidate thus far is the notion of "physiologic futility." As the guidelines on the termination of life-sustaining treatment prepared by the Hastings Center state, if a treatment is "clearly futile in achieving its physiological objective and so offer[s] no physiological benefit to the patient, the professional has no obligation to provide it."[20] For example, the physiologic objective of mechanical ventilation is to maintain adequate ventilation and oxygenation in the presence of respiratory failure, and the physiologic objective of CPR is to maintain adequate cardiac output and respiration in the presence of cardiorespiratory failure. The New York State Task Force on Life and the Law mistakenly concludes that CPR is physiologically futile when it will "be unsuccessful in restoring cardiac and respiratory function or [when] the patient will experience repeated arrest in a short time period before death occurs."[21] CPR is physiologically futile only when it is impossible to perform effective cardiac massage and ventilation (such as in the presence of cardiac rupture or severe outflow obstruction). Saying that CPR is physiologically futile when it will be unsuccessful in restoring cardiac function is like saying that mechanical ventilation is physiologically futile if it cannot restore respiratory function. The immediate physiologic effect of the intervention differs from the broader and more uncertain question of prognosis.

Physiologic futility, understood in narrow terms, comes close to providing a value-free understanding of futility. Unfortunately, it applies to a very small number of real cases involving CPR. Similarly, since in the case of Mrs. Wanglie mechanical ventilation could maintain adequate oxygenation and ventilation, her treatment could not be considered futile in the physiologic sense. Even the use of extracorporeal membrane oxygenation in terminally ill patients cannot be considered physiologically futile, since it can maintain circulation and ventilation. The concept of physiologic futility therefore falls short of providing guidance in most cases resembling those described above.

FUTILITY AND STATISTICAL UNCERTAINTY

In most medical situations, there is no such thing as never. Futility is almost always a matter of probability. But what statistical cutoff point should be chosen as the threshold for determining futility? The statement from the Council on Ethical and Judicial Affairs of the AMA concludes that physicians have no obligation to provide futile CPR, but it fails to specify any level of statistical certainty at which the judgment is warranted.[8] The AMA statement fails to acknowledge that this is even an issue. Should each physician decide independently what probability of success should be considered to indicate futility?

Even if we could agree on a statistical cutoff point for determining futility, physicians are often highly unreliable in estimating the likelihood of success of a therapeutic intervention. Psychological research[22, 23] has shown that estimates of probability are susceptible to "severe and systematic errors."[22] Empirical studies have corroborated the limitations of clinical assessment in estimating both prognosis[24] and diagnosis.[25] Even in theory, statistical inferences about what might happen to groups of patients do not permit accurate predictions of what will happen to the next such patient. In addition, the tendency to remember cases that are unusual or bizarre predisposes physicians to make decisions on the basis of their experiences with "miraculous" cures or unexpected tragedies.

Schneiderman and colleagues recently argued that a treatment should be considered futile when 100 consecutive patients do not respond to it.[19] But how similar must the patients be? In assessing the efficacy of mechanical ventilation to treat pneumonia, for example, is it sufficient simply to recall the 100 most recent patients who received artificial ventilation for pneumonia? Or must this group be stratified according to age, etiologic organism, or coexisting illness? Clearly, many of these factors will make an important difference.

FUTILITY AND RESOURCE ALLOCATION

Although medical practice has increasingly emphasized patients' autonomy, there is growing pressure on physicians to slow the increase in health care costs by foreclosing some options. Thus, we have a tension between the value of autonomy, exercised in the form of consent to use or omit various interventions, and the desirability of a more Spartan approach to the consumption of medical resources. We promote patients' freedom to request whatever the medical menu has to offer, but we also require that interventions be guided by considerations of cost and the likelihood of benefit.[26] Unfortunately, there is no consensus about what constitutes a just method of balancing the preferences of individual patients against the diverse needs of society.

To some, the concept of futility provides at least a partial solution to this dilemma: it offers a reason to limit therapy without the need to define a fair procedure for allocating resources. This approach allows treatments to be denied on the grounds that they are simply not indicated, apart from the matter of cost. Despite its attractions, there are good reasons why we should not use this concept to solve problems of allocation.

First, arguments based on the futility concept conceal many statistical and value-laden assumptions, whereas strategies based on resource allocation force these assumptions to be stated explicitly. Societies may choose to limit the use of therapies that may be of value and have a reasonable likelihood of success in some cases. For example, the much discussed Oregon plan for allocating Medicaid funds[27] seeks to reflect community values in ranking various health care goals (placing preventive care ahead of cosmetic surgery, for example). Since rationing policies make explicit the values and probabilities that futility-based arguments leave implicit, it is clearly preferable to develop and adopt them rather than use futility arguments as a cover for limiting the availability of scarce and expensive resources.

Another problem with invoking the idea of futility in the debate over allocation is that we have no reason to believe that it is applicable in enough cases to make a difference in the scarcity of medical resources. Although it may be true that beds in the intensive care unit (especially those used for extracorporeal membrane oxygenation) are relatively scarce, it seems unlikely that patients similar to Helga Wanglie occupy an important fraction of those beds, let alone account for a major proportion of the cost of medical care in the United States. From a macroeconomic perspective at least, we must remain skeptical that an appeal to the idea of futility will get us very far.

MOVING BEYOND FUTILITY

Our rejection of futility as a useful concept does not imply that we endorse patients' unrestricted demands for interventions such as those described in our prototypical scenarios. On the contrary, when providers oppose such demands they are usually acting from a profound sense that further treatment would be fundamentally wrong. Our task is to take account of that sense of wrongness without resorting to unilateral, provider-initiated declarations of futility.

In many of the situations in which questions of futility arise, providers believe that the treatment in question would not be in the patient's interests, even from the patient's perspective, and that any insistence by the patient (or surrogate) on further interventions is based on faulty reasoning, unrealistic expectations, or psychological factors, such as denial or guilt. In these circumstances, providers are obligated to make every effort to clarify precisely what the patient intends to achieve with continued treatment. If the patient's goals appear to reflect unrealistic expectations about the probable course of the underlying illness or the probable effect of medical interventions, providers should attempt to correct those impressions. Because inadequate or insensitive communication by providers probably accounts for a substantial proportion of unrealistic requests, such discussions will successfully resolve many conflicts.[14, 28] Empirical studies of ethics consultations have demonstrated precisely this point.[29, 30]

Although this appeal to the patient's interests may seem to contain some of the same ambiguities as arguments using the concept of futility, there is a subtle but important distinction between the two. Judgments about what is in the patient's interest are properly grounded in the patient's perspective, whereas judgments cast in the language of futility falsely assume that there is an objective and dispassionate standard for determining benefits and burdens. Nevertheless, even after providers make sustained attempts to clarify patients' preferences, some patients or surrogates will continue to demand life-sustaining interventions when the care givers feel deeply troubled about providing them. In many such cases, unrestrained deference to the wishes of the patient or surrogate conflicts with two other values that do not require a unilateral judgment of the futility of treatment: professional ideals and social consensus.

The ideals of medical professionals include respect for patients' wishes, to be sure, but they also include other values, such as compassionate action and the minimization of suffering. Consider, for example, a bedridden victim of multiple strokes who has contractures and bedsores and who "communicates" only by moaning or grimacing when she is touched. Physicians asked to perform chest compressions, institute mechanical ventilation, or use other life-sustaining interventions in such a patient may regard these actions as cruel and inhumane.[31] Moreover, physicians and other care givers have a legitimate interest in seeing that their knowledge and skills are used wisely and effectively. For example, if surgeons were repeatedly pressured to perform operations that they believed to be inappropriate, they would certainly suffer a loss of dignity and sense of purpose. Although appealing to professional ideals can serve as a convenient means of protecting the interests of physicians at the expense of patients' values, these ideals are legitimate factors to weigh against other values. To dismiss

this perspective as irrelevant in decision making is to deny an essential part of what it means to practice medicine.

Although we believe that health care professionals should not be required to take part in care that violates their own morals, the law in this area remains uncertain. On the one hand, courts have upheld a state interest in protecting the ethical integrity of the medical profession. This may provide some basis for protecting doctors who wish to refrain from cruel or inhumane treatment, despite the wishes of the patient or surrogate.[32] On the other hand, in the two cases that have led to court decisions (those of Helga Wanglie[3] and of Jane Doe in Atlanta[33]) the judges upheld the surrogates' decision-making authority. Clearly, this area of the law remains to be defined.

Finally, social consensus is yet another expression of the values at stake in some medical decisions. In a pluralistic society, differences in personal values and interests occasionally run so deep that they cannot be resolved by the introduction of additional facts or by further private debate. At certain critical junctures, the resolution of these conflicts may require an explicit public process of social decision making.[34] Social consensus has been sought, for example, to address the issue of fair allocation of resources.[27] The involvement of society is also essential when the most highly charged questions of morality are at stake, as in the increasingly heated debate over euthanasia.[35]

In the prototypical scenarios described at the outset of this article, an ongoing attempt to achieve social consensus is perhaps most conspicuous with regard to the prolongation of life for patients in a persistent vegetative state. From a legal perspective, the relevant decisions began with the case of Karen Quinlan[36] and have extended through that of Nancy Cruzan.[37] These cases have increased awareness of the ethical issues raised by the situation of patients in a persistent vegetative state and have helped to consolidate the view that it is acceptable to withdraw life-sustaining treatment from patients in such a state. Controversy does remain about who has the ultimate authority to make these decisions. Some hold that the choice must remain with the patient or surrogate, whereas others believe that under some circumstances this prerogative may be overridden. For example, the Hastings Center[38] and the Society of Critical Care Medicine[39] have concluded that providing intensive care to patients in a persistent vegetative state is generally a misuse of resources, and the President's Commission stated that such patients should be removed from life support if such action is necessary to benefit another patient who is not in a persistent vegetative state.[40] It is unclear how this debate will conclude, but the confluence of medical, legal, and ethical thinking about the persistent vegetative state is an example of how social consensus may evolve.

In summary, the Wanglie case demonstrates how the resolution of these conflicts must proceed on many levels. Most such cases will benefit from sustained attempts to clarify the patient's values and the likelihood of the various relevant outcomes, and to improve communication with patients or their surrogates. When this approach fails, physicians and other care givers should ask themselves whether the care requested is consistent with their professional ethics and ideals. When these ideals appear to be violated, either alternative venues for such care should be found or the broader review could be provided through institutional mechanisms, such as the hospital's ethics committee, or by the courts. The public scrutiny that attends such cases will further the debate over the appropriate use of medical resources and foster the development of consensus through legislation and public policy.

CONCLUSION

In outlining the perspectives of the principal stakeholders—patients and their surrogates, physicians, and society—we have avoided the construction of a rigid formula for resolving conflicts over interventions frequently regarded as futile. Because of clinical heterogeneity, pluralistic values, and the evolutionary nature of social consensus, most clinical decision making on behalf of critically ill patients defies reduction to universally applicable principles.

The notion of futility generally fails to provide an ethically coherent ground for limiting life-sustaining treatment, except in circumstances in which narrowly defined physiologic futility can be plausibly invoked. Futility has been conceptualized as an objective entity independent of the patient's or surrogate's perspective, but differences in values and the variable probabilities of clinical outcomes undermine its basis. Furthermore, assertions of futility may camouflage judgments of comparative worth that are implicit in debates about the allocation of resources. In short, the problem with futility is that its promise of objectivity can rarely be fulfilled. The rapid advance of the language of futility into the jargon of bioethics should be followed by an equally rapid retreat.

Notes

1. *Jacobellis v. State of Ohio*, 84 S Ct 1676 (1964).
2. Hippocrates. The art. In: Reiser SJ, Dyck AJ, Curran WJ. eds. *Ethics in medicine: historical perspectives and contemporary concerns*. Cambridge. Mass.: MIT Press, 1977; 6–7.
3. Capron AM. In re Helga Wanglie. *Hastings Cent Rep* 1991; 21(5):26–8.
4. Lantos JD, Singer PA, Walker RM, et al. The illusion of futility in clinical practice. *Am J Med* 1989; 87:81–4.
5. Standards for cardiopulmonary resuscitation (CPR) and emergency cardiac care (ECC). V. Medicolegal considerations and recommendations. *JAMA* 1974; 227:Suppl:864–6.
6. Appendix A: the proposed legislation. In: *Do not resuscitate orders: the proposed legislation and report of the New York State Task Force on Life and the Law*. 2nd ed. New York: The Task Force, 1986; 83.
7. 1984 Amendments to the Child Abuse Prevention and Treatment Act. Pub Law 98-457. 1984.
8. Council on Ethical and Judicial Affairs. American Medical Association. Guidelines for the appropriate use of do-not-resuscitate orders. *JAMA* 1991; 265:1868–71.

9. Miles SH. Informed demand for "non-beneficial" medical treatment. *N Engl J Med* 1991; 325:512–5.

10. Brain-damaged woman at center of lawsuit over life-support dies. *New York Times*. July 5, 1991:A8.

11. Paris JJ, Crone RK, Reardon F. Physicians' refusal of requested treatment: the case of Baby L. *N Engl J Med* 1990; 322:1012–5.

12. Blackhall LJ. Must we always use CPR? *N Engl J Med* 1987; 317:1281–5.

13. Hackler JC, Hiller PC. Family consent to orders not to resuscitate: reconsidering hospital policy. *JAMA* 1990; 264:1281–3.

14. Murphy DJ. Do-not-resuscitate orders: time for reappraisal in long-term–care institutions. *JAMA* 1988; 260:2098–101.

15. Bedell SE, Delbanco TL, Cook EF, Epstein FH. Survival after cardiopulmonary resuscitation in the hospital. *N Engl J Med* 1983; 309:569–76.

16. Danis M, Gerrity MS, Southerland LI, Patrick DL. A comparison of patient, family, and physician assessments of the value of medical intensive care. *Crit Care Med* 1988; 16:594–600.

17. Danis M, Jarr SL, Southerland LI, Nocella RS, Patrick DL. A comparison of patient, family, and nurse evaluations of the usefulness of intensive care. *Crit Care Med* 1987; 15:138–43.

18. Danis M, Patrick DL, Southerland LI, Green ML. Patients' and families' preferences for medical intensive care. *JAMA* 1988; 260:797–802.

19. Schneiderman LJ, Jecker NS, Jonsen AR. Medical futility: its meaning and ethical implications. *Ann Intern Med* 1990; 112:949–54.

20. The Hastings Center. *Guidelines on the termination of life-sustaining treatment and the care of the dying*. Bloomington: Indiana University Press 1987:32.

21. Appendix C: New York Public Health Law Article 29-B — orders not to resuscitate. In: *Do not resuscitate orders: the proposed legislation and report of the New York State Task Force on Life and the Law*. 2nd ed. New York: The Task Force, 1986:96.

22. Tversky A, Kahneman D. Judgment under uncertainty: heuristics and biases. *Science* 1974; 185:1124–31.

23. Elstein AS. Clinical judgment: psychological research and medical practice. *Science* 1976; 194:696–700.

24. Poses RM, Bekes C, Copare FJ, Scott WE. The answer to "What are my chances, doctor?" depends on whom is asked: prognostic desagreement and inaccuracy for critically ill patients. *Crit Care Med* 1989; 17:827–33.

25. Poses RM, Cebul RD, Collins M, Fager SS. The accuracy of experienced physicians' probability estimates for patients with sore throats: implications for decision making. *JAMA* 1985; 254:925–9.

26. Aaron H, Schwartz WB. Rationing health care the choice before us. *Science* 1990; 247:418–22.

27. Eddy DM. What's going on in Oregon. *JAMA* 1991; 266:417–20.

28. Youngner SJ. Who defines futility? *JAMA* 1988; 260:2094–5.

29. Brennan TA. Ethics committees and decisions to limit care: the experience at the Massachusetts General Hospital. *JAMA* 1988; 260:803–7.

30. La Puma J. Consultations in clinical ethics — issues and questions in 27 cases. *West J Med* 1987; 146:633–7.

31. Braithwaite S, Thomasma DC. New guidelines on foregoing life-sustaining treatment in incompetent patients: an anti-cruelty policy. *Ann Intern Med* 1986; 104:711–5.

32. Meisel A. *The right to die*. New York: John Wiley & Sons, 1989:104.

33. In re: Doe, Civil Action No. D93064 (Fulton County, GA, October 17, 1991).

34. Callahan D. Medical futility, medical necessity: the-problem-without-a-name. *Hastings Cent Rep* 1991; 21(4):30–5.

35. Misbin RI. Physicians' aid in dying. *N Engl J Med* 1991; 325:1307–11.

36. In the Matter of Karen Ann Quinlan, an alleged incompetent. 355 A.2d 647; or 70 NJ 10. March 31, 1976.

37. Annas GJ. Nancy Cruzan and the right to die. *N Engl J Med* 1990; 323:670–3.

38. The Hastings Center. *Guidelines on the termination of life-sustaining treatment and the care of the dying*. Bloomington: Indiana University Press, 1987:112.

39. Task Force on Ethics of the Society of Critical Care Medicine. Consensus report on the ethics of foregoing life-sustaining treatments in the critically ill. *Crit Care Med* 1990; 18:1435–9.

40. President's Commission for the Study of Ethical Problems in Medicine and Biomedical and Behavioral Research. *Deciding to forego life-sustaining treatment: ethical, medical, and legal issues in treatment decisions*. Washington, D.C.: Government Printing Office, 1983:188–9.

Voluntary Active Euthanasia

Dan W. Brock

Since the case of Karen Quinlan first seized public attention fifteen years ago, no issue in biomedical ethics has been more prominent than the debate about forgoing life-sustaining treatment. Controversy continues regarding some aspects of that debate, such as forgoing life-sustaining nutrition and hydration, and relevant law varies some from state to state. Nevertheless, I believe it is possible to identify an emerging consensus that competent patients, or the surrogates of incompetent patients, should be permitted to weigh the benefits and burdens of alternative treatments, including the alternative of no treatment, according to the patient's values, and either to refuse any treatment or to select from among available alternative treatments. This consensus is reflected in bioethics scholarship, in reports of prestigious bodies such as the President's Commission for the Study of Ethical Problems in Medicine, The Hastings Center, and the American Medical Association, in a large body of judicial decisions in courts around the country, and finally in the beliefs and practices of health care professionals who care for dying patients.[1]

More recently, significant public and professional attention has shifted from life-sustaining treatment to euthanasia—more specifically, voluntary active euthanasia—and to physician-assisted suicide. Several factors have contributed to the increased interest in euthanasia. In the Netherlands, it has been openly practiced by physicians for several years with the acceptance of the country's highest court.[2] In 1988 there was an unsuccessful attempt to get the question of whether it should be made legally permissible on the ballot in California. In November 1991 voters in the state of Washington defeated a widely publicized referendum proposal to legalize both voluntary active euthanasia and physician-assisted suicide. Finally, some cases of this kind, such as "It's Over, Debbie," described in the *Journal of the American Medical Association,* the "suicide machine" of Dr. Jack Kevorkian, and the cancer patient "Diane" of Dr. Timothy Quill, have captured wide public and professional attention.[3] Unfortunately, the first two of these cases were sufficiently problematic that even most supporters of euthanasia or assisted suicide did not defend the physicians' actions in them. As a result, the subsequent debate they spawned has often shed more heat than light. My aim is to increase the light, and perhaps as well to reduce the heat, on this important subject by formulating and evaluating the central ethical arguments for and against voluntary active euthanasia and physician-assisted suicide. My evaluation of the arguments leads me, with reservations to be noted, to support permitting both practices. My primary aim, however, is not to argue for euthanasia, but to identify confusions in some common arguments, and problematic assumptions and claims that need more defense or data in others. The issues are considerably more complex than either supporters or opponents often make out; my hope is to advance the debate by focusing attention on what I believe the real issues under discussion should be.

In the recent bioethics literature some have endorsed physician-assisted suicide but not euthanasia.[4] Are they sufficiently different that the moral arguments for one often do not apply to the other? A paradigm case of physician-assisted suicide is a patient's ending his or her life with a lethal dose of a medication requested of and provided by a physician for that purpose. A paradigm case of voluntary active euthanasia is a physician's administering the lethal dose, often because the patient is unable to do so. The only difference that need exist between the two is the person who actually administers the lethal dose—the physician or the patient. In each, the physician plays an active and necessary causal role.

In physician-assisted suicide the patient acts last (for example, Janet Adkins herself pushed the button after Dr. Kevorkian hooked her up to his suicide machine), whereas in euthanasia the physician acts last by performing the physical equivalent of pushing the button. In both cases, however, the choice rests fully with the patient. In both the patient acts last in the sense of retaining the right to change his or her mind until the point at which the lethal process becomes irreversible. How could there be a substantial moral difference between the two based only on this small difference in the part played by the physician in the causal process resulting in death? Of course, it might be held that the moral difference is clear and important—in euthanasia the physician kills the patient whereas in physician-assisted suicide the patient kills him- or herself. But this is misleading at best. In assisted suicide the physician and patient together kill the patient. To see this, suppose a physician supplied a lethal dose to a patient with the knowledge and intent that the patient will wrongfully administer it to another. We would have no difficulty in morality or the law recognizing this as a case of joint action to kill for which both are responsible.

If there is no significant, intrinsic moral difference between the two, it is also difficult to see why public or legal policy should permit one but not the other; worries about abuse or about giving anyone dominion over the lives of others apply equally to either. As a result, I will take the arguments evaluated below to apply to both and will focus on euthanasia.

My concern here will be with *voluntary* euthanasia only—that is, with the case in which a clearly competent patient makes a fully voluntary and persistent request for aid in dying. Involuntary euthanasia, in which a competent patient explicitly refuses or opposes receiving euthanasia, and nonvoluntary euthanasia, in which a patient is incompetent and unable to express his or her wishes about euthanasia, will

be considered here only as potential unwanted side-effects of permitting voluntary euthanasia. I emphasize as well that I am concerned with *active* euthanasia, notwithholding or withdrawing life-sustaining treatment, which some commentators characterize as "passive euthanasia." Finally, I will be concerned with euthanasia where the motive of those who perform it is to respect the wishes of the patient and to provide the patient with a "good death," though one important issue is whether a change in legal policy could restrict the performance of euthanasia to only those cases.

A last introductory point is that I will be examining only secular arguments about euthanasia, though of course many people's attitudes to it are inextricable from their religious views. The policy issue is only whether euthanasia should be permissible, and no one who has religious objections to it should be required to take any part in it, though of course this would not fully satisfy some opponents.

THE CENTRAL ETHICAL ARGUMENT FOR VOLUNTARY ACTIVE EUTHANASIA

The central ethical argument for euthanasia is familiar. It is that the very same two fundamental ethical values supporting the consensus on patient's rights to decide about life-sustaining treatment also support the ethical permissibility of euthanasia. These values are individual self-determination or autonomy and individual well-being. By self-determination as it bears on euthanasia, I mean people's interest in making important decisions about their lives for themselves according to their own values or conceptions of a good life, and in being left free to act on those decisions. Self-determination is valuable because it permits people to form and live in accordance with their own conception of a good life, at least within the bounds of justice and consistent with others doing so as well. In exercising self-determination people take responsibility for their lives and for the kinds of persons they become. A central aspect of human dignity lies in people's capacity to direct their lives in this way. The value of exercising self-determination presupposes some minimum of decisionmaking capacities or competence, which thus limits the scope of euthanasia supported by self-determination; it cannot justifiably be administered, for example, in cases of serious dementia or treatable clinical depression.

Does the value of individual self-determination extend to the time and manner of one's death? Most people are very concerned about the nature of the last stage of their lives. This reflects not just a fear of experiencing substantial suffering when dying, but also a desire to retain dignity and control during this last period of life. Death is today increasingly preceded by a long period of significant physical and mental decline, due in part to the technological interventions of modern medicine. Many people adjust to these disabilities and find meaning and value in new activities and ways. Others find the impairments and burdens in the last stage of their lives at some point sufficiently great to make life no longer worth living. For many patients near death, maintaining the quality of one's life, avoiding great suffering, maintaining one's dignity, and insuring that others remember us as we wish them to become of paramount importance and outweigh merely extending one's life. But there is no single, objectively correct answer for everyone as to when, if at all, one's life becomes all things considered a burden and unwanted. If self-determination is a fundamental value, then the great variability among people on this question makes it especially important that individuals control the manner, circumstances, and timing of their dying and death.

The other main value that supports euthanasia is individual well-being. It might seem that individual well-being conflicts with a person's self-determination when the person requests euthanasia. Life itself is commonly taken to be a central good for persons, often valued for its own sake, as well as necessary for pursuit of all other goods within a life. But when a competent patient decides to forgo all further life-sustaining treatment then the patient, either explicitly or implicitly, commonly decides that

the best life possible for him or her with treatment is of sufficiently poor quality that it is worse than no further life at all. Life is no longer considered a benefit by the patient, but has now become a burden. The same judgment underlies a request for euthanasia: continued life is seen by the patient as no longer a benefit, but now a burden. Especially in the often severely compromised and debilitated states of many critically ill or dying patients, there is no objective standard, but only the competent patient's judgment of whether continued life is no longer a benefit.

Of course, sometimes there are conditions, such as clinical depression, that call into question whether the patient has made a competent choice, either to forgo life-sustaining treatment or to seek euthanasia, and then the patient's choice need not be evidence that continued life is no longer a benefit for him or her. Just as with decisions about treatment, a determination of incompetence can warrant not honoring the patient's choice; in the case of treatment, we then transfer decisional authority to a surrogate, though in the case of voluntary active euthanasia a determination that the patient is incompetent means that choice is not possible.

The value or right of self-determination does not entitle patients to compel physicians to act contrary to their own moral or professional values. Physicians are moral and professional agents whose own self-determination or integrity should be respected as well. If performing euthanasia became legally permissible, but conflicted with a particular physician's reasonable understanding of his or her moral or professional responsibilities, the care of a patient who requested euthanasia should be transferred to another.

Most opponents do not deny that there are some cases in which the values of patient self-determination and well-being support euthanasia. Instead, they commonly offer two kinds of arguments against it that on their view outweigh or override this support. The first kind of argument is that in any individual case where considerations of the patient's self-determination and well-being do support euthanasia, it is nevertheless always ethically wrong or impermissible. The second kind of argument grants that in some individual cases euthanasia may *not* be ethically wrong, but maintains nonetheless that public and legal policy should never permit it. The first kind of argument focuses on features of any individual case of euthanasia, while the second kind focuses on social or legal policy. In the next section I consider the first kind of argument.

EUTHANASIA IS THE DELIBERATE KILLING OF AN INNOCENT PERSON

The claim that any individual instance of euthanasia is a case of deliberate killing of an innocent person is, with only minor qualifications, correct. Unlike forgoing life-sustaining treatment, commonly understood as allowing to die, euthanasia is clearly killing, defined as depriving of life or causing the death of a living being. While providing morphine for pain relief at doses where the risk of respiratory depression and an earlier death may be a foreseen but unintended side effect of treating the patient's pain, in a case of euthanasia the patient's death is deliberate or intended even if in both the physician's ultimate end may be respecting the patient's wishes. If the deliberate killing of an innocent person is wrong, euthanasia would be nearly always impermissible.

In the context of medicine, the ethical prohibition against deliberately killing the innocent derives some of its plausibility from the belief that nothing in the currently accepted practice of medicine is deliberate killing. Thus, in commenting on the "It's Over, Debbie" case, four prominent physicians and bioethicists could entitle their paper "Doctors Must Not Kill."[5] The belief that doctors do not in fact kill requires the corollary belief that forgoing life-sustaining treatment, whether by not starting or by stopping treatment, is allowing to die, not killing. Common though this view is, I shall argue that it is confused and mistaken.

Why is the common view mistaken? Consider the case of a patient terminally ill with ALS disease. She is completely respirator dependent with no hope of ever being weaned. She is unquestionably competent but finds her condition intolerable and persistently requests to be removed from the respirator and allowed to die. Most people and physicians would agree that the patient's physician should respect the patient's wishes and remove her from the respirator, though this will certainly cause the patient's death. The common understanding is that the physician thereby allows the patient to die. But is that correct?

Suppose the patient has a greedy and hostile son who mistakenly believes that his mother will never decide to stop her life-sustaining treatment and that even if she did her physician would not remove her from the respirator. Afraid that his inheritance will be dissipated by a long and expensive hospitalization, he enters his mother's room while she is sedated, extubates her, and she dies. Shortly thereafter the medical staff discovers what he has done and confronts the son. He replies, "I didn't kill her, I merely allowed her to die. It was her ALS disease that caused her death." I think this would rightly be dismissed as transparent sophistry—the son went into his mother's room and deliberately killed her. But, of course, the son performed just the same physical actions, did just the same thing, that the physician would have done. If that is so, then doesn't the physician also kill the patient when he extubates her?

I underline immediately that there are important ethical differences between what the physician and the greedy son do. First, the physician acts with the patient's consent whereas the son does not. Second, the physician acts with a good motive—to respect the patient's wishes and self-determination—whereas the son acts with a bad motive—to protect his own inheritance. Third, the physician acts in a social role through which he is legally authorized to carry out the patient's wishes regarding treatment whereas the son has no such authorization. These and perhaps other ethically important differences show that what the physician did was morally justified whereas what the son did was morally wrong. What they do *not* show, however, is that the son killed while the physician allowed to die. One can either kill or allow to die with or without consent, with a good or bad motive, within or outside of a social role that authorizes one to do so.

The difference between killing and allowing to die that I have been implicitly appealing to here is roughly that between acts and omissions resulting in death.[6] Both the physician and the greedy son act in a manner intended to cause death, do cause death, and so both kill. One reason this conclusion is resisted is that on a different understanding of the distinction between killing and allowing to die, what the physician does is allow to die. In this account, the mother's ALS is a lethal disease whose normal progression is being held back or blocked by the life-sustaining respirator treatment. Removing this artificial intervention is then viewed as standing aside and allowing the patient to die of her underlying disease. I have argued elsewhere that this alternative account is deeply problematic, in part because it commits us to accepting that what the greedy son does is to allow to die, not kill.[7] Here, I want to note two other reasons why the conclusion that stopping life support is killing is resisted.

The first reason is that killing is often understood, especially within medicine, as unjustified causing of death; in medicine it is thought to be done only accidentally or negligently. It is also increasingly widely accepted that a physician is ethically justified in stopping life support in a case like that of the ALS patient. But if these two beliefs are correct, then what the physician does cannot be killing, and so must be allowing to die. Killing patients is not, to put it flippantly, understood to be part of physicians' job description. What is mistaken in this line of reasoning is the assumption that all killings are *unjustified* causings of death. Instead, some killings are ethically justified, including many instances of stopping life support.

Another reason for resisting the conclusion that stopping life support is often killing is that it is psychologically uncomfortable. Suppose the physician had stopped the ALS patient's respirator and had made the son's claim, "I didn't kill her, I merely allowed her to die. It was her ALS disease that caused her death." The clue to the psychological role here is how naturally the "merely" modifies "allowed her to die." The characterization as allowing to die is meant to shift felt responsibility away from the agent—the physician—and to the lethal disease process. Other language common in death and dying contexts plays a similar role; "letting nature take its course" or "stopping prolonging the dying process" both seem to shift responsibility from the physician who stops life support to the fatal disease process. However psychologically helpful these conceptualizations may be in making the difficult responsibility of a physician's role in the patient's death bearable, they nevertheless are confusions. Both physicians and family members can instead be helped to understand that it is the patient's decision and consent to stopping treatment that limits their responsibility for the patient's death and that shifts that responsibility to the patient.

Many who accept the difference between killing and allowing to die as the distinction between acts and omissions resulting in death have gone on to argue that killing is not in itself morally different from allowing to die.[8] In this account, very roughly, one kills when one performs an action that causes the death of a person (we are in a boat, you cannot swim, I push you overboard, and you drown), and one allows to die when one has the ability and opportunity to prevent the death of another, knows this, and omits doing so, with the result that the person dies (we are in a boat, you cannot swim, you fall overboard, I don't throw you an available life ring, and you drown). Those who see no moral difference between killing and allowing to die typically employ the strategy of comparing cases that differ in these and no other potentially morally important respects. This will allow people to consider whether the mere difference that one is a case of killing and the other of allowing to die matters morally, or whether instead it is other features that make most cases of killing worse than most instances of allowing to die. Here is such a pair of cases:

Case 1. A very gravely ill patient is brought to a hospital emergency room and sent up to the ICU. The patient begins to develop respiratory failure that is likely to require intubation very soon. At that point the patient's family members and long-standing physician arrive at the ICU and inform the ICU staff that there had been extensive discussion about future care with the patient when he was unquestionably competent. Given his grave and terminal illness, as well as his state of debilitation, the patient had firmly rejected being placed on a respirator under any circumstances, and the family and physician produce the patient's advance directive to that effect. The ICU staff do not intubate the patient, who dies of respiratory failure.

Case 2. The same as Case 1 except that the family and physician are slightly delayed in traffic and arrive shortly after the patient has been intubated and placed on the respirator. The ICU staff extubate the patient, who dies of respiratory failure.

In Case 1 the patient is allowed to die, in Case 2 he is killed, but it is hard to see why what is done in Case 2 is significantly different morally than what is done in Case 1. It must be other factors that make most killings worse than most allowings to die, and if so, euthanasia cannot be wrong simply because it is killing instead of allowing to die.

Suppose both my arguments are mistaken. Suppose that killing is worse than allowing to die and that withdrawing life support is not killing, although euthanasia is. Euthanasia still need not for that reason be morally wrong. To see this, we need to determine the basic principle for the moral evaluation of killing persons. What is it that makes paradigm cases of wrongful killing wrongful? One very plausible answer is that killing denies the victim something that he or she values greatly—continued life or a future. Moreover, since continued life is necessary for

pursuing any of a person's plans and purposes, killing brings the frustration of all of these plans and desires as well. In a nutshell, wrongful killing deprives a person of a valued future, and of all the person wanted and planned to do in that future.

A natural expression of this account of the wrongness of killing is that people have a moral right not to be killed.[9] But in this account of the wrongness of killing, the right not to be killed, like other rights, should be waivable when the person makes a competent decision that continued life is no longer wanted or a good, but is instead worse than no further life at all. In this view, euthanasia is properly understood as a case of a person having waived his or her right not to be killed.

This rights view of the wrongness of killing is not, of course, universally shared. Many people's moral views about killing have their origins in religious views that human life comes from God and cannot be justifiably destroyed or taken away, either by the person whose life it is or by another. But in a pluralistic society like our own with a strong commitment to freedom of religion, public policy should not be grounded in religious beliefs which many in that society reject. I turn now to the general evaluation of public policy on euthanasia.

WOULD THE BAD CONSEQUENCES OF EUTHANASIA OUTWEIGH THE GOOD?

The argument against euthanasia at the policy level is stronger than at the level of individual cases, though even here I believe the case is ultimately unpersuasive, or at best indecisive. The policy level is the place where the main issues lie, however, and where moral considerations that might override arguments in favor of euthanasia will be found, if they are found anywhere. It is important to note two kinds of disagreement about the consequences for public policy of permitting euthanasia. First, there is empirical or factual disagreement about what the consequences would be. This disagreement is greatly exacerbated by the lack of firm data on the issue. Second, since on any reasonable assessment there would be both good and bad consequences, there are moral disagreements about the relative importance of different effects. In addition to these two sources of disagreement, there is also no single, well-specified policy proposal for legalizing euthanasia on which policy assessments can focus. But without such specification, and especially without explicit procedures for protecting against well-intentioned misuse and ill-intentioned abuse, the consequences for policy are largely speculative. Despite these difficulties, a preliminary account of the main likely good and bad consequences is possible. This should help clarify where better data or more moral analysis and argument are needed, as well as where policy safeguards must be developed.

Potential Good Consequences of Permitting Euthanasia. What are the likely good consequences? First, if euthanasia were permitted it would be possible to respect the self-determination of competent patients who want it, but now cannot get it because of its illegality. We simply do not know how many such patients and people there are. In the Netherlands, with a population of about 14.5 million (in 1987), estimates in a recent study were that about 1,900 cases of voluntary active euthanasia or physician-assisted suicide occur annually. No straightforward extrapolation to the United States is possible for many reasons, among them, that we do not know how many people here who want euthanasia now get it, despite its illegality. Even with better data on the number of persons who want euthanasia but cannot get it, significant moral disagreement would remain about how much weight should be given to any instance of failure to respect a person's self-determination in this way.

One important factor substantially affecting the number of persons who would seek euthanasia is the extent to which an alternative is available. The widespread acceptance in the law, social policy, and medical practice of the right of a competent patient to forgo life-sustaining treatment suggests that the number of

competent persons in the United States who would want euthanasia if it were permitted is probably relatively small.

A second good consequence of making euthanasia legally permissible benefits a much larger group. Polls have shown that a majority of the American public believes that people should have a right to obtain euthanasia if they want it.[10] No doubt the vast majority of those who support this right to euthanasia will never in fact come to want euthanasia for themselves. Nevertheless, making it legally permissible would reassure many people that if they ever do want euthanasia they would be able to obtain it. This reassurance would supplement the broader control over the process of dying given by the right to decide about life-sustaining treatment. Having fire insurance on one's house benefits all who have it, not just those whose houses actually burn down, by reassuring them that in the unlikely event of their house burning down, they will receive the money needed to rebuild it. Likewise, the legalization of euthanasia can be thought of as a kind of insurance policy against being forced to endure a protracted dying process that one has come to find burdensome and unwanted, especially when there is no life-sustaining treatment to forgo. The strong concern about losing control of their care expressed by many people who face serious illness likely to end in death suggests that they give substantial importance to the legalization of euthanasia as a means of maintaining this control.

A third good consequence of the legalization of euthanasia concerns patients whose dying is filled with severe and unrelievable pain or suffering. When there is a life-sustaining treatment that, if forgone, will lead relatively quickly to death, then doing so can bring an end to these patients' suffering without recourse to euthanasia. For patients receiving no such treatment, however, euthanasia may be the only release from their otherwise prolonged suffering and agony. This argument from mercy has always been the strongest argument for euthanasia in those cases to which it applies.[11]

The importance of relieving pain and suffering is less controversial than is the frequency with which patients are forced to undergo untreatable agony that only euthanasia could relieve. If we focus first on suffering caused by physical pain, it is crucial to distinguish pain that *could* be adequately relieved with modern methods of pain control, though it in fact is not, from pain that is relievable only by death.[12] For a variety of reasons, including some physicians' fear of hastening the patient's death, as well as the lack of a publicly accessible means for assessing the amount of the patient's pain, many patients suffer pain that could be, but is not, relieved.

Specialists in pain control, as for example the pain of terminally ill cancer patients, argue that there are very few patients whose pain could not be adequately controlled, though sometimes at the cost of so sedating them that they are effectively unable to interact with other people or their environment. Thus, the argument from mercy in cases of physical pain can probably be met in a large majority of cases by providing adequate measures of pain relief. This should be a high priority, whatever our legal policy on euthanasia—the relief of pain and suffering has long been, quite properly, one of the central goals of medicine. Those cases in which pain could be effectively relieved, but in fact is not, should only count significantly in favor of legalizing euthanasia if all reasonable efforts to change pain management techniques have been tried and have failed.

Dying patients often undergo substantial psychological suffering that is not fully or even principally the result of physical pain.[13] The knowledge about how to relieve this suffering is much more limited than in the case of relieving pain, and efforts to do so are probably more often unsuccessful. If the argument from mercy is extended to patients experiencing great and unrelievable psychological suffering, the numbers of patients to which it applies are much greater.

One last good consequence of legalizing euthanasia is that once death has been accepted, it is often more humane to end life quickly and peacefully, when that is what the patient wants. Such a death will often be seen as better than a more prolonged one. People who suffer a sudden and unexpected death, for example by dying quickly or in their sleep from a heart attack or stroke, are often considered lucky to have died in this way. We care about how we die in part because we care about how others remember us, and we hope they will remember us as we were in "good times" with them and not as we might be when disease has robbed us of our dignity as human beings. As with much in the treatment and care of the dying, people's concerns differ in this respect, but for at least some people, euthanasia will be a more humane death than what they have often experienced with other loved ones and might otherwise expect for themselves.

Some opponents of euthanasia challenge how much importance should be given to any of these good consequences of permitting it, or even whether some would be good consequences at all. But more frequently, opponents cite a number of bad consequences that permitting euthanasia would or could produce, and it is to their assessment that I now turn.

Potential Bad Consequences of Permitting Euthanasia. Some of the arguments against permitting euthanasia are aimed specifically against physicians, while others are aimed against anyone being permitted to perform it. I shall first consider one argument of the former sort. Permitting physicians to perform euthanasia, it is said, would be incompatible with their fundamental moral and professional commitment as healers to care for patients and to protect life. Moreover, if euthanasia by physicians became common, patients would come to fear that a medication was intended not to treat or care, but instead to kill, and would thus lose trust in their physicians. This position was forcefully stated in a paper by Willard Gaylin and his colleagues:

> The very soul of medicine is on trial … This issue touches medicine at its moral center; if this moral center collapses, if

physicians become killers or are even licensed to kill, the profession—and, therewith, each physician—will never again be worthy of trust and respect as healer and comforter and protector of life in all its frailty.

These authors go on to make clear that, while they oppose permitting anyone to perform euthanasia, their special concern is with physicians doing so:

We call on fellow physicians to say that they will not deliberately kill. We must also say to each of our fellow physicians that we will not tolerate killing of patients and that we shall take disciplinary action against doctors who kill. And we must say to the broader community that if it insists on tolerating or legalizing active euthanasia, it will have to find nonphysicians to do its killing.[14]

If permitting physicians to kill would undermine the very "moral center" of medicine, then almost certainly physicians should not be permitted to perform euthanasia. But how persuasive is this claim? Patients should not fear, as a consequence of permitting *voluntary* active euthanasia, that their physicians will substitute a lethal injection for what patients want and believe is part of their care. If active euthanasia is restricted to cases in which it is truly voluntary, then no patient should fear getting it unless she or he has voluntarily requested it. (The fear that we might in time also come to accept nonvoluntary, or even involuntary, active euthanasia is a slippery slope worry I address below.) Patients' trust of their physicians could be increased, not eroded, by knowledge that physicians will provide aid in dying when patients seek it.

Might Gaylin and his colleagues nevertheless be correct in their claim that the moral center of medicine would collapse if physicians were to become killers? This question raises what at the deepest level should be the guiding aims of medicine, a question that obviously

cannot be fully explored here. But I do want to say enough to indicate the direction that I believe an appropriate response to this challenge should take. In spelling out above what I called the positive argument for voluntary active euthanasia, I suggested that two principal values—respecting patients' self-determination and promoting their well-being—underlie the consensus that competent patients, or the surrogates of incompetent patients, are entitled to refuse any life-sustaining treatment and to choose from among available alternative treatments. It is the commitment to these two values in guiding physicians' actions as healers, comforters, and protectors of their patients' lives that should be at the "moral center" of medicine, and these two values support physicians' administering euthanasia when their patients make competent requests for it.

What should not be at that moral center is a commitment to preserving patients' lives as such, without regard to whether those patients want their lives preserved or judge their preservation a benefit to them. Vitalism has been rejected by most physicians, and despite some statements that suggest it, is almost certainly not what Gaylin and colleagues intended. One of them, Leon Kass, has elaborated elsewhere the view that medicine is a moral profession whose proper aim is "the naturally given end of health," understood as the wholeness and well-working of the human being; "for the physician, at least, human life in living bodies commands respect and reverence—*by its very nature*." Kass continues, "the deepest ethical principle restraining the physician's power is not the autonomy or freedom of the patient; neither is it his own compassion or good intention. Rather, it is the dignity and mysterious power of human life itself."[15] I believe Kass is in the end mistaken about the proper account of the aims of medicine and the limits on physicians' power, but this difficult issue will certainly be one of the central themes in the continuing debate about euthanasia.

A second bad consequence that some foresee is that permitting euthanasia would weaken society's commitment to provide optimal care for dying patients. We live at a time in which the control of health care costs has become, and is likely to continue to be, the dominant focus of health care policy. If euthanasia is seen as a cheaper alternative to adequate care and treatment, then we might become less scrupulous about providing sometimes costly support and other services to dying patients. Particularly if our society comes to embrace deeper and more explicit rationing of health care, frail, elderly, and dying patients will need to be strong and effective advocates for their own health care and other needs, although they are hardly in a position to do this. We should do nothing to weaken their ability to obtain adequate care and services.

This second worry is difficult to assess because there is little firm evidence about the likelihood of the feared erosion in the care of dying patients. There are at least two reasons, however, for skepticism about this argument. The first is that the same worry could have been directed at recognizing patients' or surrogates' rights to forgo life-sustaining treatment, yet there is no persuasive evidence that recognizing the right to refuse treatment has caused a serious erosion in the quality of care of dying patients. The second reason for skepticism about this worry is that only a very small proportion of deaths would occur from euthanasia if it were permitted. In the Netherlands, where euthanasia under specified circumstances is permitted by the courts, though not authorized by statute, the best estimate of the proportion of overall deaths that result from it is about 2 percent.[16] Thus, the vast majority of critically ill and dying patients will not request it, and so will still have to be cared for by physicians, families, and others. Permitting euthanasia should not diminish people's commitment and concern to maintain and improve the care of these patients.

A third possible bad consequence of permitting euthanasia (or even a public discourse in which strong support for euthanasia is evident) is to threaten the progress made in securing the rights of patients or their surrogates to decide about and to refuse life-sustaining treatment.[17] This progress has been made against the backdrop of a clear and firm legal prohibition of euthanasia, which has provided a relatively bright line limiting the dominion of others over patients' lives. It has therefore been an important reassurance to concerns about how the authority to take steps ending life might be misused, abused, or wrongly extended.

Many supporters of the right of patients or their surrogates to refuse treatment strongly oppose euthanasia, and if forced to choose might well withdraw their support of the right to refuse treatment rather than accept euthanasia. Public policy in the last fifteen years has generally let life-sustaining treatment decisions be made in health care settings between physicians and patients or their surrogates, and without the involvement of the courts. However, if euthanasia is made legally permissible greater involvement of the courts is likely, which could in turn extend to a greater court involvement in life-sustaining treatment decisions. Most agree, however, that increased involvement of the courts in these decisions would be undesirable, as it would make sound decisionmaking more cumbersome and difficult without sufficient compensating benefits.

As with the second potential bad consequence of permitting euthanasia, this third consideration too is speculative and difficult to assess. The feared erosion of patients' or surrogates' rights to decide about life-sustaining treatment, together with greater court involvement in those decisions, are both possible. However, I believe there is reason to discount this general worry. The legal rights of competent patients and, to a lesser degree, surrogates of incompetent patients to decide about treatment are very firmly embedded in a long line of informed consent and life-sustaining treatment cases, and are not likely to be eroded by a debate over, or even acceptance of, euthanasia. It will not be accepted without safeguards that reassure the public about abuse, and if that debate shows the need for similar safeguards for some life-sustaining treatment decisions they should be adopted there as well. In neither case are the only possible safeguards greater court involvement, as the recent growth of institutional ethics committees shows.

The fourth potential bad consequence of permitting euthanasia has been developed by David Velleman and turns on the subtle point that making a new option or choice available to people can sometimes make them worse off, even if once they have the choice they go on to choose what is best for them.[18] Ordinarily, people's continued existence is viewed by them as given, a fixed condition with which they must cope. Making euthanasia available to people as an option denies them the alternative of staying alive by default. If people are offered the option of euthanasia, their continued existence is now a choice for which they can be held responsible and which they can be asked by others to justify. We care, and are right to care, about being able to justify ourselves to others. To the extent that our society is unsympathetic to justifying a severely dependent or impaired existence, a heavy psychological burden of proof may be placed on patients who think their terminal illness or chronic infirmity is not a sufficient reason for dying. Even if they otherwise view their life as worth living, the opinion of others around them that it is not can threaten their reason for living and make euthanasia a rational choice. Thus the existence of the option becomes a subtle pressure to request it.

This argument correctly identifies the reason why offering some patients the option of euthanasia would not benefit then. Velleman takes it not as a reason for opposing all euthanasia, but for restricting it to circumstances where there are "unmistakable and overpowering reasons for persons to want the option of euthanasia," and for denying the option in all other cases. But there are at least three reasons why such restriction may not be warranted. First, polls and other evidence support that most Americans believe euthanasia should be permitted (though the recent defeat of the referendum to permit it in the state of Washington raises some doubt about this support). Thus, many more people seem to want the choice than would be made worse off by getting it. Second, if giving people the option of ending their life really makes them worse off, then we should not only prohibit euthanasia, but also take back from people the right they now have to decide about life-sustaining treatment. The feared harmful effect should already have occurred from securing people's right to refuse life-sustaining treatment, yet there is no evidence of any such widespread harm or any broad public desire to rescind that right. Third, since there is a wide range of conditions in which reasonable people can and do disagree about whether they would want continued life, it is not possible to restrict the permissibility of euthanasia as narrowly as Velleman suggests without thereby denying it to most persons who would want it; to permit it only in cases in which virtually everyone would want it would be to deny it to most who would want it.

A fifth potential bad consequence of making euthanasia legally permissible is that it might weaken the general legal prohibition of homicide. This prohibition is so fundamental to civilized society, it is argued, that we should do nothing that erodes it. If most cases of stopping life support are killing, as I have already argued, then the court cases permitting such killing have already in effect weakened this prohibition. However, neither the courts nor most people have seen these cases as killing and so as challenging the prohibition of homicide. The courts have usually grounded patients' or their surrogates' rights to refuse life-sustaining treatment in rights to privacy, liberty, self-determination, or bodily integrity, not in exceptions to homicide laws.

Legal permission for physicians or others to perform euthanasia could not be grounded in patients' rights to decide about medical treatment. Permitting euthanasia would require qualifying, at least in effect, the legal prohibition against homicide, a prohibition that in general does not allow the consent of the victim to justify or excuse the act. Nevertheless, the very same fundamental basis of the right to decide about life-sustaining treatment—respecting a person's self-determination—does support euthanasia as well. Individual self-determination has long been a well-entrenched and fundamental value in the law, and so extending it to euthanasia would not require appeal to novel legal values or principles. That suicide or attempted suicide is no longer a criminal offense in virtually all states indicates an acceptance of individual self-determination in the taking of one's own life analogous to that required for voluntary active euthanasia. The legal prohibition (in most states) of assisting in suicide and the refusal in the law to accept the consent of the victim as a possible justification of homicide are both arguably a result of difficulties in the legal process of establishing the consent of the victim after the fact. If procedures can be designed that clearly establish the voluntariness of the person's request for euthanasia, it would under those procedures represent a carefully circumscribed qualification on the legal prohibition of homicide. Nevertheless, some remaining worries about this weakening can be captured in the final potential bad consequence, to which I will now turn.

This final potential bad consequence is the central concern of many opponents of euthanasia and, I believe, is the most serious objection to a legal policy permitting it. According to this "slippery slope" worry, although active euthanasia may be morally permissible in cases in which it is unequivocally voluntary and the patient finds his or her condition unbearable, a legal policy permitting euthanasia would inevitably lead to active euthanasia being performed in many other cases in which it would be morally wrong. To prevent those other wrongful cases of euthanasia we should not permit even morally justified performance of it.

Slippery slope arguments of this form are problematic and difficult to evaluate.[19] From one perspective, they are the last refuge of conservative defenders of the status quo. When all the opponent's objections to the wrongness of euthanasia itself have been met, the opponent then shifts ground and acknowledges both that it is not in itself wrong and that a legal policy which resulted only in its being performed would not be bad. Nevertheless, the opponent maintains, it should still not be permitted because doing so would result in its being performed in other cases in which it is not voluntary and would be wrong. In this argument's most extreme form, permitting euthanasia is the first and fateful step down the

slippery slope to Nazism. Once on the slope we will be unable to get off.

Now it cannot be denied that it is *possible* that permitting euthanasia could have these fateful consequences, but that cannot be enough to warrant prohibiting it if it is otherwise justified. A similar *possible* slippery slope worry could have been raised to securing competent patients' rights to decide about life support, but recent history shows such a worry would have been unfounded. It must be relevant how likely it is that we will end with horrendous consequences and an unjustified practice of euthanasia. How *likely* and *widespread* would the abuses and unwarranted extensions of permitting it be? By abuses, I mean the performance of euthanasia that fails to satisfy the conditions required for voluntary active euthanasia, for example, if the patient has been subtly pressured to accept it. By unwarranted extensions of policy, I mean later changes in legal policy to permit not just voluntary euthanasia, but also euthanasia in cases in which, for example, it need not be fully voluntary. Opponents of voluntary euthanasia on slippery slope grounds have not provided the data or evidence necessary to turn their speculative concerns into well-grounded likelihoods.

It is at least clear, however, that both the character and likelihood of abuses of a legal policy permitting euthanasia depend in significant part on the procedures put in place to protect against them. I will not try to detail fully what such procedures might be, but will just give some examples of what they might include:

1. The patient should be provided with all relevant information about his or her medical condition, current prognosis, available alternative treatments, and the prognosis of each.
2. Procedures should ensure that the patient's request for euthanasia is stable or enduring (a brief waiting period could be required) and fully voluntary (an advocate for the patient might be appointed to ensure this).
3. All reasonable alternatives must have been explored for improving the patient's quality of life and relieving any pain or suffering.

4. A psychiatric evaluation should ensure that the patient's request is not the result of a treatable psychological impairment such as depression.[20]

These examples of procedural safeguards are all designed to ensure that the patient's choice is fully informed, voluntary, and competent, and so a true exercise of self-determination. Other proposals for euthanasia would restrict its permissibility further—for example, to the terminally ill—a restriction that cannot be supported by self-determination. Such additional restrictions might, however, be justified by concern for limiting potential harms from abuse. At the same time, it is important not to impose procedural or substantive safeguards so restrictive as to make euthanasia impermissible or practically infeasible in a wide range of justified cases.

These examples of procedural safeguards make clear that it is possible to substantially reduce, though not to eliminate, the potential for abuse of a policy permitting voluntary active euthanasia. Any legalization of the practice should be accompanied by a well-considered set of procedural safeguards together with an ongoing evaluation of its use. Introducing euthanasia into only a few states could be a form of carefully limited and controlled social experiment that would give us evidence about the benefits and harms of the practice. Even then firm and uncontroversial data may remain elusive, as the continuing controversy over what has taken place in the Netherlands in recent years indicates.[21]

The Slip into Nonvoluntary Active Euthanasia. While I believe slippery slope worries can largely be limited by making necessary distinctions both in principle and in practice, one slippery slope concern is legitimate. There is reason to expect that legalization of voluntary active euthanasia might soon be followed by strong pressure to legalize some nonvoluntary euthanasia of incompetent patients unable to express their own wishes. Respecting a person's self-determination and recognizing that continued life is not always of value to a person can support not only voluntary active euthanasia, but

some nonvoluntary euthanasia as well. These are the same values that ground competent patients' right to refuse life-sustaining treatment. Recent history here is instructive. In the medical ethics literature, in the courts since Quinlan, and in norms of medical practice, that right has been extended to incompetent patients and exercised by a surrogate who is to decide as the patient would have decided in the circumstances if competent.[22] It has been held unreasonable to continue life-sustaining treatment that the patient would not have wanted just because the patient now lacks the capacity to tell us that. Life-sustaining treatment for incompetent patients is today frequently forgone on the basis of a surrogate's decision, or less frequently on the basis of an advance directive executed by the patient while still competent. The very same logic that has extended the right to refuse life-sustaining treatment from a competent patient to the surrogate of an incompetent patient (acting with or without a formal advance directive from the patient) may well extend the scope of active euthanasia. The argument will be, Why continue to force unwanted life on patients just because they have now lost the capacity to request euthanasia from us?

A related phenomenon may reinforce this slippery slope concern. In the Netherlands, what the courts have sanctioned has been clearly restricted to voluntary euthanasia. In itself, this serves as some evidence that permitting it need *not* lead to permitting the nonvoluntary variety. There is some indication, however, that for many Dutch physicians euthanasia is no longer viewed as a special action, set apart from their usual practice and restricted only to competent persons.[23] Instead, it is seen as one end of a spectrum of caring for dying patients. When viewed in this way it will be difficult to deny euthanasia to a patient for whom it is seen as the best or most appropriate form of care simply because that patient is now incompetent and cannot request it.

Even if voluntary active euthanasia should slip into nonvoluntary active euthanasia, with surrogates acting for incompetent patients, the ethical evaluation is more complex than many opponents of euthanasia allow. Just as in the case of surrogates' decisions to forgo life-sustaining treatment for incompetent patients, so also surrogates' decisions to request euthanasia for incompetent persons would often accurately reflect what the incompetent person would have wanted and would deny the person nothing that he or she would have considered worth having. Making nonvoluntary active euthanasia legally permissible, however, would greatly enlarge the number of patients on whom it might be performed and substantially enlarge the potential for misuse and abuse. As noted above, frail and debilitated elderly people, often demented or otherwise incompetent and thereby unable to defend and assert their own interests, may be especially vulnerable to unwanted euthanasia.

For some people, this risk is more than sufficient reason to oppose the legalization of voluntary euthanasia. But while we should in general be cautious about inferring much from the experience in the Netherlands to what our own experience in the United States might be, there may be one important lesson that we can learn from them. One commentator has noted that in the Netherlands families of incompetent patients have less authority than do families in the United States to act as surrogates for incompetent patients in making decisions to forgo life-sustaining treatment.[24] From the Dutch perspective, it may be we in the United States who are *already* on the slippery slope in having given surrogates broad authority to forgo life-sustaining treatment for incompetent persons. In this view, the more important moral divide, and the more important with regard to potential for abuse, is not between forgoing life-sustaining treatment and euthanasia, but instead between voluntary and nonvoluntary performance of either. If this is correct, then the more important issue is ensuring the appropriate principles and procedural safeguards for the exercise of decisionmaking authority by surrogates for incompetent persons in *all* decisions at the end of life. This may be the correct response to slippery slope worries about euthanasia.

I have cited both good and bad consequences that have been thought likely from a policy change permitting voluntary active euthanasia, and have tried to evaluate their likelihood and relative importance. Nevertheless, as I noted earlier, reasonable disagreement remains both about the consequences of permitting euthanasia and about which of these consequences are more important. The depth and strength of public and professional debate about whether, all things considered, permitting euthanasia would be desirable or undesirable reflects these disagreements. While my own view is that the balance of considerations supports permitting the practice, my principal purpose here has been to clarify the main issues.

THE ROLE OF PHYSICIANS

If euthanasia is made legally permissible, should physicians take part in it? Should only physicians be permitted to perform it, as is the case in the Netherlands? In discussing whether euthanasia is incompatible with medicine's commitment to curing, caring for, and comforting patients, I argued that it is not at odds with a proper understanding of the aims of medicine, and so need not undermine patients' trust in their physicians. If that argument is correct, then physicians probably should not be prohibited, either by law or by professional norms, from taking part in a legally permissible practice of euthanasia (nor, of course, should they be compelled to do so if their personal or professional scruples forbid it). Most physicians in the Netherlands appear not to understand euthanasia to be incompatible with their professional commitments.

Sometimes patients who would be able to end their lives on their own nevertheless seek the assistance of physicians. Physician involvement in such cases may have important benefits to patients and others beyond simply assuring the use of effective means. Historically, in the United States suicide has carried a strong negative stigma that many today believe unwarranted. Seeking a physician's assistance, or what can almost seem a physician's blessing, may be a way of trying to remove that stigma and show others that the decision for suicide was made with due seriousness and was justified under the circumstances. The physician's involvement provides a kind of social approval, or more accurately helps counter what would otherwise be unwarranted social disapproval.

There are also at least two reasons for restricting the practice of euthanasia to physicians only. First, physicians would inevitably be involved in some of the important procedural safeguards necessary to a defensible practice, such as seeing to it that the patient is well-informed about his or her condition, prognosis, and possible treatments, and ensuring that all reasonable means have been taken to improve the quality of the patient's life. Second, and probably more important, one necessary protection against abuse of the practice is to limit the persons given authority to perform it, so that they can be held accountable for their exercise of that authority. Physicians, whose training and professional norms give some assurance that they would perform euthanasia responsibly, are an appropriate group of persons to whom the practice may be restricted.

Acknowledgments

Earlier versions of this paper were presented at the American Philosophical Association Central Division meetings (at which David Velleman provided extremely helpful comments), Massachusetts General Hospital, Yale University School of Medicine, Princeton University, Brown University, and as the Brin Lecture at The Johns Hopkins School of Medicine. I am grateful to the audiences on each of these occasions, to several anonymous reviewers, and to Norman Daniels for helpful comments. The paper was completed while I was a Fellow in the Program in Ethics and the Professions at Harvard University.

Notes

1. President's Commission for the Study of Ethical Problems in Medicine and Biomedical and Behavioral Research, *Deciding to Forego Life-Sustaining Treatment* (Washington, D.C.: U.S. Government Printing Office, 1983); The Hastings Center, *Guidelines on the Termination of Life-Sustaining Treatment and Care of the Dying* (Bloomington: Indiana University Press, 1987); *Current Opinions of the Council on Ethical and Judicial Affairs of the American Medical Association—1989: Withholding or Withdrawing Life-Prolonging Treatment* (Chicago: American Medical Association, 1989); George Annas and Leonard Glantz, "The Right of Elderly Patients to Refuse Life-Sustaining Treatment," *Millbank Memorial Quarterly* 64, suppl. 2 (1986): 95–162; Robert F. Weir, *Abating Treatment with Critically Ill Patients* (New York: Oxford University Press, 1989); Sidney J. Wanzer et al., "The Physician's Responsibility toward Hopelessly Ill Patients," *NEJM* 310 (1984): 955–59.

2. M.A.M. de Wachter, "Active Euthanasia in the Netherlands," *JAMA* 262, no. 23 (1989): 3315–19.

3. Anonymous, "It's Over, Debbie," *JAMA* 259 (1988): 272; Timothy E. Quill, "Death and Dignity," *NEJM* 322 (1990): 1881–83.

4. Wanzer et al., "The Physician's Responsibility toward Hopelessly Ill Patients: A Second Look," *NEJM* 320 (1989): 844–49.

5. Willard Gaylin, Leon R. Kass, Edmund D. Pellegrino, and Mark Siegler, "Doctors Must Not Kill," *JAMA* 259 (1988): 2139–40.

6. Bonnie Steinbock, ed., *Killing and Allowing to Die* (Englewood Cliffs, NJ.: Prentice Hall, 1980).

7. Dan W. Brock, "Forgoing Food and Water: Is It Killing?" in *By No Extraordinary Means: The Choice to Forgo Life-Sustaining Food and Water,* ed, Joanne Lynn (Bloomington: Indiana University Press, 1986), pp. 117–31.

8. James Rachels, "Active and Passive Euthanasia," *NEJM* 292 (1975): 78–80; Michael Tooley, *Abortion and Infanticide* (Oxford: Oxford University Press, 1983). In my paper, "Taking Human Life," *Ethics* 95 (1985): 851–65, I argue in more detail that killing in itself is not morally different from allowing to die and defend the strategy of argument employed in this and the succeeding two paragraphs in the text.

9. Dan W. Brock, "Moral Rights and Permissible Killing," in *Ethical Issues Relating to Life and Death*, ed. John Ladd (New York: Oxford University Press, 1979), pp. 94–117.

10. P. Painton and E. Taylor, "Love or Let Die," *Time,* 19 March 1990, pp. 62–71; *Boston Globe*/Harvard University Poll, *Boston Globe,* 3 November 1991.

11. James Rachels, *The End of Life* (Oxford: Oxford University Press, 1986).

12. Marcia Angell, "The Quality of Mercy," *NEJM* 306 (1982): 98–99; M. Donovan, P. Dillon, and

L. Mcguire, "Incidence and Characteristics of Pain in a Sample of Medical-Surgical Inpatients," *Pain* 30 (1987): 69–78.

13. Eric Cassell, *The Nature of Suffering and the Goals of Medicine* (New York: Oxford University Press, 1991).

14. Gaylin et al., "Doctors Must Not Kill."

15. Leon R. Kass, "Neither for Love Nor Money: Why Doctors Must Not Kill," *The Public Interest* 94 (1989): 25–46; cf. also his *Toward a More Natural Science: Biology and Human Affairs* (New York: The Free Press, 1985), chs. 6–9.

16. Paul J. Van der Maas et al., "Euthanasia and Other Medical Decisions Concerning the End of Life," *Lancet* 338 (1991): 669–74.

17. Susan M. Wolf, "Holding the Line on Euthanasia," Special Supplement, *Hastings Center Report* 19, no. 1 (1989): 13–15.

18. My formulation of this argument derives from David Velleman's statement of it in his commentary on an earlier version of this paper delivered at the American Philosophical Association Central Division meetings; a similar point was made to me by Elisha Milgram in discussion on another occasion. For more general development of the point see Thomas Schelling, *The Strategy of Conflict*

(Cambridge, Mass.: Harvard University Press, 1960); and Gerald Dworkin, "Is More Choice Better Than Less?" in *The Theory and Practice of Autonomy* (Cambridge: Cambridge University Press, 1988).

19. Frederick Schauer, "Slippery Slopes," *Harvard Law Review* 99 (1985): 361–83; Wibren van der Burg, "The Slippery Slope Argument," *Ethics* 102 (October 1991): 42–65.

20. There is evidence that physicians commonly fail to diagnose depression. See Robert I. Misbin, "Physicians Aid in Dying," *NEJM* 325 (1991): 1304–7.

21. Richard Fenigsen, "A Case against Dutch Euthanasia," Special Supplement, *Hastings Center Report* 19, no. 1 (1989): 22–30.

22. Allen E. Buchanan and Dan W. Brock, *Deciding for Others: The Ethics of Surrogate Decisionmaking* (Cambridge: Cambridge University Press, 1989).

23. Van der Maas et al., "Euthanasia and Other Medical Decisions."

24. Margaret P. Battin, "Seven Caveats Concerning the Discussion of Euthanasia in Holland," *American Philosophical Association Newsletter on Philosophy and Medicine* 89, no. 2 (1990).

When Self-Determination Runs Amok

Daniel Callahan

The euthanasia debate is not just another moral debate, one in a long list of arguments in our pluralistic society. It is profoundly emblematic of three important turning points in Western thought. The first is that of the legitimate conditions under which one person can kill another. The acceptance of voluntary active euthanasia would morally sanction what can only be called "consenting adult killing." By that term I mean the killing of one person by another in the name of their mutual right to be killer and killed if they freely agree to play those roles. This turn flies in the face of a longstanding effort to limit the circumstances under which one person can take the life of another, from efforts to control the free

flow of guns and arms, to abolish capital punishment, and to more tightly control warfare. Euthanasia would add a whole new category of killing to a society that already has too many excuses to indulge itself in that way.

The second turning point lies in the meaning and limits of self-determination. The acceptance of euthanasia would sanction a view of autonomy holding that individuals may, in the name of their own private, idiosyncratic view of the good life, call upon others, including such institutions as medicine, to help them pursue that life, even at the risk of harm to the common good. This works against the idea that the meaning and scope of our own right to lead our own lives must be conditioned by, and be compatible with, the good of the community, which is more than an aggregate of self-directing individuals.

The third turning point is to be found in the claim being made upon medicine: it should be prepared to make its skills available to individuals to help them achieve their private vision of the good life. This puts medicine in the business of promoting the individualistic pursuit of general human happiness and well-being. It would overturn the traditional belief that medicine should limit its domain to promoting and preserving human health, redirecting it instead to the relief of that suffering which stems from life itself, not merely from a sick body.

I believe that, at each of these three turning points, proponents of euthanasia push us in the wrong direction. Arguments in favor of euthanasia fall into four general categories, which I will take up in turn: (1) the moral claim of individual self-determination and well-being; (2) the moral irrelevance of the difference between killing and allowing to die; (3) the supposed paucity of evidence to show likely harmful consequences of legalized euthanasia; and (4) the compatibility of euthanasia and medical practice.

SELF-DETERMINATION

Central to most arguments for euthanasia is the principle of self-determination. People are presumed to have an interest in deciding for themselves, according to their own beliefs about what makes life good, how they will conduct their lives. That is an important value, but the question in the euthanasia context is, What does it mean and how far should it extend? If it were a question of suicide, where a person takes her own life without assistance from another, that principle might be pertinent, at least for debate. But euthanasia is not that limited a matter. The self-determination in that case can only be effected by the moral and physical assistance of another. Euthanasia is thus no longer a matter only of self-determination, but of a mutual, social decision between two people, the one to be killed and the other to do the killing.

How are we to make the moral move from my right of self-determination to some doctor's right to kill me—from my right to his right? Where does the doctor's moral warrant to kill come from? Ought doctors to be able to kill anyone they want as long as permission is given by competent persons? Is our right to life just like a piece of property, to be given away or alienated if the price (happiness, relief of suffering) is right? And then to be destroyed with our permission once alienated?

In answer to all those questions, I will say this: I have yet to hear a plausible argument why it should be permissible for us to put this kind of power in the hands of another, whether a doctor or anyone else. The idea that we can waive our right to life, and then give to another the power to take that life, requires a justification yet to be provided by anyone.

Slavery was long ago outlawed on the ground that one person should not have the right to own another, even with the other's permission. Why? Because it is a fundamental moral wrong for one person to give over his life and fate to another, whatever the good consequences, and no less a wrong for another person to have that kind of total, final power. Like slavery, dueling was long ago banned on similar grounds: even free, competent individuals should not have the power to kill each other, whatever their motives, whatever the circumstances. Consenting adult killing, like consenting adult slavery or degradation, is a strange route to human dignity.

There is another problem as well. If doctors, once sanctioned to carry out euthanasia, are to be themselves responsible moral agents—not simply hired hands with lethal injections at the ready—then they must have their own independent moral grounds to kill those who request such services. What do I mean? As those who favor euthanasia are quick to point out, some people want it because their life has become so burdensome it no longer seems worth living.

The doctor will have a difficulty at this point. The degree and intensity to which people suffer from their diseases and their dying, and whether they find life more of a burden than a benefit, has very little directly to do with the nature or extent of their actual physical condition. Three people can have the same condition, but only one will find the suffering unbearable. People suffer, but suffering is as much a function of the values of individuals as it is of the physical causes of that suffering. Inevitably in that circumstance, the doctor will in effect be treating the patient's values. To be responsible, the doctor would have to share those values. The doctor would have to decide, on her own, whether the patient's life was "no longer worth living."

But how could a doctor possibly know that or make such a judgment? Just because the patient said so? I raise this question because, while in Holland at the euthanasia conference reported by Maurice de Wachter elsewhere in this issue, the doctors present agreed that there is no objective way of measuring or judging the claims of patients that their suffering is unbearable. And if it is difficult to measure suffering, how much more difficult to determine the value of a patient's statement that her life is not worth living?

However one might want to answer such questions, the very need to ask them, to inquire into the physician's responsibility and grounds for medical and moral judgment, points out the social nature of the decision. Euthanasia is not a private matter of self-determination. It is an act that requires two people to make it possible, and a complicit society to make it acceptable.

KILLING AND ALLOWING TO DIE

Against common opinion, the argument is sometimes made that there is no moral difference between stopping life-sustaining treatment and more active forms of killing, such as lethal injection. Instead I would contend that the notion that there is no morally significant difference between omission and commission is just wrong. Consider in its broad implications what the eradication of the distinction implies: that death from disease has been banished, leaving only the actions of physicians in terminating treatment as the cause of death. Biology, which used to bring about death, has apparently been displaced by human agency. Doctors have finally, I suppose, thus genuinely become gods, now doing what nature and the deities once did.

What is the mistake here? It lies in confusing causality and culpability, and in failing to note the way in which human societies have overlaid natural causes with moral rules and interpretations. Causality (by which I mean the direct physical causes of death) and culpability (by which I mean our attribution of moral responsibility to human actions) are confused under three circumstances.

They are confused, first, when the action of a physician in stopping treatment of a patient with an underlying lethal disease is construed as *causing* death. On the contrary, the physician's omission can only bring about death on the condition that the patient's disease will kill him in the absence of treatment. We may hold the physician morally responsible for the death, if we have morally judged such actions wrongful omissions. But it confuses reality and moral judgment to see an omitted action as having the same causal status as one that directly kills. A lethal injection will kill both a healthy person and a sick person. A physician's omitted treatment will have no effect on a healthy person. Turn off the machine on me, a healthy person, and nothing will happen. It will only, in contrast, bring the life of a sick person to an end because of an underlying fatal disease.

Causality and culpability are confused, second, when we fail to note that judgments of moral responsibility and culpability are human constructs. By that I mean that we human beings, after moral reflection, have decided to call some actions right or wrong, and to devise moral rules to deal with them. When physicians could do nothing to stop death, they were not held responsible for it. When, with medical progress, they began to have some power over death—but only its timing and circumstances, not its ultimate inevitability—moral rules were devised to set forth their obligations. Natural causes of death were not thereby banished. They were, instead, overlaid with a medical ethics designed to determine moral culpability in deploying medical power.

To confuse the judgments of this ethics with the physical causes of death—which is the connotation of the word kill—is to confuse nature and human action. People will, one way or another, die of some disease; death will have dominion over all of us. To say that a doctor "kills" a patient by allowing this to happen should only be understood as a moral judgment about the licitness of his omission, nothing more. We can, as a fashion of speech only, talk about a doctor killing a patient by omitting treatment he should have provided. It is a fashion of speech precisely because it is the underlying disease that brings death when treatment is omitted; that is its cause, not the physician's omission. It is a misuse of the word *killing* to use it when a doctor stops a treatment he believes will no longer benefit the patient—when, that is, he steps aside to allow an eventually inevitable death to occur now rather than later. The only deaths that human beings invented are those that come from direct killing—when, with a lethal injection, we both cause death and are morally responsible for it. In the case of omissions, we do not cause death even if we may be judged morally responsible for it.

This difference between causality and culpability also helps us see why a doctor who has omitted a treatment he should have provided has "killed" that patient while another doctor—performing precisely the same act of omission on another patient in different circumstances—does not kill her, but only allows her to die. The difference is that we have come, by moral convention and conviction, to classify unauthorized or illegitimate omissions as acts of "killing." We call them "killing" in the expanded sense of the term: a culpable action that permits the real cause of death, the underlying disease, to proceed to its lethal conclusion. By contrast, the doctor who, at the patient's request, omits or terminates unwanted treatment does not kill at all. Her underlying disease, not his action, is the physical cause of death; and we have agreed to consider actions of that kind to be morally licit. He thus can truly be said to have "allowed" her to die.

If we fail to maintain the distinction between killing and allowing to die, moreover, there are some disturbing possibilities. The first would be to confirm many physicians in their already too-powerful belief that, when patients die or when physicians stop treatment because of the futility of continuing it, they are somehow both morally and physically responsible for the deaths that follow. That notion needs to be abolished, not strengthened. It needlessly and wrongly burdens the physician, to whom should not be attributed the powers of the gods. The second possibility would be that, in every case where a doctor judges medical treatment no longer effective in prolonging life, a quick and direct killing of the patient would be seen as the next, most reasonable step, on grounds of both humaneness and economics. I do not see how that logic could easily be rejected.

CALCULATING THE CONSEQUENCES

When concerns about the adverse social consequences of permitting euthanasia are raised, its advocates tend to dismiss them as unfounded and overly speculative. On the contrary; recent data about the Dutch experience suggests that such concerns are right on target. From my own discussions in Holland, and from the articles on that subject in this issue and elsewhere, I believe we can now fully see most of the likely consequences of legal euthanasia.

Three consequences seem almost certain, in this or any other country: the inevitability of some abuse of the law; the difficulty of precisely writing, and then enforcing, the law; and the inherent slipperiness of the moral reasons for legalizing euthanasia in the first place.

Why is abuse inevitable? One reason is that almost all laws on delicate, controversial matters are to some extent abused. This happens because not everyone will agree with the law as written and will bend it, or ignore it, if they can get away with it. From explicit admissions to me by Dutch proponents of euthanasia, and from the corroborating information provided by the Remmelink Report and the outside studies of Carlos Gomez and John Keown, I am convinced that in the Netherlands there are a substantial number of cases of nonvoluntary euthanasia, that is, euthanasia undertaken without the explicit permission of the person being killed. The other reason abuse is inevitable is that the law is likely to have a low enforcement priority in the criminal justice system. Like other laws of similar status, unless there is an unrelenting and harsh willingness to pursue abuse, violations will ordinarily be tolerated. The worst thing to me about my experience in Holland was the casual, seemingly indifferent attitude toward abuse. I think that would happen everywhere.

Why would it be hard to precisely write, and then enforce, the law? The Dutch speak about the requirement of "unbearable" suffering, but admit that such a term is just about indefinable, a highly subjective matter admitting of no objective standards. A requirement for outside opinion is nice, but it is easy to find complaisant colleagues. A requirement that a medical condition be "terminal" will run aground on the notorious difficulties of knowing when an illness is actually terminal.

Apart from those technical problems there is a more profound worry. I see no way, even in principle, to write or enforce a meaningful law that can guarantee effective procedural safeguards. The reason is obvious yet almost always overlooked. The euthanasia transaction will ordinarily take place within the boundaries of the private and confidential doctor-patient relationship. No one can possibly know what takes place in that context unless the doctor chooses to reveal it. In Holland, less than 10 percent of the physicians report their acts of euthanasia and do so with almost complete legal impunity. There is no reason why the situation should be any better elsewhere. Doctors will have their own reasons for keeping euthanasia secret, and some patients will have no less a motive for wanting it concealed.

I would mention, finally, that the moral logic of the motives for euthanasia contain within them the ingredients of abuse. The two standard motives for euthanasia and assisted suicide are said to be our right of self-determination, and our claim upon the mercy of others, especially doctors, to relieve our suffering. These two motives are typically spliced together and presented as a single justification. Yet if they are considered independently—and there is no inherent reason why they must be linked—they reveal serious problems. It is said that a competent, adult person should have a right to euthanasia for the relief of suffering. But why must the person be suffering? Does not that stipulation already compromise the principle of self-determination? How can self-determination have any limits? Whatever the person's motives may be, why are they not sufficient?

Consider next the person who is suffering but not competent, who is perhaps demented or mentally retarded. The standard argument would deny euthanasia to that person. But why? If a person is suffering but not competent, then it would seem grossly unfair to deny relief solely on the grounds of incompetence. Are the incompetent less entitled to relief from suffering than the competent? Will it only be affluent, middle-class people, mentally fit and savvy about working the medical system, who can qualify? Do the incompetent suffer less because of their incompetence?

Considered from these angles, there are no good moral reasons to limit euthanasia once the principle of taking life for that purpose has been legitimated. If we really believe in self-determination, then any competent person should have a right to be killed by a doctor for any reason that suits him. If we believe in the relief of suffering, then it seems cruel and capricious to deny it to the incompetent. There is, in short, no reasonable or logical stopping point once the turn has been made down the road to euthanasia, which could soon turn into a convenient and commodious expressway.

EUTHANASIA AND MEDICAL PRACTICE

A fourth kind of argument one often hears both in the Netherlands and in this country is that euthanasia and assisted suicide are perfectly compatible with the aims of medicine. I would note at the very outset that a physician who participates in another person's suicide already abuses medicine. Apart from depression (the main statistical cause of suicide), people commit suicide because they find life empty, oppressive, or meaningless. Their judgment is a judgment about the value of continued life, not only about health (even if they are sick). Are doctors now to be given the right to make judgments about the kinds of life worth living and to give their blessing to suicide for those they judge wanting? What conceivable competence, technical or moral, could doctors claim to play such a role? Are we to medicalize suicide, turning judgments about its worth and value into one more clinical issue? Yes, those are rhetorical questions.

Yet they bring us to the core of the problem of euthanasia and medicine. The great temptation of modern medicine, not always resisted, is to move beyond the promotion and preservation of health into the boundless realm of general human happiness and well-being. The root problem of illness and mortality is both medical and philosophical or religious. "Why must I die?" can be asked as a technical, biological question or as a question about the meaning of life. When medicine tries to respond to the latter, which it is always under pressure to do, it moves beyond its proper role.

It is not medicine's place to lift from us the burden of that suffering which turns on the meaning we assign to the decay of the body and its eventual death. It is not medicine's place to determine when lives are not worth living or when the burden of life is too great to be borne. Doctors have no conceivable way of evaluating

such claims on the part of patients, and they should have no right to act in response to them. Medicine should try to relieve human suffering, but only that suffering which is brought on by illness and dying as biological phenomena, not that suffering which comes from anguish or despair at the human condition.

Doctors ought to relieve those forms of suffering that medically accompany serious illness and the threat of death. They should relieve pain, do what they can to allay anxiety and uncertainty, and be a comforting presence. As sensitive human beings, doctors should be prepared to respond to patients who ask why they must die, or die in pain. But here the doctor and the patient are at the same level. The doctor may have no better an answer to those old questions than anyone else; and certainly no special insight from his training as a physician. It would be terrible for physicians to forget this, and to think that in a swift, lethal injection, medicine has found its own answer to the riddle of life. It would be a false answer, given by the wrong people. It would be no less a false answer for patients. They should neither ask medicine to put its own vocation at risk to serve their private interests, nor think that the answer to suffering is to be killed by another. The problem is precisely that, too often in human history, killing has seemed the quick, efficient way to put aside that which burdens us. It rarely helps, and too often simply adds to one evil still another. That is what I believe euthanasia would accomplish. It is self-determination run amok.

Is It Time to Abandon Brain Death?

Robert D. Troug

Over the past several decades, the concept of brain death has become well entrenched within the practice of medicine. At a practical level, this concept has been successful in delineating

widely accepted ethical and legal boundaries for the procurement of vital organs for transplantation. Despite this success, however, there have been persistent concerns over whether the con-

End of Life Issues

cept is theoretically coherent and internally consistent.[1] Indeed, some have concluded that the concept is fundamentally flawed, and that it represents only a "superficial and fragile consensus."[2] In this analysis I will identify the sources of these inconsistencies, and suggest that the best resolution to these issues may be to abandon the concept of brain death altogether.

DEFINITIONS, CONCEPTS, AND TESTS

In its seminal work "Defining Death," the President's Commission for the Study of Ethical Problems in Medicine and Biomedical and Behavioral Research articulated a formulation of brain death that has come to be known as the "whole-brain standard."[3] In the Uniform Determination of Death Act, the President's Commission specified two criteria for determining death: (1) irreversible cessation of circulatory and respiratory functions, or (2) irreversible cessation of all functions of the entire brain, including the brainstem."

Neurologist James Bernat has been influential in defending and refining this standard. Along with others, he has recognized that analysis of the concept of brain death must begin by differentiating between three distinct levels. At the most general level, the concept must involve a *definition*. Next, *criteria* must be specified to determine when the definition has been fulfilled. Finally, *tests* must be available for evaluating whether the criteria have been satisfied.[4] As clarified by Bernat and colleagues, therefore, the concept of death under the whole-brain formulation can be outlined as follows: [5]

> *Definition of Death*: The "permanent cessation of functioning of the organism as a whole."
>
> *Criterion for Death*: The "permanent cessation of functioning of the entire brain."
>
> *Tests for death*: Two distinct sets of tests are available and acceptable for determining that the criterion is fulfilled:

(1) The cardiorespiratory standard is the traditional approach for determining death and relies upon documenting the prolonged absence of circulation or respiration. These tests fulfill the criterion, according to Bernat, since the prolonged absence of these vital signs is diagnostic for the permanent loss of all brain function.

(2) The neurological standard consists of a battery of tests and procedures, including establishment of an etiology sufficient to account for the loss of all brain functions, diagnosing the presence of coma, documenting apnea and the absence of brainstem reflexes, excluding reversible conditions, and showing the persistence of these findings over a sufficient period of time.[6]

CRITIQUE OF THE CURRENT FORMULATION OF BRAIN DEATH

Is this a coherent account of the concept of brain death? To answer this question, one must determine whether each level of analysis is consistent with the others. In other words, individuals who fulfill the tests must also fulfill the criterion, and those who satisfy the criterion must also satisfy the definition.[7]

First, regarding the tests-criterion relationship, there is evidence that many individuals who fulfill all of the tests for brain death do not have the "permanent cessation of functioning of the entire brain." In particular, many of these individuals retain clear evidence of integrated brain function at the level of the brainstem and midbrain, and may have evidence of cortical function.

For example, many patients who fulfill the tests for the diagnosis of brain death continue to exhibit intact neurohumoral function. Between

22 percent and 100 percent of brain-dead patients in different series have been found to retain free-water homeostasis through the neurologically mediated secretion of arginine vasopressin, as evidenced by serum hormonal levels and the absence of diabetes insipidus.[8] Since the brain is the only source of the regulated secretion of arginine vasopressin, patients without diabetes insipidus do not have the loss of all brain function. Neurologically regulated secretion of other hormones is also quite common.[9]

In addition, the tests for the diagnosis of brain death require the patient not to be hypothermic.[10] This caveat is a particularly confusing Catch 22, since the absence of hypothermia generally indicates the continuation of neurologically mediated temperature homeostasis. The circularity of this reasoning can be clinically problematic, since hypothermic patients cannot be diagnosed as brain-dead but the absence of hypothermia is itself evidence of brain function.

Furthermore, studies have shown that many patients (20 percent in one series) who fulfill the tests for brain death continue to show electrical activity on their electroencephalograms.[11] While there is no way to determine how often this electrical activity represents true "function" (which would be incompatible with the criterion for brain death), in at least some cases the activity observed seems fully compatible with function.[12]

Finally, clinicians have observed that patients who fulfill the tests for brain death frequently respond to surgical incision at the time of organ procurement with a significant rise in both heart rate and blood pressure. This suggests that integrated neurological function at a supraspinal level may be present in at least some patients diagnosed as brain-dead.[13] This evidence points to the conclusion that there is a significant disparity between the standard tests used to make the diagnosis of brain death and the criterion these tests are purported to fulfill. Faced with these facts, even supporters of the current statutes acknowledge that the criterion of "whole-brain" death is only an "approximation."[14]

If the tests for determining brain death are incompatible with the current criterion, then one way of solving the problem would be to require tests that always correlate with the "permanent cessation of functioning of the entire brain." Two options have been considered in this regard. The first would require tests that correlate with the actual destruction of the brain, since complete destruction would, of course, be incompatible with any degree of brain function. Only by satisfying these tests, some have argued, could we be assured that all functions of the entire brain have totally and permanently ceased.[15] But is there a constellation of clinical and laboratory tests that correlate with this degree of destruction? Unfortunately, a study of over 500 patients with both coma and apnea (including 146 autopsies for neuropathologic correlation) showed that "it was not possible to verify that a diagnosis made prior to cardiac arrest by any set or subset of criteria would invariably correlate with a diffusely destroyed brain."[16] On the basis of these data, a definition that required total brain destruction could only be confirmed at autopsy. Clearly, a condition that could only be determined after death could never be a requirement for declaring death.

Another way of modifying the tests to conform with the criterion would be to rely solely upon the cardiorespiratory standard for determining death. This standard would certainly identify the permanent cessation of all brain function (thereby fulfilling the criterion), since it is well established by common knowledge that prolonged absence of circulation and respiration results in the death of the entire brain (and every other organ). In addition, fulfillment of these tests would also convincingly demonstrate the cessation of function of the organism as a whole (thereby fulfilling the definition). Unfortunately, this approach for resolving the problem would also make it virtually impossible to obtain vital organs in a viable condition for transplantation, since under current laws it is generally necessary for these organs to be removed from a heart-beating donor.

These inconsistencies between the tests and the criterion are therefore not easily resolvable. In addition to these problems, there are also inconsistencies between the criterion and the definition. As outlined above, the whole-brain concept assumes that the "permanent cessation of functioning of the entire brain" (the criterion) necessarily implies the "permanent cessation of functioning of the organism as a whole" (the definition). Conceptually, this relationship assumes the principle that the brain is responsible for maintaining the body's homeostasis, and that without brain function the organism rapidly disintegrates. In the past, this relationship was demonstrated by showing that individuals who fulfilled the tests for the diagnosis of brain death inevitably had a cardiac arrest within a short period of time, even if they were provided with mechanical ventilation and intensive care.[17] Indeed, this assumption had been considered one of the linchpins in the ethical justification for the concept of brain death.[18] For example, in the largest empirical study of brain death ever performed, a collaborative group working under the auspices of the National Institutes of Health sought to specify the necessary tests for diagnosing brain death by attempting to identify a constellation of neurological findings that would inevitably predict the development of a cardiac arrest within three months, regardless of the level or intensity of support provided.[19]

This approach to defining brain death in terms of neurological findings that predict the development of cardiac arrest is plagued by both logical and scientific problems, however. First, it confuses a prognosis with a diagnosis. Demonstrating that a certain class of patients will suffer a cardiac arrest within a defined period of time certainly proves that they are *dying,* but it says nothing about whether they are *dead.*[20] This conceptual mistake can be clearly appreciated if one considers individuals who are dying of conditions not associated with severe neurological impairment. If a constellation of tests could identify a subgroup of patients with metastatic cancer who invariably suffered a cardiac arrest within a short period of time, for example, we would certainly be comfortable in concluding that they were dying, but we clearly could not claim that they were already dead.

Second, this view relies upon the intuitive notion that the brain is the principal organ of the body, the "integrating" organ whose functions cannot be replaced by any other organ or by artificial means. Up through the early 1980s, this view was supported by numerous studies showing that almost all patients who fulfilled the usual battery of tests for brain death suffered a cardiac arrest within several weeks.[21]

The loss of homeostatic equilibrium that is empirically observed in brain-dead patients is almost certainly the result of their progressive loss of integrated neurohumoral and autonomic function. Over the past several decades, however, intensive care units (ICUs) have become increasingly sophisticated "surrogate brainstems," replacing both the respiratory functions as well as the hormonal and other regulatory activities of the damaged neuraxis.[22] This technology is presently utilized in those tragic cases in which a pregnant woman is diagnosed as brain-dead and an attempt is made to maintain her somatic existence until the fetus reaches a viable gestation, as well as for prolonging the organ viability of brain-dead patients awaiting organ procurement.[23] Although the functions of the brainstem are considerably more complex than those of the heart or the lungs, in theory (and increasingly in practice) they are entirely replaceable by modern technology. In terms of maintaining homeostatic functions, therefore, the brain is no more irreplaceable than any of the other vital organs. A definition of death predicated upon the "inevitable" development of a cardiac arrest within a short period of time is therefore inadequate, since this empirical "fact" is no longer true. In other words, cardiac arrest is inevitable only if it is allowed to occur, just as respiratory arrest in brain-dead patients is inevitable only if they are not provided with mechanical ventilation. This gradual development in technical expertise has unwittingly undermined one of the central ethical justifications for the whole-brain criterion of death.

In summary, then, the whole-brain concept is plagued by internal inconsistencies in both the tests-criterion and the criterion-definition relationships, and these problems cannot be easily solved. In addition, there is evidence that this lack of conceptual clarity has contributed to misunderstandings about the concept among both clinicians and laypersons. For example, Stuart Youngner and colleagues found that only 35 percent of physicians and nurses who were likely to be involved in organ procurement for transplantation correctly identified the legal and medical criteria for determining death.[24] Indeed, most of the respondents used inconsistent concepts of death, and a substantial minority misunderstood the criterion to be the permanent loss of consciousness, which the President's Commission had specifically rejected, in part because it would have classified anencephalic newborns and patients in a vegetative state as dead. In other words, medical professionals who were otherwise knowledgeable and sophisticated were generally confused about the concept of brain death. In an editorial accompanying this study, Dan Wikler and Alan Weisbard claimed that this confusion was "appropriate," given the lack of philosophical coherence in the concept itself.[25] In another study, a survey of Swedes found that laypersons were more willing to consent to autopsies than to organ donation for themselves or a close relative. In seeking an explanation for these findings, the authors reported that "the fear of not being dead during the removal of organs, reported by 22 percent of those undecided toward organ donation, was related to the uncertainty surrounding brain death."[26]

On one hand, these difficulties with the concept might be deemed to be so esoteric and theoretical that they should play no role in driving the policy debate about how to define death and procure organs for transplantation. This has certainly been the predominant view up to now. In many other circumstances, theoretical issues have taken a back seat to practical matters when it comes to determining public policy. For example, the question of whether tomatoes should be considered a vegetable or a fruit for purposes of taxation was said to hinge little upon the biological facts of the matter, but to turn primarily upon the political and economic issues at stake.[27] If this view is applied to the concept of brain death, then the best public policy would be that which best served the public's interest, regardless of theoretical concerns.

On the other hand, medicine has a long and respected history of continually seeking to refine the theoretical and conceptual underpinnings of its practice. While the impact of scientific and philosophical views upon social policy and public perception must be taken seriously, they cannot be the sole forces driving the debate. Given the evidence demonstrating a lack of coherence in the whole-brain death formulation and the confusion that is apparent among medical professionals, there is ample reason to prompt a look at alternatives to our current approach.

ALTERNATIVE APPROACHES TO THE WHOLE-BRAIN FORMULATION

Alternatives to the whole-brain death formulation fall into two general categories. One approach is to emphasize the overriding importance of those functions of the brain that support the phenomenon of consciousness and to claim that individuals who have permanently suffered the loss of all consciousness are dead. This is known as the "higher-brain" criterion. The other approach is to return to the traditional tests for determining death, that is, the permanent loss of circulation and respiration. As noted above, this latter strategy could fit well with Bernat's formulation of the definition of death, since adoption of the cardiorespiratory standard as the test for determining death is consistent with both the criterion and the definition. The problem with this potential solution is that it would virtually eliminate the possibility of procuring vital organs from heart-beating donors under our present system of law and ethics, since current requirements insist that organs be removed only from individuals who have been declared dead (the "dead-donor rule").[28] Consideration of this latter view would therefore be feasible only if it could be linked to fundamental changes in the permissible limits of organ procurement.

The Higher-Brain Formulation. The higher-brain criterion for death holds that maintaining the potential for consciousness is the critical function of the brain relevant to questions of life and death. Under this definition, all individuals who are permanently unconscious would be considered to be dead. Included in this category would be (1) patients who fulfill the cardiorespiratory standard, (2) those who fulfill the current tests for whole-brain death, (3) those diagnosed as being in a permanent vegetative state, and (4) newborns with anencephaly. Various versions of this view have been defended by many philosophers, and arguments have been advanced from moral as well as ontological perspectives.[29] In addition, this view correlates very well with many commonsense opinions about personal identity. To take a stock philosophical illustration, for example, consider the typical reaction of a person who has undergone a hypothetical "brain switch" procedure, where one's brain is transplanted into another's body, and vice versa. Virtually anyone presented with this scenario will say that "what matters" for their existence now resides in the new body, even though an outside observer would insist that it is the person's old body that "appears" to be the original person. Thought experiments like this one illustrate that we typically identify ourselves with our experience of consciousness, and this observation forms the basis of the claim that the permanent absence of consciousness should be seen as representing the death of the person.

Implementation of this standard would present certain problems, however. First, is it possible to diagnose the state of permanent unconsciousness with the high level of certainty required for the determination of death? More specifically, is it currently possible to definitively diagnose the permanent vegetative state and anencephaly? A Multi-Society Task Force recently outlined guidelines for diagnosis of permanent vegetative state and claimed that sufficient data are now available to make the diagnosis of permanent vegetative state in appropriate patients with a high degree of certainty.[30] On the other hand, case reports of patients who met these criteria but who later recovered a higher degree of neurological functioning suggest that use of the term "permanent" may be overstating the degree of diagnostic certainty that is currently possible. This would be an especially important issue in the context of diagnosing death, where false positive diagnoses would be particularly problematic.[31] Similarly, while the Medical Task Force on Anencephaly has concluded that most cases of anencephaly can be diagnosed by a competent clinician without significant uncertainty, others have emphasized the ambiguities inherent in evaluating this condition.[32]

Another line of criticism is that the higher-brain approach assumes the definition of death should reflect the death of the *person,* rather than the death of the *organism.*[33] By focusing on the person, this theory does not account for what is common to the death of all organisms, such as humans, frogs, or trees. Since we do not know what it would mean to talk about the permanent loss of consciousness of frogs or trees, then this approach to death may appear to be idiosyncratic. In response, higher-brain theorists believe that it is critical to define death within the context of the specific subject under consideration. For example, we may speak of the death of an ancient civilization, the death of a species, or the death of a particular system of belief. In each case, the definition of death will be different, and must be appropriate to the subject in order for the concept to make any sense. Following this line of reasoning, the higher-brain approach is correct precisely because it seeks to identify what is uniquely relevant to the death of a person.

Aside from these diagnostic and philosophical concerns, however, perhaps the greatest objections to the higher brain formulation emerge from the implications of treating breathing patients as if they are dead. For example, if patients in a permanent vegetative state were considered to be dead, then they should logically be considered suitable for burial. Yet all of these patients breathe, and some of them "live" for many years.[34] The thought of burying or cremating a breathing individual, even if unconscious, would be unthinkable for many people, creating a significant barrier to acceptance of this view into public policy.[35]

One way of avoiding this implication would be to utilize a "lethal injection" before cremation or burial to terminate cardiac and respiratory function. This would not be euthanasia, since the individual would be declared dead before the injection. The purpose of the injection would be purely "aesthetic." This practice could even be viewed as simply an extension of our current protocols, where the vital functions of patients diagnosed as brain-dead are terminated prior to burial, either by discontinuing mechanical ventilation or by removing their heart and/or lungs during the process of organ procurement. While this line of argumentation has a certain logical persuasiveness, it nevertheless fails to address the central fact that most people find it counterintuitive to perceive a breathing patient as "dead." Wikler has suggested that this attitude is likely to change over time, and that eventually society will come to accept that the body of a patient in a permanent vegetative state is simply that person's "living remains."[36] This optimism about higher-brain death is reminiscent of the comments by the President's Commission regarding whole-brain death: "Although undeniably disconcerting for many people, the confusion created in personal perception by a determination of 'brain death' does not … provide a basis for an ethical objection to discontinuing medical measures on these dead bodies any more than on other dead bodies."[37] Nevertheless, at the present time any inclination toward a higher-brain death standard remains primarily in the realm of philosophers and not policymakers.

Return to the Traditional Cardiorespiratory Standard. In contrast to the higher-brain concept of death, the other main alternative to our current approach would involve moving in the opposite direction and abandoning the diagnosis of brain death altogether. This would involve returning to the traditional approach to determining death, that is, the cardiorespiratory standard. In evaluating the wisdom of "turning back the clock," it

is helpful to retrace the development of the concept of brain death back to 1968 and the conclusions of the Ad Hoc Committee that developed the Harvard Criteria for the diagnosis of brain death. They began by claiming:

> There are two reasons why there is need for a definition [of brain death]: (1) Improvements in resuscitative and supportive measures have led to increased efforts to save those who are desperately injured. Sometimes these efforts have only partial success so that the result is an individual whose heart continues to beat but whose brain is irreversibly damaged. The burden is great on patients who suffer permanent loss of intellect, on their families, and on those in need of hospital beds already occupied by these comatose patients. (2) Obsolete criteria for the definition of death can lead to controversy in obtaining organs for transplantation.[38]

These two issues can be subdivided into at least four distinct questions:

1) When is it permissible to withdraw life support from patients with irreversible neurological damage for the benefit of the patient?
2) When is it permissible to withdraw life support from patients with irreversible neurological damage for the benefit of society, where the benefit is either in the form of economic savings or to make an ICU bed available for someone with a better prognosis?
3) When is it permissible to remove organs from a patient for transplantation?
4) When is a patient ready to be cremated or buried?

The Harvard Committee chose to address all of these questions with a single answer, that is, the determination of brain death. Each of these questions involves unique theoretical issues, however, and each raises a different set of concerns. By analyzing the concept of brain death in terms of the separate questions that led to its development, alternatives to brain death may be considered.

Withdrawal of life support. The Harvard Committee clearly viewed the diagnosis of brain death as a necessary condition for the withdrawal of life support: "It should be emphasized that we recommend the patient be declared dead before any effort is made to take him off a respirator … [since] otherwise, the physicians would be turning off the respirator on a person who is, in the present strict, technical application of law, still alive" (p. 339).

The ethical and legal mandates that surround the withdrawal of life support have changed dramatically since the recommendations of the Harvard Committee. Numerous court decisions and consensus statements have emphasized the rights of patients or their surrogates to demand the withdrawal of life-sustaining treatments, including mechanical ventilation. In the practice of critical care medicine today, patients are rarely diagnosed as brain-dead solely for the purpose of discontinuing mechanical ventilation. When patients are not candidates for organ transplantation, either because of medical contraindications or lack of consent, families are informed of the dismal prognosis, and artificial ventilation is withdrawn. While the diagnosis of brain death was once critical in allowing physicians to discontinue life-sustaining treatments, decision-making about these important questions is now appropriately centered around the patient's previously stated wishes and judgments about the patient's best interest. Questions about the definition of death have become virtually irrelevant to these deliberations.

Allocation of scarce resources. The Harvard Committee alluded to its concerns about having patients with a hopeless prognosis occupying ICU beds. In the years since that report, this issue has become even more pressing. The diagnosis of brain death, however, is of little significance in helping to resolve these issues. Even considering the unusual cases where families refuse to have the ventilator removed from a brain-dead patient, the overall impact of the diagnosis of brain death upon scarce ICU resources is minimal. Much more important to the current debate over the just allocation of ICU resources are patients with less severe degrees of neurological dysfunction, such as patients in a permanent vegetative state or individuals with advanced dementia. Again, the diagnosis of brain death is of little relevance to this central concern of the Harvard Committee.

Organ transplantation. Without question, the most important reason for the continued use of brain death criteria is the need for transplantable organs. Yet even here, the requirement for brain death may be doing more harm than good. The need for organs is expanding at an ever-increasing rate, while the number of available organs has essentially plateaued. In an effort to expand the limited pool of organs, several attempts have been made to circumvent the usual restrictions of brain death on organ procurement.

At the University of Pittsburgh, for example, a new protocol allows critically ill patients or their surrogates to offer their organs for donation after the withdrawal of life-support, even though the patients never meet brain death criteria.[39] Suitable patients are taken to the operating room, where intravascular monitors are placed and the patient is "prepped and draped" for surgical incision. Life-support is then withdrawn, and the patient is monitored for the development of cardiac arrest. Assuming this occurs within a short period of time, the attending physician waits until there has been two minutes of pulselessness, and then pronounces the patient dead. The transplant team then enters the operating room and immediately removes the organs for transplantation.

This novel approach has a number of problems when viewed from within the traditional framework. For example, after the patient is pronounced dead, why should the team rush to remove the organs? If the Pittsburgh team truly believes that the patient is dead, why not begin chest compressions and mechanical ventilation, insert cannulae to place the patient on full cardiopulmonary bypass, and remove the organs in a more controlled fashion? Presumably, this is not done because two minutes of pulselessness is almost certainly not long enough to ensure the development of brain death.[40] It is even conceivable that patients managed in this way could regain consciousness during the process of organ procurement while supported with cardiopulmonary bypass, despite having already been diagnosed as "dead." In other words, the reluctance of the Pittsburgh team to extend their protocol in ways that would be acceptable for dead patients could be an indication that the patients may really not be dead after all.

A similar attempt to circumvent the usual restrictions on organ procurement was recently attempted with anencephalic newborns at Loma Linda University. Again, the protocol involved manipulation of the dying process, with mechanical ventilation being instituted and maintained solely for the purpose of preserving the organs until criteria for brain death could be documented. The results were disappointing, and the investigators concluded that "it is usually not feasible, with the restrictions of current law, to procure solid organs for transplantation from anencephalic infants."[41]

Why do these protocols strike many commentators as contrived and even somewhat bizarre? The motives of the individuals involved are certainly commendable: they want to offer the benefits of transplantable organs to individuals who desperately need them. In addition, they are seeking to obtain organs only from individuals who cannot be harmed by the procurement and only in those situations where the patient or a surrogate requests the donation. The problem with these protocols lies not with the motive, but with the method and justification. By manipulating both the process and the definition of death, these protocols give the appearance that the physicians involved are only too willing to draw the boundary between life and death wherever it happens to maximize the chances for organ procurement.

How can the legitimate desire to increase the supply of transplantable organs be reconciled with the need to maintain a clear and simple distinction between the living and the dead? One way would be to abandon the requirement for the death of the donor prior to organ procurement and, instead, focus upon alternative and perhaps more fundamental ethical criteria to constrain the procurement of organs, such as the principles of consent and nonmaleficence.[42]

For example, policies could be changed such that organ procurement would be permitted only with the consent of the donor or appropriate surrogate and only when doing so would not harm the donor. Individuals who could not be harmed by the procedure would include those who are permanently and irreversibly unconscious (patients in a persistent vegetative state or newborns with anencephaly) and those who are imminently and irreversibly dying.

The American Medical Association's Council on Ethical and Judicial Affairs recently proposed (but has subsequently retracted) a position consistent with this approach.[43] The council stated that, "It is ethically permissible to consider the anencephalic as a potential organ donor, although still alive under the current definition of death," if, among other requirements, the diagnosis is certain and the parents give their permission. The council concluded, "It is normally required that the donor be legally dead before removal of their life-necessary organs ... The use of the anencephalic neonate as a live donor is a limited exception to the general standard because of the fact that the infant has never experienced, and will never experience, consciousness" (pp. 1617–18).

This alternative approach to organ procurement would require substantial changes in the law. The process of organ procurement would have to be legitimated as a form of justified killing, rather than just as the dissection of a corpse. There is certainly precedent in the law for recognizing instances of justified killing. The concept is also not an anathema to the public, as evidenced by the growing support for euthanasia, another practice that would have to be legally construed as a form of justified killing. Even now, surveys show that one-third of physicians and nurses do not believe brain-dead patients are actually dead, but feel comfortable with the process of organ procurement because the patients are permanently unconscious and/or imminently dying.[44] In other words, many clinicians already seem to justify their actions on the basis of nonmaleficence and consent, rather than with the belief that the patients are actually dead.

This alternative approach would also eliminate the need for protocols like the one being used at the University of Pittsburgh, with its contrived and perhaps questionable approach to declaring death prior to organ procurement. Under the proposed system, qualified individuals who had given their consent could simply have their organs removed under general anesthesia, without first undergoing an orchestrated withdrawal of life support. Anencephalic newborns whose parents requested organ donation could likewise have the organs removed under general anesthesia, without the need to wait for the diagnosis of brain death.

The diagnosis of death. Seen in this light, the concept of brain death may have become obsolete. Certainly the diagnosis of brain death has been extremely useful during the last several decades, as society has struggled with a myriad of issues that were never encountered before the era of mechanical ventilation and organ transplantation. As society emerges from this transitional period, and as many of these issues are more clearly understood as questions that are inherently unrelated to the distinction between life and death, then the concept of brain death may no longer be useful or relevant. If this is the case, then it may be preferable to return to the traditional standard and limit tests for the determination of death to those based solely upon the permanent cessation of respiration and circulation. Even today we uniformly regard the cessation of respiration and circulation as the standard for determining when patients are ready to be cremated or buried.

Another advantage of a return to the traditional approach is that it would represent a "common denominator" in the definition of death that virtually all cultural groups and religious traditions would find acceptable.[45] Recently both New Jersey and New York have enacted statutes that recognize the objections of particular religious views to the concept of brain death. In New Jersey, physicians are prohibited from declaring brain death in persons who come from religious traditions that do not accept the concept.[46] Return to a cardiorespiratory standard would eliminate problems with these objections.

Linda Emanuel recently proposed a "bounded zone" definition of death that shares some features with the approach outlined here.[47] Her proposal would adopt the cardiorespiratory standard as a "lower bound" for determining death that would apply to all cases, but would allow individuals to choose a definition of death that encompassed neurologic dysfunction up to the level of the permanent vegetative state (the "higher bound"). The practical implications of such a policy would be similar to some of those discussed here, in that it would (1) allow patients and surrogates to request organ donation when and if the patients were diagnosed with whole-brain death, permanent vegetative state, or anencephaly, and (2) it would permit rejection of the diagnosis of brain death by patients and surrogates opposed to the concept. Emanuel's proposal would not permit organ donation from terminal and imminently dying patients, however, prior to the diagnosis of death.

Despite these similarities, these two proposals differ markedly in the justifications used to support their conclusions. Emanuel follows the President's Commission in seeking to address several separate questions by reference to the diagnosis of death, whereas the approach suggested here would adopt a single and uniform definition of death, and then seek to resolve questions around organ donation on a different ethical and legal foundation.

Emanuel's proposal also provides another illustration of the problems encountered when a variety of diverse issues all hinge upon the definition of death. Under her scheme, some individuals would undoubtedly opt for a definition of death based on the "higher bound" of the permanent vegetative state in order to permit the donation of their vital organs if they should develop this condition. However, few of these individuals would probably agree to being cremated while still breathing, even if they were vegetative. Most likely, they would not want to be cremated until after they had sustained a cardiorespiratory arrest. Once again, this creates the awkward and confusing necessity of diagnosing death for one purpose (organ donation) but not for another (cremation). Only by abandoning the concept of brain death is it possible to adopt a definition of death that is valid for all purposes, while separating questions of organ donation from dependence upon the life/death dichotomy.

TURNING BACK

The tension between the need to maintain workable and practical standards for the procurement of transplantable organs and our desire to have a conceptually coherent account of death is an issue that must be given serious attention. Resolving these inconsistencies by moving toward a higher-brain definition of death would most likely create additional practical problems regarding accurate diagnosis as well as introduce concepts that are highly counterintuitive to the general public. Uncoupling the link between organ transplantation and brain death, on the other hand, offers a number of advantages. By shifting the ethical foundations for organ donation to the principles of nonmaleficence and consent, the pool of potential donors may be substantially increased. In addition, by reverting to a simpler and more traditional definition of death, the long-standing debate over fundamental inconsistencies in the concept of brain death may finally be resolved.

The most difficult challenge for this proposal would be to gain acceptance of the view that killing may sometimes be a justifiable necessity for procuring transplantable organs. Careful attention to the principles of consent and nonmaleficence should provide an adequate bulwark against slippery slope concerns that this practice would be extended in unforeseen and unacceptable ways. Just as the euthanasia debate often seems to turn less upon abstract theoretical concerns and more upon the empirical question of whether guidelines for assisted dying would be abused, so

the success of this proposal could also rest upon factual questions of societal acceptance and whether this approach would erode respect for human life and the integrity of clinicians. While the answers to these questions are not known, the potential benefits of this proposal make it worthy of continued discussion and debate.

Acknowledgments

The author thanks numerous friends and colleagues for critical readings of the manuscript, with special acknowledgments to Dan Wikler and Linda Emanuel.

Notes

1. Some of the more notable critiques include Robert M. Veatch, "The Whole Brain-Oriented Concept of Death. An Outmoded Philosophical Formulation," *Journal of Thanatology* 3 (1975): 13–30; Michael B. Green and Daniel Wikler, "Brain Death and Personal Identity," *Philosophy and Public Affairs* 9 (1980): 105–33; Stuart J. Youngner and Edward T. Bartlett, "Human Death and High Technology: The Failure of the Whole-Brain Formulations," *Annals of Internal Medicine* 99 (1983): 25258; Amir Halevy and Baruch Brody, "Brain Death: Reconciling Definitions, Criteria, and Tests," *Annals of Internal Medicine* 119 (1993): 519–25.

2. Stuart J. Youngner, "Defining Death: A Superficial and Fragile Consensus," *Archives of Neurology* 49 (1992): 570–72.

3. President's Commission for the Study of Ethical Problems in Medicine and Biomedical and Behavioral Research, *Defining Death* (Washington, D.C.: Government Printing Office, 1981).

4. Karen Gervais has been especially articulate in defining these levels. See Karen G. Gervais, *Redefining Death* (New Haven: Yale University Press, 1986); "Advancing the Definition of Death: A Philosophical Essay," *Medical Humanities Review* 3, no. 2 (1989): 7–19.

5. James L. Bernat, Charles M. Culver, and Bernard Gert, "On the Definition and Criterion of Death," *Annals of Internal Medicine* 94 (1981): 389–94; James L. Bernat, "How Much of the Brain Must Die in Brain Death?" *Journal of Clinical Ethics* 3 (1992): 21–26.

6. Report of the Medical Consultants on the Diagnosis of Death, "Guidelines for the Determination of Death," *JAMA* 246 (1981): 2184–86.

7. Aspects of this analysis have been explored previously in Robert D. Truog and James C. Fackler, "Rethinking Brain Death," *Critical Care Medicine* 20 (1992): 1705–13; Halevy and Brody, "Brain Death."

8. H. Schrader et al., "Changes of Pituitary Hormones in Brain Death," *Acta Neurochirurgica* 52 (1980): 239–48; Kristen M. Outwater and Mark A. Rockoff, "Diabetes Insipidus Accompanying Brain Death in Children," *Neurology* 34 (1984): 1243–46; James C. Fackler, Juan C. Troncoso, and Frank R. Gioia, "Age-Specific Characteristics of Brain Death in Children," *American Journal of Diseases of Childhood* 142 (1988): 999–1003.

9. Schrader et al., "Changes of Pituitary Hormones in Brain Death"; H. J. Gramm et al., "Acute Endocrine Failure after Brain Death," *Transplantation* 54 (1992): 851–57.

10. Report of Medical Consultants on the Diagnosis of Death, "Guidelines for the Determination of Death," p. 339.

11. Madeleine M. Grigg et al., "Electroencephalographic Activity after Brain Death," *Archives of Neurology* 44 (1987): 948–54; A. Earl Walker, *Cerebral Death,* 2nd ed. (Baltimore: Urban & Schwarzenberg, 1981), pp. 89-90; and Christopher Pallis, "ABC of Brain Stem Death. The Arguments about the EEG," *British Medical Journal [Clinical Research]* 286 (1983): 284–87.

12. Ernst Rodin et al., "Brainstem Death," *Clinical Electroencephalography* 16 (1985): 63–71.

13. Randall C. Wetzel et al., "Hemodynamic Responses in Brain Dead Organ Donor Patients," *Anesthesia and Analgesia* 64 (1985): 125–28; S. H. Pennefather, J. H. Dark, and R. E. Bullock, "Haemodynamic Responses to Surgery in Brain-Dead Organ Donors," *Anaesthesia* 48 (1993): 1034–38; and D. J. Hill, R. Munglani, and D. Sapsford, "Haemodynamic Responses to Surgery in Brain-Dead Organ Donors," *Anaesthesia* 49 (1994): 835–36.

14. Bernat, "How Much of the Brain Must Die in Brain Death?"

15. Paul A Byrne, Sean O'Reilly, and Paul M. Quay, "Brain Death—An Opposing Viewpoint," *JAMA* 242 (1979): 1985–90.

16. Gaetano F. Molinari, "The NINCDS Collaborative Study of Brain Death: A Historical Perspective," in U.S. Department of Health and Human Services, NINCDS monograph No. 24. NIH publication No. 81-2286 (1980): 1–32.

17. Pallis, "ABC of Brain Stem Death," pp. 123–24; Bryan Jennett and Catherine Hessett, "Brain Death in Britain as Reflected in Renal Donors," *British Medical Journal* 283 (1981): 359–62; Peter M. Black, "Brain Death (first of two parts)," *NEJM* 299 (1978): 338–44.

18. President's Commission, *Defining Death.*

19. "An Appraisal of the Criteria of Cerebral Death, A Summary Statement: A Collaborative Study," *JAMA* 237 (1977): 982–86.

20. Green and Wikler, "Brain Death and Personal Identity."

21. President's Commission, *Defining Death.*

22. Green and Wikler, "Brain Death and Personal Identity"; Daniel Wikler, "Brain Death: A Durable Consensus?" *Bioethics* 7 (1993): 239–46.

23. David R. Field et al., "Maternal Brain Death During Pregnancy: Medical and Ethical issues," *JAMA* 260 (1988): 816–22; Masanobu Washida et al., "Beneficial Effect of Combined 3,5,3'-Triiodothyronine and Vasopressin Administration on Hepatic Energy Status and Systemic Hemodynamics after Brain Death," *Transplantation* 54 (1992): 44–49.

24. Stuart J. Youngner et al., "'Brain Death' and Organ Retrieval: A Cross-Sectional Survey of Knowledge and Concepts among Health Professionals," *JAMA* 261 (1989): 2205–10.

25. Daniel Wikler and Alan J. Weisbard, "Appropriate Confusion over 'Brain Death,'" *JAMA* 261 (1989): 2246.

26. Margareta Sanner, "A Comparison of Public Attitudes toward Autopsy Organ Donation, and Anatomic Dissection: A Swedish Survey," *JAMA* 271 (1994): 284–88, at 287.

27. Green and Wikler, "Brain Death and Personal Identity."

28. Robert M. Arnold and Stuart J. Youngner, "The Dead Donor Rule: Should We Stretch It, Bend It, or Abandon It?" *Kennedy Institute of Ethics Journal* 3 (1993): 263–78.

29. Some of the many works defending this view include: Green and Wikler, "Brain Death and Personal Identity"; Gervais, *Redefining Death*; Truog and Fackler, "Rethinking Brain Death"; and Robert M. Veatch, *Death, Dying, and the Biological Revolution* (New Haven: Yale University Press, 1989).

30. The Multi-Society Task Force on PVS, "Medical Aspects of the Persistent Vegetative State," *NEJM* 330 (1994): 1499–1508 and 1572–79; D. Alan Shewmon, "Anencephaly: Selected Medical Aspects," *Hastings Center Report* 18, no. 5 (1988): 11–19.

31. Nancy L. Childs and Walt N. Mercer, "Brief Report: Late Improvement in Consciousness after

Post-Traumatic Vegetative State," *NEJM* 334 (1996): 24–25; James L. Bernat, "The Boundaries of the Persistent Vegetative State," *Journal of Clinical Ethics* 3 (1992): 176–80.

32. Medical Task Force on Anencephaly, "The Infant with Anencephaly," *NEJM* 322 (1990): 669–74; Shewmon, "Anencephaly: Selected Medical Aspects."

33. Jeffrey R Botkin and Stephen G. Post, "Confusion in the Determination of Death: Distinguishing Philosophy from Physiology," *Perspectives in Biology and Medicine* 36 (1993): 129–38.

34. The Multi-Society Task Force on PVS, "Medical Aspects of the Persistent Vegetative State."

35. Marcia Angell, "After Quinlan: The Dilemma of the Persistent Vegetative State," *NEJM* 330 (1994): 1524–25.

36. Wikler, "Brain Death: A Durable Consensus?"

37. President's Commission, *Defining Death,* p. 84.

38. Report of the Ad Hoc Committee of the Harvard Medical School to Examine the Definition of Brain Death, "A Definition of Irreversible Coma," *JAMA* 205 (1968): 337–40.

39. "University of Pittsburgh Medical Center Policy and Procedure Manual: Management of Terminally Ill Patients Who May Become Organ Donors after Death," *Kennedy Institute of Ethics Journal* 3 (1993): A1–A15; Stuart Youngner and Robert Arnold, "Ethical, Psychosocial, and Public Policy Implications of Procuring Organs from Non-Heart-Beating Cadaver Donors," *JAMA* 269 (1993): 2769–74. Of note, the June 1993 issue of the *Kennedy Institute of Ethics Journal* is devoted to this topic in its entirety.

40. Joanne Lynn, "Are the Patients Who Become Organ Donors Under the Pittsburgh Protocol for 'Non-Heart-Beating Donors' Really Dead?"

Kennedy Institute of Ethics Journal 3 (1993): 167–78.

41. Joyce L. Peabody, Janet R. Emery, and Stephen Ashwal, "Experience with Anencephalic Infants as Prospective Organ Donors," *NEJM* 321 (1989): 344–50.

42. See for example, Norman Fost, "The New Body Snatchers: On Scott's 'The Body as Property,' " *American Bar Foundation Research Journal* 3 (1983): 718-32; John A. Robertson, "Relaxing the Death Standard for Organ Donation in Pediatric Situations," in *Organ Substitution Technology: Ethical, Legal, and Public Policy Issues,* ed. D. Mathieu (Boulder, Col.: Westview Press, 1988), pp. 69–76; Arnold and Youngner, "The Dead Donor Rule."

43. AMA Council on Ethical and Judicial Affairs, "The Use of Anencephalic Neonates as Organ Donors," *JAMA* 273 (1995): 1614–18. After extensive debate among AMA members, the Council retracted this position statement. See Charles W. Plows, "Reconsideration of AMA Opinion on Anencephalic Neonates as Organ Donors," *JAMA* 275 (1996): 443–44.

44. Youngner et al., "'Brain Death' and Organ Retrieval."

45. Jiro Nudeshima, "Obstacles to Brain Death and Organ Transplantation in Japan," *Lancet* 338 (1991): 1063–64.

46. Robert S. Olick, "Brain Death, Religious Freedom, and Public Policy: New Jersey's Landmark Legislative Initiative," *Kennedy Institute of Ethics Journal* 1 (1991): 275–88.

47. Linda L. Emanuel, "Reexamining Death: The Asymptotic Model and a Bounded Zone Definition," *Hastings Center Report* 25, no. 4 (1995): 27–35.

Malette v. Shulman (1987), 72 O.R. (2d) 417 (C.A.)

Summary prepared by Lisa Shields

The plaintiff, Mrs. Malette, was seriously injured in an automobile accident. She arrived at the hospital unconscious. The attending emergency room physician, Dr. Shulman, diagnosed Mrs. Malette as suffering from shock and severe blood loss requiring a transfusion of blood. Without the transfusion, Dr. Shulman did not think that Mrs. Malette would survive.

Before any blood was administered, a nurse discovered a card in Mrs. Malette's purse that stated that she did not consent to blood transfusions under any circumstances because of her religious beliefs as a Jehovah's Witness and that she understood the consequences of this refusal. Despite being made aware of the existence of this card by the nurse, Dr. Shulman proceeded to administer blood transfusions to Mrs. Malette. He felt that his decision was appropriate given the necessity of the blood transfusions and his duty as a physician to provide the best possible care to his patient. Dr. Shulman also had reservations about withholding blood transfusions because the signature on the card was neither witnessed nor dated. These factors led Dr. Shulman to consider the possibility that Mrs. Malette's wishes may have changed since she had signed the card and to question whether Mrs. Malette had received sufficient information on the effects of a decision to refuse all blood transfusions so as to constitute an informed refusal of a necessary medical treatment.

Mrs. Malette recovered from her injuries and brought an action against Dr. Shulman, the attending nurses, the hospital where the transfusions took place, and its executive director for negligence, assault, and battery. The Court found no wrongdoing on the part of the nurses, the hospital, or its executive director. Furthermore, the Court determined that Dr. Shulman's diagnosis and treatment had been in accordance with the requisite standard of care and as such there was no negligence in his medical treatment of Mrs. Malette. The treatment, specifically the blood transfusions, may well have been responsible for saving Mrs. Malette's life.

Nonetheless, the Court found that Dr. Shulman had committed the tort of battery by administering medical treatment to Mrs. Malette without her consent. Mrs. Malette was awarded $20,000 in damages.

According to the Court, all medical treatment requires informed consent from the patient (or a surrogate decision-maker). This requirement recognizes the fundamental principle of the right of a person to control his or her own body. Without informed consent, medical treatment is intentional, non-consensual touching of a person's body, or battery. The only exception to the informed consent rule is in an emergency situation when consent is not practicable. In that context, under the doctrine of necessity, a physician may proceed with appropriate medical treatment without the consent of the patient. Although this case involved an emergency medical situation, the patient had already expressed her wishes regarding the specific treatment through the use of the Jehovah's Witness card. The physician had no legitimate reason to doubt that the card was an accurate, current reflection of Mrs. Malette's wishes. Furthermore, Dr. Shulman had no reason to believe that Mrs. Malette did not understand the consequences of her decision or that her beliefs would be any different in a situation where a blood transfusion was required to save her life. If there had been any reason to doubt the validity of the card, Dr. Shulman would have been justified in proceeding with the administration of the blood transfusions.

Although the state has an interest in preserving the lives and health of its citizens, the Court found, the right of an adult to refuse medically necessary treatment prevails. In this case, Mrs. Malette had chosen an appropriate method for ensuring that her wishes would be known if she was ever to be in an emergency situation where she could not otherwise express her refusal. Dr. Shulman should not have given her the transfusion.

Fleming v. Reid (1991), 4 O.R. (3d) 74 (C.A.)

Summary prepared by Fiona McDonald

George Reid and Kenneth Gallagher were found not guilty of criminal offences by reason of insanity (both had schizophrenia) and were confined as involuntary patients in a psychiatric facility.

Although Mr. Reid and Mr. Gallagher were detained in a psychiatric hospital through criminal justice processes, Ontario's *Mental Health Act 1980* granted them the same rights as other involuntary patients. Involuntary patients have the right to refuse treatment and, if an involuntary patient is considered incompetent to make decisions about care, then a substitute decision-maker makes decisions for them, guided by the patient's past competent decisions.

In September 1987, Dr. Fleming formed the view that the severity of Mr. Reid's illness meant that he was not competent to give or withhold consent to psychiatric treatment which, in Dr. Fleming's opinion, would improve his deteriorating condition. Dr. Fleming reached a similar conclusion with regard to Mr. Gallagher in the spring of 1988.

Dr. Fleming wanted to treat Mr. Reid and Mr. Gallagher with neuroleptic drugs that are commonly used to treat mental disorders, such as schizophrenia. Mr. Reid and Mr. Gallagher had previously taken neuroleptic drugs and believed that these drugs were non-beneficial and possibly harmful. They had both previously refused to take neuroleptic drugs. As they were judged not competent to make treatment decisions, their substitute decision-maker was asked to give consent. The substitute decision-maker refused consent because Mr. Reid and Mr. Gallagher had previously (when competent) refused neuroleptic drugs.

Dr. Fleming asked the Psychiatric Review Board to overturn this refusal and authorize him to treat Mr. Reid and Mr. Gallagher with neuroleptic drugs. The Ontario *Mental Health Act 1980* allows a Psychiatric Review Board to authorize the attending physician to administer treatment to an involuntary incompetent psychiatric patient, despite the substitute decision-maker's refusal to consent even where the refusal is based on the patient's prior competent refusal of the proposed treatment. The Board granted an order authorizing Dr. Fleming to administer neuroleptic drugs to Mr. Reid and Mr. Gallagher.

Mr. Reid and Mr. Gallagher sought a court order declaring that the *Mental Health Act* deprived them, and others in the same circumstances, of their right to security of the person guaranteed by section 7 of the *Charter of Rights and Freedoms* and asked the court to overturn the Board's order. Section 7 of the *Charter of Rights and Freedoms* guarantees everyone the right to life, liberty, and security of the person and the right not to be deprived of that right except in accordance with the principles of fundamental justice.

The Ontario Court of Appeal noted that neuroleptic drugs are generally effective as they act to alleviate the symptoms of the disorder but that the drugs do not work in every case. The Court also noted that neuroleptic drugs carry the risk of a number of serious and unpredictable side effects, both short and long term.

The Court noted that the right to determine what shall or shall not be done to one's own body and to be free from non-consensual medical treatment is deeply rooted in law. The patient ultimately must decide if treatment is to be administered. The fact that the patient's decision to refuse treatment may result in serious risks or consequences for the patient does not remove the patient's rights. The patient may specify in advance the patient's refusal of a particular treatment for a time when the patient is unable to make this decision. The doctor is not able to disregard such an advance directive, even in an emergency. These rights extend to patients in psychiatric facilities, whether the patient is a voluntary or involuntary patient, as, although ill, the patient may be competent to make decisions about medical care or may have been competent to make decisions in the past.

The Court stated that the right to bodily integrity and personal autonomy is so entrenched in the traditions of the law as to be ranked as fundamental and deserving of the highest protection. It stated that few medical procedures can be more intrusive than the forcible injection of powerful mind-altering drugs, which may result in severe and sometimes irreversible side effects. The Court concluded that to deprive involuntary patients of any right to make an advance directive about treatment and to force them to be treated despite their previously expressed competent wishes and without the consent of their substitute decision-maker infringes *Charter* rights to the security of the person.

The Court said that the state's power to care for those unable to care for themselves is not intended to be used by the state to overrule a treatment decision made by a competent patient, regardless of whether the patient's decision is considered not to be in the patient's best interests. Nor can it be used to authorize the medical treatment of an incompetent patient, who, while competent, had made an advance directive refusing to consent to a particular form of treatment. The Court stated that after creating a substitute decision-making system to recognize the prior competent wishes of incompetent patients and to ensure that those wishes are respected, the Act then proceeds to render those wishes, and the substitute decision-maker's decision based on those wishes, meaningless, by allowing the Review Board to overrule that decision. The Court concluded that this is contrary to the principles of fundamental justice and said that, while the right to be free from non-consensual psychiatric treatment is not absolute, the state needs to demonstrate a reason to remove patients' rights, in their "best interests," without hearing or review in contravention of their expressed wishes. The Court declared that the challenged sections of Ontario's *Mental Health Act* were inoperative and granted an order that Mr. Reid and Mr. Gallagher should not be given neuroleptic drugs.

B. (N.) v. Hotel-Dieu de Québec (1992), 86 D.L.R. (4th) 385 (C.S.)

Summary prepared by Fiona McDonald

Nancy B. became ill in June 1989. She was admitted to the Hotel-Dieu de Québec, diagnosed with Guillian-Barré syndrome, intubated, and placed on a respirator. Guillian-Barré syndrome causes ascending motor paralysis but the patient's intellectual faculties remain intact. In December 1990, the hospital's chief neurologist reported that Nancy B.'s motor nerves had degenerated to a point that bordered on complete denervation and allowed her little, or no, ability to move. In January 1991, Nancy B was advised that her condition was irreversible. By this time respiratory support was essential to keep Nancy B. alive, as she was unable to breathe without mechanical assistance since her respiratory muscles had atrophied. Respiratory support had already prolonged her life well beyond her estimated life expectancy if it had not been available. If the respirator was removed or failed, Nancy B. would die very shortly afterwards.

Nancy B. decided that she wanted the respirator to be removed to allow her irreversible disease to take its course. She was aware that she would die shortly after the respirator was removed. Nancy B. discussed her decision with a number of doctors. Nancy B.'s mental competence was assessed by a psychiatrist, who concluded that she was in good mental health and was able to make and understand the consequences of her decisions.

Nancy B. withdrew her consent to continuing with respiratory support and sought an injunction from the Court to require the hospital and her doctor to remove the respirator, as she was in no physical condition to remove it herself.

The judge noted that, following the *Civil Code of Quebec*, a patient's consent must be freely given and must be informed. Article 19.1 of the *Code* states that "no person may be made to undergo care of any nature, whether for examination, specimen taking, removal of tissue, treatment or any other act, except with his consent."

The judge decided that respiratory support is a life-sustaining technique and that the definition of treatment in the *Civil Code* could include a third person placing a respirator on a patient.

The judge said that the logical corollary of the right to consent is the right not to consent—to refuse treatment or to stop treatment when it has begun. Putting a patient on a respirator and constantly keeping the patient on it without the patient's consent constitutes intrusion and interference that violates the patient's person. The judge determined that Nancy B. was competent to make autonomous choices about treatment. She had withdrawn her consent to the use of the respirator and requested that it be removed and her decision was freely given and informed. Therefore Nancy B. was entitled to have her personal autonomy and her right to self-determination respected and the respirator removed as she requested.

Nancy B. needed assistance to remove the respirator as she could not do it herself. The judge stated that a person who removed a respirator at the patient's request, in the circumstances of this case, would not be vulnerable to criminal prosecution or sanction, as that person was allowing a disease to take its natural course (providing for a natural death), rather than assisting the patient to commit suicide or intentionally killing the patient.

Rodriguez v. British Columbia (Attorney General), [1993] 3 S.C.R. 519

Summary prepared by Josephine Johnston

At the time of her appeal to the Supreme Court of Canada, Sue Rodriguez was a 42-year-old woman living in British Columbia. She had been diagnosed with amyotrophic lateral sclerosis, also known as Lou Gehrig's disease. As a result of this disease, Ms. Rodriguez's health was rapidly deteriorating such that she would soon be unable to swallow, speak, walk, or move without assistance. She would eventually lose the ability to breathe without a respirator or eat without a surgically placed feeding tube. She knew that she would soon die (at the time of appeal, her life expectancy was estimated at between 2 and 14 months). Ms. Rodriguez did not wish to die while she could still enjoy her life. However, she wanted the option of ending her life at a time of her choosing and with the aid of a physician before she died naturally. To this end, she went to court to challenge the *Criminal Code* prohibition on assisted suicide.

Section 241(b) of the *Criminal Code* states that every person who "aids or abets a person to commit suicide" is guilty of an offence and liable for 14 years imprisonment. Under the section, any physician who set up technological means by which Ms. Rodriguez could end her life, if and when she chose to, would be guilty of aiding her to commit suicide. In light of this potential criminal liability, Ms. Rodriguez sought an order declaring section 241(b) of the *Criminal Code* invalid on the ground that it breached the *Canadian Charter of Rights and Freedoms*. Specifically, she argued that the criminal prohibition infringed her section 7 right to "life, liberty and security of the person," her section 12 right "not to be subjected to cruel and unusual treatment," and her section 15 rights to be "equal before and under the law" and to "the

equal protection and equal benefit of the law without discrimination." She further argued that section 241(b) of the *Code* was not saved by section 1 of the *Charter* because infringement of these rights was not "demonstrably justified in a free and democratic society."

The Supreme Court of Canada dismissed Ms. Rodriguez's appeal by a five to four majority. The majority judgment, delivered by Justice Sopinka, stated that even though section 241(b) of the *Code* had the effect of impinging Ms. Rodriguez's *Charter* rights, such infringement was either in accordance with the principles of fundamental justice or could be excused under section 1 of the *Charter*.

Justice Sopinka began by defining the section 7 right to security of the person to include "control over one's bodily integrity free from state interference." He found that the prohibition on assisted suicide deprived Ms. Rodriguez of autonomy over her person, as well as causing her physical pain and psychological distress. However, section 7 rights can be limited so long as the limits are in accordance with the principles of fundamental justice. In assessing the principles of fundamental justice, Justice Sopinka considered the history of Canada's legislative and social policy in the area of suicide and assisted suicide. He noted the lack of a successful movement to decriminalize assisted suicide, the reluctance of the English House of Lords and the Law Commission of Canada to condone deliberate acts to cut short the life of terminally ill patients, and the predominance among Western democracies of legislative provisions similar to section 241(b) prohibiting assisting suicide. In particular, he noted that, despite a recognition of the suffering caused by a blanket ban on assisted suicide, such a ban appeared to be preferable to a law that may not adequately prevent abuse. In light of this consensus, Justice Sopinka did not feel able to conclude that any fundamental aspects of justice were violated, even though Ms. Rodriguez's right to security of the person was infringed.

In dismissing Ms. Rodriguez's claim under section 12 of the *Charter*, Justice Sopinka found that the ban on assisting suicide did not amount to "cruel and unusual treatment or punishment." Although he accepted that "treatment" in section 12 may refer to actions by the state outside the penal or quasi-penal context, he did not accept that a mere prohibition on certain action could constitute treatment at the hands of the state. He held that there must be a more active state process, involving an exercise of state action, before the state's control can come within section 12.

Finally, Justice Sopinka dismissed Ms. Rodriguez's section 15 *Charter* claim without considering whether section 241(b) of the *Code* was discriminatory. Regardless of whether section 15 was breached in this case, he felt that any breach would be saved by section 1 of the *Charter* because any breach could be "demonstrably justified in a free and democratic society." The Justice's reasons were similar to those he gave when considering the issue of fundamental justice in his section 7 analysis. That is, that the government had both a pressing and substantial reason for legislating against assisting suicide (the preservation of the sanctity of life) and a reasonable basis for concluding that the prohibition on assisted suicide minimally impaired the rights of Canadians.

> This protection is grounded on a substantial consensus … that in order to effectively protect life and those who are vulnerable in society, a prohibition without exception on the giving of assistance to commit suicide is the best approach. Attempts to fine tune this approach by creating exceptions have been unsatisfactory and have tended to support the theory of the "slippery slope." The formulation of safeguards to prevent excesses has been unsatisfactory and has failed to allay fears that a relaxation of the clear standard set by the law will undermine the protection of life and will lead to abuses of the exception.

Three separate dissenting judgments were delivered, each allowing the appeal on slightly different grounds. Chief Justice Lamer found that section 241(b) of the *Code* infringed section 15(1) of the *Charter*. He stated that unlike able-bodied individuals, some people with physical disabilities are, or would become, unable to end their lives without the assistance of others. The criminal prohibition against assisting suicide deprived these persons with disabilities of choosing suicide, an option available to the remainder of Canadians. The Chief Justice held that this deprivation was discriminatory because it created an inequality based on "physical disability," a personal characteristic listed in section 15.

He further held that this discrimination was not justifiable under section 1 of the *Charter*. With the abolition of the crime of attempted suicide, self-determination had become the paramount factor in state regulation of suicide. Despite accepting that the purpose of the section 241 crime was to protect persons who may be vulnerable to the influence of others when deciding whether to terminate their lives, he found that the section overreached this purpose when it arbitrarily robbed some physically disabled individuals of the self-determination available to other people. He was not persuaded by the respondents' arguments that decriminalizing assisted suicide could lead to persons with disabilities being manipulated by others (a so-called slippery slope argument), or that it was not possible to design legislation to protect persons against abuse while still allowing assisted suicide in some cases.

The Chief Justice suggested a declaration that section 241(b) of the *Criminal Code* was of no force or effect, with such declaration being suspended for one year to allow Parliament to address the issue. In view of the one-year suspension, he declared that a personal remedy should be made available to Ms. Rodriguez, whereby a constitutional exemption would be made to allow a physician to help her commit suicide without fear of criminal prosecution. The exemption would be subject to a number of conditions, including that Ms. Rodriquez be certified competent by a treating physician and an independent psychiatrist at the time arrangements were put in place to allow her to terminate her life, and that the act of causing death must be that of Ms. Rodriguez herself.

The other substantial dissenting judgment was delivered by Justice McLachlin (as she then was) on behalf of herself and Justice L'Hereux-Dubé. Justice McLachlin thought that the case was not at heart about discrimination, but rather about the manner and extent of the state's interference with Ms. Rodriguez's decisions about her body. Like the majority, she agreed that section 241(b) of the *Criminal Code* infringed the section 7 *Charter* right to security of the person. However, Justice McLachlin found that the infringement was not in accordance with principles of fundamental justice, and that it was not "demonstrably necessary in a free and democratic society" under section 1 of the *Charter*.

Citing the majority judgment in *R v. Morgentaler*, Justice McLachlin concluded that the prohibition on assisting suicide had the effect of preventing Ms. Rodriguez from dealing with her body as she would have chosen. Further, this prohibition was arbitrary. Parliament had not shown an absolute intention to protect the sanctity of human life, so sanctity-of-life arguments were of little assistance in justifying the prohibition. Also, the prohibition's legislative purpose of preventing the killing of disabled or vulnerable people, although practical and reasonable, disproportionately infringed on Ms. Rodriguez's right to security of the person. Justice McLachlin did not believe that "a law which infringes the principles of fundamental justice can be found to be reasonable and demonstrably justified on the sole ground that crimes other than those which it prohibits may become more frequent." She pointed to the laws against culpable homicide as adequate protection and ruled that this existing law, supplemented by the conditions of the constitutional exemption detailed by the Chief Justice, satisfied fears of false consent.

In his brief judgment Justice Cory expressed agreement with the reasoning given by the Chief Justice. In addition, he agreed with Justice McLachlin that section 241(b) of the *Criminal Code* was in contravention of section 7 of the *Charter* because it deprived Ms Rodriguez of security of the person by denying her the right to choose death.

R. v. Latimer, [2001] 1 S.C.R. 3

Summary prepared by Maegen Giltrow

On Sunday, October 24, 1993, while Tracy Latimer's mother and siblings were at church, her father, Robert Latimer, sat Tracy in the cab of his pickup truck and siphoned exhaust into the cab. Tracy died of carbon monoxide poisoning. Mr. Latimer was found guilty at trial and on appeal of the second degree murder of his 12-year-old daughter. Despite the mandatory minimum sentence of 10 years before eligibility for parole, at trial the jury suggested a period of one year before parole eligibility in Mr. Latimer's case. The trial judge granted Mr. Latimer a constitutional exemption to the mandatory minimum sentence, sentencing him to one year in prison, with one year of parole. On appeal the mandatory minimum sentence for second degree murder of life imprisonment with no eligibility for parole for ten years was imposed.

Tracy had suffered a severe form of cerebral palsy; she was quadriplegic and immobile. She was said to have the mental capacity of a four-month-old baby, with the concomitant ability to communicate through facial expressions, laughter, and crying. She suffered five to six seizures daily, and it was thought that she experienced a great deal of pain. The pain could not be reduced through medication, as pain medication conflicted with her anti-epileptic medication, and because she had difficulty swallowing. The Latimers had rejected a feeding-tube option as being both intrusive, and as a first step toward preserving Tracy's life artificially.

Mr. Latimer made the decision to end Tracy's life when another in a long line of surgeries for Tracy had been scheduled. This one was to address her dislocated hip, and, it was hoped, to lessen her constant pain. The Latimers were told that the surgery, wherein Tracy's upper thighbone would be removed and her leg left connected only by soft tissue, would cause Tracy pain. They were also told that future surgery would be required in the future to relieve the pain Tracy felt in various joints of her body. Both of Tracy's parents felt that further surgery would be a mutilation of Tracy. Mr. Latimer concluded that Tracy's death was an alternative favourable to constant surgery and constant pain, the future that Tracy faced.

On appeal to the Supreme Court of Canada (SCC) were essentially three issues. First, had the trial judge erred in preventing the jury from considering the defence of necessity? Second, did the trial judge render Mr. Latimer's trial unfair because of trial procedures that might have lessened the chance of jury nullification? And finally, would the imposition of the mandatory minimum sentence for second degree murder constitute cruel and unusual punishment, contrary to section 12 of the *Charter*, in this particular case?

The SCC described the defence of necessity as one that rests upon a "realistic assessment of human weakness," that bestows upon the accused in some circumstances not praise, but pardon. The SCC emphasized however, that this defence is a strict and narrow one, restricted to cases of true involuntariness. The SCC found

that the trial judge was right to prevent the jury from considering the defence—that there was no "air of reality" to the defence. While a defence can fail the "air of reality" test if *any* component of the defence cannot be met by the facts, in this case, the SCC found that *none* of the components of the defence could be met on the facts.

Of particular note was the SCC's discussion surrounding the component of proportionality—that the harm avoided and the harm inflicted must, at a minimum, be of comparable gravity. The SCC held that this component of the defence must be measured on a purely objective basis, "since evaluating the gravity of the act is a matter of community standards infused with constitutional considerations (such as, in this case, the s. 15 equality rights of the disabled)," and not of the accused's perception of the harms at issue. While the SCC left open the question of whether a case of homicide could *ever* meet this proportionality requirement, it found that in this case, it certainly did not. Death was a harm far greater than the non–life-threatening pain Mr. Latimer sought to avoid on Tracy's behalf.

Just as the defence of necessity serves to pardon some guilty acts that are determined to be of a lower moral culpability, degrees of moral culpability are also inherent in sentencing. First, second degree murder is less morally culpable than first degree murder, and the minimum sentence for each crime reflects this. Second, beyond the minimum sentence, those whose circumstances mitigate their moral culpability can meet a parole eligibility requirement less severe that those without such mitigating factors. Mr. Latimer wanted to go beyond these inherent considerations of moral culpability in our law by seeking a constitutional exemption to the mandatory minimum sentence.

The SCC weighed the contextual factors in Mr. Latimer's case, and found the aggravating and mitigating factors to cancel each other out. Thus there was no basis for a constitutional exemption to the minimum sentence. It is interesting to note that one of the aggravating factors in Mr. Latimer's case was his lack of remorse. That is, his principled conviction that what he did for Tracy was the right thing in fact weakened his argument that, given his and Tracy's circumstances, he should be granted a constitutional exemption to the minimum sentence. The SCC held instead that the collective symbolic statement society makes denunciating murder through a mandatory minimum sentence is one that is of particular importance in the case of a vulnerable victim—for instance, in the case of a disabled victim. Tracy's disability was not, therefore, a mitigating factor, but rather an aggravating one in the sentencing of Mr. Latimer.

Finally, Mr. Latimer argued that, whatever our law is, and however his actions are culpable and unpardonable in law, the jury should not be undermined by trial procedures in its power to decide simply not to apply the law to his case.

The SCC recognizes jury nullification as "the citizen's ultimate protection against oppressive laws and the oppressive enforcement of the law," and that it is a "safety valve" for exceptional cases. The SCC found, however, that while it should be recognized that nullification happens, it is not a legal process to be encouraged or even supported by the courts. That is, there is no constitutional right to a trial that does not undermine the power of the jury to nullify.

The SCC, however, recognized that there might be something different about Mr. Latimer's case, even if it wasn't a legal difference. It was in the recognition of this possibility that the SCC referred, at the end of its decision, to the executive's power to respond to any sentence it deems unjust through the royal prerogative of mercy.

Useful Resources in Bioethics

Romanow Report

The Commission on the Future of Health Care in Canada. *Building on Values: The Future of Health Care in Canada,* 2002.
http://www.hc-sc.gc.ca/english/care/romanow/index.html

Professional Groups' Codes of Ethics

Baylis F, Downie J, Dewhirst K (eds.). *Codes of Ethics: Ethics Codes, Standards and Guidelines for Professionals Working in a Health Care Setting in Canada.* 2nd ed. Toronto: Department of Bioethics, The Hospital for Sick Children, 1999, 192 pp.

Canadian Medical Association Code of Ethics

CMA policy on the rights and responsibilities of physicians and patients. CMA's comprehensive guide to ethical conduct and behavior for its members.
http://www.cma.ca/cma/common/displayPage.do?pageId=/staticContent/HTML/N0/l2/inside/policybase/1996/10-15.htm

Canadian Nurses Association Code of Ethics for Registered Nurses

Provides guidance and education for decision-making concerning ethical matters, also serves as a means for self-evaluation and reflection regarding ethical nursing practice.
http://www.cna-nurses.ca/pages/ethics/ethics.htm

ETHICS GUIDELINES FOR HEALTH RESEARCH

Tri-Council Policy Statement: Ethical Conduct for Research Involving Humans

Describes the standards and procedures for research involving humans adopted by the three major sources of Canadian federal funding for research: The Canadian Institutes of Health Research (CIHR), the Natural Sciences and Engineering Research Council (NSERC), and the Social Sciences and Humanities Research Council (SSHRC).
http://www.nserc.ca/programs/ethics/english/policy.htm

Human Pluripotent Stem Cell Research: Guidelines for CIHR-Funded Research

Canadian Institutes of Health Research developed this framework to ensure ethical and scientific oversight of publicly funded research. Addresses the following: Guiding Principles, oversight, review, funding, commercial interests, and ineligible research.
http://www.cihr-irsc.gc.ca/e/publications/1487.shtml#?

Protecting Human Research Subjects: Case-based Learning for Canadian Research Ethics Boards and Researchers

Baylis F, Ireland A, Kaufman D, Weijer C. *Protecting Human Research Subjects: Case-based Learning for Canadian Research Ethics Boards and Researchers.* Ottawa: National Council on Ethics in Human Research. 2000, 110pp.
Available from the National Council on Ethics in Human Research.
http://www.ncehr-cnerh.org/

The Belmont Report: Ethical Principles and Guidelines for the Protection of Human Subjects

Influential report of The (U.S.) National Commission for the Protection of Human Subjects of Biomedical and Behavioral Research (1979).
http://ohsr.od.nih.gov/mpa/belmont.php3

U.S. Code of Federal Regulations Title 45, Part 46 Protection of Human Subjects

Title 45, CFR, Part 46 Common Rule is federal human research subject protection policy, as mandated by the Executive Branch of the United States (revised as of October 1, 1999).
http://pw1.netcom.com/~alalli/BillSite_Documents/CommonRule.html

Council for International Organizations of Medical Sciences (CIOMS)

In coordination with the United Nations, CIOMS facilitates and promotes international activities in the field of biomedical sciences and serves the scientific interest of the biomedical community through initiating and coordinating long-term projects in the following fields: bioethics, health policy, ethics and human values, drug development and use, and international nomenclature of diseases.
http://www.cioms.ch/

International Ethical Guidelines for Biomedical Research Involving Human Subjects *(CIOMS)*

The 2002 CIOMS Guidelines are designed to be of use to countries in defining national policies on the ethics of biomedical research involving human subjects, applying ethical standards in local circumstances, and establishing or improving ethical review mechanisms. A particular aim is to reflect the conditions and the needs of low-resource countries, and the implications for multinational or transnational research in which they may be partners.
http://www.cioms.ch/frame_guidelines_nov_2002.htm

Declaration of Helsinki

The World Medical Association's statement intended to provide ethical guidance to physicians and other participants in medical research involving human subjects.
http://www.wma.net/e/policy/b3.htm

INTERNET RESOURCES

Bioethics Online

Brown R. *Bioethics Online: A Guide to Bioethical Resources on the Internet.* New York, Writers Club Press, 2002.

National Reference Center for Bioethics Literature: Bioethics Resources on the Web (Scope Note 38)

This page offers links to databases, electronic journals, full-text documents, news, and teaching resources in bioethics.
http://www.georgetown.edu/research/nrcbl/scopenotes/sn38.htm

PubMed

PubMed is a useful search engine that now includes *Bioethicsline.*
http://www.pubmedcentral.nih.gov/

Bioethics.net "What's Written?"

This site provides links to the Tables of Contents of most bioethics journals.
http://www.bioethics.net/wiw

BioethicsWeb

Wellcome Library, BioethicsWeb offers free access to a searchable catalogue of Internet sites and resources covering biomedical ethics.
http://bioethicsweb.ac.uk

Canadian Bioethics Society (CBS)

CBS has a number of useful links to Canadian bioethics resources.
http://www.bioethics.ca/

Canadian Institutes of Health Research Ethics Useful Links

The CIHR website's ethics section provides links divided into four categories: Guidelines for Health Research, Relevant Agencies and Organizations, Academic Bioethics and Health Law Centers/Institutes, and Bioethics Information Resources on the Web.
http://www.cihr-irsc.gc.ca/e/about/6427.shtml

University of Toronto Joint Centre for Bioethics: Bioethics Resources

This site provides a collection of full-text documents organized by topics such as child health, organizational ethics, research ethics, and global ethics.
http://www.utoronto.ca/jcb/Resources/resources.html

HumGen

The HumGen website provides a selective bibliography of literature related to ethics and policy issues in human genetics.
http://www.humgen.umontreal.ca/en/

American Society for Bioethics and Humanities Resource Links

ASBH has an extensive list of links divided into groups such as academic centers, organizations and networks, and government offices for science and technology.
http://www.asbh.org/resources/links/index.htm

U.S. National Institutes of Health Bioethics Resources on the Web

The brief annotations in this directory are divided into the five categories: Bioethics at NIH, General Resources, Organizations, Federal Bioethics Resources, and Specific Topics (Research Ethics, Genetics, and Medicine and Health Care).
http://www.nih.gov/sigs/bioethics

Bioethics Institute, Johns Hopkins University

The Phoebe R. Berman Bioethics Institute home page features a list of recent news stories in bioethics with links to electronic versions of these stories in the newspapers where they have been published. The citations and links for these articles are retained in the Archives section of the site.
http://www.med.jhu.edu/bioethics_institute/

The United Kingdom's Human Fertilisation and Embryology Authority (HFEA)

The HFEA was established by the passage of the Human Fertilisation and Emrbyology Act of 1990, among the first and most influential pieces of bioethics legislation. The site contains information about current Authority members as well as links to policy statements, public consultations, and the 1990 Act.
http://www.hfea.gov.uk

World Health Organization Links to Bioethics Resources on the Web

The WHO website's ethics section provides links divided into five categories: Collaborating Centres in Bioethics, United Nations Organizations, International Organizations, Regional and National Organizations, and Related Health Topics.
http://www.who.int/ethics/links/en/

ENCYCLOPEDIAS

Chadwick R (ed). *Encyclopedia of Applied Ethics* Four Volumes. New York: Academic Press, 1998.

Cooper D (ed). *Nature Encyclopedia of the Human Genome* Five Volumes. Hampshire, England: Nature Publishing Group, Macmillan, 2003.

Reich WT (ed). *Encyclopedia of Bioethics* Five Volumes. New York: London; Toronto: Macmillan: Simon & Schuster Macmillan; Prentice Hall International, 1995. (Third edition is in press, Steven Post is the editor.)

Mitcham C (ed). *Encyclopedia of Science, Technology and Ethics* Four Volumes. Toronto: Macmillan, forthcoming.

Credits

The editors wish to thank the publishers and copyright holders for permission to reprint the selections in this book, which are listed below in order of their appearance.

Chapter 1

Peter Singer, *Practical Ethics*, Second Edition (New York: Cambridge University Press, 1993), pp. 8–13. Copyright © 1993 Peter Singer. Reprinted with the permission of Cambridge University Press.

Ruth Faden and Tom L. Beauchamp, *The History and Theory of Informed Consent*, pp. 3–22, copyright © 1986 by Oxford University Press. Used by permission of Oxford University Press, Inc.

James F. Childress, "Metaphor and Analogy in Bioethics" from *Practical Reasoning in Bioethics* (Bloomington, IN: Indiana University Press, 1997), pp. 3–24. Reprinted with permission. Much of the material appeared earlier in "Metaphor and Analogy" in *Encyclopedia of Bioethics*, Second Edition, ed. Warren T. Reich (New York: Simon & Schuster Macmillan, 1995), vol. 3, pp. 1765–73.

Margaret Olivia Little, "Why a Feminist Approach to Bioethics?" *Kennedy Institute of Ethics Journal* 6, no. 1 (1996): 1–18. © The Johns Hopkins University Press. Reprinted with permission of the Johns Hopkins University Press.

Chapter 2

Jill Klessig, "The Effect of Values and Culture on Life-Support Decisions," *The Western Journal of Medicine* 157, no. 3 (1992): 316–322. Reproduced with permission from the BMJ Publishing Group.

Carolyn Ells and Donna Caniano, "The Impact of Culture on the Patient–Surgeon Relationship." Reprinted from *Journal of the American College of Surgeons* 195, no. 4:520–30. Copyright © 2002, with permission from American College of Surgeons.

Antonella Surbone, "Truth Telling to the Patient," *The Journal of the America Medical Association* 268, no. 13 (October 7, 1992): 1661–62. Copyright © 1992 American Medical Association. Reprinted by permission.

Jonathan H. Ellerby, et. al., "Bioethics for Clinicians: 18. Aboriginal Cultures" reprinted from *CMAJ* 163, no. 7 (October 3, 2000): 845–50, by permission of the publisher. © 2000 Canadian Medical Association.

Neil Levy, "Deafness, Culture and Choice," *The Journal of Medical Ethics* 28, no. 5 (2002): 284–85. Reproduced with permission from the BMJ Publishing Group.

Chapter 3

Royal Commission on the Future of Health Care in Canada, *Building on Values: The Future of Health Care in Canada*, pp. 1–44, © 2002. Reproduced with the permission of the Minister of Public Works and Government Services, 2003, and Courtesy of the Privy Council Office.

Jeremiah Hurley, "Ethics, Economics, and Public Financing of Health Care," *The Journal of Medical Ethics* 27 (2001): 234–39. Reproduced with permission from the BMJ Publishing Group.

Giacomini et al., "The Many Meanings of Deinsuring a Health Service: The Case of in Vitro Fertiliziation in Ontario," reprinted from *Social Science and Medicine* 50, no. 10 (2000): 1485–1500, copyright 2000, with permission from Elsevier.

Chapter 4

George J. Annas, "The Prostitute, the Playboy, and the Poet: Rationing Schemes for Organ Transplantation," *American Journal of Public Health* 75, no. 2 (February 1985): 187–89, copyright 1985 American Public Health Association. Reprinted with permission.

Chapter 5

Chapter 6

Chapter 7

Carl Elliot, "Nothing Matters: Depression and Competence in Clinical Research," Copyright © 1999 from *A Philosophical Disease: Bioethics, Culture and Identity* by Carl Elliot. Reprinted by permission of Routledge/Taylor & Francis Books, Inc.

Louis C. Charland, "Cynthia's Dilemma: Consenting to Heroin Prescription," *American Journal of Bioethics* 2, no. 2 (Spring 2002): 37–47. © 2002 by The MIT Press. Reprinted with permission.

Carl Elliott, "Who Holds the Leash?" *American Journal of Bioethics* 2, no. 2 (Spring 2002): 48. © 2002 by The MIT Press. Reprinted with permission.

Chapter 8

Charles Weijer and James A. Anderson, "Placebo-controlled Trials in Schizophrenia: Are They Ethical? Are They Necessary?" reprinted from *Schizophrenia Research* 35 (1999): 211–18. Copyright © 1999, with permission from Elsevier.

Franklin G. Miller and Howard Brody, "A Critique of Clinical Equipoise: Therapeutic Misconception in the Ethics of Clinical Trials," *The Hastings Report* 33, no. 3 (2003): 19–28. Reproduced by permission. © The Hastings Center.

Barry F. Brown, "Proxy Consent for Research on the Incompetent Elderly." Reprinted with permission of the publisher from *Ethics and Aging* by James E. Thornton and Earl R. Winkler © University of British Columbia Press 1988. All rights reserved by the publisher.

Anna Mastroianni and Jeffrey Kahn, "Swinging on the Pendulum: Shifting Views of Justice in Human Subjects Research," *Hastings Center Report* 31, no. 3 (May/June 2001): 21–28. Reproduced by permission. © The Hastings Center.

Søren Holm, "Going to the Roots of the Stem Cell Controversy," *Bioethics* 16, no. 6 (November 2002): 493–507. Reprinted with permission of Blackwell Publishing Ltd.

Steven Lewis et. al. "Dancing with the Porcupine: Rules for Governing the University-Industry Relationship" reprinted from *CMAJ* 165, no. 6 (18 Sept 2001): 783–85. By permission of the publisher. © 2001, Canadian Medical Association.

Chapter 9

L.W. Sumner, "A Third Way," from L.W. Sumner, *Abortion and Moral Theory*. Copyright 1981 by PUP. Reprinted by permission of Princeton University Press.

Christine Overall, "Selective Termination of Pregnancy and Women's Reproductive Autonomy," *Hastings Center Report* 20, no. 3 (May/June 1990): 6–11. Reproduced by permission. © The Hastings Center.

Susan Sherwin, "Normalizing Reproductive Technolgies and the Implicatons for Autonomy" From *Globalizing Feminist Bioethics: Crosscultural Perspectives* by Rosemarie Tong. Copyright © 2000 by Westview Press. Reprinted by permission of Westview Press, a member of Perseus Books, L.L.C.

Royal Commission on New Reproductive Technologies. "Judicial Intervention in Pregnancy and Birth." *Proceed with Care: Final Report of the Royal Commission on New Reproductive Technologies*, vol. 2, pp. 949–65, The Commission, © 1993. Reproduced with the permission of the Minister of Public Works and Government Services, 2003, and Courtesy of the Privy Council Office.

Suzanne Rozell Scorsone, "Annex: Judicial Intervention in Pregnancy." Royal Commission on New Reproductive Technologies. *Proceed with Care: Final Report of the Royal Commission on New Reproductive Technologies*, vol. 2, pp. 1123–43, The Commission, © 1993. Reproduced with the permission of the Minister of Public Works and Government Services, 2003, and Courtesy of the Privy Council Office.

Chapter 10

A. Lippman, "Prenatal Genetic Testing and Screening: Constructing Needs and Reinforcing Inequities," *American Journal of Law & Medicine* 17, nos. 1&2 (1991): 15–50. © 1991. Reprinted with the permission of the American Society of Law, Medicine & Ethics and Boston University. All rights reserved.

Dorothy C. Wertz and John C. Fletcher, "A Critique of Some Feminist Challenges to Prenatal Diagnosis," *Journal of Women's Health* 2, no. 2 (1993): 173–88. Copyright © 1993 Dorothy C. Wertz and John C. Fletcher. Reprinted by permission of Mary Ann Liebert, Inc. Publishers.

D.J. Willison and S.M. MacLeod, "Patenting of Genetic Material: Are the Benefits to Society Being Realized?" reprinted from *CMAJ* 167, no. 3 (August 6, 2002): 259–62. By permission of the publisher, © 2002 Canadian Medical Association.

Patricia Baird, "Will Genetics Be Used Wisely?" *ISUMA* 2, no. 1 (2002): 94–101. Reprinted with permission.

Françoise Baylis, "Human Cloning: Three Mistakes and an Alternative," *Journal of Medicine and Philosophy* 27, no. 3 (2002): 319–37. © Swets & Zeitlinger. Reprinted with permission.

Françoise Baylis and Jason Scott Robert, "The Inevitability of Genetic Enhancement Technologies," *Bioethics*, forthcoming. Reprinted with permission of Blackwell Publishing Ltd.

Chapter 11

Robert D. Truog, Allan S. Brett, and Joel Frader, "The Problem with Futility," *New England Journal of Medicine* 326, no. 23 (June 4, 1992): 1560–64. Copyright © 1987 Massachusetts Medical Society. All rights reserved.

Dan W. Brock, "Voluntary Active Euthanasia," *Hastings Center Report* 22, no. 2 (March/April 1992): 10–22. Reproduced by permission. © The Hastings Center.

Daniel Callahan, "When Self-Determination Runs Amok," *Hastings Center Report* 22, no. 2 (March/April 1992): 52–55. Reproduced by permission. © The Hastings Center.

Robert Truog, "Is It Time to Abandon Brain Death?" *Hastings Center Report* 27, no. 1 (January/February 1997): 29–37. Reproduced by permission. © The Hastings Center.